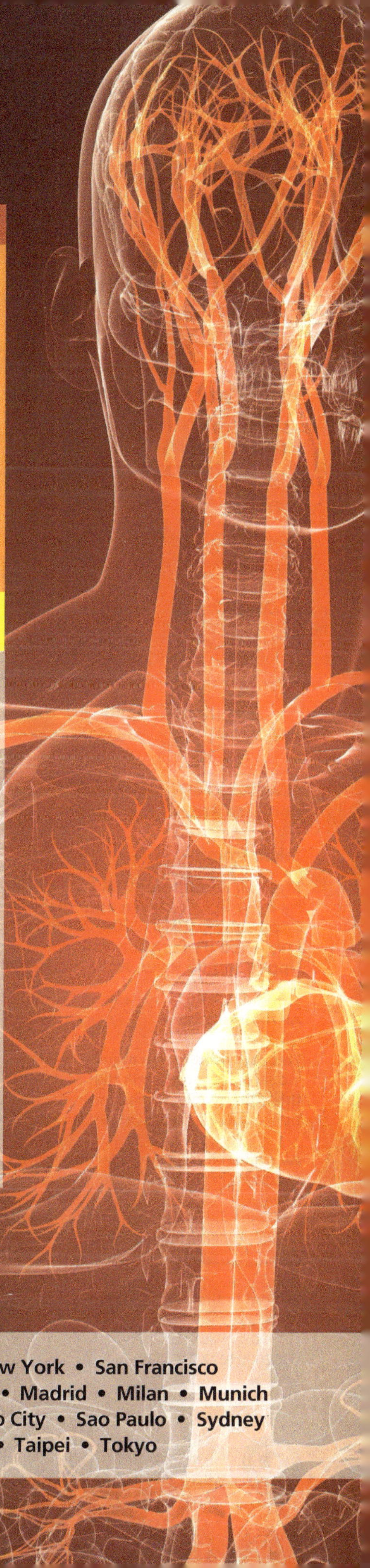

Second Edition

MEDICAL TERMINOLOGY

A LIVING LANGUAGE

Bonnie F. Fremgen, PhD

Suzanne S. Frucht, PhD
Associate Professor Emeritus
Northwest Missouri State University
Maryville, MO

TENNESSEE

Tennessee Edition

Pearson

Boston • Columbus • Indianapolis • New York • San Francisco
Amsterdam • Cape Town • Dubai • London • Madrid • Milan • Munich
Paris • Montreal • Toronto • Delhi • Mexico City • Sao Paulo • Sydney
Hong Kong • Seoul • Singapore • Taipei • Tokyo

Cover Art: Courtesy of Michael Taylor/Shutterstock, Africa Studio/Shutterstock, Sebastin Kaulitzki/Shutterstock, Stefanolunardi/Shutterstock, and Keithley & Associates, Inc.

Taken from:

Medical Terminology: A Living Language
by Bonnie F. Fremgen and Suzanne S. Frucht
Copyright © 2013, 2009, 2005, 2002, 1997 by Pearson Education, Inc.
Published by Prentice Hall
Upper Saddle River, New Jersey 07458

Pearson Learning Solutions, 501 Boylston Street, Suite 900, Boston, MA 02116
A Pearson Education Company
www.pearsoned.com

Printed in the United States of America
1 16

000200010271847074
RP

ISBN 10: 0-13-470250-6
ISBN 13: 978-0-13-470250-6

Welcome!

Welcome to the fascinating study of medical language—a vital part of your preparation for a career as a health professional. We are glad that you have joined us. Throughout your career, in a variety of settings, you will use medical terminology to communicate with co-workers and patients. Employing a carefully constructed learning system, Medical Terminology: A Living Language has helped thousands of readers gain a successful grasp of medical language within a real-world context.

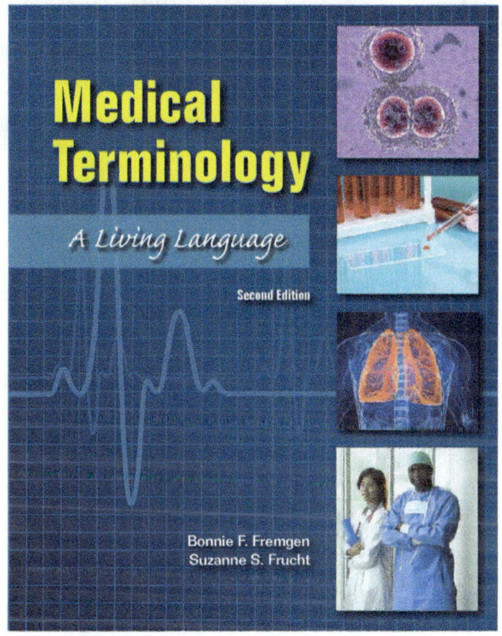

In developing this book we had six goals in mind:

1. To provide a clear introduction to the basic rules of using word parts to form medical terms.
2. To use phonetic pronunciations that will help you easily pronounce terms by spelling out the word part according to the way it sounds.
3. To help you understand medical terminology within the context of the human body systems. Realizing that this book is designed for a terminology course and not an anatomy & physiology course, we have aimed to stick to only the basics.
4. To help you develop a full range of Latin and Greek word parts used to build medical terms so that you will be able to interpret unfamiliar terms you encounter in the future.
5. To help you visualize medical language with an abundance of real-life photographs and accurate illustrations.
6. To provide you with a wealth of practice applications at the end of each chapter to help you review and master the content as you go along.

Please turn the page to get a visual glimpse of what makes this book an ideal guide to your exploration of medical terminology.

A Guide to What Makes This Book Special

Streamlined Content

Fourteen chapters and only the most essential anatomy & physiology coverage makes this book a perfect mid-sized fit for students new to medical terminology.

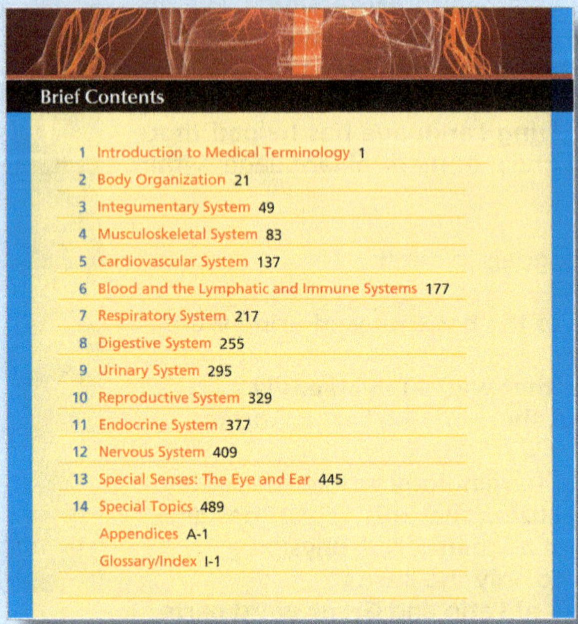

Brief Contents

Chapter-Opening Page Spreads

"At a Glance" and "Illustrated" pages begin each chapter, providing a quick, visual snapshot of what's covered.

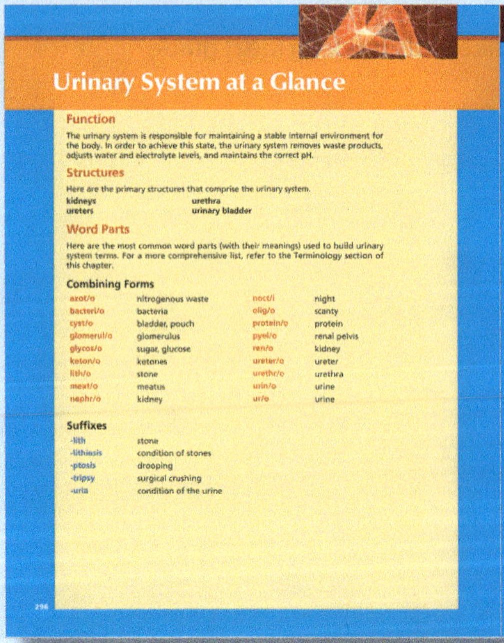

Urinary System at a Glance

Function

The urinary system is responsible for maintaining a stable internal environment for the body. In order to achieve this state, the urinary system removes waste products, adjusts water and electrolyte levels, and maintains the correct pH.

Structures

Here are the primary structures that comprise the urinary system.

kidneys	**urethra**
ureters	**urinary bladder**

Word Parts

Here are the most common word parts (with their meanings) used to build urinary system terms. For a more comprehensive list, refer to the Terminology section of this chapter.

Combining Forms

azot/o	nitrogenous waste	noct/i	night
bacteri/o	bacteria	olig/o	scanty
cyst/o	bladder, pouch	protein/o	protein
glomerul/o	glomerulus	pyel/o	renal pelvis
glycos/o	sugar, glucose	ren/o	kidney
keton/o	ketones	ureter/o	ureter
lith/o	stone	urethr/o	urethra
meat/o	meatus	urin/o	urine
nephr/o	kidney	ur/o	urine

Suffixes

-lith	stone
-lithiasis	condition of stones
-ptosis	drooping
-tripsy	surgical crushing
-uria	condition of the urine

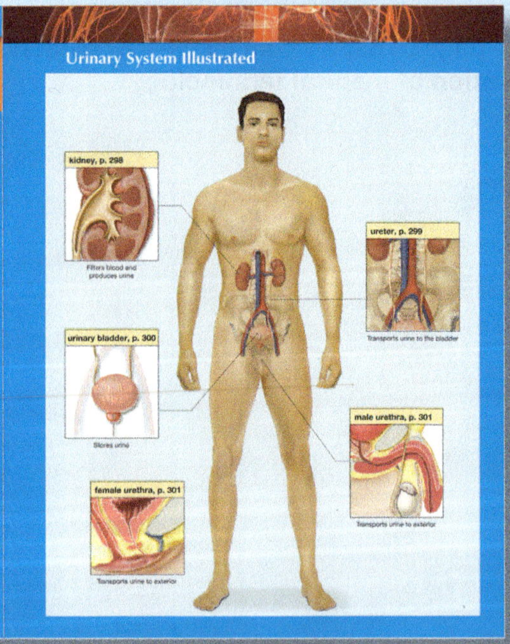

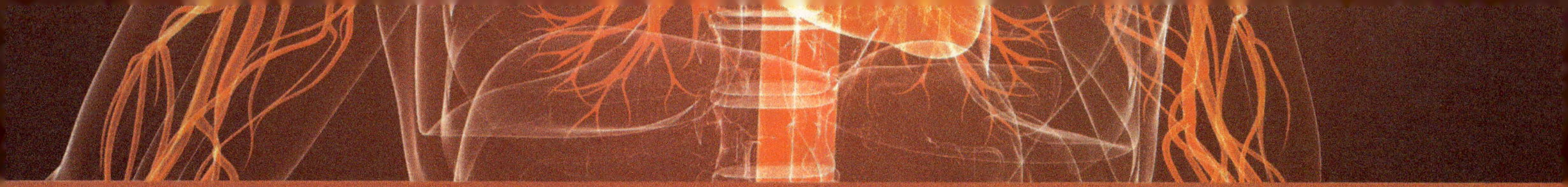

Key Terms and Pronunciations

Every subsection starts with a list of key terms and pronunciations for those words that will be covered in that section. This sets the stage for comprehension and mastery.

Med Term Tips

This popular feature offers tidbits of noteworthy information about medical terms that engage learners.

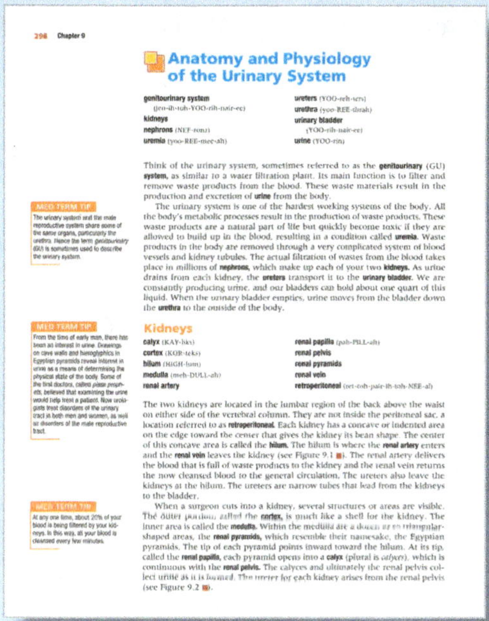

298 Chapter 9

Anatomy and Physiology of the Urinary System

genitourinary system (jen-ih-toh-YOO-rih-nair-ee)
kidneys
nephrons (NEF-ronz)
uremia (yoo-REE-mee-ah)
ureters (YOO-reh-ters)
urethra (yoo-REE-thrah)
urinary bladder (YOO-rih-nair-ee)
urine (YOO-rin)

Think of the urinary system, sometimes referred to as the **genitourinary** (GU) **system**, as similar to a water filtration plant. Its main function is to filter and remove waste products from the blood. These waste materials result in the production and excretion of **urine** from the body.

The urinary system is one of the hardest working systems of the body. All the body's metabolic processes result in the production of waste products. These waste products are a natural part of life but quickly become toxic if they are allowed to build up in the blood, resulting in a condition called **uremia**. Waste products in the body are removed through a very complicated system of blood vessels and kidney tubules. The actual filtration of wastes from the blood takes place in millions of **nephrons**, which make up each of your two **kidneys**. As urine drains from each kidney, the **ureters** transport it to the **urinary bladder**. We are constantly producing urine, and our bladders can hold about one quart of this liquid. When the urinary bladder empties, urine moves from the bladder down the **urethra** to the outside of the body.

MED TERM TIP

The urinary system and the male reproductive system share some of the same organs, particularly the urethra. Hence the term *genitourinary* (GU) is sometimes used to describe the urinary system.

Kidneys

calyx (KAY-liks)
cortex (KOR-teks)
hilum (HIGH-lum)
medulla (meh-DULL-ah)
renal artery
renal papilla (pah-PILL-ah)
renal pelvis
renal pyramids
renal vein
retroperitoneal (ret-roh-pair-ih-toh-NEE-al)

The two kidneys are located in the lumbar region of the back above the waist on either side of the vertebral column. They are not inside the peritoneal sac, a location referred to as **retroperitoneal**. Each kidney has a concave or indented area on the edge toward the center that gives the kidney its bean shape. The center of this concave area is called the **hilum**. The hilum is where the **renal artery** enters and the **renal vein** leaves the kidney (see Figure 9.1). The renal artery delivers the blood that is full of waste products to the kidney and the renal vein returns the now cleansed blood to the general circulation. The ureters also leave the kidneys at the hilum. The ureters are narrow tubes that lead from the kidneys to the bladder.

When a surgeon cuts into a kidney, several structures or areas are visible. The outer portion, called the **cortex**, is much like a shell for the kidney. The inner area is called the **medulla**. Within the medulla are a dozen or so triangular-shaped areas, the **renal pyramids**, which resemble their namesake, the Egyptian pyramids. The tip of each pyramid points inward toward the hilum. At its tip, called the **renal papilla**, each pyramid opens into a **calyx** (plural is *calyces*), which is continuous with the **renal pelvis**. The calyces and ultimately the renal pelvis collect urine as it is formed. The ureter for each kidney arises from the renal pelvis (see Figure 9.2).

MED TERM TIP

From the time of early man, there has been an interest in urine. Drawings on cave walls and hieroglyphics in Egyptian pyramids reveal interest in urine as a means of determining the physical state of the body. Some of the first doctors, called *pisse prophets*, believed that examining the urine would help treat a patient. Now urologists treat disorders of the urinary tract in both men and women, as well as disorders of the male reproductive tract.

MED TERM TIP

At any one time, about 20% of your blood is being filtered by your kidneys. In this way, all your blood is cleansed every few minutes.

Medically-Accurate Illustrations

Concepts come to life with vibrant, clear, consistent, and scientifically precise images.

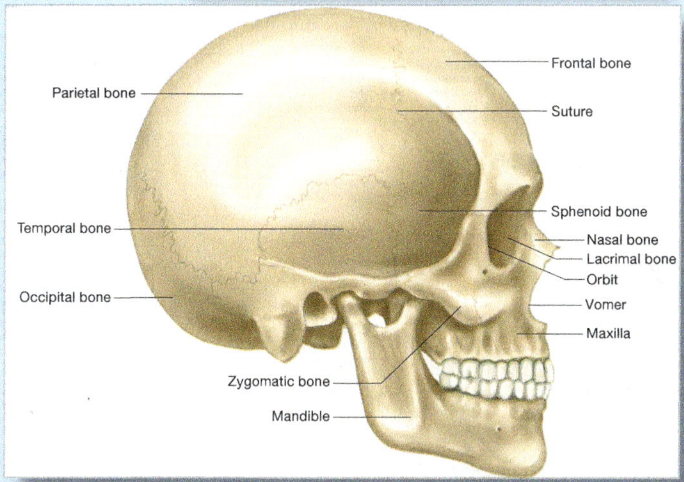

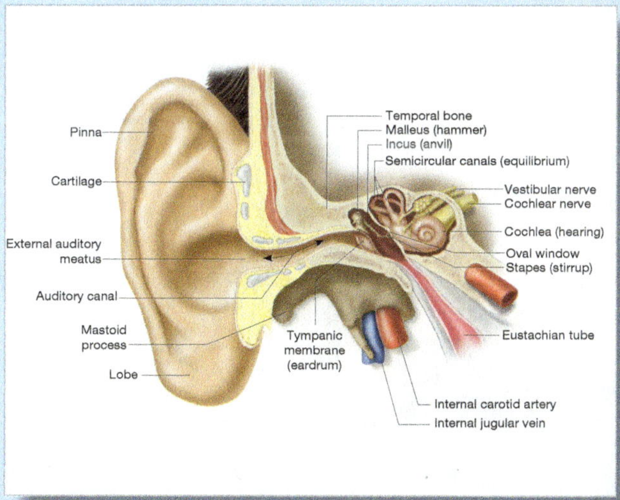

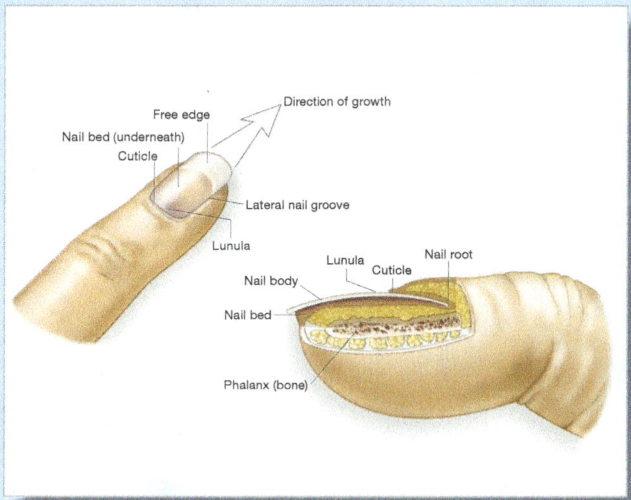

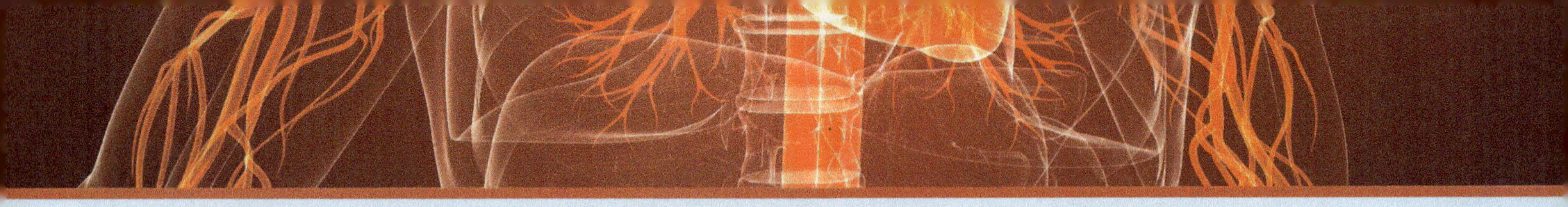

Word Tables

Study lists are categorized and presented in a clear, logical, color-coded format that eases the learning process.

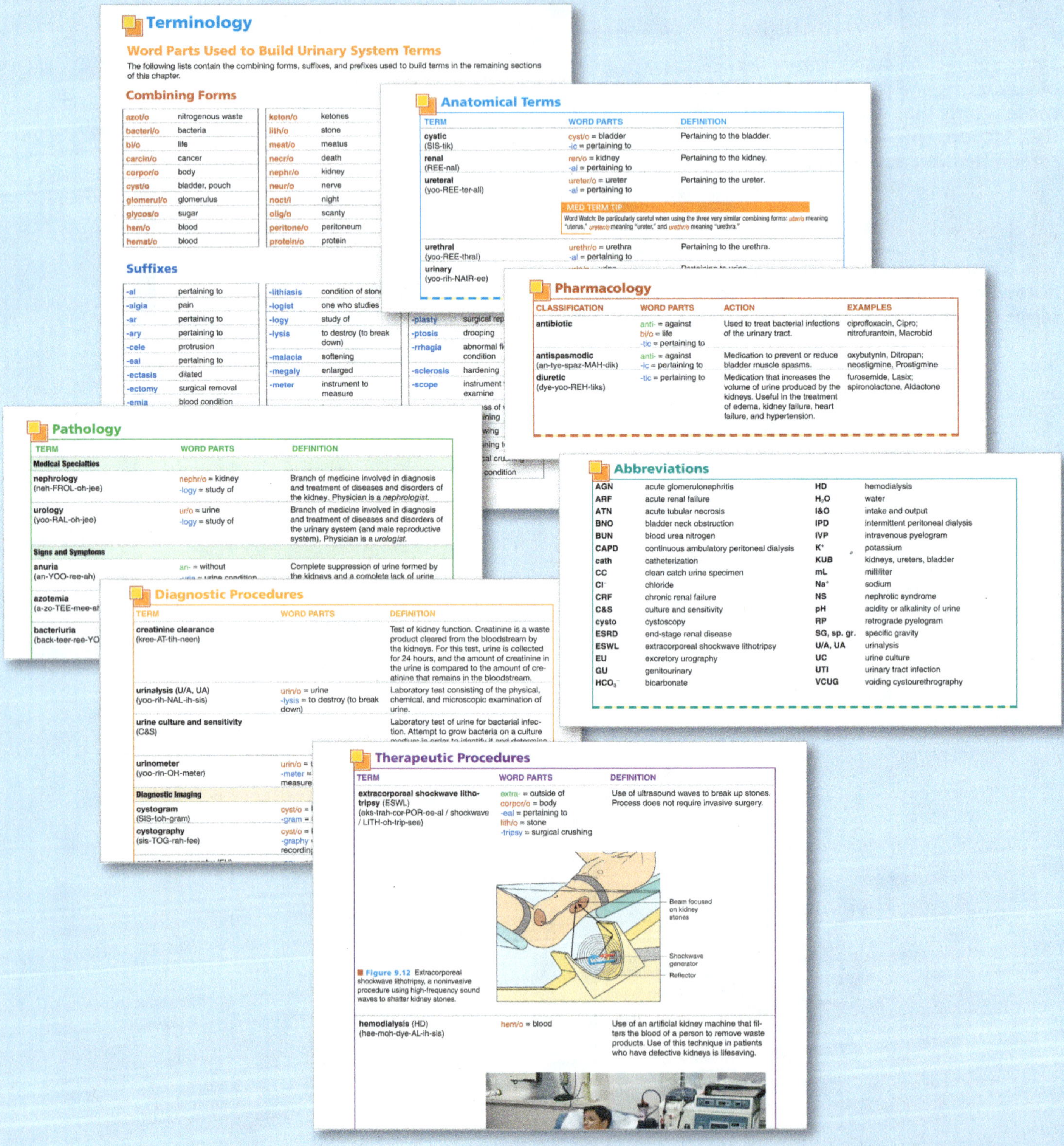

Workbook Sections

A wide array of exercises at the end of each chapter serve as a fun and challenging study review. Here are some examples:

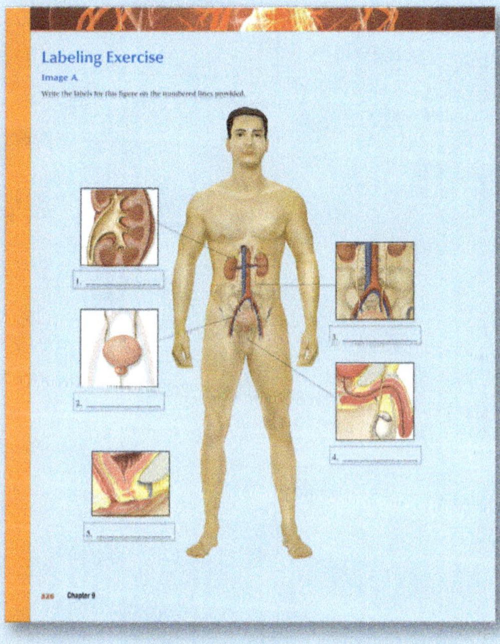

Labeling Exercise

Image A

Labeling Exercises—A visual challenge to reinforce students' grasp of anatomy & physiology concepts.

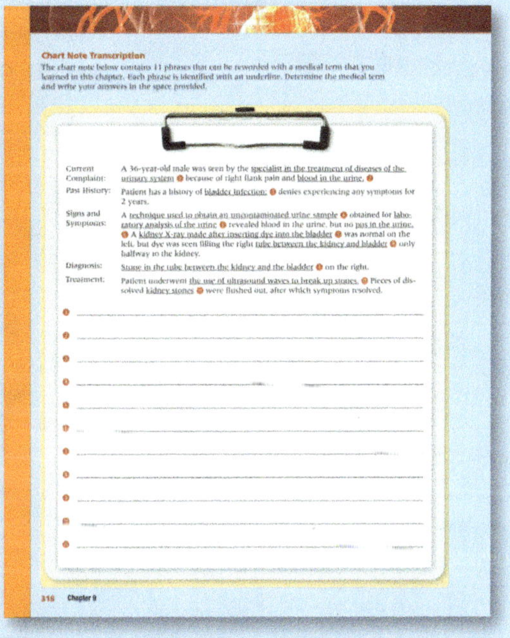

Chart Note Transcription

Chart Note Transcription—Slice-of-real-life exercise that asks students to replace lay terms in a medical chart with the proper medical term.

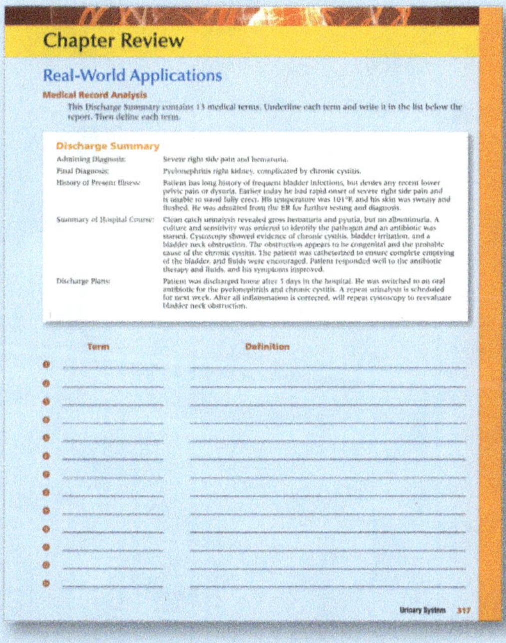

Chapter Review

Real-World Applications

Medical Record Analysis

Discharge Summary

Medical Record Analysis—Exercises that challenge students to read examples of real medical records and then to apply their medical terminology knowledge in answering related questions.

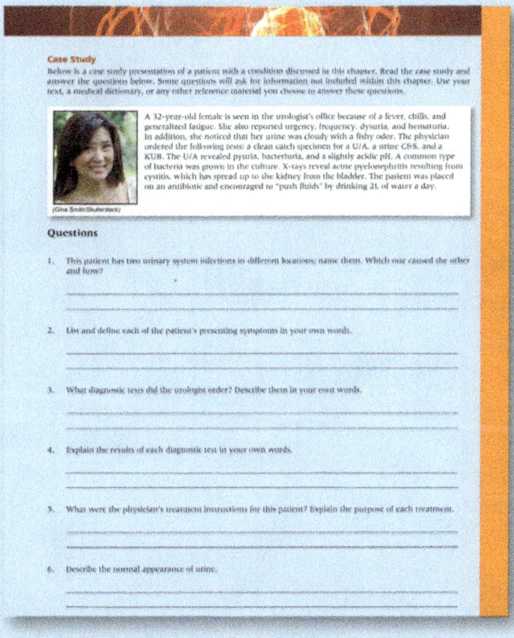

Case Study

Questions

Case Study—Scenarios that use critical thinking questions to help students develop a firmer understanding of the terminology in context.

Preface

Since the first edition of Medical Terminology: A Living Language was published it has been noted for its "clean" and logical format that promotes learning. In this revised edition, we have built upon this strength by enhancing many features to make this text an ideal choice for semester-or quarter-length courses.

Features of this Edition

This new second edition contains features that facilitate student mastery, while maintaining the best aspects of previous editions. Each chapter is arranged in a similar format and the content is organized with an emphasis on maintaining consistency and accuracy. All terms have been evaluated to ensure they remain in current use and reflect the newest technologies and procedures.

We have revised Medical Terminology: A Living Language so that it provides for an even more valuable teaching and learning experience. Here are the enhancements we have made:

- The Terminology section includes a comprehensive list of all combining forms, suffixes, and prefixes used to build terms in the remaining sections of the chapter.
- The Signs and Symptoms subsection within the Pathology table contains disease-related terms grouped by organ. This allows terms to be categorized into smaller groups, therefore making learning easier.
- Improved three-column format in the word building sections allows for the term (with pronunciation and/or abbreviation), word parts (if appropriate), and definitions to be displayed. The Pharmacology table also includes word parts in a new fourth column.
- The Anatomical Terms section includes anatomical terms as well as adjective forms of organs.
- Color-coded word parts—red combining forms, blue suffixes, and green prefixes allow for quick recognition throughout the book.
- The Real World Applications section now contains three critical thinking activities (Medical Record Analysis, Chart Note Transcription, and a new Case Study) to allow readers to apply their knowledge to real world situations.

Organization of the Book

Introductory Chapter

Chapter 1 contains information necessary for an understanding of how medical terms are formed. This includes learning about word roots, combining forms, prefixes, and suffixes, and general rules for building medical terms. Readers will also learn about terminology for medical records and the different health care settings. Chapter 2 presents terminology relating to the body organization, including organs and body systems. Here readers will first encounter word building tables, a feature found in each remaining chapter that lists medical terms and their respective word parts.

Anatomy and Physiology Chapters

Chapters 3 through 13 are organized by body system. Each chapter begins with a System At A Glance which lists combining forms, prefixes, and/or suffixes with their meanings and is followed by System Illustrated overview of the organs in the system. The anatomy and physiology section is divided into the various components of the system, and each subsection begins with a list of key medical terms accompanied by a pronunciation guide. Key terms are boldfaced the first time they appear in the narrative. The Terminology section of each chapter begins with a list of all word parts used within the chapter. For ease of learning, the medical terms are divided into five separate sections: anatomical terms, pathology, diagnostic procedures, therapeutic procedures, and pharmacology. The word parts used to build terms are highlighted within each table. An abbreviations section then follows to complete the chapter.

Special Topics Chapter

Chapter 14 contains timely information and appropriate medical terms relevant to the following medical specialties: pharmacology, mental health, diagnostic imaging, rehabilitation services, surgery, and oncology. Knowledge of these topics is necessary for the well-rounded health care worker.

Appendices

The appendices contain helpful reference lists of word parts and definitions. This information is intended for quick access. There are three word part/definition appendices: Word Parts Arranged Alphabetically and Defined, Word Parts Arranged Alphabetically by Definition and Abbreviations. All of the key terms appear again in the glossary/index at the end of the text. In addition, there is a Common Core Connection appendix that relates English Language Arts and Math Common Core standards back to the text.

About the Authors

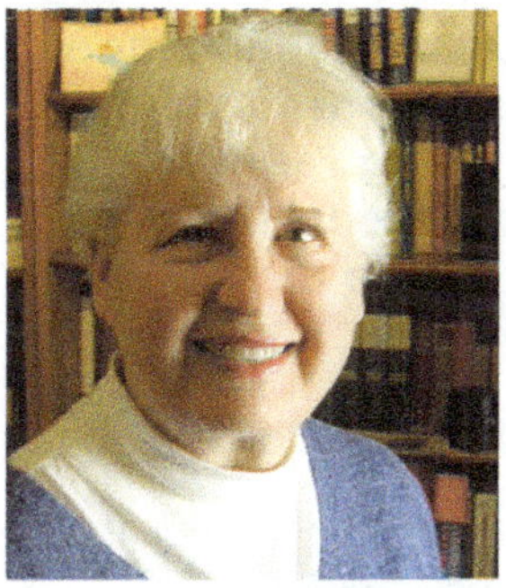

Bonnie F. Fremgen

Bonnie F. Fremgen is a former associate dean of the Allied Health Program at Robert Morris College. She has taught medical law and ethics courses as well as clinical and administrative topics. In addition, she has served as an advisor for students' career planning. She has broad interests and experiences in the health care field, including hospitals, nursing homes, and physicians' offices.

Dr. Fremgen holds a nursing degree as well as a master's in health care administration. She received her PhD from the College of Education at the University of Illinois. She has performed postdoctoral studies in Medical Law at Loyola University Law School in Chicago. She has authored five textbooks with Pearson.

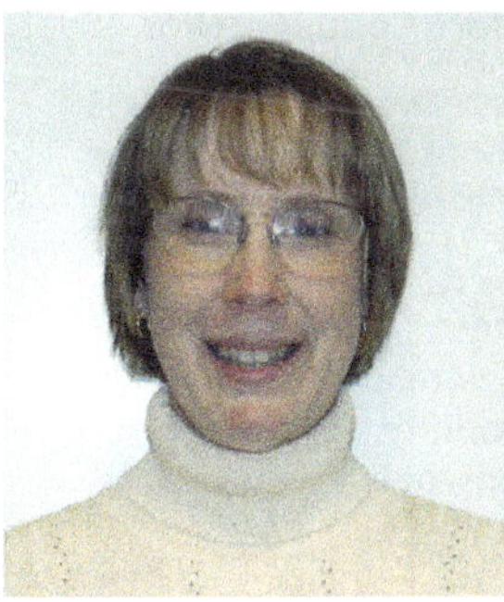

Suzanne S. Frucht

Suzanne S. Frucht is an Associate Professor Emeritus of Anatomy and Physiology at Northwest Missouri State University (NWMSU). She holds baccalaureate degrees in biological sciences and physical therapy from Indiana University, an MS in biological sciences at NWMSU, and a PhD in molecular biology and biochemistry from the University of Missouri-Kansas City.

For 14 years she worked full-time as a physical therapist in various health care settings, including acute care hospitals, extended care facilities, and home health. Based on her educational and clinical experience she was invited to teach medical terminology part-time in 1988 and became a full-time faculty member three years later as she discovered her love for the challenge of teaching. She taught a variety of courses including medical terminology, human anatomy, human physiology, and animal anatomy and physiology. She received the Governor's Award for Excellence in Teaching in 2003. After retiring from teaching in 2008, she continues to be active in student learning through writing medical terminology texts and anatomy and physiology laboratory manuals.

About the Illustrators

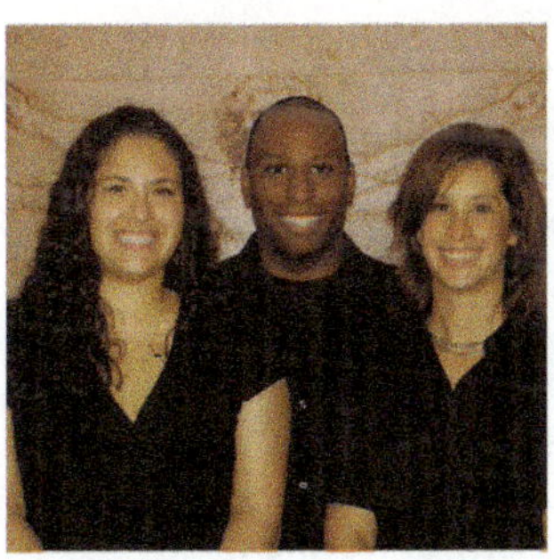

Marcelo Oliver is president and founder of Body Scientific International LLC. He holds an MFA degree in Medical and Biological Illustration from University of Michigan. For the past 15 years, his passion has been to condense complex anatomical information into visual education tools for students, patients, and medical professionals. For seven years he worked as a medical illustrator and creative director developing anatomical charts used for student and patient education. In the years that followed, he created educational and marketing tools for medical device companies prior to founding Body Scientific International, LLC.

Body Scientific's lead artists in this publication were medical illustrators Liana Bauman and Katie Burgess. Both hold an Master of Science degrees in Biomedical Visualization degree from the University of Illinois at Chicago. Their contribution in the publication was key in the creation and editing of artwork throughout.

Our Development Team

We would like to express deep gratitude to our 105 colleagues from schools across the country that have provided us with hundreds of hours of their time over the years to help us tailor this book to suit the dynamic needs of instructors and students. These individuals have reviewed manuscript chapters and illustrations for content, accuracy, level, and utility. We sincerely thank you and feel that Medical Terminology: A Living Language has benefited immeasurably from your efforts, insights, encouragement, and selfless willingness to share your expertise as educators. Thanks also to Beverly Campbell, President, BECGroup Consulting, for her development of the Common Core Connection appendix.

Reviewers of the 5th Edition

Dr. Pam Besser Ph.D
Jefferson Community and Technical College
Louisville, Kentucky

Jeannie Bower, BS, NRCAMA
Central Penn College
Summerdale, Pennsylvania

Karen R. Hardney, M.S. Ed
Chicago State University
Chicago, Illinois

Holly Jodon, MPAS, PA-C
Gannon University
Erie, Pensylvania

Francesca L. Langlow, BS
Delgado Community College
New Orleans, Louisiana

Bridgit R. Moore, EdD, MT(ASCP), CPC
McLennan Community College
Waco, Texas

Christine J. Moore, M Ed
Armstrong Atlantic State University
Savannah, Georgia

Lisa J. Pierce, MSA, RRT
Augusta Technical College
Augusta, Georgia

Georgette Rosenfeld, Ph.D, RRT, RN
Indian River State College
Fort Pierce, Florida

Donna J. Slovensky, PhD, RHIA, FAHIMA
University of Alabama at Birmingham
Birmingham, Alabama

Jodi Taylor, A.A.S, LPN, RMA
Terra State Community College
Fremont, Ohio

Scott Throneberry, BS, NREMTP
Calhoun Community College
Decatur, Alabama

Patricia A. Slachta, PhD, RN, ACNS-BC, CWOCN
Technical College of the Lowcountry
Beaufort, South Carolina

Lenette Thompson, CST, AS
Piedmont Technical College
Greenwood, South Carolina

Carole A. Zeglin, MSEd, BS, MT, RMA (AMT)
Westmoreland County Community College
Youngwood, Pennsylvania

Reviewers of Earlier Editions

Yvonne Alles, MBA, RMT
Davenport University
Grand Rapids, Michigan

Rachael C. Alstatter, Program Director
Southern Ohio College
Fairfield, Ohio

Steve Arinder, BS, MPH
Meridian Community College
Meridian, Mississippi

K. William Avery, BSMT, JD, PhD
City College
Gainesville, Florida

Beverly A. Baker, DA, CST
Western Iowa Technical Community College
Sioux City, Iowa

Michael Battaglia, MS
Greenville Technical College
Taylors, South Carolina

Nancy Ridinger Bean, Health Assistant Instructor
Wythe County Vocational School
Wytheville, Virginia

Deborah J. Bedford, CMA, AAS
North Seattle Community College
Seattle, Washington

Barbara J Behrens, PTA, MS
Mercer County Community College
Trenton, New Jersey

Pam Besser, Ph.D.
Jefferson Community College
Louisville, Kentucky

Norma J Bird, M.Ed., BS, CMA
Idaho State University College of Technology
Pocatello, Idaho

Trina Blaschko, RHIT
Chippewa Valley Technical College
Eau Claire, Wisconsin

Richard T. Boan, PhD
Midlands Technical College
Columbia, South Carolina

Susan W. Boggs, RN, BSN, CNOR
Piedmont Technical College
Greenwood, South Carolina

Bradley S. Bowden, PhD
Alfred University
Alfred, New York

Joan Walker Brittingham
Sussex Tech Adult Division
Georgetown, Delaware

Phyills J. Broughton, Curriculum Coordinator
Pitt Community College
Greenville, North Carolina

Barbara Bussard, Instructor
Southwestern Michigan College
Dowagiac, Michigan

Toni Cade, MBA, RHIA, CCS
University of Louisiana at Lafayette
Lafayette, Louisiana

Gloria H. Coats, RN, MSN
Modesto Junior College
Modesto, California

Lyndal M. Curry, M.A., R.P.
University of South Alabama
Mobile, Alabama

Nancy Dancs, P.T.
Waukesha County Technical College
Pewaukee, Wisconsin

Antoinette Deshaies, RN, BSPA
Glendale Community College
Glendale, Arizona

Theresa H. deBeche, RN, MN, CNS
Louisiana State University at Eunice
Eunice, Louisiana

Bonnie Deister, MS, BSN, CMA-C
Broome Community College
Binghamton, New York

Carol Eckert, RN, MSN
Southwestern Illinois College
Belleville, Illinois

Jamie Erskine, Ph.D., R.D.
University of Northern Colorado
Greeley, Colorado

Mildred K. Fuller, Ph.D., MT(ASCP), CLS(NCA)
Norfolk State University
Norfolk, Virginia

Deborah Galanski-Maciak
Davenport University
Grand Rapids, Michigan

Debra Getting, Practical Nursing Instructor
Norwest Iowa Community College
Sheldon, Iowa

Ann Queen Giles, MHS, CMA
Western Piedmont Community College
Morganton, North Carolina

Brenda L. Gleason, MSN
Iowa Central Community College
Fort Dodge, Iowa

Steven B. Goldschmidt, DC, CCFC
North Hennepin Community College
Brooklyn Park, Minnesota

Linda S. Gott, RN, MS
Pensacola High School
Pensacola, Florida

Martha Grove, Staff Educator
Mercy Regional Health System
Cincinnati, Ohio

Kathryn Gruber
Globe College
Oakdale, Minnesota

Karen R. Hardney, M.S., Ed.
Chicago State University
Chicago, Illinois

Mary Hartman, MS, OTR/L
Genesee Community College
Batavia, New York

Joyce B. Harvey, Ph.D, RHIA
Norfolk State University
Norfolk, Virginia

Beulah A. Hofmann, RN, BSN, MSN, CMA
Ivy Tech Community College of Indiana
Greencastle, Indiana

Kimberley Hontz , RN
Antonelli Medical and Professional Institute
Pottstown, Pennsylvania

Pamela S. Huber, M.S., MT(ASCP)
Erie Community College
Williamsville, New York

Eva I. Irwin
Ivy Tech State College
Indianapolis, Indiana

Susan Jackson, EdS
Valdosta Technical College
Valdosta, Georgia

Mark Jaffe, DPM, MHSA
Nova Southeastern University
Ft. Lauderdale, Florida

Carol Lee Jarrell, MLT,AHI
Brown Mackie College
Merrillville, Indiana

Virginia J. Johnson, CMA
Lakeland Academy
Minneapolis, Minnesota

Marcie C. Jones, BS, CMA
Gwinnett Technical Institute
Lawrenceville, Georgia

Robin Jones, RHIA
Meridian Community College
Meridian, Mississippi

Gertrude A. Kenny, BSN, RN, CMA
Baker College of Muskegon
Muskegon, Michigan

Dianne K. Kuiti, RN
Duluth Business University
Duluth, Minnesota

Andrew La Marca, EMT-P
Mobile Life Support Services
Middletown, New York

Julie A. Leu, CPC
Creighton University
Omaha, Nebraska

Norma Longoria, BS, COI
South Texas Community College
McAllen, Texas

Jeanne W. Lovelock, RN, MSN
Piedmont Virginia Community College
Charlottesville, Virginia

Jan Martin, R.T.(R)
Ogeechee Tech College
Statesboro, Georgia

Leslie M. Mazzola, MA
Cuyahoga Community College
Parma, Ohio

Michelle C. McCranie, CPhT
Ogeechee Technical College
Statesboro, Georgia

Lola McGourty, MSN, RN
Bossier Parish Community College
Bossier City, Louisiana

Connie Morgan
Ivy Tech State College
Kokomo., Indiana

Katrina B. Myricks
Holmes Community College
Ridgeland, Mississippi

Patricia Moody, RN
Athens Technical College
Athens, Georgia

Catherine Moran, Ph.D.
Breyer State University
Birmingham, Alabama

Pam Ncu, CMA
International Business College
Fort Wayne, Indiana

Judy Ortiz MHS, MS, PA-C
Pacific University
Hillsboro, Oregon

Tina M. Peer, BSN, RN
College of Southern Idaho
Twin Falls, ID
Sylvania, Ohio

Dave Peruski, RN, MSA, MSN
Delta College
University Center, Michigan

Sister Marguerite Polcyn, OSF, PhD
Lourdes College
Sylvania, Ohio

Vicki Prater, CMA, RMA, RAHA
Concorde Career Institute
San Bernardino, California

Carolyn Ragsdale CST, BS
Parkland College
Champaign, Illinois

LuAnn Reicks, RNC, BS, MSN
Iowa Central Community College
Fort Dodge, Iowa

Linda Reigel
Glenville State College
Glenville, West Virginia

Ellen Rosen, RN, MN
Glendale Community College
Glendale, California

Georgette Rosenfeld, Ph.D., RN, RRT
Indian River Community College
Fort Pierce, Florida

Brian L. Rutledge, MHSA
Hinds Community College
Jackson, Mississippi

Sue Shibley, M.Ed., CMT, CCS-P, CPC
North Idaho College
Coeur d'Alene, Idaho

Misty Shuler, RHIA
Asheville Buncombe Technical Community College
Asheville, North Carolina

Connie Smith, RPh
University of Louisiana at Monroe School of Pharmacy
Monroe, Louisiana

Karen Snipe, CPhT, ASBA, MAEd
Trident Technical College
Charleston, South Carolina

Donna Stern
University of California San Diego Extension
La Jolla, California

Janet Stehling, RHIA
McLennan College
Lorena, Texas

Annmary Thomas, MEd, NREMT-P
Community College of Philadelphia
Philadelphia, Pennsylvania

Marilyn Turner, RN, CMA
Ogeechee Technical College
Statesboro, Georgia

Joan Ann Verderame, RN, MA
Bergen Community College
Paramus, New Jersey

Kathy Wallington
Phillips Junior College
Campbell, California

Twila Wallace, MEd
Central Community College
Columbus, Nebraska

Linda Walter, RN, MSN
Northwestern Michigan College
Traverse City, Michigan

Jean Watson, PhD
Clark College
Vancouver, Washington

Twila Weiszbrod, MPA
College of the Sequoias
Visalia, California

Sara J. Wellman, RHIT
Indiana University Northwest
Gary, Indiana

Leesa Whicker, BA, CMA
Central Piedmont Community College
Charlotte, NC

Lynn C. Wimett, RN, ANP, EdD
Regis University
Denver, Colorado

Kathy Zaiken, Pharm.D.
Massachusetts College of Pharmacy and Health Sciences
Boston, Massachusetts

Common Core Connection Appendix

Beverly Campbell, President
BECGroup Consulting
Cameron Park, California

A Commitment to Accuracy

As a student embarking on a career in health care you probably already know how critically important it is to be precise in your work. Patients and co-workers will be counting on you to avoid errors on a daily basis. Likewise, we owe it to you—the reader—to ensure accuracy in this book. We have gone to great lengths to verify that the information provided in Medical Terminology: A Living Language is complete and correct. To this end, here are the steps we have taken:

1. Editorial Review—We have assembled a large team of developmental consultants (listed on the preceding pages) to critique every word and every image in this book. No fewer than 10 content experts have read each chapter for accuracy.
2. Medical Illustrations—A team of medically-trained illustrators was hired to prepare each piece of art that graces the pages of this book. These illustrators have a higher level of scientific education than the artists for most textbooks, and they worked directly with the authors and members of our development team to make sure that their work was clear, correct, and consistent with what is described in the text.
3. Accurate Ancillaries—Realizing that the teaching and learning ancillaries are often as vital to instruction as the book itself, we took extra steps to ensure accuracy and consistency within these components. We assigned some members of our development team to specifically focus on critiquing every bit of content that comprises the instructional ancillary resources to confirm accuracy.

While our intent and actions have been directed at creating an error-free text, we have established a process for correcting any mistakes that may have slipped past our editors. Pearson takes this issue seriously and therefore welcomes any and all feedback that you can provide along the lines of helping us enhance the accuracy of this text. If you identify any errors that need to be corrected in a subsequent printing, please send them to:

Pearson Health Editorial
Medical Terminology Corrections
One Lake Street
Upper Saddle River, NJ 07458

Thank you for helping Pearson to reach its goal of providing the most accurate medical terminology textbooks available.

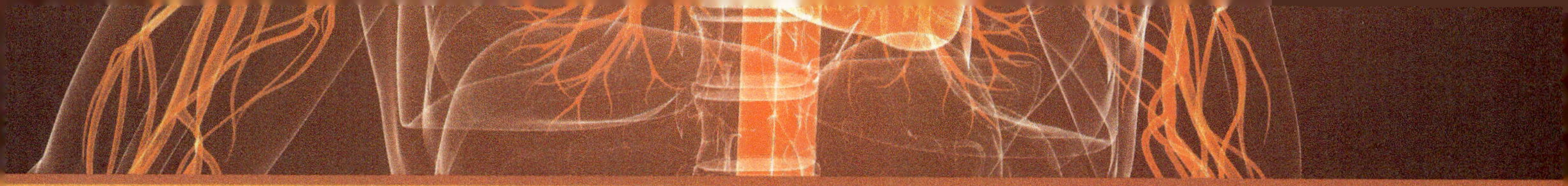

Contents

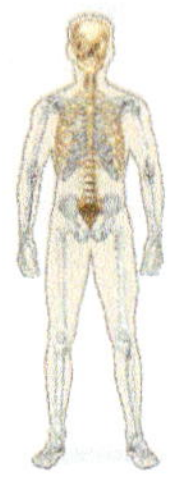

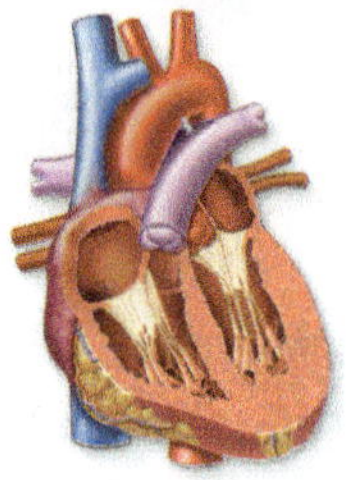

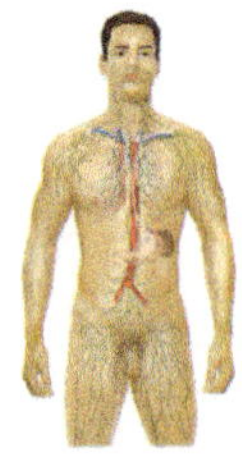

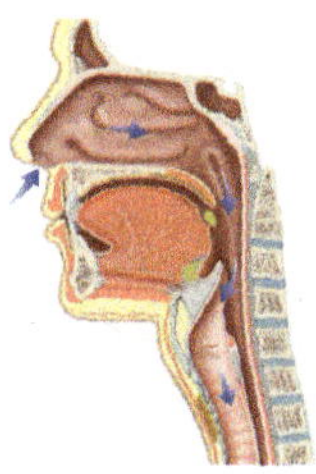

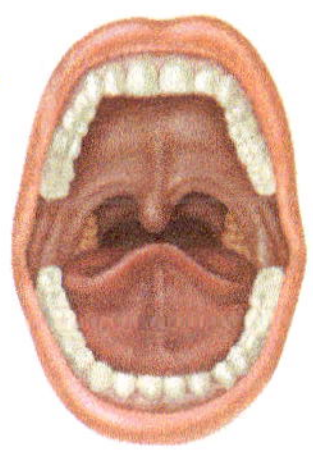

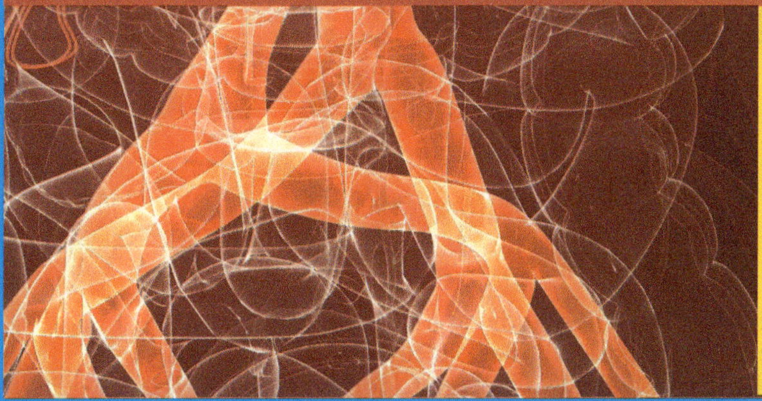

1

INTRODUCTION TO MEDICAL TERMINOLOGY

Learning Objectives

Upon completion of this chapter, you will be able to

- Discuss the four parts of medical terms.
- Recognize word roots and combining forms.
- Identify the most common prefixes and suffixes.
- Define word building and describe a strategy for translating medical terms.
- State the importance of correct spelling of medical terms.
- State the rules for determining singular and plural endings.
- Discuss the importance of using caution with abbreviations.
- Recognize the documents found in a medical record.
- Recognize the different healthcare settings.
- Understand the importance of confidentiality.

Medical Terminology at a Glance

Learning medical terminology can initially seem like studying a strange new language. However, once you understand some of the basic rules about how medical terms are formed using word building, it will become much like piecing together a puzzle. The general guidelines for forming words; an understanding of word roots, combining forms, prefixes, and suffixes; pronunciation; and spelling are discussed in this chapter. In addition, "Med Term Tips" are sprinkled throughout to assist in clarifying some of the material. New medical terms discussed in each section are listed separately at the beginning of the section, and each chapter contains numerous pathological, diagnostic, treatment, and surgical terms. You can use these lists as an additional study tool for previewing and reviewing terms.

Understanding medical terms requires you being able to put words together or build words from their parts. It is impossible to memorize thousands of medical terms; however, once you understand the basics, you can distinguish the meaning of medical terms by analyzing their prefixes, suffixes, and word roots. Remember that there will always be some exceptions to every rule, and medical terminology is no different. We attempt to point out these exceptions where they exist. Most medical terms, however, do follow the general rule that there is a **word root** or fundamental meaning for the word, a **prefix** and a **suffix** that modify the meaning of the word root, and sometimes a **combining vowel** to connect other word parts. You will be amazed at the seemingly difficult words you will be able to build and understand when you follow the simple steps in word building (see Figure 1.1 ■).

The ancient Greeks were considered the first to study the field of medicine and to develop a useful vocabulary and represent the starting point of the Greek era of the language of medicine. It is estimated that three quarters of our medical terminology is of Greek origin. Importantly, use of the classical roots form an *international language* that is easily understood by anyone responsible for health care practices and procedures.

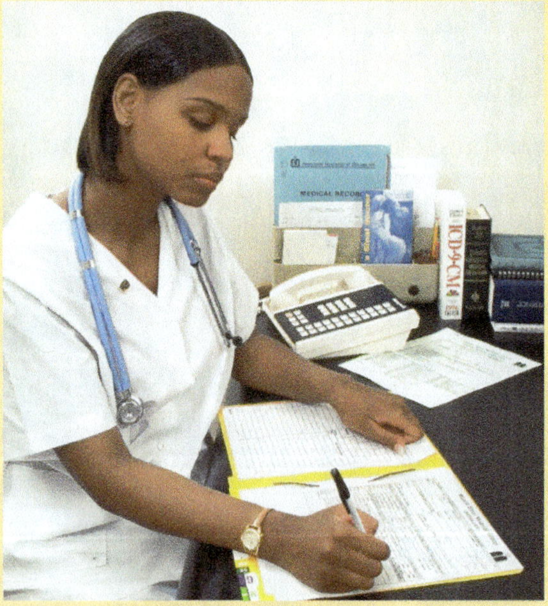

■ **Figure 1.1** Nurse completing a patient report. Healthcare workers use medical terminology in order to accurately and efficiently communicate patient information to each other.

Building Medical Terms from Word Parts

Four different word parts or elements can be used to construct medical terms:

1. The **word root** is the foundation of the word. — **cardi**ogram = record of the heart
2. A **prefix** is at the beginning of the word. — **peri**cardium = around the heart
3. A **suffix** is at the end of the word. — card**itis** = inflammation of the heart
4. The **combining vowel** is a vowel (usually *o*) that links the word root to another word root or a suffix. — cardi**o**my**o**pathy = disease of the heart muscle

The following sections on word roots, combining vowels and forms, prefixes, and suffixes will consider each of these word parts in more detail and present examples of some of those most commonly used.

MED TERM TIP

Medical terms are built from word parts:

Word Building Part	Example (Meaning)
1. Word root	*cardi* (heart)
2. Prefix	*peri-* (around)
3. Suffix	*-itis* (inflammation)

When these components are put together, the word *pericarditis* is formed, meaning inflammation around the heart.

Word Roots

The word root is the foundation of a medical term and provides the general meaning of the word. The word root often indicates the body system or part of the body being discussed, such as *cardi* for heart. At other times the word root may be an action. For example, the word root *cis* means to cut (as in incision).

A term may have more than one word root. For example, **osteoarthritis** (oss-tee-oh-ar-THRY-tis) combines the word root *oste* meaning bone and *arthr* meaning the joints. When the suffix *-itis*, meaning inflammation, is added, we have the entire word, meaning an inflammation involving bone at the joints.

MED TERM TIP

Several root words you will recognize as you become familiar with medical terminology.

Greek root words, pertaining to:
derma (skin)
trauma (wound)

Latin root words, pertaining to:
cranialis (skull)
dorsalis (back)

Combining Vowel/Form

To make it possible to pronounce long medical terms with ease and to combine several word parts, a combining vowel is used. This is most often the vowel *o*. Combining vowels are utilized in two places: between a word root and a suffix or between two word roots.

To decide whether or not to use a combining vowel between a word root and a suffix, first look at the suffix. If it begins with a vowel, do not use the combining vowel. If, however, the suffix begins with a consonant, then use a combining vowel. For example: To combine *arthr* with *-scope* will require a combining vowel: **arthroscope** (AR-throh-scope). But to combine *arthr* with *-itis* does not require a combining vowel: **arthritis** (ar-THRY-tis).

The combining vowel is typically kept between two word roots, even if the second word root begins with a vowel. For example, in forming the term **gastroenteritis** (gas-troh-en-ter-EYE-tis) the combining vowel is kept between the two word roots *gastr* and *enter* (gastrenteritis is incorrect). As you can tell from pronouncing these two terms, the combining vowel makes the pronunciation easier.

When writing a word root by itself, its **combining form** is typically used. This consists of the word root and its combining vowel written in a word root/vowel form, for example, *cardi/o*. Since it is often simpler to pronounce word roots when they appear in their combining form, this format is used throughout this text.

MED TERM TIP

Remember to break down every word into its components (prefix, word root/combining form, and suffix) when learning medical terminology. Do not try to memorize every medical term. Instead, figure out how the word is formed from its components. In a short time you will be able to do this automatically when seeing a new term.

Common Combining Forms

Some commonly used word roots in their combining form, their meaning, and examples of their use follow. Review the examples to observe when a combining vowel was kept and when it was dropped according to the rules presented on the preceding page.

COMBINING FORM	MEANING	EXAMPLE (DEFINITION)
aden/o	gland	adenopathy (gland disease)
carcin/o	cancer	carcinoma (cancerous tumor)
cardi/o	heart	cardiac (pertaining to the heart)
chem/o	chemical	chemotherapy (treatment with chemicals)
cis/o	to cut	incision (process of cutting into)
dermat/o	skin	dermatology (study of the skin)
enter/o	small intestine	enteric (pertaining to the small intestine)
gastr/o	stomach	gastric (pertaining to the stomach)
gynec/o	female	gynecology (study of females)
hemat/o	blood	hematic (pertaining to the blood)
hydr/o	water	hydrocele (protrusion of water [in the scrotum])
immun/o	immunity	immunology (study of immunity)
laryng/o	voice box	laryngeal (pertaining to the voice box)
nephr/o	kidney	nephromegaly (enlarged kidney)
neur/o	nerve	neural (pertaining to a nerve)
ophthalm/o	eye	ophthalmic (pertaining to the eye)
ot/o	ear	otic (pertaining to the ear)
path/o	disease	pathology (study of disease)
pulmon/o	lung	pulmonary (pertaining to the lungs)
rhin/o	nose	rhinoplasty (surgical repair of the nose)

Prefixes

A new medical term is formed when a prefix is added to the front of the term. Prefixes frequently give information about the location of an organ, the number of parts, or the time (frequency). For example, the prefix *bi-* stands for two of something, such as **bilateral** (bye-LAH-ter-al), meaning to have two sides. However, not every term will have a prefix.

Common Prefixes

Some of the more common prefixes, their meanings, and examples of their use follow. When written by themselves, prefixes are followed by a hyphen.

PREFIX	MEANING	EXAMPLE (DEFINITION)
a-	without, away from	aphasia (without speech)
an-	without	anoxia (without oxygen)
ante-	before, in front of	antepartum (before birth)
anti-	against	antibiotic (against life)
auto-	self	autograft (a graft from one's own body)
brady-	slow	bradycardia (slow heartbeat)
contra-	against	contraception (against conception)
de-	without	depigmentation (without pigment)
dys-	painful, difficult, abnormal	dyspnea (difficulty breathing)
endo-	within, inner	endoscope (instrument to view within)
epi-	upon, over	epigastric (upon or over the stomach)
eso-	inward	esotropia (inward turning)
eu-	normal, good	eupnea (normal breathing)
ex-	external, outward	exostosis (condition of external bone)
exo-	outward	exotropia (outward turning)
extra-	outside of	extracorporeal (outside of the body)
hetero-	different	heterograft (graft [like a skin graft] from another species)
homo-	same	homograft (graft [like a skin graft] from the same species)
hydro-	water	hydrotherapy (water therapy)
hyper-	over, above	hypertrophy (overdevelopment)
hypo-	under, below	hypodermic (under the skin)
in-	not; inward	infertility (not fertile); inhalation (to breathe in)
inter-	among, between	intervertebral (between the vertebrae)
intra-	within, inside	intravenous (inside, within a vein)
macro-	large	macrotia (having large ears)
micro-	small	microtia (having small ears)
myo-	to shut	myopia (to shut eyes/squint)
neo-	new	neonatology (study of the newborn)
pan-	all	pansinusitis (inflammation of all the sinuses)
para-	beside, near; abnormal; two like parts of a pair	paranasal (beside the nose); paresthesia (abnormal sensation); paraplegia (paralysis of two like parts of a pair/the legs)
per-	through	percutaneous (through the skin)
peri-	around	pericardial (around the heart)
post-	after	postpartum (after birth)
pre-	before, in front of	preoperative (before a surgical operation)
pro-	before	prolactin (before milk)
pseudo-	false	pseudocyesis (false pregnancy)

MED TERM TIP

Be very careful with prefixes; many have similar spellings but very different meanings. For example:

anti- means "against"; *ante-* means "before"

inter- means "between"; *intra-* means "inside"

per- means "through"; *peri-* means "around"

PREFIX	MEANING	EXAMPLE (DEFINITION)
retro-	backward, behind	retroperitoneal (behind the peritoneum)
sub-	below, under	subcutaneous (under, below the skin)
supra-	above	suprapubic (above the pubic bone)
tachy-	rapid, fast	tachycardia (fast heartbeat)
trans-	through, across	transurethral (across the urethra)
ultra-	beyond, excess	ultrasound (high-frequency sound waves)
un-	not	unconscious (not conscious)

Number Prefixes

Some common prefixes pertaining to the number of items or measurement, their meanings, and examples of their use follow.

PREFIX	MEANING	EXAMPLE (DEFINITION)
bi-	two	bilateral (two sides)
hemi-	half	hemiplegia (paralysis of one side/half of the body)
mono-	one	monoplegia (paralysis of one extremity)
multi-	many	multigravida (woman pregnant more than once)
nulli-	none	nulligravida (woman with no pregnancies)
poly-	many	polyuria (large amounts of urine)
primi-	first	primigravida (first pregnancy)
quadri-	four	quadriplegia (paralysis of all four limbs)
semi-	partial, half	semiconscious (partially conscious)
tetra-	four	tetraplegia (paralysis of all four limbs)
tri-	three	triceps (muscle with three heads)

Suffixes

A suffix is attached to the end of a word to add meaning, such as a condition, disease, or procedure. For example, the suffix *-itis,* meaning inflammation, when added to *cardi-* forms the new word **carditis** (car-DYE-tis), meaning inflammation of the heart. Every medical term *must* have a suffix. Most often the suffix is added to a word root, as in carditis above; however, terms can also be built from a suffix added directly to a prefix, without a word root. For example, the term **dystrophy** (DIS-troh-fee), meaning abnormal development, is built from the prefix *dys-* (meaning abnormal) and the suffix *-trophy* (meaning development).

MED TERM TIP

Remember, if a suffix begins with a vowel, the combining vowel is dropped; for example, *mastitis* rather than *mast**o**itis.*

Common Suffixes

Some common suffixes, their meanings, and examples of their use follow. When written by themselves, suffixes are preceded by a hyphen.

SUFFIX	MEANING	EXAMPLE (DEFINITION)
-algia	pain	gastralgia (stomach pain)
-cele	hernia, protrusion	cystocele (protrusion of the bladder)

SUFFIX	MEANING	EXAMPLE (DEFINITION)
-cyte	cell	erythrocyte (red cell)
-dynia	pain	cardiodynia (heart pain)
-ectasis	dilation	bronchiectasis (dilated bronchi)
-gen	that which produces	pathogen (that which produces disease)
-genesis	produces, generates	spermatogenesis (produces sperm)
-genic	producing, produced by	carcinogenic (producing cancer)
-ia	state, condition	bradycardia (condition of slow heart)
-iasis	abnormal condition	lithiasis (abnormal condition of stones)
-iatry	medical treatment	podiatry (medical treatment for the foot)
-ism	state of	hypothyroidism (state of low thyroid)
-itis	inflammation	dermatitis (inflammation of skin)
-logist	one who studies	cardiologist (one who studies the heart)
-logy	study of	cardiology (study of the heart)
-lysis	destruction	hemolysis (blood destruction)
-lytic	destruction	thrombolytic (clot destruction)
-malacia	abnormal softening	chondromalacia (abnormal cartilage softening)
-megaly	enlargement, large	cardiomegaly (enlarged heart)
-oid	resembling	fibroid (resembling fibers)
-oma	tumor, mass, swelling	carcinoma (cancerous tumor)
-osis	abnormal condition	cyanosis (abnormal condition of being blue)
-pathy	disease	myopathy (muscle disease)
-phobia	fear	photophobia (fear of light)
-plasia	development, growth	hyperplasia (excessive development)
-plasm	formation, development	neoplasm (new formation)
-ptosis	drooping	blepharoptosis (drooping eyelid)
-rrhage	excessive, abnormal flow	hemorrhage (excessive bleeding)
-rrhagia	abnormal flow condition	cystorrhagia (abnormal flow from the bladder)
-rrhea	discharge, flow	rhinorrhea (discharge from the nose)
-rrhexis	rupture	hysterorrhexis (ruptured uterus)
-sclerosis	hardening	arteriosclerosis (hardening of an artery)
-stenosis	narrowing	angiostenosis (narrowing of a vessel)
-therapy	treatment	chemotherapy (treatment with chemicals)
-trophy	nourishment, development	hypertrophy (excessive development)
-ule	small	venule (small vein)

Adjective Suffixes

The following suffixes are used to convert a word root into an adjective. These suffixes usually are translated as *pertaining to.*

SUFFIX	MEANING	EXAMPLE (DEFINITION)
-ac	pertaining to	cardiac (pertaining to the heart)
-al	pertaining to	duodenal (pertaining to the duodenum)
-an	pertaining to	ovarian (pertaining to the ovary)
-ar	pertaining to	ventricular (pertaining to a ventricle)
-ary	pertaining to	pulmonary (pertaining to the lungs)
-atic	pertaining to	lymphatic (pertaining to lymph)
-eal	pertaining to	esophageal (pertaining to the esophagus)
-iac	pertaining to	chondriac (pertaining to cartilage)
-ic	pertaining to	gastric (pertaining to the stomach)
-ile	pertaining to	penile (pertaining to the penis)
-ine	pertaining to	uterine (pertaining to the uterus)
-ior	pertaining to	superior (pertaining to above)
-nic	pertaining to	embryonic (pertaining to an embryo)
-ory	pertaining to	auditory (pertaining to hearing)
-ose	pertaining to	adipose (pertaining to fat)
-ous	pertaining to	intravenous (pertaining to within a vein)
-tic	pertaining to	acoustic (pertaining to hearing)

Surgical Suffixes

The following suffixes indicate surgical procedures.

MED TERM TIP

Surgical suffixes have very specific meanings:

-otomy means "to cut into"
-ostomy means "to create a new opening"
-ectomy means "to cut out" or "remove"

SUFFIX	MEANING	EXAMPLE (DEFINITION)
-centesis	puncture to withdraw fluid	arthrocentesis (puncture to withdraw fluid from a joint)
-ectomy	surgical removal	gastrectomy (surgically remove the stomach)
-ostomy	surgically create an opening	colostomy (surgically create an opening for the colon [through the abdominal wall])
-otomy	cutting into	thoracotomy (cutting into the chest)
-pexy	surgical fixation	nephropexy (surgical fixation of a kidney)
-plasty	surgical repair	dermatoplasty (surgical repair of the skin)
-rrhaphy	suture	myorrhaphy (suture together muscle)

Procedural Suffixes

The following suffixes indicate procedural processes or instruments.

SUFFIX	MEANING	EXAMPLE (DEFINITION)
-gram	record or picture	electrocardiogram (record of heart's electricity)
-graph	instrument for recording	electrocardiograph (instrument for recording the heart's electrical activity)

SUFFIX	MEANING	EXAMPLE (DEFINITION)
-graphy	process of recording	electrocardiography (process of recording the heart's electrical activity)
-meter	instrument for measuring	audiometer (instrument to measure hearing)
-metry	process of measuring	audiometry (process of measuring hearing)
-scope	instrument for viewing	gastroscope (instrument to view stomach)
-scopy	process of visually examining	gastroscopy (process of visually examining the stomach)

Word Building

Word building consists of putting together two or more word elements to form a variety of terms. Prefixes and suffixes may be added to a combining form to create a new descriptive term. For example, adding the prefix *hypo-* (meaning below) and the suffix *-ic* (meaning pertaining to) to the combining form *derm/o* (meaning skin) forms **hypodermic** (high-poh-DER-mik), pertaining to below the skin.

Interpreting Medical Terms

The following strategy is a reliable method for puzzling out the meaning of an unfamiliar medical term.

STEP	EXAMPLE
1. Divide the term into its word parts.	gastr/o/enter/o/logy
2. Define each word part.	gastr = stomach
	o = combining vowel, no meaning
	enter = small intestine
	o = combining vowel, no meaning
	-logy = study
3. Combine the meaning of the word parts.	stomach, small intestine, study of

MED TERM TIP

To gain a quick understanding of a term, it may be helpful to you to read from the end of the word (or the suffix) back to the beginning (the prefix), and then pick up the word root. For example, *pericarditis* reads inflammation (*-itis*) surrounding (*peri-*) the heart (*cardi/o*).

Pronunciation

You will hear different pronunciations for the same terms depending on where people were born or educated. As long as it is clear which term people are discussing, differing pronunciations are acceptable. Some people are difficult to understand over the telephone or on a transcription tape. If you have any doubt about a term being discussed, ask for the term to be spelled. For example, it is often difficult to hear the difference between the terms **abduction** and **adduction.** However, since the terms refer to opposite directions of movement, it is very important to double-check if there is any question about which term was used.

Each new term in this text is introduced in boldface type, with the phonetic or "sounds like" pronunciation in parentheses immediately following. The part of the word that should receive the greatest emphasis during pronunciation appears in capital letters: for example, **pericarditis** (per-ih-car-DYE-tis).

Spelling

Although you will hear differing pronunciations of the same term, there will be only one correct spelling. If you have any doubt about the spelling of a term or of its meaning, always look it up in a medical dictionary. If only one letter of the word is changed, it could make a critical difference for the patient. For example, imagine the problem that could arise if you note for insurance purposes that a portion of a patient's **ileum,** or small intestine, was removed when in reality he had surgery for removal of a piece of his **ilium,** or hip bone.

> **MED TERM TIP**
> If you have any doubt about the meaning or spelling of a word, look it up in your medical dictionary. Even experienced medical personnel still need to look up a few words.

Some words have the same beginning sounds but are spelled differently. Examples include:

Sounds like *si*

psy	**psychiatry** (sigh-KIGH-ah-tree)
cy	**cytology** (sigh-TALL-oh-gee)

Sounds like *dis*

dys	**dyspepsia** (dis-PEP-see-ah)
dis	**dislocation** (dis-low-KAY-shun)

Singular and Plural Endings

Many medical terms originate from Greek and Latin words. The rules for forming the singular and plural forms of some words follow the rules of these languages rather than English. For example, the heart has a left atrium and a right atrium for a total of two *atria,* not two *atriums.* Other words, such as *virus* and *viruses,* are changed from singular to plural by following English rules. Each medical term needs to be considered individually when changing from the singular to the plural form. The following examples illustrate how to form plurals.

Words ending in	Singular	Plural
-a	vertebra	vertebrae
-ax	thorax	thoraces
-ex or -ix	appendix	appendices
-is	metastasis	metastases
-ma	sarcoma	sarcomata
-nx	phalanx	phalanges
-on	ganglion	ganglia
-us	nucleus	nuclei
-um	ovum	ova
-y	biopsy	biopsies

Abbreviations

Abbreviations are commonly used in the medical profession as a way of saving time. However, some abbreviations can be confusing, such as *SM* for simple mastectomy and *sm* for small. Use of the incorrect abbreviation can result in problems for a patient, as well as with insurance records and processing. If you have any concern that you will confuse someone by using an abbreviation, spell out the word instead. It is never acceptable to use made-up abbreviations. All types of healthcare facilities will have a list of approved abbreviations, and it is extremely important that you become familiar with this list and follow it closely.

The Medical Record

The **medical record** or chart documents the details of a patient's hospital stay. Each healthcare professional who has contact with the patient in any capacity completes the appropriate report of that contact and adds it to the medical chart. This results in a permanent physical record of the patient's day-to-day condition, when and what services he or she received, and the response to treatment. Each institution adopts a specific format for each document and its location within the chart. This is necessary because each healthcare professional must be able to locate quickly and efficiently the information he or she needs in order to provide proper care for the patient. The medical record is also a legal document. Therefore, it is essential that all chart components be completely filled out and signed. Each page must contain the proper patient identification information: the patient's name, age, gender, physician, admission date, and identification number.

While the patient is still in the hospital, a unit clerk is usually responsible for placing documents in the proper place. After discharge, the medical records department ensures that all documents are present, complete, signed, and in the correct order. If a person is readmitted, especially for the same diagnosis, parts of this previous chart can be pulled and added to the current chart for reference (see Figure 1.2 ■). Physicians' offices and other outpatient care providers such as clinics and therapists also maintain a medical record detailing each patient's visit to their facility.

The digital revolution has also impacted healthcare with the increasing use of the **Electronic Medical Record** (EMR). A software program is used to enter patient information into a computer which then organizes and stores the information. Information may be entered either at a centralized workstation or by using mobile devices at the point of care. Once digitally stored, the information may be analyzed and monitored to detect and prevent potential errors. Since the records are digitally stored, they can be easily accessed and shared between healthcare providers which will reduce repeating tests unnecessarily and inadvertent medication errors. The following list includes the most common elements of a paper chart with a brief description.

History and Physical—Written or dictated by admitting physician; details patient's history, results of physician's examination, initial diagnoses, and physician's plan of treatment

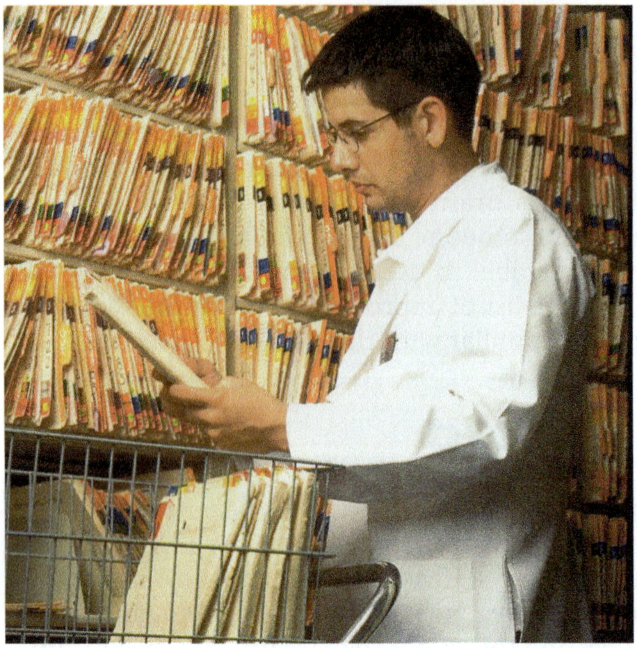

Figure 1.2 Health information professionals maintain accurate, orderly, and permanent patient records. Medical records are securely stored and available for future reference.

Physician's Orders—Complete list of care, medications, tests, and treatments physician orders for patient

Nurse's Notes—Record of patient's care throughout the day; includes vital signs, treatment specifics, patient's response to treatment, and patient's condition

Physician's Progress Notes—Physician's daily record of patient's condition, results of physician's examinations, summary of test results, updated assessment and diagnoses, and further plans for patient's care

Consultation Reports—Reports given by specialists whom physician has asked to evaluate patient

Ancillary Reports—Reports from various treatments and therapies patient has received, such as rehabilitation, social services, or respiratory therapy

Diagnostic Reports—Results of diagnostic tests performed on patient, principally from clinical lab (e.g., blood tests) and medical imaging (e.g., X-rays and ultrasound)

Informed Consent—Document voluntarily signed by patient or a responsible party that clearly describes purpose, methods, procedures, benefits, and risks of a diagnostic or treatment procedure

Operative Report—Report from surgeon detailing an operation; includes pre- and postoperative diagnosis, specific details of surgical procedure itself, and how patient tolerated procedure

Anesthesiologist's Report—Relates details regarding substances (such as medications and fluids) given to patient, patient's response to anesthesia, and vital signs during surgery

Pathologist's Report—Report given by pathologist who studies tissue removed from patient (e.g., bone marrow, blood, or tissue biopsy)

Discharge Summary—Comprehensive outline of patient's entire hospital stay; includes condition at time of admission, admitting diagnosis, test results, treatments and patient's response, final diagnosis, and follow-up plans

Healthcare Settings

The use of medical terminology is widespread. It provides healthcare professionals with a precise and efficient method of communicating very specific patient information to one another, regardless of whether they are in the same type of facility (see Figure 1.3 ■). Descriptions follow of the different types of settings where medical terminology is used.

Acute Care or General Hospitals—Provide services to diagnose (laboratory, diagnostic imaging) and treat (surgery, medications, therapy) diseases for a short period of time; in addition, they usually provide emergency and obstetrical care

Specialty Care Hospitals—Provide care for very specific types of diseases; for example, a psychiatric hospital

Nursing Homes or Long-Term Care Facilities—Provide long-term care for patients needing extra time to recover from illness or injury before returning home, or for persons who can no longer care for themselves

Ambulatory Care Centers, Surgical Centers, or Outpatient Clinics—Provide services not requiring overnight hospitalization; services range from simple surgeries to diagnostic testing or therapy

Physicians' Offices—Provide diagnostic and treatment services in a private office setting

Health Maintenance Organization (HMO)—Provides wide range of services by a group of primary-care physicians, specialists, and other healthcare professionals in a prepaid system

Home Health Care—Provides nursing, therapy, personal care, or housekeeping services in patient's own home

Rehabilitation Centers—Provide intensive physical and occupational therapy; includes inpatient and outpatient treatment

Hospices—Provide supportive treatment to terminally ill patients and their families

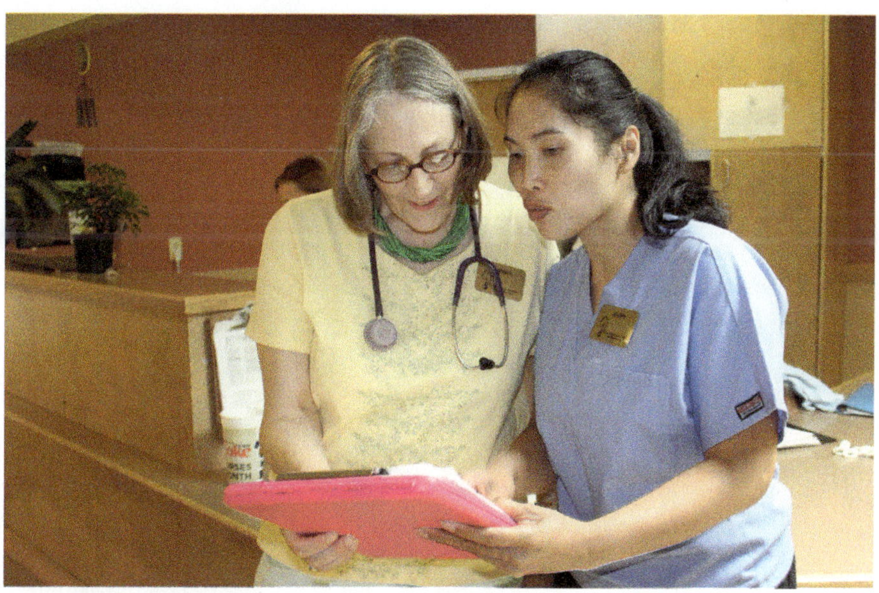

■ **Figure 1.3** A nurse and medical assistant review a patient's chart and plan his or her daily care.

Confidentiality

Anyone working with medical terminology and involved in the medical profession must have a firm understanding of confidentiality. Any information or record relating to a patient must be considered privileged. This means that you have a moral and legal responsibility to keep all information about the patient confidential. If you are asked to supply documentation relating to a patient, the proper authorization form must be signed by the patient. Give only the specific information that the patient has authorized. The Health Insurance Portability and Accountability Act of 1996 (HIPAA) set federal standards providing patients with more protection of their medical records and health information, better access to their own records, and greater control over how their health information is used and to whom it is disclosed.

Chapter Review

Practice Exercises

A. Complete the Statement

1. The combination of a word root and the combining vowel is called a(n) ______________________.

2. The vowel that connects two word roots or a suffix with a word root is usually a(n) ______________________.

3. A word part used at the end of a word root to change the meaning of the word is called a(n) ______________________.

4. A(n) ______________________ is used at the beginning of a word to indicate number, location, or time.

5. Although the pronunciation of medical terms may differ slightly from one person to another, the ______________________ must never change.

6. The four components of a medical term are ______________________, ______________________, ______________________, and ______________________.

B. Terminology Matching

Match each definition to its term.

	Definition		Term
1.	________ Provides services for a short period of time	a.	rehabilitation center
2.	________ Complete outline of a patient's entire hospital stay	b.	nurse's notes
3.	________ Describes purpose, methods, benefits, and risks of procedure	c.	ancillary report
4.	________ Contains updated assessment, diagnoses, and further plans for care	d.	hospice
5.	________ Provides supportive care to terminally ill patients and families	e.	discharge summary
6.	________ Written by the admitting physician	f.	physician's progress notes
7.	________ Reports results from study of tissue removed from the patient	g.	ambulatory care center
8.	________ Written by the surgeon	h.	diagnostic report
9.	________ Provides services not requiring overnight hospital stay	i.	long-term care facility
10.	________ Report given by a specialist	j.	informed consent
11.	________ Record of a patient's care through the day	k.	history and physical
12.	________ Clinical lab and medical imaging reports	l.	acute care hospital
13.	________ Provides intensive physical and occupational therapy	m.	pathologist's report
14.	________ Report of treatment/therapy the patient received	n.	consultation report
15.	________ Provides care for patients who need more time to recover	o.	operative report

C. Define the Suffix

1. **-plasty** ______
2. **-stenosis** ______
3. **-itis** ______
4. **-al** ______
5. **-algia** ______
6. **-otomy** ______
7. **-megaly** ______
8. **-ectomy** ______
9. **-rrhage** ______
10. **-centesis** ______
11. **-gram** ______
12. **-ac** ______
13. **-malacia** ______
14. **-ism** ______
15. **-rrhaphy** ______
16. **-ostomy** ______
17. **-pexy** ______
18. **-rrhea** ______
19. **-scopy** ______
20. **-oma** ______

D. Combining Form and Suffix Practice

Join a combining form and a suffix to form words with the following meanings.

1. study of lungs ______
2. pain relating to a nerve ______
3. nose discharge or flow ______
4. abnormal softening of a kidney ______
5. enlarged heart ______
6. cutting into the stomach ______
7. inflammation of the skin ______

8. surgical removal of the voice box ______________________________

9. surgical repair of a joint ______________________________

10. gland disease ______________________________

E. Name That Prefix

1. within, inside ______________________________

2. large ______________________________

3. before, in front of ______________________________

4. around ______________________________

5. new ______________________________

6. without ______________________________

7. half ______________________________

8. painful, difficult ______________________________

9. above ______________________________

10. over, above ______________________________

11. many ______________________________

12. slow ______________________________

13. self ______________________________

14. across ______________________________

15. two ______________________________

F. Prefix Practice

Circle the prefixes in the following terms and define in the space provided.

1. tachycardia ______________________________

2. pseudocyesis ______________________________

3. hypoglycemia ______________________________

4. intercostal ______________________________

5. eupnea ______________________________

6. postoperative ______________________________

7. monoplegia ______________________________

8. subcutaneous ______________________________

G. Make It Plural

Change the following singular terms to plural terms.

1. metastasis ______________________________
2. ovum ______________________________
3. diverticulum ______________________________
4. atrium ______________________________
5. diagnosis ______________________________
6. vertebra ______________________________

H. Name That Term

Use the suffix **-ology** to write a term for each medical specialty.

1. heart ______________________________
2. stomach ______________________________
3. skin ______________________________
4. eye ______________________________
5. immunity ______________________________
6. kidney ______________________________
7. blood ______________________________
8. female ______________________________
9. nerve ______________________________
10. disease ______________________________

I. Metric Prefixes

In the United States, most everyday measurements are made using standard units such as ounces, pounds, and feet. In the medical industry, however, many measurements are made using metric units, examples include measuring and weighing medications, physical therapy angles, and intake and output recording. The meter (m), gram (g), and liter (L) are basic metric units. The metric system is a system of measurement that is based on 10, which greatly simplifies calculations. By multiplying or dividing by 10, a new metric unit can be reached.

Different metric units can be identified by their prefixes. If you recognize the prefix, you immediately know information about the given measurement.

For example, 1 kilometer equals 1,000 meters, while 1 millimeter equals 1/1000 of a meter. You may often need to convert from one unit to another. Converting between units is accomplished by moving the decimal point. Look at the decimal relationships in the chart. For example, suppose you are given a measurement of 1.5 kilograms, but you need the measurement in grams.

To convert from kilograms to grams, move the decimal three places to the right. So 1.5 kilograms is equal to 1,500 grams.

Prefix	Symbol	Exponent Form	Decimal Equivalent
kilo-	k	103	1000
hecto-	h	102	100
deka-	da	10	10
—	—	—	—
deci-	d	10^{-1}	0.1
centi-	c	10^{-2}	0.01
milli-	m	10^{-3}	0.001

How many milliliters are in 25 liters? Determine a medical process or procedure that uses metric measures. Choose a level of accuracy appropriate for the selected process or procedure measurement.

J. Building Medical Terms

Build a medical term by combining the word parts requested in each question.

For example, use the combining form for *spleen* with the suffix meaning *enlargement* to form a word meaning *enlargement of the spleen* (answer: *splenomegaly*).

1. combining form for *heart* ____________
   suffix meaning *abnormal softening* ____________
   term meaning *softening of the heart* ____________
2. word root form for *stomach* ____________
   suffix meaning *to surgically create an opening* ____________
   term meaning *creating an opening into the stomach* ____________
3. combining form for *nose* ____________
   suffix meaning *surgical repair* ____________
   term meaning *surgical repair of the nose* ____________
4. prefix meaning *over, above* ____________
   suffix meaning *nourishment, development* ____________
   term meaning *overdevelopment* ____________
5. combining form meaning *disease* ____________
   suffix meaning *the study of* ____________
   term meaning *the study of disease* ____________
6. word root meaning *gland* ____________
   suffix for *tumor/mass* ____________
   term meaning *gland tumor or mass* ____________
7. combining form meaning *stomach* ____________
   combining form meaning *small intestine* ____________
   suffix meaning *study of* ____________
   term meaning *study of stomach and small intestine* ____________
8. word root meaning *ear* ____________
   suffix meaning *inflammation* ____________
   term meaning *ear inflammation* ____________
9. prefix meaning *water* ____________
   suffix meaning *treatment* ____________
   term meaning *water treatment* ____________
10. combining form meaning *cancer* ____________
    suffix meaning *that which produces* ____________
    term meaning *that which produces cancer* ____________

K. Define the Combining Form

1. **aden/o** ______________________
2. **carcin/o** ______________________
3. **cardi/o** ______________________
4. **chem/o** ______________________
5. **cis/o** ______________________
6. **dermat/o** ______________________
7. **enter/o** ______________________
8. **gastr/o** ______________________
9. **gynec/o** ______________________
10. **hemat/o** ______________________
11. **hydr/o** ______________________
12. **immun/o** ______________________
13. **laryng/o** ______________________
14. **path/o** ______________________
15. **nephr/o** ______________________
16. **neur/o** ______________________
17. **ophthalm/o** ______________________
18. **ot/o** ______________________
19. **pulmon/o** ______________________
20. **rhin/o** ______________________

L. Professionalism

If you exhibit a professional look and demeanor, your clients and colleagues will have more confidence in you. Why is this? Give specific examples of positive and negative behaviors and appearance factors.

M. Career Exploration

Using nursing careers as the example:

- Identify the organization that grants credentialing for registering nurses and examine the specific preparation required for receiving a registered nurse designation, e.g., education, internship, examination, etc.
- Identify the state or national organization that grants certification for nurse assistants and examine the specific preparation required for receiving the certification, e.g., education, internship, examination, etc.
- Examine the role of the professional organization in the governance of registered nurse credentialing, including maintaining a current license and potential causes for having the license revoked.
- Examine the role of the organization or agency in the governance of nurse assistant certification, including maintaining a current license and potential causes for having the license revoked.

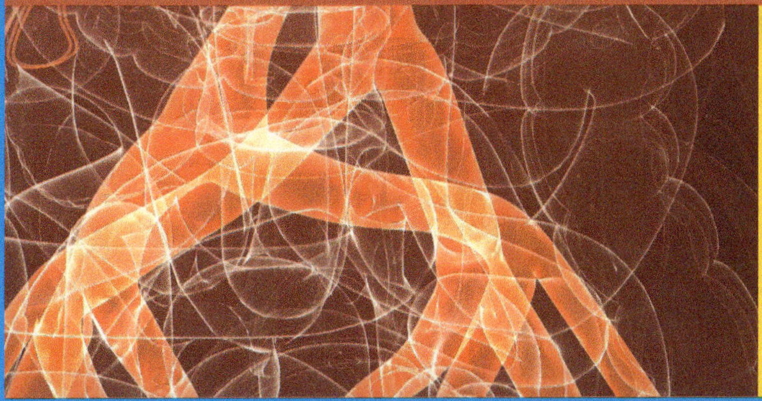

2

BODY ORGANIZATION

Learning Objectives

Upon completion of this chapter, you will be able to

- Recognize the combining forms introduced in this chapter.
- Correctly spell and pronounce medical terms and anatomical structures relating to body structure.
- Discuss the organization of the body in terms of cells, tissues, organs, and systems.
- Describe the common features of cells.
- Define the four types of tissues.
- List the major organs found in the 12 organ systems.
- Describe the anatomical position.
- Define the body planes.
- Identify regions of the body.
- Define directional and positional terms.
- List the body cavities and their contents.
- Locate and describe the nine anatomical and four clinical divisions of the abdomen.
- Build body organization medical terms from word parts.
- Interpret abbreviations associated with body organization.

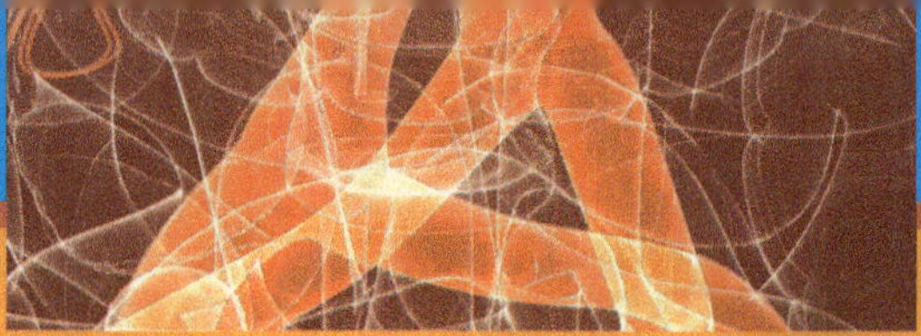

Body Organization at a Glance

Arrangement

The body is organized into levels; each is built from the one below it. In other words, the body as a whole is composed of systems, a system is composed of organs, an organ is composed of tissues, and tissues are composed of cells.

Levels

cells   tissues   organs   systems   body

Word Parts

Presented here are some of the more common combining forms used to build body organizational terms. For a list of the prefixes and suffixes used, refer to the Terminology section of this chapter.

Combining Forms

abdomin/o	abdomen
adip/o	fat
anter/o	front
brachi/o	arm
cardi/o	heart
caud/o	tail
cephal/o	head
cervic/o	neck
chondr/o	cartilage
crani/o	skull
crin/o	to secrete
crur/o	leg
cyt/o	cell
dermat/o	skin
dist/o	away from
dors/o	back of body
enter/o	small intestine
epitheli/o	epithelium
gastr/o	stomach
glute/o	buttock
gynec/o	woman
hemat/o	blood
hist/o	tissue
immun/o	protection
infer/o	below
laryng/o	larynx
later/o	side
lumb/o	loin
lymph/o	lymph
medi/o	middle
muscul/o	muscles
nephr/o	kidney
neur/o	nerve
ophthalm/o	eye
ot/o	ear
pelv/o	pelvis
peritone/o	peritoneum
pleur/o	pleura
poster/o	back
proct/o	rectum and anus
proxim/o	near to
pub/o	genital region
pulmon/o	lung
rhin/o	nose
spin/o	spine
super/o	above
thorac/o	chest
ur/o	urine
vascul/o	blood vessel
ventr/o	belly
vertebr/o	vertebra
viscer/o	internal organ

Body Organization Illustrated

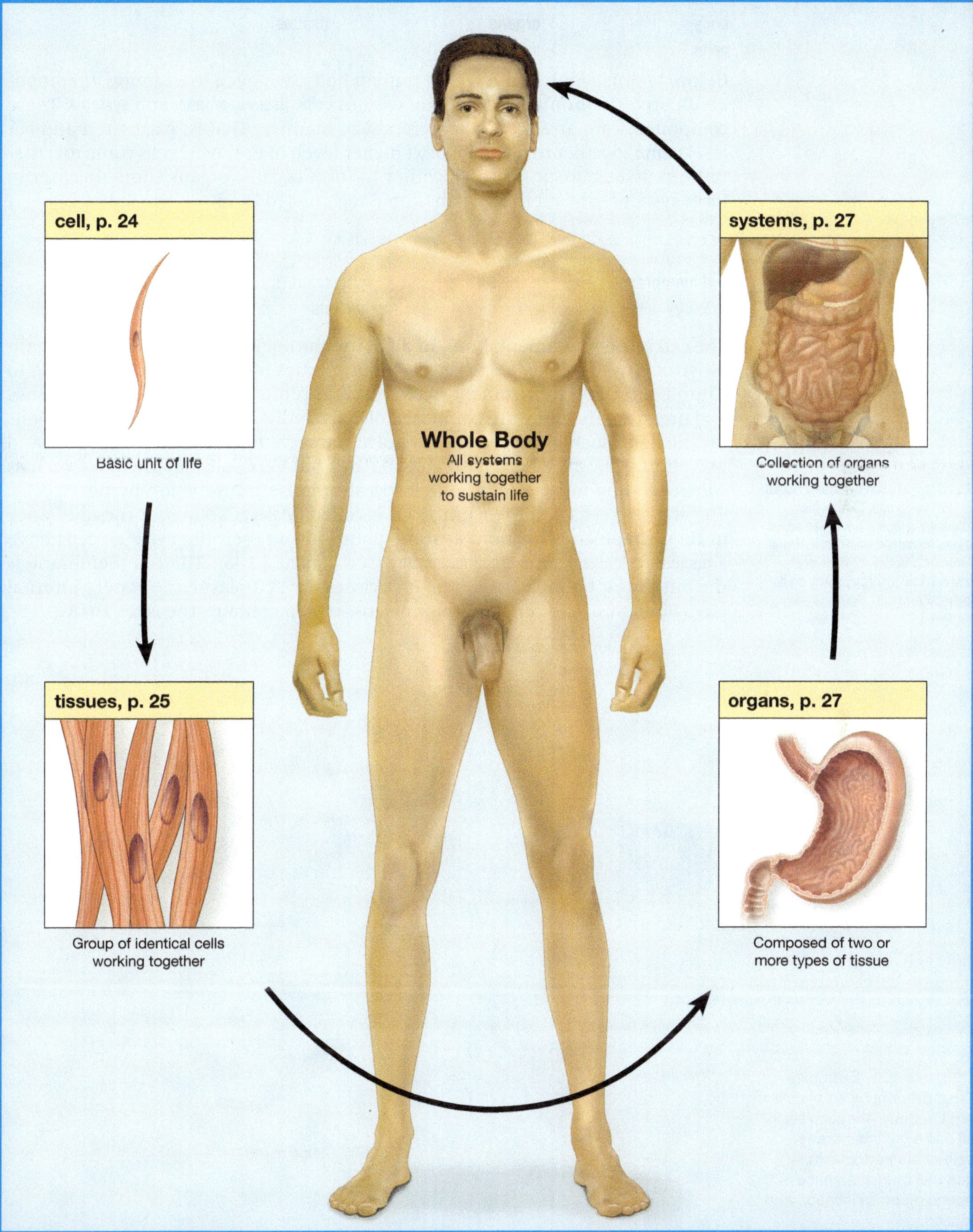

Levels of Body Organization

body **organs** **tissues**
cells **systems**

Before taking a look at the whole human body, we need to examine its component parts. The human **body** is composed of **cells, tissues, organs,** and **systems.** These components are arranged in a hierarchical manner. That is, parts from a lower level come together to form the next higher level. In that way, cells come together to form tissues, tissues come together to form organs, organs come together to form systems, and all the systems come together to form the whole body.

Cells

cell membrane **cytoplasm** (SIGH-toh-plazm)
cytology (sigh-TALL-oh-jee) **nucleus**

The cell is the fundamental unit of all living things. That is to say, it is the smallest structure of a body that has all the properties of being alive: responding to stimuli, engaging in metabolic activities, and reproducing itself. All the tissues and organs in the body are composed of cells. Individual cells perform functions for the body such as reproduction, hormone secretion, energy production, and excretion. Special cells are also able to carry out very specific functions, such as contraction by muscle cells and electrical impulse transmission by nerve cells. The study of cells and their functions is called **cytology.** No matter the difference in their shape and function, at some point during their life cycle all cells have a **nucleus, cytoplasm,** and a **cell membrane** (see Figure 2.1 ■). The cell membrane is the outermost boundary of a cell. It encloses the cytoplasm, the watery internal environment of the cell, and the nucleus, which contains the cell's DNA.

MED TERM TIP

Cells were first seen by Robert Hooke over 300 years ago. To him, the rectangular shapes looked like prison cells, so he named them cells. It was a common practice for early anatomists to name an organ solely on its appearance.

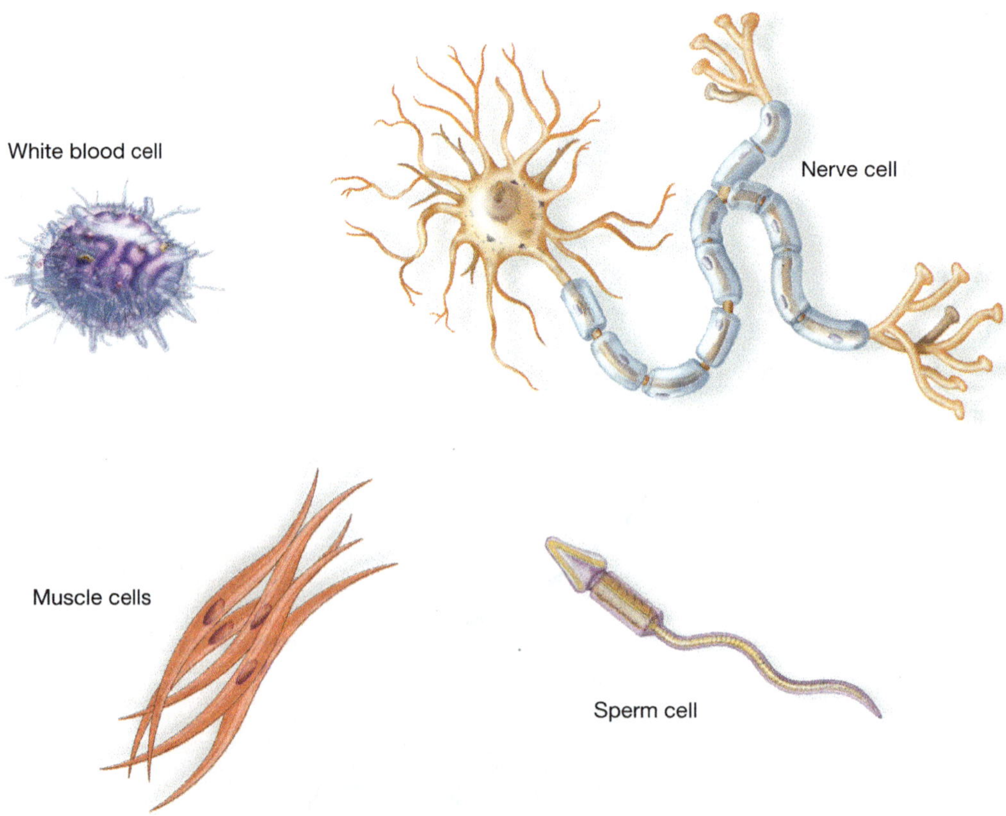

■ **Figure 2.1** Examples of four different types of cells from the body. Although each cell has a cell membrane, nucleus, and cytoplasm, each has a unique shape depending on its location and function.

Tissues

connective tissue
epithelial tissue (ep-ih-THEE-lee-al)
histology (hiss-TALL-oh-jee)
muscle tissue
nervous tissue

Histology is the study of tissue. A tissue is formed when like cells are grouped together and function together to perform a specific activity. The body has four types of tissue: **muscle tissue, epithelial tissue, connective tissue,** and **nervous tissue** (see Figure 2.2 ■).

Muscle Tissue

cardiac muscle
smooth muscle
muscle fibers
skeletal muscle

Muscle tissue produces movement in the body through contraction, or shortening in length, and is composed of individual muscle cells called **muscle fibers**. Muscle tissue forms one of three basic types of muscles: **skeletal muscle, smooth muscle,** or **cardiac muscle.** Skeletal muscle is attached to bone. Smooth muscle is found in internal organs such as the intestine, uterus, and blood vessels. Cardiac muscle is found only in the heart.

Epithelial Tissue

epithelium (ep-ih-THEE-lee-um)

Epithelial tissue, or **epithelium,** is found throughout the body and is composed of close-packed cells that form the covering for and lining of body structures. For example, both the top layer of skin and the lining of the stomach are epithelial tissue (see Figure 2.2). In addition to forming a protective barrier, epithelial tissue may be specialized to absorb substances (such as nutrients from the intestine), secrete substances (such as sweat glands), or excrete wastes (such as the kidney tubules).

MED TERM TIP

The term *epithelium* comes from the prefix *epi-* meaning "on top of" and the combining form *theli/o* meaning "nipple" (referring to any projection from the surface).

Connective Tissue

adipose (ADD-ih-pohs)
bone
cartilage (CAR-tih-lij)
tendons

Connective tissue is the supporting and protecting tissue in body structures. Because connective tissue performs many different functions depending on its location, it appears in many different forms so that each is able to perform the task required at that location. For example, **bone** provides structural support for the whole body. **Cartilage** is the shock absorber in joints. **Tendons** tightly connect skeletal muscles to bones. **Adipose** provides protective padding around body structures (see Figure 2.2).

Nervous Tissue

brain
nerves
neurons
spinal cord

Nervous tissue is composed of cells called **neurons** (see Figure 2.2). This tissue forms the **brain, spinal cord,** and a network of **nerves** throughout the entire body, allowing for the conduction of electrical impulses to send information between the brain and the rest of the body.

Figure 2.2 The appearance of different types of tissues—muscle, epithelial, nervous, connective—and their location within the body.

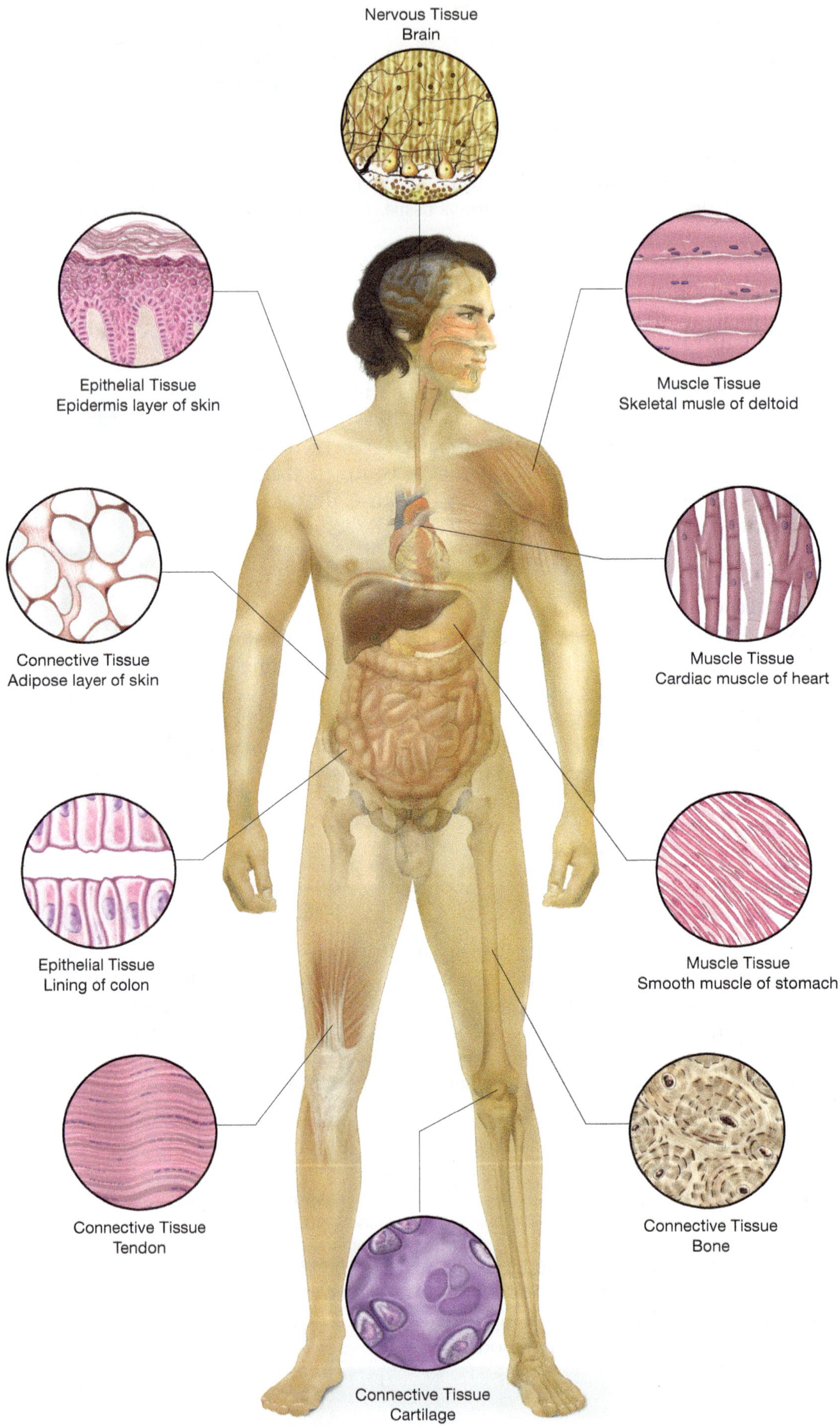

Organs and Systems

Organs are composed of several different types of tissue that work as a unit to perform special functions. For example, the stomach contains smooth muscle tissue, nervous tissue, and epithelial tissue that allow it to contract to mix food with digestive juices.

A system is composed of several organs working in a coordinated manner to perform a complex function or functions. To continue our example, the stomach plus the other digestive system organs—the oral cavity, esophagus, liver, pancreas, small intestine, and colon—work together to ingest, digest, and absorb our food.

Table 2.1 ■ presents the organ systems that are discussed in this text along with the major organs found in each system, the system functions, and the medical specialties that treat conditions of that system.

Table 2.1 Organ Systems of the Human Body

SYSTEM/MEDICAL SPECIALTY	STRUCTURES		FUNCTIONS
Integumentary System (in-teg-you-MEN-tah-ree) **dermatology** (der-mah-TALL-oh-jee)	• skin • hair • nails • sweat glands • sebaceous glands	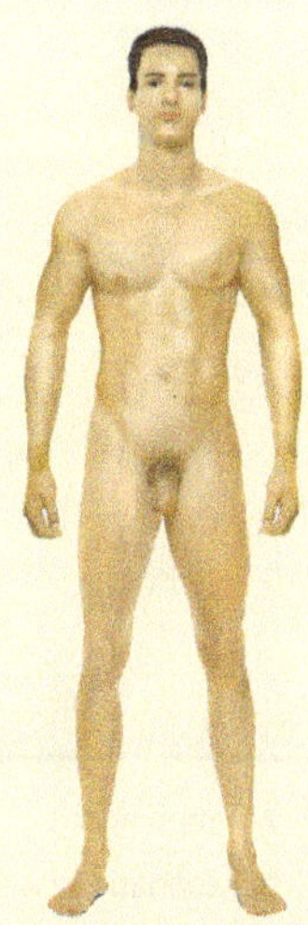	Forms protective two-way barrier and aids in temperature regulation.
Musculoskeletal System (MS) (mus-qu-low-SKEL-et-all) **orthopedics** (or-thoh-PEE-diks) **orthopedic surgery** (or-the-PEE-dik)	• bones • joints • muscles	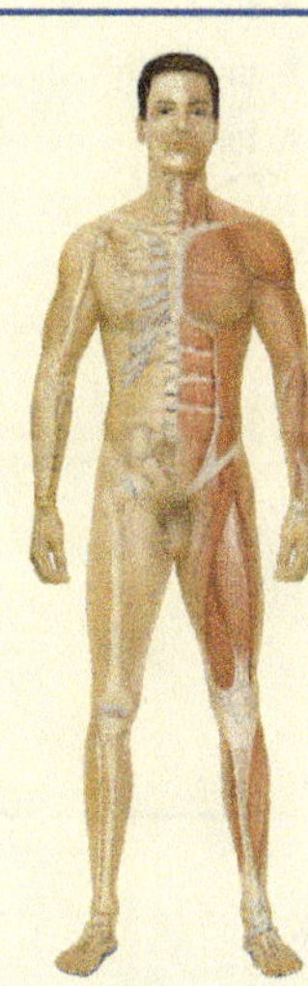	Skeleton supports and protects the body, forms blood cells, and stores minerals. Muscles produce movement.

(Continued)

Table 2.1 Organ Systems of the Human Body (continued)

SYSTEM/MEDICAL SPECIALTY	STRUCTURES	FUNCTIONS
Cardiovascular System (CV) (car-dee-oh-VAS-kew-lar) **cardiology** (car-dee-ALL-oh-jee)	• heart • arteries • veins 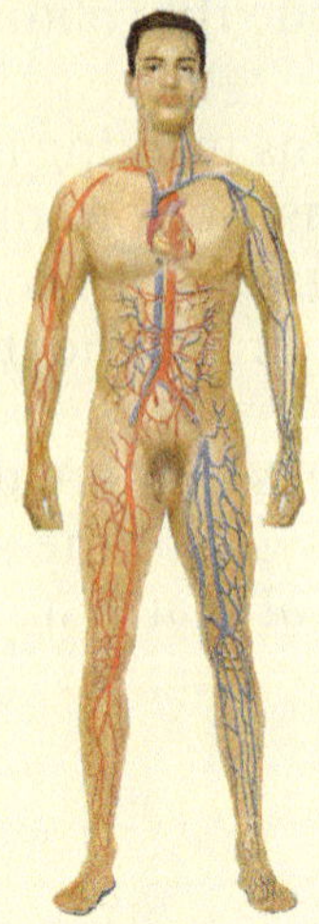	Pumps blood throughout the entire body to transport nutrients, oxygen, and wastes.
Blood (Hematic System) (he-MAT-tik) **hematology** (hee-mah-TALL-oh-jee)	• plasma • erythrocytes • leukocytes • platelets 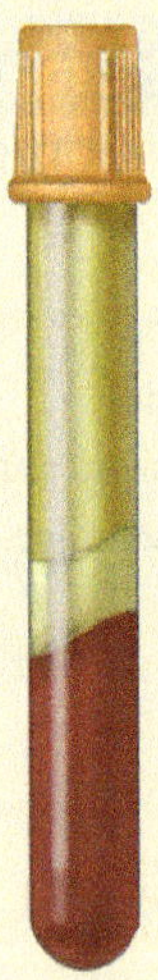	Transports oxygen, protects against pathogens, and controls bleeding.
Lymphatic System (lim-FAT-ik) **immunology** (im-yoo-NALL-oh-jee)	• lymph nodes • lymphatic vessels • spleen • thymus gland • tonsils 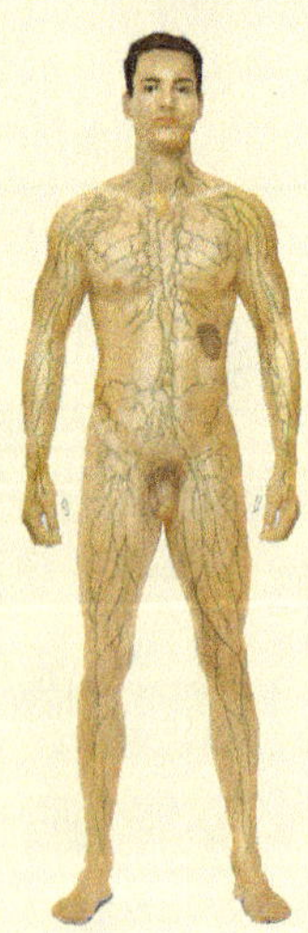	Protects the body from disease and invasion from pathogens.

Table 2.1 Organization Systems of the Human Body (continued)

SYSTEM/MEDICAL SPECIALTY	STRUCTURES	FUNCTIONS
Respiratory System **otorhinolaryngology** (ENT) (oh-toh-rye-noh- lair-ing-GALL-oh-jee) **pulmonology** (pull-mon-ALL-oh-jee) **thoracic surgery** (tho-RASS-ik)	• nasal cavity • pharynx • larynx • trachea • bronchial tubes • lungs 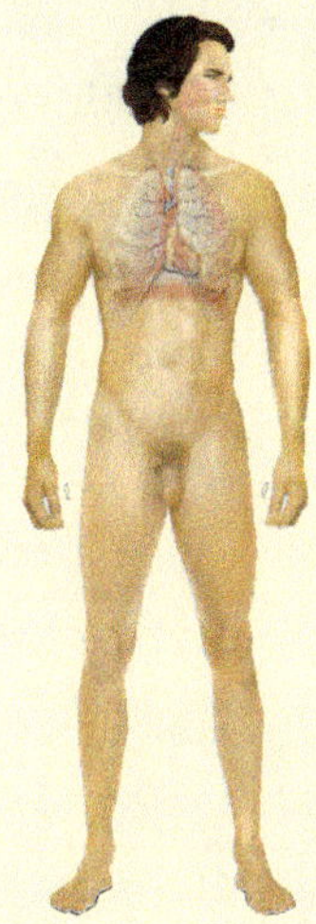	Obtains oxygen and removes carbon dioxide from the body.
Digestive or **Gastrointestinal System** (GI) **gastroenterology** (gas-troh-en-ter-ALL-oh-jee) **proctology** (prok-TOL-oh-jee)	• oral cavity • pharynx • esophagus • stomach • small intestine • colon • liver • gallbladder • pancreas • salivary glands 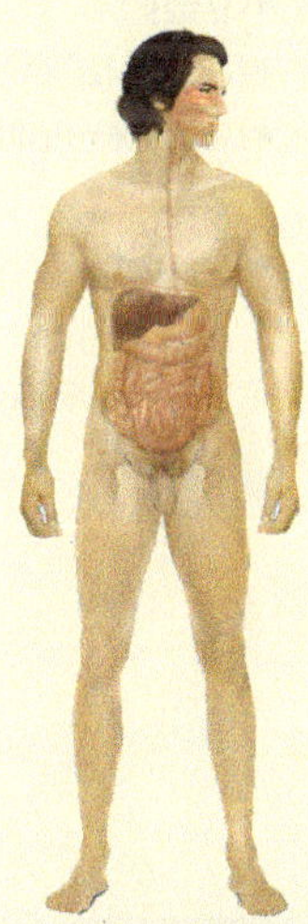	Ingests, digests, and absorbs nutrients for the body.
Urinary System (YOO-rih-nair-ee) **nephrology** (neh-FROL-oh-jee) **urology** (yoo-RALL-oh-jee)	• kidneys • ureters • urinary bladder • urethra 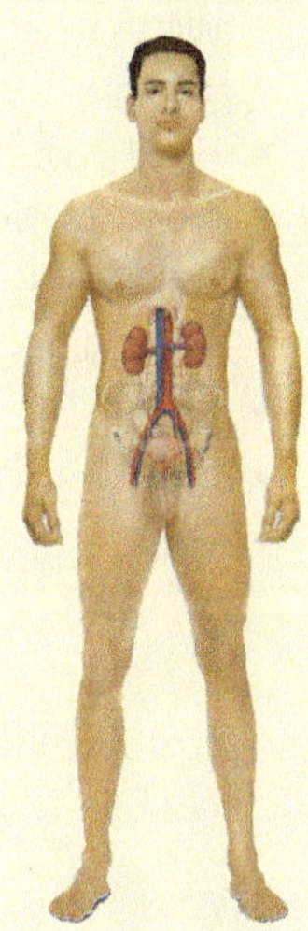	Filters waste products out of the blood and removes them from the body.

(Continued)

Table 2.1 Organ Systems of the Human Body (continued)

SYSTEM/MEDICAL SPECIALTY	STRUCTURES	FUNCTIONS
Female Reproductive System **gynecology** (GYN) (gigh-neh-KOL- oh-jee) **obstetrics** (OB) (ob-STET-riks)	• ovary • fallopian tubes • uterus • vagina • vulva • breasts 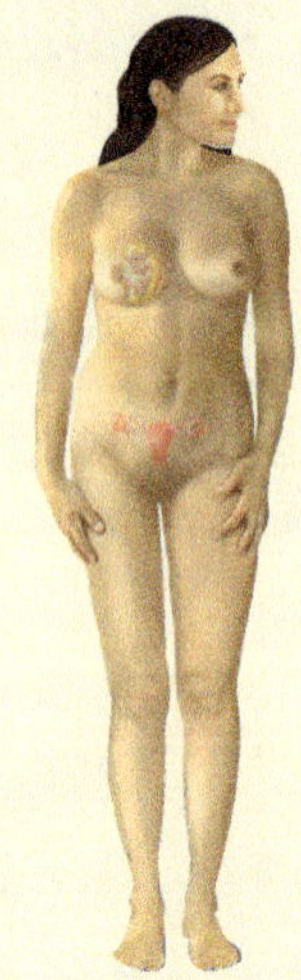	Produces eggs for reproduction and provides place for growing baby.
Male Reproductive System **urology** (yoo-RALL-oh-jee)	• testes • epididymis • vas deferens • penis • seminal vesicles • prostate gland • bulbourethral gland 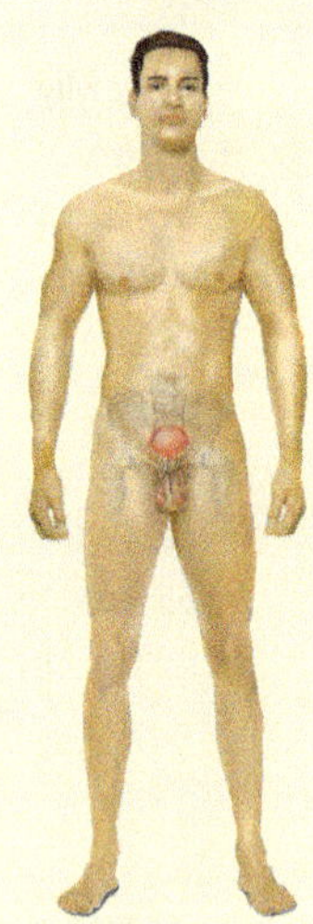	Produces sperm for reproduction.
Endocrine System (EN-doh-krin) **endocrinology** (en-doh-krin-ALL-oh-jee)	• pituitary gland • pineal gland • thyroid gland • parathyroid glands • thymus gland • adrenal glands • pancreas • ovaries • testes 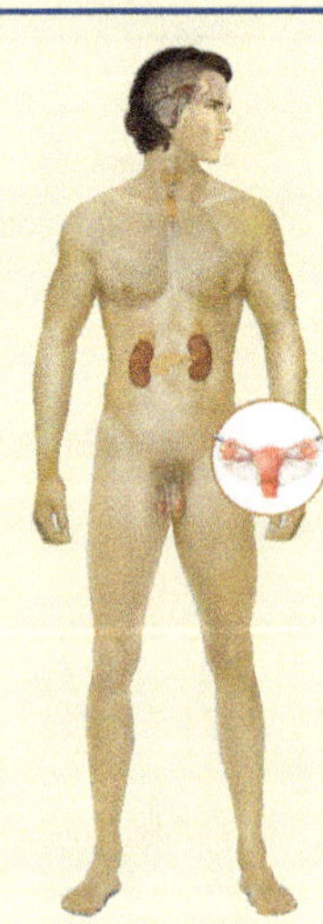	Regulates metabolic activities of the body.

Table 2.1 Organ Systems of the Human Body (continued)

SYSTEM/MEDICAL SPECIALTY	STRUCTURES	FUNCTIONS
Nervous System **neurology** (noo-RAL-oh-jee) **neurosurgery** (noo-roh-SIR-jer-ee)	• brain • spinal cord • nerves 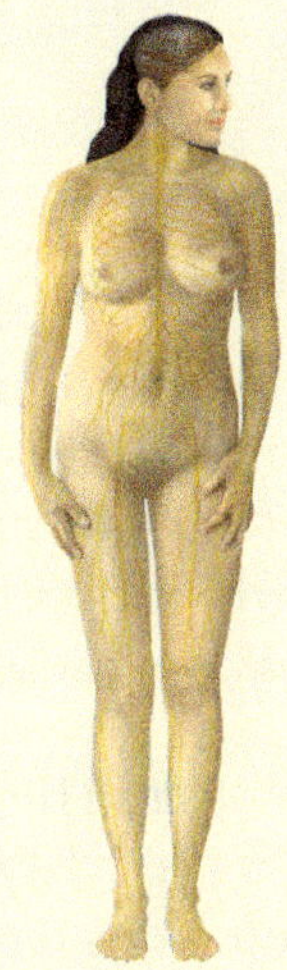	Receives sensory information and coordinates the body's response.
Special Senses **ophthalmology** (off-thal-MALL-oh-jee)	• eye 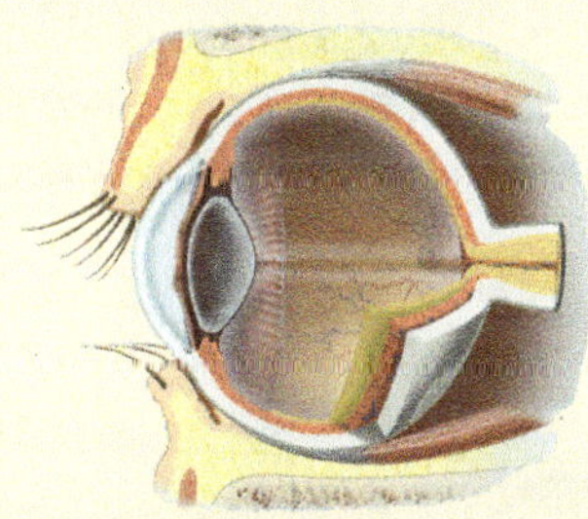	Vision
otorhinolaryngology (ENT) (oh-toh-rye-noh-lair- ing-GALL-oh-jee)	• ear 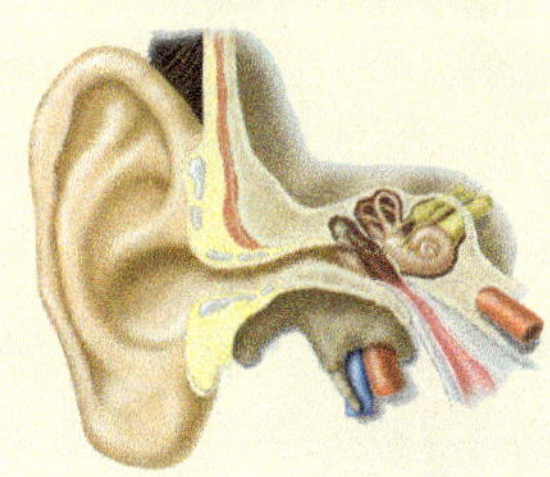	Hearing and balance

Body

anatomical position

As seen from the previous sections, the body is the sum of all the systems, organs, tissues, and cells found in it. It is important to learn the anatomical terminology that applies to the body as a whole in order to correctly identify specific locations and directions when dealing with patients. The **anatomical position** is used when describing the positions and relationships of structures in the human body. A body in the anatomical position is standing erect with the arms at the sides of the body, the palms of the hands facing forward, and the eyes looking straight ahead. In addition, the legs are parallel with the feet, and the toes are pointing forward (see Figure 2.3 ■). For descriptive purposes the assumption is always that the person is in the anatomical position even if the body or parts of the body are in any other position.

Body Planes

coronal plane (kor-RONE-al)
coronal section
cross-section
frontal plane
frontal section
horizontal plane
longitudinal section
median plane
sagittal plane (SAJ-ih-tal)
sagittal section
transverse plane
transverse section

The terminology for body planes is used to assist medical personnel in describing the body and its parts. To understand body planes, imagine cuts slicing through the body at various angles. This imaginary slicing allows us to use more specific language when describing parts of the body. These body planes, illustrated in Figure 2.4 ■, include the following:

1. **Sagittal plane:** This vertical plane runs lengthwise from front to back and divides the body or any of its parts into right and left portions. The right and left sides do not have to be equal. If the sagittal plane passes through the middle of the body, thus dividing it into equal right and left halves, it is called a **midsagittal** or **median plane.** A cut along the sagittal plane yields a **sagittal section** view of the inside of the body.

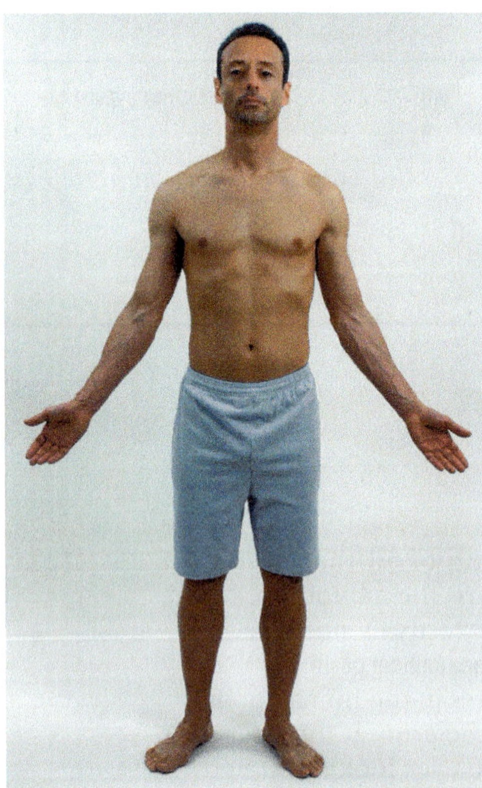

■ **Figure 2.3** The anatomical position: standing erect, gazing straight ahead, arms down at sides, palms facing forward, fingers extended, legs together, and toes pointing forward.

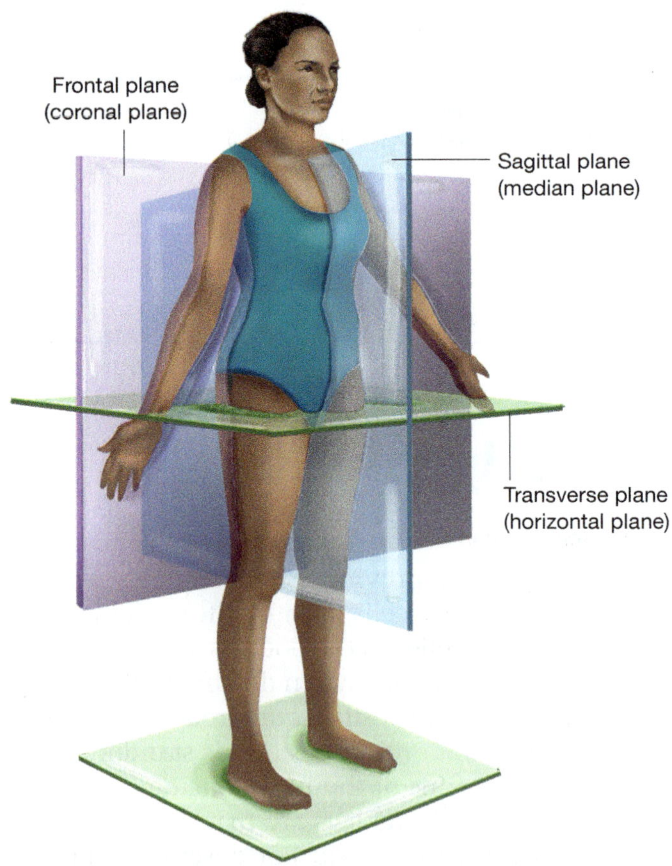

■ **Figure 2.4** The planes of the body. The sagittal plane is vertical from front to back, the frontal plane is vertical from left to right, and the transverse plane is horizontal.

2. **Frontal plane:** The frontal, or **coronal plane,** divides the body into front and back portions; a vertical lengthwise plane is running from side to side. A cut along the frontal plane yields a **frontal** or **coronal section** view of the inside of the body.
3. **Transverse plane:** The transverse, or **horizontal plane,** is a crosswise plane that runs parallel to the ground. This imaginary cut would divide the body or its parts into upper and lower portions. A cut along the transverse plane yields a **transverse section** view of the inside of the body.

The terms **cross-section** and **longitudinal section** are frequently used to describe internal views of structures. A longitudinal section is produced by a lengthwise slice along the long axis of a structure. A cross-section view is produced by a slice perpendicular to the long axis of the structure.

Body Regions

abdominal region (ab-DOM-ih-nal)
brachial region (BRAY-kee-all)
cephalic region (she-FAL-ik)
cervical region (SER-vih-kal)
crural region (KREW-ral)
dorsum (DOOR-sum)
gluteal region (GLOO-tee-all)
lower extremities
pelvic region (PELL-vik)
pubic region (PEW-bik)
thoracic region (tho-RASS-ik)
trunk
upper extremities
vertebral region (VER-tee-bral)

The body is divided into large regions that can easily be identified externally. The **cephalic region** is the entire head. The neck is the **cervical region** and connects the head to the **trunk** (the torso). The trunk is further subdivided into different anterior and posterior regions. The anterior side consists of the **thoracic** (the chest), **abdominal, pelvic,** and **pubic** (genital) **regions.** The posterior side consists of the **dorsum** (the back), **vertebral region,** and **gluteal** (buttock) **region.** The **upper extremities** (UE) and **lower extremities** (LE) are attached to the trunk. The upper extremities or **brachial regions** are the arms. The lower extremities or **crural regions** are the legs. See Figure 2.5 ■ to locate each region on the body.

MED TERM TIP

As you learn medical terminology, it is important that you remember not to use common phrases and terms any longer. Many people commonly use the term *stomach* (an organ) when they actually mean *abdomen* (a body region).

Regions of the body

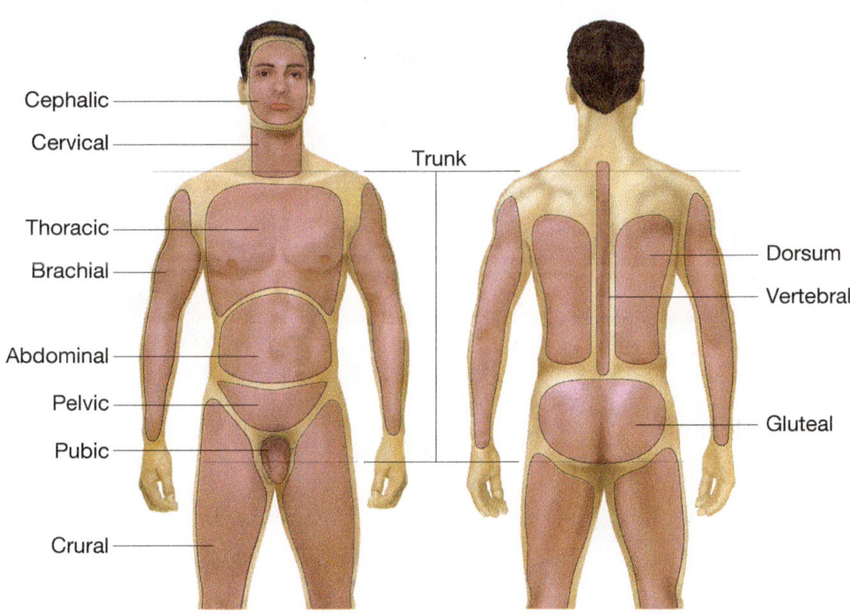

■ **Figure 2.5** Anterior and posterior views of the body illustrating the location of various body regions.

Body Cavities

abdominal cavity
abdominopelvic cavity (ab-dom-ih-noh-PELL-vik)
cranial cavity (KRAY-nee-al)
diaphragm (DYE-ah-fram)
mediastinum (mee-dee-ass-TYE-num)
parietal layer (pah-RYE-eh-tal)
parietal peritoneum
parietal pleura
pelvic cavity
pericardial cavity (pair-ih-CAR-dee-al)
peritoneum (pair-ih-toh-NEE-um)
pleura (PLOO-rah)
pleural cavity (PLOO-ral)
spinal cavity
thoracic cavity
viscera (VISS-er-ah)
visceral layer (VISS-er-al)
visceral peritoneum
visceral pleura

The body is not a solid structure; it has many open spaces or cavities. The cavities are part of the normal body structure and are illustrated in Figure 2.6 ■. We can divide the body into four major cavities—two dorsal cavities and two ventral cavities.

The dorsal cavities include the **cranial cavity,** containing the brain, and the **spinal cavity,** containing the spinal cord.

The ventral cavities include the **thoracic cavity** and the **abdominopelvic cavity.** The thoracic cavity contains the two lungs and a central region between them called the **mediastinum.** The heart, aorta, esophagus, trachea, and thymus gland are some of the structures located in the mediastinum. There is an actual physical wall between the thoracic cavity and the abdominopelvic cavity called the **diaphragm.** The diaphragm is a muscle used for breathing. The abdominopelvic cavity is generally subdivided into a superior **abdominal cavity** and an inferior **pelvic cavity.** The organs of the digestive, excretory, and reproductive systems are located in

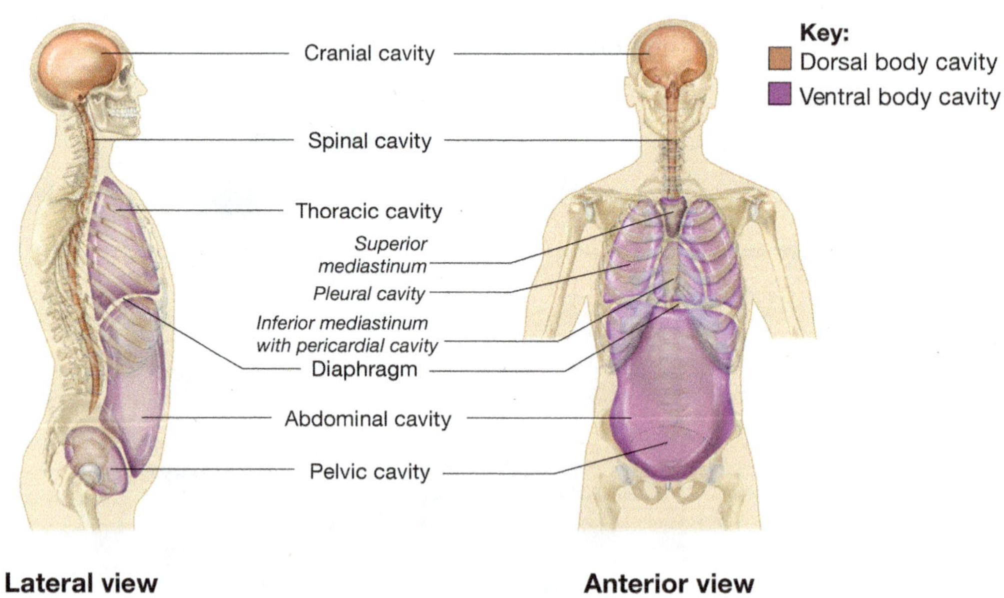

■ **Figure 2.6** The dorsal (orange) and ventral (purple) body cavities.

these cavities. The organs within the ventral cavities are referred to as a group as the internal organs or **viscera.** Table 2.2 ■ describes the body cavities and their major organs.

All of the cavities are lined by, and the viscera are encased in, a two-layer membrane called the **pleura** in the thoracic cavity and the **peritoneum** in the abdominopelvic cavity. The outer layer that lines the cavities is called the **parietal layer** (i.e., **parietal pleura** and **parietal peritoneum**), and the inner layer that encases the viscera is called the **visceral layer** (i.e., **visceral pleura** and **visceral peritoneum**).

Within the thoracic cavity, the pleura is subdivided, forming the **pleural cavity,** containing the lungs, and the **pericardial cavity,** containing the heart. The larger abdominopelvic cavity is usually subdivided into regions so different areas can be precisely referred to. Two different methods of subdividing this cavity are used: the anatomical divisions and the clinical divisions. Choose a method partly on personal preference and partly on which system best describes the patient's condition. See Table 2.3 ■ for a description of these methods for dividing the abdominopelvic cavity.

MED TERM TIP

The kidneys are the only major abdominopelvic organ located outside the sac formed by the peritoneum. Because they are found behind this sac, their position is referred to as *retroperitoneal* (retro- = behind; peritone/o = peritoneum; -al = pertaining to).

Directional and Positional Terms

Directional terms assist medical personnel in discussing the position or location of a patient's complaint. Directional or positional terms also help to describe one process, organ, or system as it relates to another. Table 2.4 ■ presents commonly used terms for describing the position of the body or its parts. They are listed in pairs that have opposite meanings; for example, superior versus inferior, anterior versus posterior, medial versus lateral, proximal versus distal, superficial versus deep, and supine versus prone. Directional terms are illustrated in Figure 2.7 ■.

MED TERM TIP

Remember when using location or direction terms, it is assumed that the patient is in the anatomical position unless otherwise noted.

Table 2.2 Body Cavities and Their Major Organs

CAVITY	MAJOR ORGANS
Dorsal cavities	
Cranial cavity	Brain
Spinal cavity	Spinal cord
Ventral cavities	
Thoracic cavity	Pleural cavity: lungs
	Pericardial cavity: heart
	Mediastinum: heart, esophagus, trachea, thymus gland, aorta
Abdominopelvic cavity	
Abdominal cavity	Stomach, spleen, liver, gallbladder, pancreas, and portions of the small intestines and colon
Pelvic cavity	Urinary bladder, ureters, urethra, and portions of the small intestines and colon
	Female: uterus, ovaries, fallopian tubes, vagina
	Male: prostate gland, seminal vesicles, portion of the vas deferens

Table 2.3 Methods of Subdividing the Abdominopelvic Cavity

Anatomical Divisions of the Abdomen

- **Right hypochondriac** (high-poh-KON-dree-ak): Right lateral region of upper row beneath the lower ribs
- **Epigastric** (ep-ih-GAS-trik): Middle area of upper row above the stomach
- **Left hypochondriac:** Left lateral region of the upper row beneath the lower ribs
- **Right lumbar:** Right lateral region of the middle row at the waist
- **Umbilical** (um-BILL-ih-kal): Central area over the navel
- **Left lumbar:** Left lateral region of the middle row at the waist
- **Right iliac** (ILL-ee-ak): Right lateral region of the lower row at the groin
- **Hypogastric** (high-poh-GAS-trik): Middle region of the lower row beneath the navel
- **Left iliac:** Left lateral region of the lower row at the groin

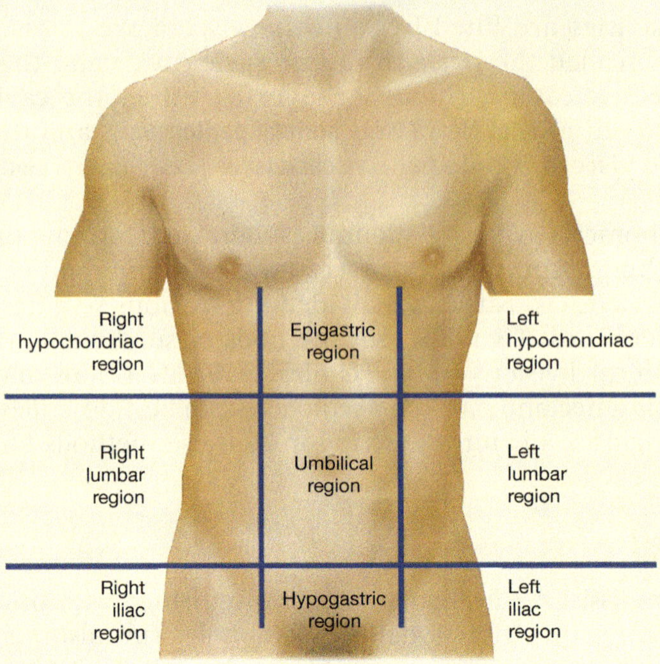

MED TERM TIP

To visualize the nine anatomical divisions, imagine a tic-tac-toe diagram over this region.

MED TERM TIP

The term *hypochondriac*, literally meaning "under the cartilage" (of the ribs), has come to refer to a person who believes he or she is sick when there is no obvious cause for illness. These patients commonly complain of aches and pains in the hypochondriac region.

Clinical Divisions of the Abdomen

- **Right upper quadrant (RUQ):** Contains majority of liver, gallbladder, small portion of pancreas, right kidney, small intestines, and colon
- **Right lower quadrant (RLQ):** Contains small intestines and colon, right ovary and fallopian tube, appendix, and right ureter
- **Left upper quadrant (LUQ):** Contains small portion of liver, spleen, stomach, majority of pancreas, left kidney, small intestines, and colon
- **Left lower quadrant (LLQ):** Contains small intestines and colon, left ovary and fallopian tube, and left ureter
- Midline organs: uterus, bladder, prostate gland

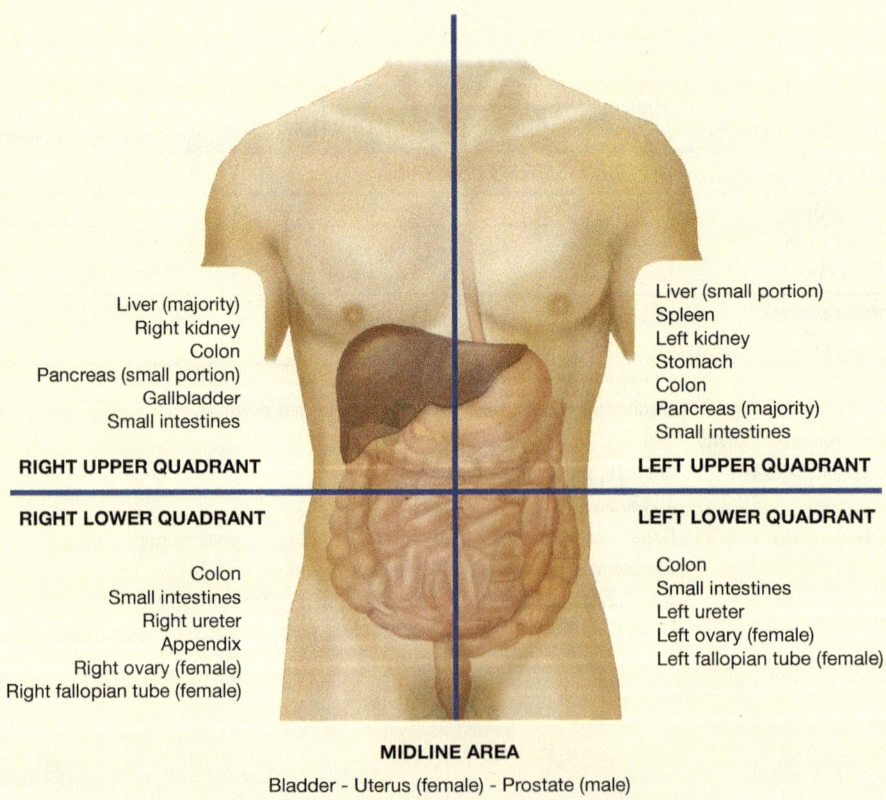

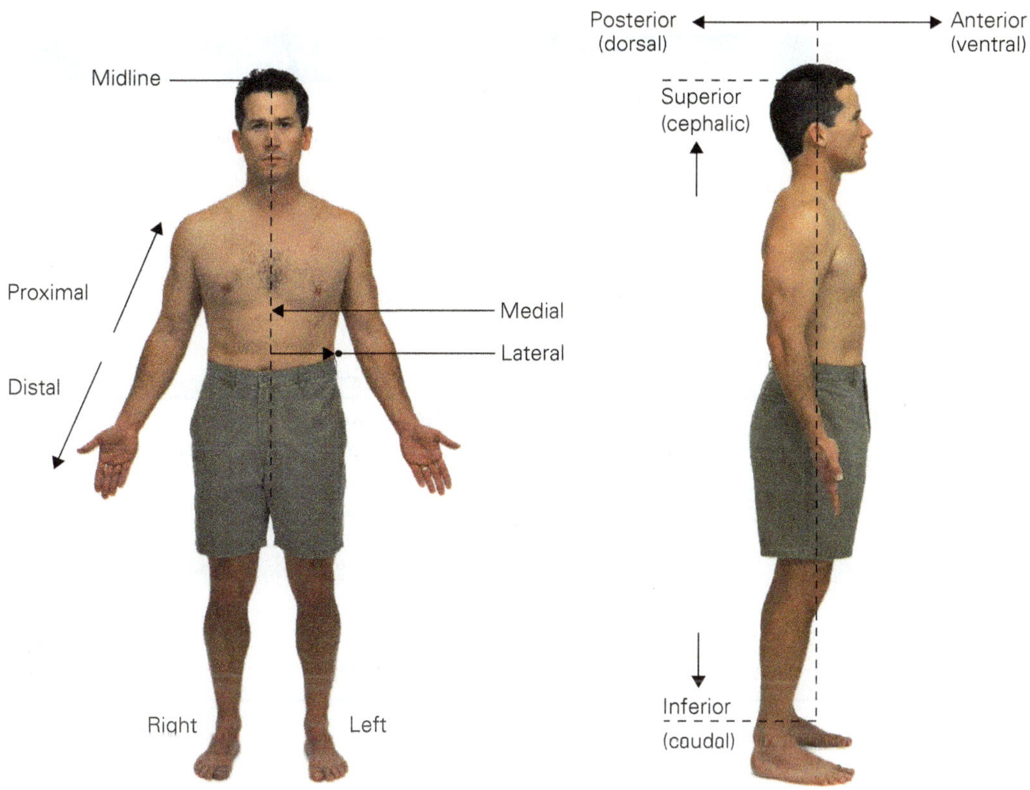

■ **Figure 2.7** Anterior and lateral views of the body illustrating directional terms.

Table 2.4	Terms for Describing Body Position
superior (soo-PEE-ree-or) or **cephalic** (seh-FAL-ik)	More toward the head, or above another structure. *Example:* The adrenal glands are superior to the kidneys.
inferior (in-FEE-ree-or) or **caudal** (KAWD-al)	More toward the feet or tail, or below another structure. *Example:* The intestine is inferior to the heart.
anterior (an-TEE-ree-or) or **ventral** (VEN-tral)	More toward the front or belly-side of the body. *Example:* The navel is located on the anterior surface of the body.
posterior (poss-TEE-ree-or) or **dorsal** (DOR-sal)	More toward the back or spinal cord side of the body. *Example:* The posterior wall of the right kidney was excised.
medial (MEE-dee-al)	Refers to the middle or near the middle of the body or the structure. *Example:* The heart is medially located in the chest cavity.
lateral (lat) (LAT-er-al)	Refers to the side. *Example:* The ovaries are located lateral to the uterus.
proximal (PROK-sim-al)	Located nearer to the point of attachment to the body. *Example:* In the anatomical position, the elbow is proximal to the hand.
distal (DISS-tal)	Located farther away from the point of attachment to the body. *Example:* The hand is distal to the elbow.
apex (AY-peks)	Tip or summit of an organ. *Example:* We hear the heart beat by listening over the apex of the heart.
base	Bottom or lower part of an organ. *Example:* On the X-ray, a fracture was noted at the base of the skull.
superficial	More toward the surface of the body. *Example:* The cut was superficial.
deep	Further away from the surface of the body. *Example:* An incision into an abdominal organ is a deep incision.

(Continued)

Table 2.4	Terms for Describing Body Position (continued)
supine (soo-PINE)	The body lying horizontally and facing upward. *Example:* The patient is in the supine position for abdominal surgery. 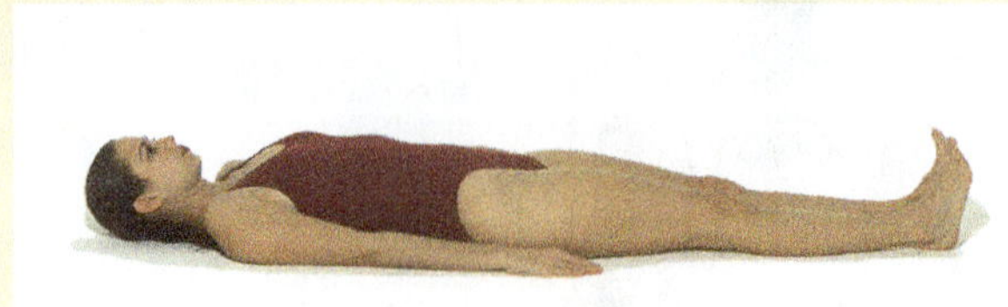 Figure 2.8A The supine position.
prone (PROHN)	The body lying horizontally and facing downward. *Example:* The patient is placed in the prone position for spinal surgery. 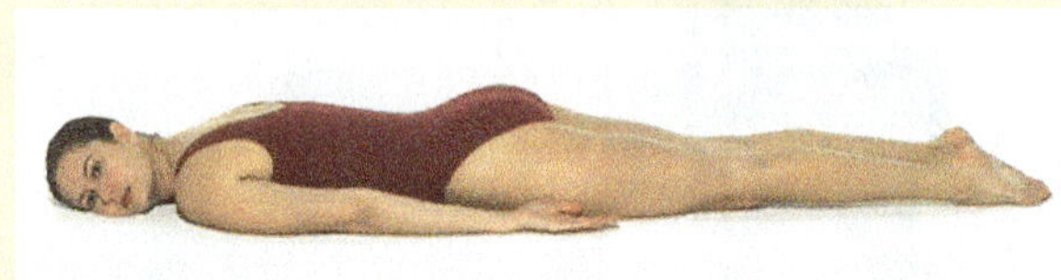 Figure 2.8B The prone position.

Terminology

The following lists contain the suffixes and prefixes used to build terms in the remaining section of this chapter. The combining forms were introduced earlier in this chapter.

Suffixes

-ac	pertaining to
-al	pertaining to
-ar	pertaining to
-ary	pertaining to
-atic	pertaining to
-iac	pertaining to
-ic	pertaining to
-ior	pertaining to
-logy	study of
-ose	resembling

Prefixes

endo-	within
epi-	above
hypo-	under
peri-	around
retro-	behind

The terms below, introduced in this chapter, are built directly from word parts following the rules given earlier. Review these terms in order to begin to familiarize yourself with how medical terms are built.

Anatomical Terms

TERM	WORD PARTS	DEFINITION
abdominal	abdomin/o = abdomen -al = pertaining to	pertaining to the abdomen
adipose	adip/o = fat -ose = resembling	resembling fat
anterior	anter/o = front -ior = pertaining to	pertaining to the front
brachial	brachi/o = arm -al = pertaining to	pertaining to the arm
cardiac	cardi/o = heart -ac = pertaining to	pertaining to the heart
cardiology	cardi/o = heart -logy = study of	study of the heart
cardiovascular	cardi/o = heart vascul/o = blood vessel -ar = pertaining to	pertaining to the heart and blood vessels
caudal	caud/o = tail -al = pertaining to	pertaining to the tail
cephalic	cephal/o = head -ic = pertaining to	pertaining to the head
cervical	cervic/o = neck -al = pertaining to	pertaining to the neck
cranial	crani/o = skull -al = pertaining to	pertaining to the skull
crural	crur/o = leg -al = pertaining to	pertaining to the leg
cytology	cyt/o = cell -logy = study of	study of the cell
dermatology	dermat/o = skin -logy = study of	study of the skin
distal	dist/o = away from -al = pertaining to	pertaining to away from
dorsal	dors/o = back of body -al = pertaining to	pertaining to the back of body
endocrinology	endo- = within crin/o = to secrete -logy = study of	study of secreting within [endocrine system]
epigastric	epi- = above gastr/o = stomach -ic = pertaining to	pertaining to above the stomach
epithelial	epitheli/o = epithelium -al = pertaining to	pertaining to the epithelium

Anatomical Terms (continued)

TERM	WORD PARTS	DEFINITION
gastroenterology	gastr/o = stomach enter/o = small intestine -logy = study of	study of the stomach and small intestine
gluteal	glute/o = buttock -al = pertaining to	pertaining to the buttocks
gynecology	gynec/o = woman -logy = study of	study of women
hematic	hemat/o = blood -ic = pertaining to	pertaining to the blood
hematology	hemat/o = blood -logy = study of	study of the blood
histology	hist/o = tissue -logy = study of	study of tissue
hypochondriac	hypo- = under chondr/o = cartilage -iac = pertaining to	pertaining to under the cartilage
hypogastric	hypo- = under gastr/o = stomach -ic = pertaining to	pertaining to under the stomach
immunology	immun/o = protection -logy = study of	study of protection [immune system]
inferior	infer/o = below -ior = pertaining to	pertaining to below
lateral	later/o = side -al = pertaining to	pertaining to the side
lumbar	lumb/o = loin -ar = pertaining to	pertaining to the loin [side and back between ribs and pelvic bones]
lymphatic	lymph/o = lymph -atic = pertaining to	pertaining to lymph
medial	medi/o = middle -al = pertaining to	pertaining to the middle
muscular	muscul/o = muscles -ar = pertaining to	pertaining to muscles
nephrology	nephr/o = kidney -logy = study of	study of the kidney
neurology	neur/o = nerve -logy = study of	study of nerves
ophthalmology	ophthalm/o = eye -logy = study of	study of the eye
otorhinolaryngology	ot/o = ear rhin/o = nose laryng/o = larynx -logy = study of	study of ear, nose, and larynx
pelvic	pelv/o = pelvis -ic = pertaining to	pertaining to the pelvis
peritoneal	peritone/o = peritoneum -al = pertaining to	pertaining to the peritoneum

Anatomical Terms *(continued)*

TERM	WORD PARTS	DEFINITION
pleural	pleur/o = pleura -al = pertaining to	pertaining to the pleura
posterior	poster/o = back -ior = pertaining to	pertaining to the back
proctology	proct/o = rectum and anus -logy = study of	study of the rectum and anus
proximal	proxim/o = near to -al = pertaining to	pertaining to near to
pubic	pub/o = genital region -ic = pertaining to	pertaining to the genital region
pulmonology	pulmon/o = lung -logy = study of	study of the lungs
spinal	spin/o = spine -al = pertaining to	pertaining to the spine
superior	super/o = above -ior = pertaining to	pertaining to above
thoracic	thorac/o = chest -ic = pertaining to	pertaining to the chest
urology	ur/o = urine -logy = study of	study of urine
ventral	ventr/o = belly -al = pertaining to	pertaining to the belly [side]
vertebral	vertebr/o = vertebra -al = pertaining to	pertaining to the vertebrae
visceral	viscer/o = internal organ -al = pertaining to	pertaining to internal organs

Abbreviations

AP	anteroposterior	**LUQ**	left upper quadrant
CV	cardiovascular	**MS**	musculoskeletal
ENT	ear, nose, and throat	**OB**	obstetrics
GI	gastrointestinal	**PA**	posteroanterior
GYN	gynecology	**RLQ**	right lower quadrant
lat	lateral	**RUQ**	right upper quadrant
LE	lower extremity	**UE**	upper extremity
LLQ	left lower quadrant		

Chapter Review

Practice Exercises

A. Complete the Statement

1. The levels of organization of the body in order from smallest to largest are: ______________________, ______________________, ______________________, ______________________, ______________________.

2. No matter its shape, all cells have a ______________________, ______________________, and ______________________.

3. ______________________ is the study of tissue.

4. ______________________ tissue lines internal organs and serves as a covering for the skin.

5. In the ______________________ position the body is standing erect with arms at sides and palms facing forward.

6. The ______________________ quadrant of the abdomen contains the appendix.

7. The dorsal cavities are the ______________________ cavity and the ______________________ cavity.

8. There are ______________________ anatomical divisions in the abdominal cavity.

9. The ______________________ region of the abdominal cavity is located in the right lower lateral region near the groin.

10. Within the thoracic cavity the lungs are found in the ______________________ cavity and the heart is found in the ______________________ cavity.

B. Body Plane Matching

Match each body plane to its definition.

1.	_______ frontal plane	a.	divides the body into right and left
2.	_______ sagittal plane	b.	divides the body into upper and lower
3.	_______ transverse plane	c.	divides the body into anterior and posterior

C. Prefix Practice

Circle the prefixes in the following terms and define in the space provided.

1. epigastric ____

2. pericardium ____

3. hypochondriac ____

4. retroperitoneal ____

D. Terminology Matching

Match each term to its definition.

1.	_______ distal	a.	away from the surface
2.	_______ prone	b.	toward the surface
3.	_______ lateral	c.	located closer to point of attachment to the body
4.	_______ inferior	d.	caudal
5.	_______ deep	e.	tip or summit of an organ
6.	_______ apex	f.	lying face down
7.	_______ base	g.	cephalic
8.	_______ posterior	h.	ventral
9.	_______ superficial	i.	dorsal
10.	_______ supine	j.	lying face up
11.	_______ anterior	k.	to the side
12.	_______ medial	l.	middle
13.	_______ proximal	m.	bottom or lower part of an organ
14.	_______ superior	n.	located further away from point of attachment to the body

E. What's the Abbreviation?

1. musculoskeletal ______________________________
2. lateral ______________________________
3. right upper quadrant ______________________________
4. cardiovascular ______________________________
5. gastrointestinal ______________________________
6. anteroposterior ______________________________
7. obstetrics ______________________________
8. left lower quadrant ______________________________

F. Build a Medical Term

Build terms for each expression using the correct prefixes, suffixes, and combining forms.

1. pertaining to spinal cord side ____________________
2. pertaining to the chest ____________________
3. pertaining to above ____________________
4. pertaining to the tail ____________________
5. pertaining to internal organs ____________________
6. pertaining to the side ____________________
7. pertaining to away from ____________________
8. pertaining to nerves ____________________
9. study of the lungs ____________________
10. pertaining to the muscles ____________________
11. pertaining to the belly side ____________________
12. pertaining to the front ____________________
13. pertaining to the head ____________________
14. pertaining to the middle ____________________

G. Define the Combining Form

1. **viscer/o** ____________________
2. **poster/o** ____________________
3. **abdomin/o** ____________________
4. **thorac/o** ____________________
5. **medi/o** ____________________
6. **ventr/o** ____________________
7. **anter/o** ____________________
8. **hist/o** ____________________
9. **epitheli/o** ____________________
10. **crani/o** ____________________
11. **cyt/o** ____________________
12. **proxim/o** ____________________
13. **cephal/o** ____________________

H. Organ System and Function Challenge

For each organ listed below, identify the name of the system it belongs to and then match it to its function.

	Organ	System		Function
1.	_______ skin	______________________	a.	supports the body
2.	_______ heart	______________________	b.	provides place for growing baby
3.	_______ stomach	______________________	c.	filters waste products from blood
4.	_______ uterus	______________________	d.	provides two-way barrier
5.	_______ bones	______________________	e.	produces movement
6.	_______ lungs	______________________	f.	produces sperm
7.	_______ kidney	______________________	g.	ingest, digest, absorb nutrients
8.	_______ testes	______________________	h.	coordinates body's response
9.	_______ brain	______________________	i.	pumps blood through blood vessels
10.	_______ muscles	______________________	j.	obtains oxygen

I. Body Region Practice

For each term below, write the corresponding body region.

1. head ____
2. genitals ____
3. leg ____
4. buttocks ____
5. neck ____
6. arm ____
7. back ____
8. chest ____

J. Terminology Matching

Match each organ to its body cavity.

1. _______ gallbladder
2. _______ appendix
3. _______ urinary bladder
4. _______ small intestines
5. _______ right kidney
6. _______ left ovary
7. _______ stomach
8. _______ colon
9. _______ right ureter
10. _______ pancreas (majority)

a. right upper quadrant
b. left upper quadrant
c. right lower quadrant
d. left lower quadrant
e. all quadrants
f. midline structure

K. Fill in the Blank

cardiology	otorhinolaryngology	urology	gynecology
ophthalmology	gastroenterology	dermatology	orthopedics

1. John is a musician who plays an electric bass guitar and is experiencing difficulty in hearing soft voices. He would consult a physician in ______________________.
2. Ruth is a stock trader with the Chicago Board of Trade. She has had a pounding and racing heartbeat. She would consult a physician specializing in ______________________.
3. Mary Ann is experiencing excessive bleeding from the uterus. She would consult a ______________________ doctor.
4. José has fractured his wrist in a fall. He would be seen for an examination by a physician in ______________________.
5. A physician who performs eye exams specializes in the field of ______________________.
6. When her daughter had repeated bladder infections, Mrs. Cortez sought the opinion of a specialist in ______________________.
7. Martha could not get rid of a persistent skin rash with over-the-counter creams. She decided to make an appointment with a specialist in ______________________.
8. After reviewing his X-ray, the specialist in ______________________ informed Mr. Sparks that he had a stomach ulcer.

L. Research Project: Stem Cells

Stem cell research has been in process for a number of years, and, though amid continual controversy, offers hope for those with conditions that have not been cured or corrected by other forms of treatment. Various agencies and organizations have studied stem cell research extensively and provide excellent resources for further review. These groups include the National Institute of Medicine (NIH), International Society for Stem Cell Research (ISSCR), Mayo Clinic, and California Institute for Regenerative Medicine (CIRM).

With this research, medical journals, and other professional publications, prepare a persuasive article that could be used to begin a debate that will encourage others to accept your view on the topic. As you prepare your article consider the following questions:

- What are stem cells and how are they obtained for research purposes?
- How can stem cells treat disease?
- Which diseases might be treated as a result of stem cell research?
- Are stem cell therapies currently available, and, if so, which conditions are treated?
- What are the risks related to stem cell therapies?
- How do scientists test stem cell therapies?
- What are the controversies against the use of stem cell therapies?

List and explain, using medical terminology as appropriate, five things to know about stem cell research, then determine your personal position for or against the use of stem cells to treat disease. Defend your position in your article documenting the concepts and perspectives that led to your conclusions. Cite all sources used in your research applying conventional citation methods. Share your article with a peer. Provide feedback and suggestions to each other; then revise your document as necessary.

Labeling Exercise

Image A

1. Write the labels for this figure on the numbered lines provided.

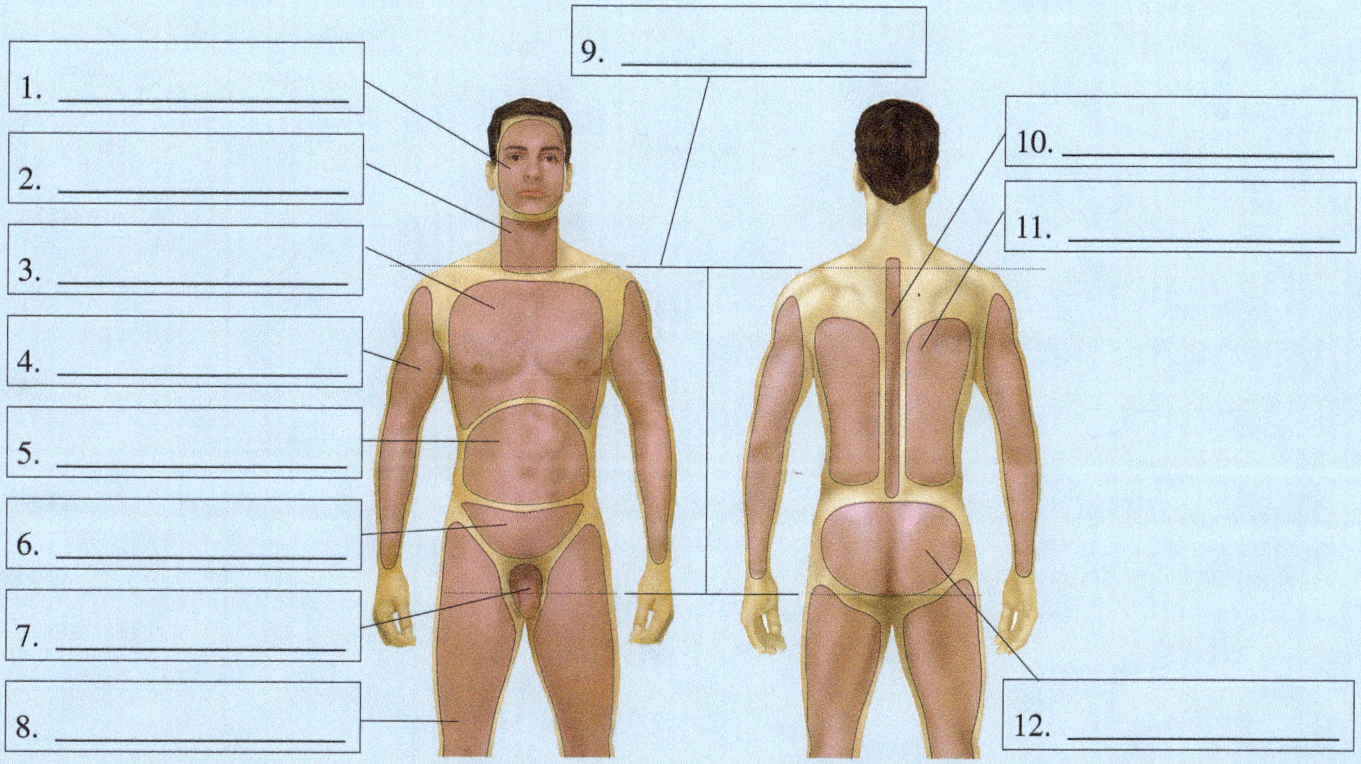

Image B

2. Write the labels for this figure on the numbered lines provided.

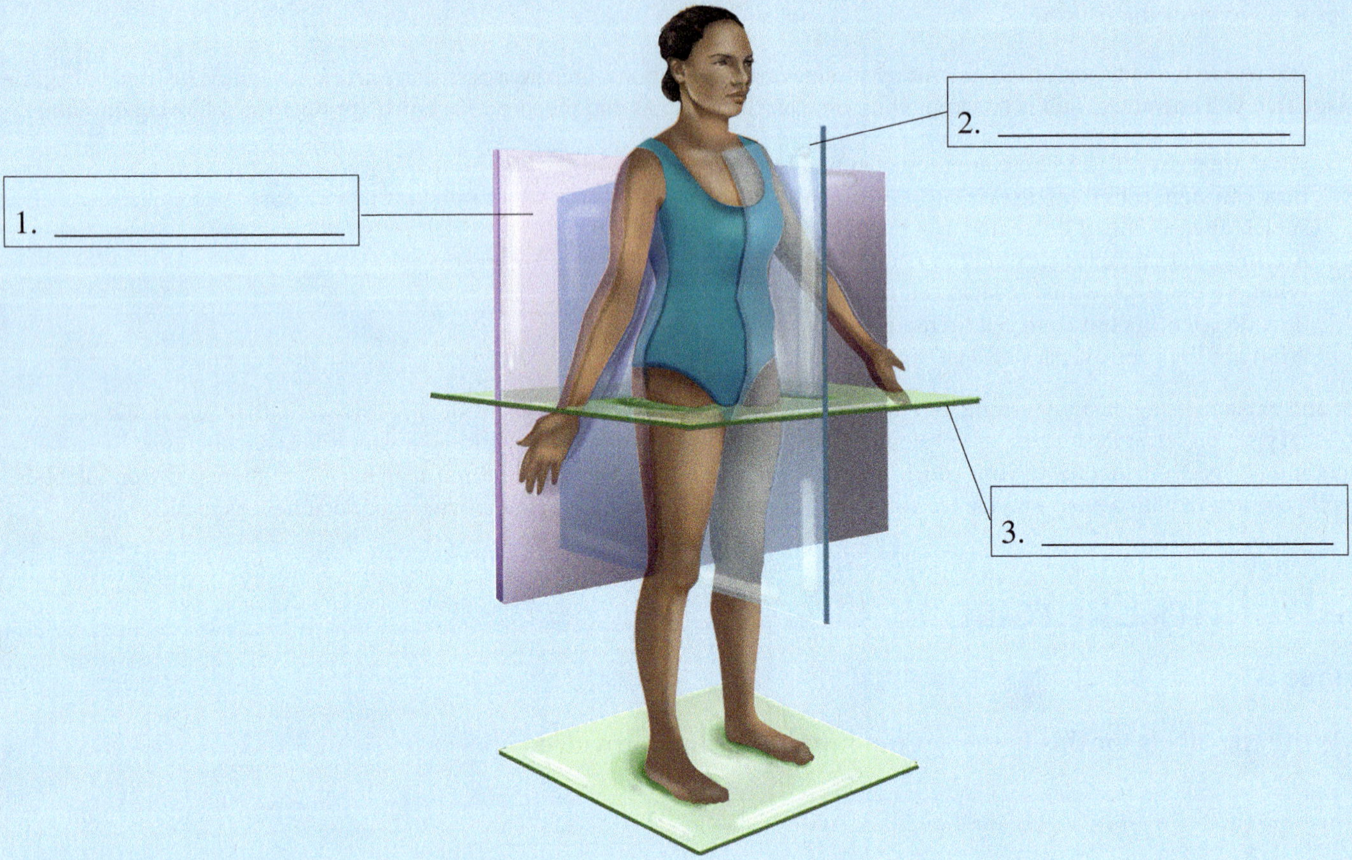

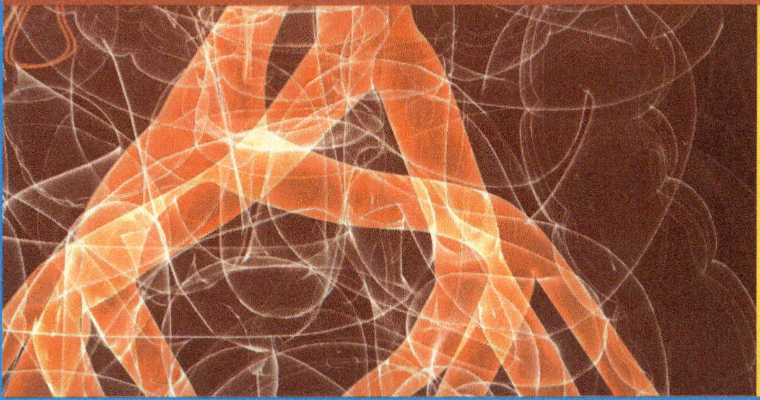

3 INTEGUMENTARY SYSTEM

Learning Objectives

Upon completion of this chapter, you will be able to

- Identify and define the combining forms, prefixes, and suffixes introduced in this chapter.
- Correctly spell and pronounce medical terms and major anatomical structures relating to the integumentary system.
- List and describe the three layers of skin and their functions.
- List and describe the four purposes of the skin.
- List and describe the accessory organs of the skin.
- Identify and define integumentary system anatomical terms.
- Identify and define selected integumentary system pathology terms.
- Identify and define selected integumentary system diagnostic procedures.
- Identify and define selected integumentary system therapeutic procedures.
- Identify and define selected medications relating to the integumentary system.
- Define selected abbreviations associated with the integumentary system.

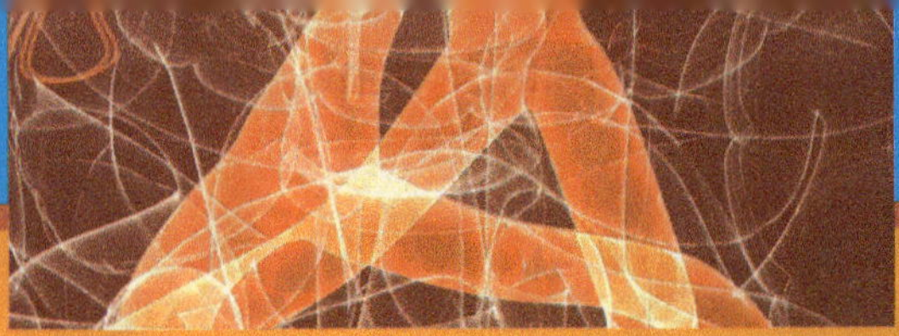

Integumentary System at a Glance

Function

The skin provides a protective two-way barrier between our internal environment and the outside world. It also plays an important role in temperature regulation, houses sensory receptors to detect the environment around us, and secretes important fluids.

Structures

Here are the primary structures that comprise the integumentary system.

skin **hair** **nails** **sebaceous glands** **sweat glands**

Word Parts

Here are the most common word parts (with their meanings) used to build integumentary system terms. For a more comprehensive list, refer to the Terminology section of this chapter.

Combining Forms

Combining Form	Meaning
albin/o	white
bi/o	life
cry/o	cold
cutane/o	skin
cyan/o	blue
derm/o	skin
dermat/o	skin
diaphor/o	profuse sweating
electr/o	electricity
erythr/o	red
hidr/o	sweat
ichthy/o	scaly, dry
kerat/o	hard, horny
leuk/o	white
lip/o	fat
melan/o	black
myc/o	fungus
necr/o	death
onych/o	nail
pedicul/o	lice
phot/o	light
py/o	pus
rhytid/o	wrinkle
scler/o	hard
seb/o	oil
trich/o	hair
ungu/o	nail
vesic/o	bladder
xer/o	dry

Suffixes

Suffix	Meaning
-derma	skin condition
-opsy	view of
-tome	instrument used to cut

Prefixes

Prefix	Meaning
allo-	other, different from usual
xeno-	strange, foreign

Integumentary System Illustrated

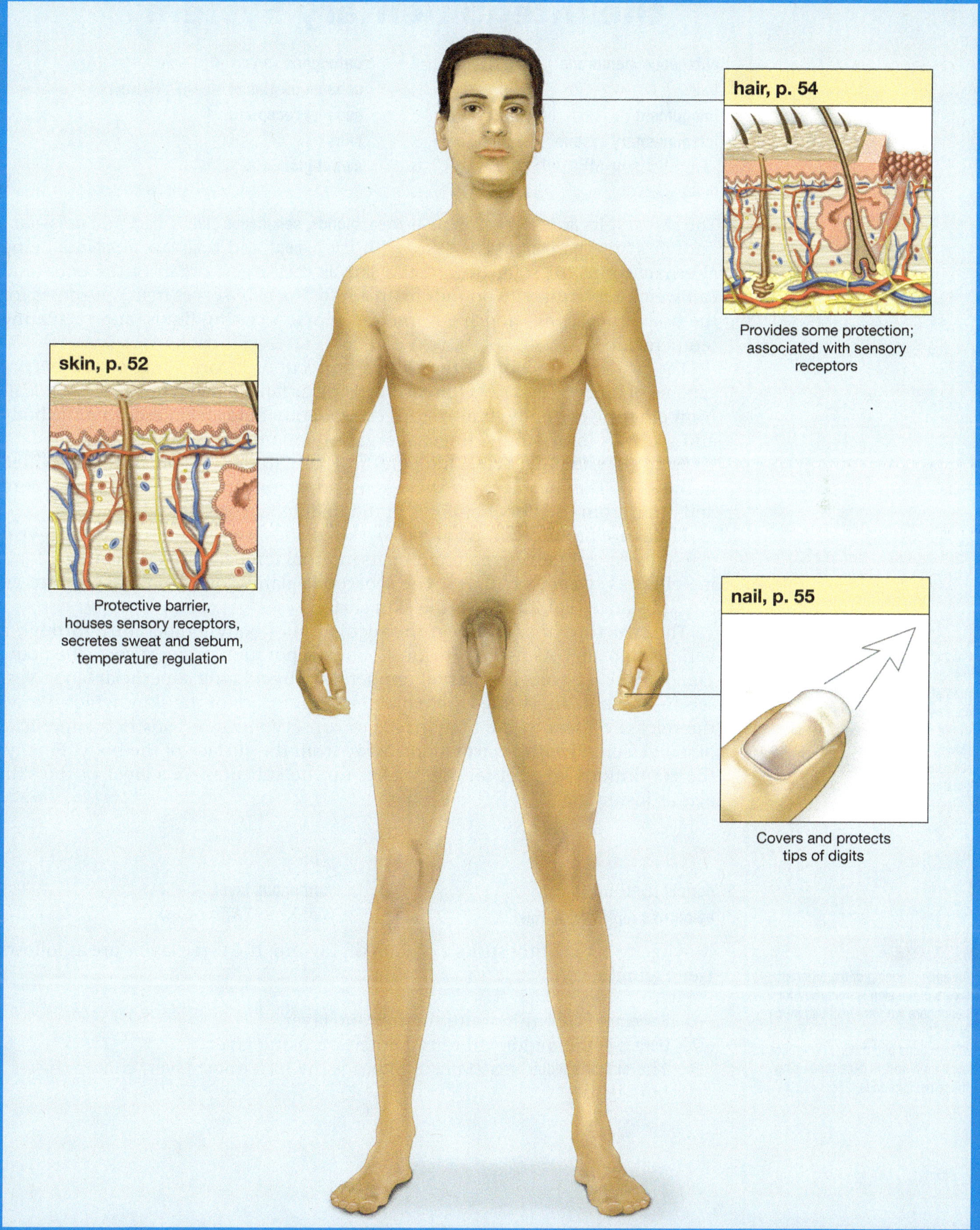

Anatomy and Physiology of the Integumentary System

cutaneous membrane (kew-TAY-nee-us)
hair
integument (in-TEG-you-mint)
integumentary system (in-teg-you-MEN-tah-ree)
nails
pathogens (PATH-oh-jenz)
sebaceous glands (see-BAY-shus)
sensory receptors
skin
sweat glands

The **skin** and its accessory organs—**sweat glands, sebaceous glands, hair,** and **nails**—are known as the **integumentary system,** with **integument** and **cutaneous membrane** being alternate terms for skin. In fact, the skin is the largest organ of the body and can weigh more than 20 pounds in an adult. The skin serves many purposes for the body: protecting, housing nerve receptors, secreting fluids, and regulating temperature.

The primary function of the skin is protection. It forms a two-way barrier capable of keeping **pathogens** (disease-causing organisms) and harmful chemicals from entering the body. It also stops critical body fluids from escaping the body and prevents injury to the internal organs lying underneath the skin.

Sensory receptors that detect temperature, pain, touch, and pressure are located in the skin. The messages for these sensations are conveyed to the spinal cord and brain from the nerve endings in the middle layer of the skin.

Fluids are produced in two types of skin glands: sweat and sebaceous. Sweat glands assist the body in maintaining its internal temperature by creating a cooling effect as sweat evaporates. The sebaceous glands, or oil glands, produce an oily substance that lubricates the skin surface.

The structure of skin aids in the regulation of body temperature through a variety of means. As noted previously, the evaporation of sweat cools the body. The body also lowers its internal temperature by dilating superficial blood vessels in the skin. This brings more blood to the surface of the skin, which allows the release of heat. If the body needs to conserve heat, it constricts superficial blood vessels, keeping warm blood away from the surface of the body. Finally, the continuous layer of fat that makes up the subcutaneous layer of the skin acts as insulation.

MED TERM TIP

Flushing of the skin, a normal response to an increase in environmental temperature or to a fever, is caused by an increased blood flow to the skin of the face and neck. However, in some people, it is also a response to embarrassment called blushing and is not easily controlled.

The Skin

dermis (DER-mis)
epidermis (ep-ih-DER-mis)
subcutaneous layer (sub-kyoo-TAY-nee-us)

Moving from the outer surface of the skin inward, the three layers are as follows (see Figure 3.1 ■):

1. **Epidermis** is the thin, outer membrane layer.
2. **Dermis** is the middle, fibrous connective tissue layer.
3. The **subcutaneous layer** (Subcu, Subq) is the innermost layer, containing fatty tissue.

MED TERM TIP

An understanding of the different layers of the skin is important for healthcare workers because much of the terminology relating to types of injections and medical conditions, such as burns, is described using these designations.

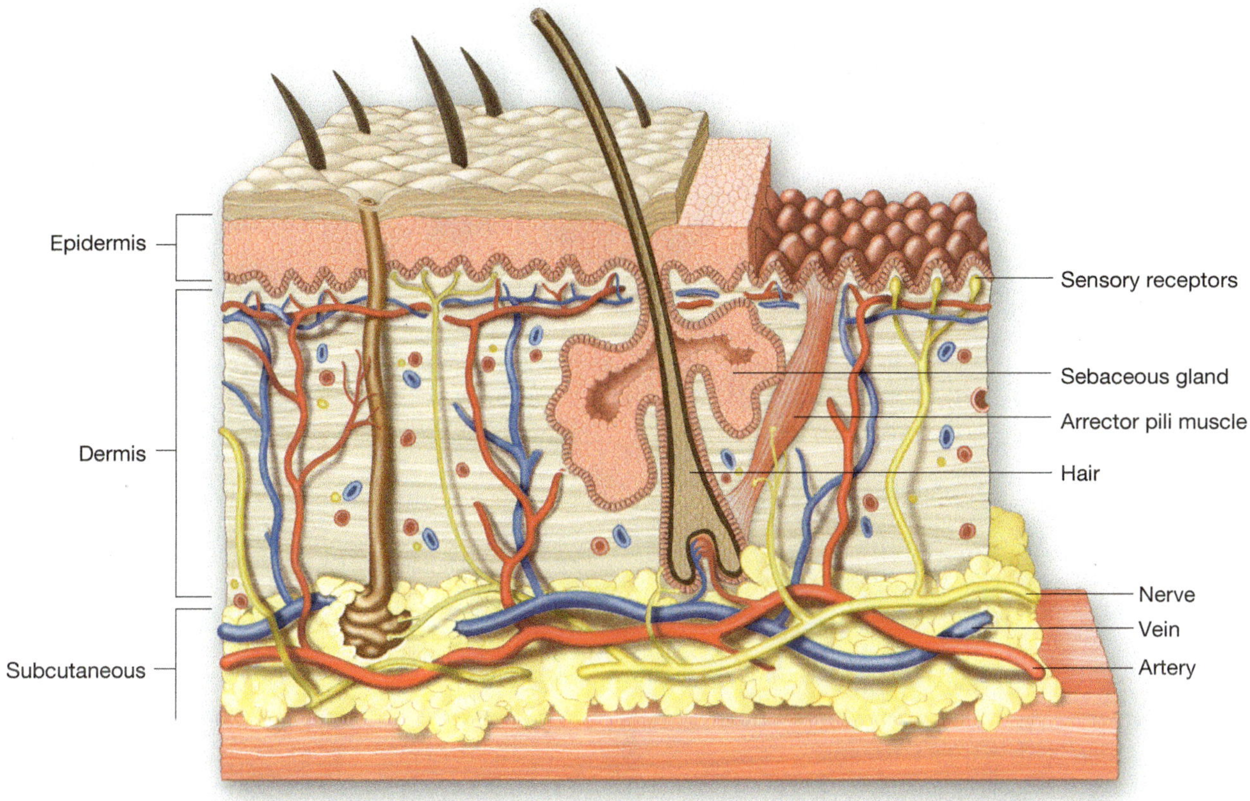

Figure 3.1 Skin structure, including the three layers of the skin and the accessory organs: sweat gland, sebaceous gland, and hair.

Epidermis

basal layer (BAY-sal)
keratin (KAIR-ah-tin)
melanin (MEL-ah-nin)
melanocytes (mel-AN-oh-sights)
stratified squamous epithelium (STRAT-ih-fyde / SKWAY-mus / ep-ih-THEE-lee-um)

The epidermis is composed of **stratified squamous epithelium** (see Figure 3.2 ■). This type of epithelial tissue consists of flat scale-like cells arranged in overlapping layers or strata. The epidermis does not have a blood supply or any connective tissue, so it is dependent for nourishment on the deeper layers of skin.

The deepest layer within the epidermis is called the **basal layer.** Cells in this layer continually grow and multiply. New cells that are forming push the old cells toward the outer layer of the epidermis. During this process the cells shrink, die, and become filled with a hard protein called **keratin.** These dead, overlapping, keratinized cells allow the skin to act as an effective barrier to infection and also make it waterproof.

The basal layer also contains special cells called **melanocytes,** which produce the black pigment **melanin.** Not only is this pigment responsible for the color of the skin, but it also protects against damage from the ultraviolet rays of the sun. This damage may be in the form of leatherlike skin and wrinkles, which are not hazardous, or it may be one of several forms of skin cancer. Dark-skinned people have more melanin and are generally less likely to get wrinkles or skin cancer.

MED TERM TIP

We lose 30,000-50,000 old, dead skin cells per minute and replace them with new, younger cells. In fact, because of this process, the epidermis is completely replaced every 25 days.

MED TERM TIP

A suntan can be thought of as a protective response to the rays of the sun. However, when the melanin in the skin is not able to absorb all the rays of the sun, the skin burns and DNA may be permanently and dangerously damaged.

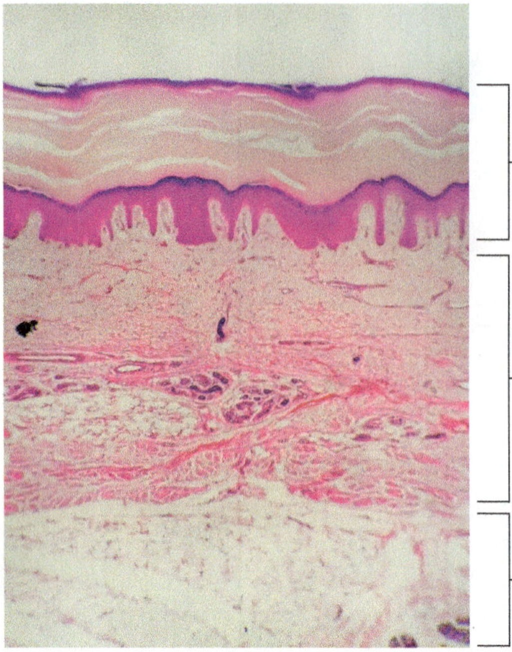

Figure 3.2 Photomicrograph showing the three layers of the skin. *(Jubal Harshaw/Shutterstock)*

Dermis

collagen fibers (KOL-ah-jen) **corium** (KOH-ree-um)

MED TERM TIP

Ridges formed in the dermis of our fingertips are what give each of us unique fingerprints. These do not change during a person's lifetime and so are a reliable means of identification. In fact, fingerprints are still visible on Egyptian mummies.

The dermis, also referred to as the **corium,** is the middle layer of skin, located between the epidermis and the subcutaneous layer (see Figure 3.2). Its name means "true skin." Unlike the thinner epidermis, the dermis is living tissue with a very good blood supply. The dermis itself is composed of connective tissue and **collagen fibers.** Collagen fibers are made from a strong, fibrous protein present in connective tissue, forming a flexible "glue" that gives connective tissue its strength. The dermis houses hair follicles, sweat glands, sebaceous glands, blood vessels, lymph vessels, sensory receptors, nerve fibers, and muscle fibers.

Subcutaneous Layer

hypodermis (high-poh-DER-mis) **lipocytes** (LIP-oh-sights)

The third and deepest layer of the skin is the subcutaneous layer, also called the **hypodermis.** This layer of tissue, composed of fat cells called **lipocytes,** protects the deeper tissues of the body and acts as insulation for heat and cold. (see Figure 3.2)

Accessory Organs

The accessory organs of the skin are the anatomical structures located within the dermis, including the hair, nails, sebaceous glands, and sweat glands.

Hair

arrector pili (ah-REK-tor / pee-lie) **hair root**
hair follicle (FALL-ikl) **hair shaft**

MED TERM TIP

Our hair turns gray as part of the normal aging process when we no longer produce melanin.

The fibers that make up hair are composed of the protein keratin, the same hard protein material that fills the cells of the epidermis. The process of hair formation is much like the process of growth in the epidermal layer of the skin. The deeper cells in the **hair root** force older keratinized cells to move upward, forming the **hair shaft.** The hair shaft grows toward the skin surface within the **hair follicle.** Melanin gives hair its color. Sebaceous glands release oil directly into the hair follicle. Each hair has a small slip of smooth muscle attached to it called the **arrector pili** muscle (see Figure 3.3 ■). When this muscle contracts the hair shaft stands up and results in "goose bumps."

Nails

cuticle (KEW-tikl)
free edge
lunula (LOO-nyoo-lah)
nail bed
nail body
nail root

Nails are a flat plate of keratin called the **nail body** that covers the ends of fingers and toes. The nail body is connected to the tissue underneath by the **nail bed.** Nails grow longer from the **nail root,** which is found at the base of the nail and is covered and protected by the soft tissue **cuticle.** The **free edge** is the exposed edge that is trimmed when nails become too long. The light-colored half-moon area at the base of the nail is the **lunula** (see Figure 3.4 ■).

MED TERM TIP

Because of its rich blood supply and light color, the nail bed is an excellent place to check patients for low oxygen levels in their blood. Deoxygenated blood is a very dark purple-red and gives skin a bluish tinge called *cyanosis.*

Sebaceous Glands

sebum

Sebaceous glands, found in the dermis, secrete the oil **sebum,** which lubricates the hair and skin, thereby helping to prevent drying and cracking. These glands secrete sebum directly into hair follicles, rather than a duct (see Figure 3.1). Secretion from the sebaceous glands increases during adolescence, playing a role in the development of acne. Sebum secretion begins to diminish as age increases. A loss of sebum in old age, along with sun exposure, can account for wrinkles and dry skin.

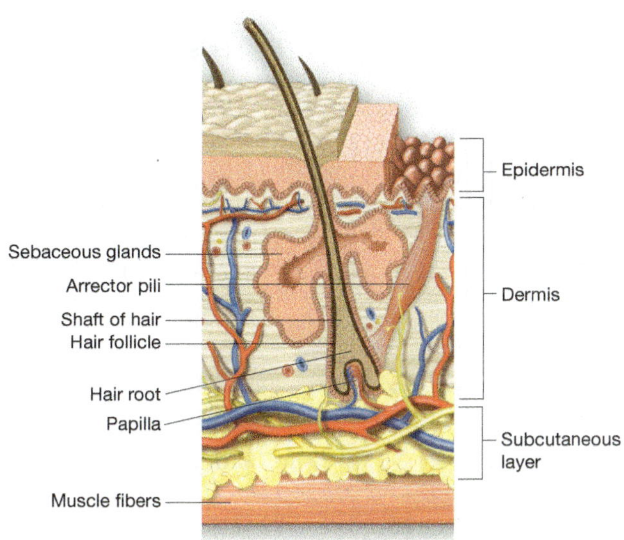

■ **Figure 3.3** Structure of a hair and its associated sebaceous gland.

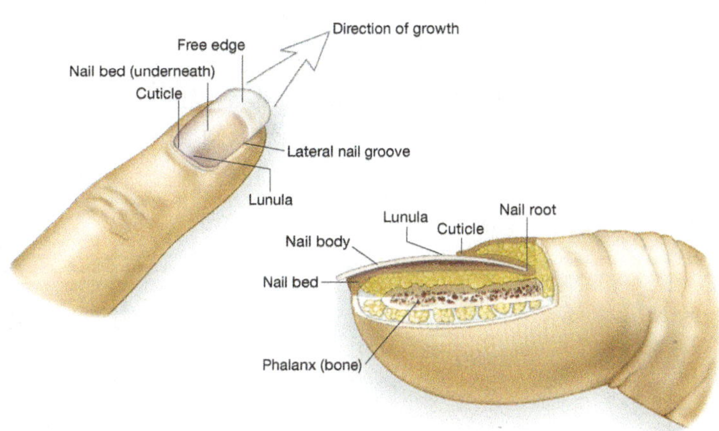

■ **Figure 3.4** External and internal structures of nails.

Sweat Glands

apocrine glands (APP-oh-krin)
perspiration
sudoriferous glands (sue-doh-RIF-er-us)
sweat duct
sweat pore

About 2 million sweat glands, also called **sudoriferous glands,** are found throughout the body. These highly coiled glands are located in the dermis. Sweat travels to the surface of the skin in a **sweat duct.** The surface opening of a sweat duct is called a **sweat pore** (see Figure 3.1).

Sweat glands function to cool the body as sweat evaporates. Sweat or **perspiration** contains a small amount of waste product but is normally colorless and odorless. However, there are sweat glands called **apocrine glands** in the pubic and underarm areas that secrete a thicker sweat, which can produce an odor when it comes into contact with bacteria on the skin. This is what we recognize as body odor.

MED TERM TIP

Word Watch: Be careful when using *hydro-* meaning "water" and *hidr/o* meaning "sweat."

Terminology

Word Parts Used to Build Integumentary System Terms

The following lists contain the combining forms, suffixes, and prefixes used to build terms in the remaining sections of this chapter.

Combining Forms

albin/o	white
angi/o	vessel
bas/o	the base
bi/o	life
carcin/o	cancer
chem/o	chemical
cis/o	to cut
cry/o	cold
cutane/o	skin
cyan/o	blue
cyt/o	cell
derm/o	skin
dermat/o	skin

diaphor/o	profuse sweating
electr/o	electricity
erythr/o	red
esthesi/o	feeling
hem/o	blood
hidr/o	sweat
ichthy/o	scaly, dry
kerat/o	hard, horny
leuk/o	white
lip/o	fat
melan/o	black
myc/o	fungus
necr/o	death

onych/o	nail
pedicul/o	lice
phot/o	light
py/o	pus
rhytid/o	wrinkle
sarc/o	flesh
scler/o	hard
seb/o	oil
system/o	system
trich/o	hair
ungu/o	nail
vesic/o	bladder
xer/o	dry

Suffixes

-al	pertaining to
-derma	skin condition
-ectomy	surgical removal
-emia	blood condition
-ia	state, condition
-ic	pertaining to
-ism	state of

-itis	inflammation
-logy	study of
-malacia	softening
-oma	mass
-opsy	to view
-osis	abnormal condition

-ous	pertaining to
-phagia	eating
-plasty	surgical repair
-rrhea	discharge
-tic	pertaining to
-tome	instrument to cut
-ule	small

Prefixes

allo-	other
an-	without
anti-	against
auto-	self

de-	without
epi-	upon
hyper-	excessive
hypo-	under

intra-	within
para-	beside
sub-	under
xeno-	strange, foreign

Anatomical Terms

TERM	WORD PARTS	DEFINITION
cutaneous (kyoo-TAY-nee-us)	cutane/o = skin -ous = pertaining to	pertaining to the skin
dermal (DER-mal)	derm/o = skin -al = pertaining to	pertaining to the skin
epidermal (ep-ih-DER-mal)	epi- = upon derm/o = skin -al = pertaining to	pertaining to upon the skin
hypodermic (high-poh-DER-mik)	hypo- = under derm/o = skin -ic = pertaining to	pertaining to under the skin
intradermal (in-trah-DER-mal)	intra- = within derm/o = skin -al = pertaining to	pertaining to within the skin
subcutaneous (sub-kyoo-TAY-nee-us)	sub- = under cutane/o = skin -ous = pertaining to	pertaining to under the skin
ungual (UNG-gwal)	ungu/o = nail -al = pertaining to	pertaining to the nails

Pathology

TERM	WORD PARTS	DEFINITION
Medical Specialties		
dermatology (Derm, derm) (der-mah-TALL-oh-jee)	dermat/o = skin -logy = study of	Branch of medicine involving diagnosis and treatment of conditions and diseases of the integumentary system. Physician is a *dermatologist.*
plastic surgery		Surgical specialty involved in repair, reconstruction, or improvement of body structures such as the skin that are damaged, missing, or misshapen. Physician is a *plastic surgeon.*
Signs and Symptoms		
abrasion (ah-BRAY-zhun)		A scraping away of the skin surface by friction.
anhidrosis (an-hi-DROH-sis)	an- = without hidr/o = sweat -osis = abnormal condition	Abnormal condition of no sweat.
comedo (KOM-ee-do)		Collection of hardened sebum in hair follicle. Also called a *blackhead.*
contusion		Injury caused by a blow to the body; causes swelling, pain, and bruising. The skin is not broken.
cyanosis (sigh-ah-NOH-sis)	cyan/o = blue -osis = abnormal condition	Bluish tint to the skin caused by deoxygenated blood.

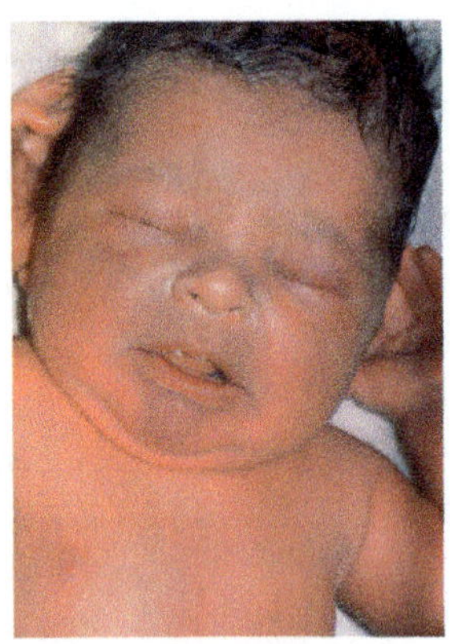

■ **Figure 3.5** A cyanotic infant. Note the bluish tinge to the skin around the lips, chin, and nose. *(St. Bartholomew's Hospital, London/Photo Researchers, Inc.)*

TERM	WORD PARTS	DEFINITION
cyst (SIST)		Fluid-filled sac under the skin.

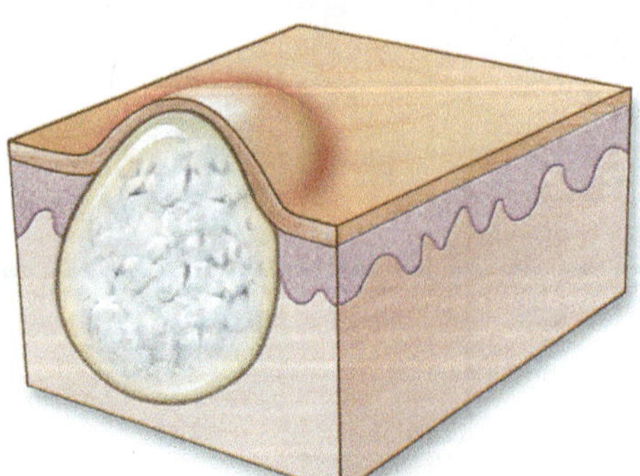

■ **Figure 3.6** Cyst.

Pathology *(continued)*

TERM	WORD PARTS	DEFINITION
depigmentation (dee-pig-men-TAY-shun)	de- = without	Loss of normal skin color or pigment.
diaphoresis (dye-ah-for-REE-sis)	diaphor/o = profuse sweating	Profuse sweating.
ecchymosis (ek-ih-MOH-sis)	-osis = abnormal condition	Skin discoloration caused by blood collecting under the skin following blunt trauma to the skin. A bruise.

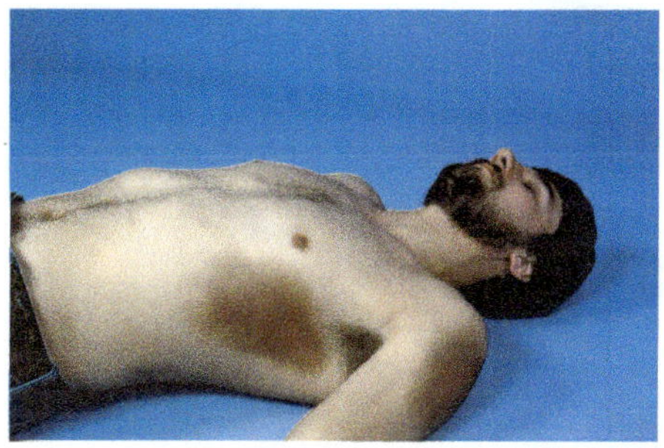

■ **Figure 3.7** Male lying supine with large ecchymosis on lateral rib cage and shoulder.

TERM	WORD PARTS	DEFINITION
erythema (er-ih-THEE-mah)	erythr/o = red hem/o = blood	Redness or flushing of the skin.
erythroderma (eh-rith-roh-DER-mah)	erythr/o = red -derma = skin condition	The condition of having reddened or flushed skin.
eschar (ES-kar)		A thick layer of dead tissue and tissue fluid that develops over a deep burn area.
fissure (FISH-er)		Crack-like lesion or groove on the skin.

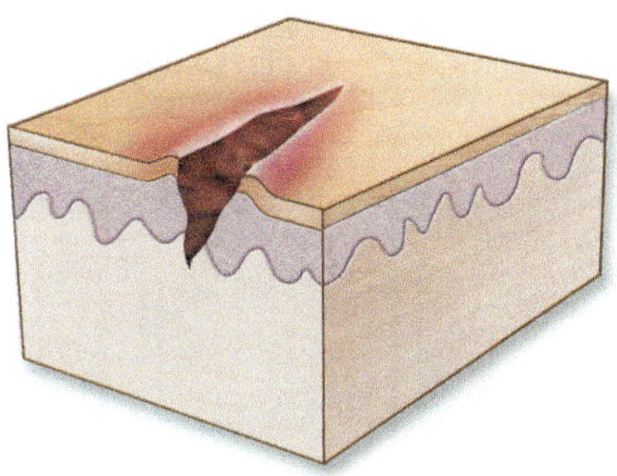

■ **Figure 3.8** Fissure.

TERM	WORD PARTS	DEFINITION
hirsutism (HER-soot-izm)		Excessive hair growth over the body.
hyperemia (high-per-EE-mee-ah)	hyper- = excessive -emia = blood condition	Redness of the skin due to increased blood flow.
hyperhidrosis (high-per-hi-DROH-sis)	hyper- = excessive hidr/o = sweat -osis = abnormal condition	Abnormal condition of excessive sweat.
hyperpigmentation (high-per-pig-men-TAY-shun)	hyper- = excessive	Abnormal amount of pigmentation in the skin.
ichthyoderma (ick-thee-oh-DER-mah)	ichthy/o = scaly, dry -derma = skin condition	The condition of having scaly and dry skin.

Pathology *(continued)*

TERM	WORD PARTS	DEFINITION
lesion (LEE-shun)		A general term for a wound, injury, or abnormality.
leukoderma (loo-koh-DER-mah)	leuk/o = white -derma = skin condition	Having skin that appears white because the normal skin pigment is absent. May be all the skin or just in some areas.
lipoma (lip-OH-mah)	lip/o = fat -oma = mass	Fatty mass.
macule (MACK-yool)	-ule = small	Flat, discolored area that is flush with the skin surface. An example would be a freckle or a birthmark.

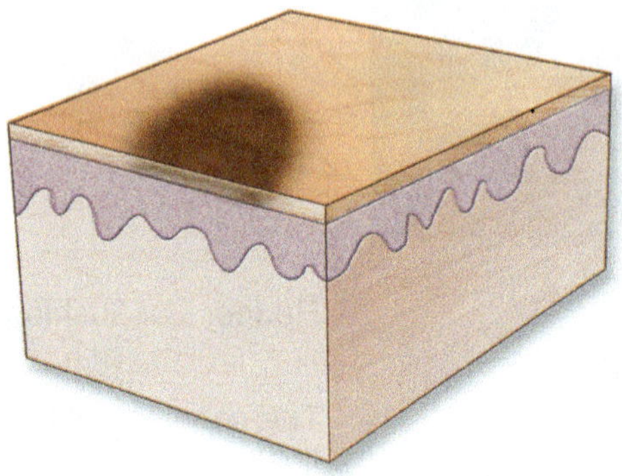

■ **Figure 3.9** Macule.

TERM	WORD PARTS	DEFINITION
necrosis (neh-KROH-sis)	necr/o = death -osis = abnormal condition	Abnormal condition of death.
nevus (NEV-us)		Pigmented skin blemish, birthmark, or mole. Usually benign but may become cancerous.
nodule (NOD-yool)	-ule = small	Firm, solid mass of cells in the skin larger than 0.5 cm in diameter.

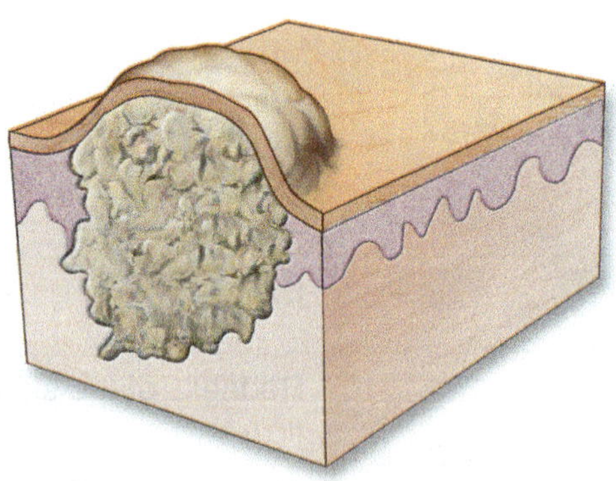

■ **Figure 3.10** Nodule.

TERM	WORD PARTS	DEFINITION
onychomalacia (on-ih-koh-mah-LAY-she-ah)	onych/o = nail -malacia = softening	Softening of the nails.
pallor (PAL-or)		Abnormal paleness of the skin.

Pathology *(continued)*

TERM	WORD PARTS	DEFINITION
papule (PAP-yool)	-ule = small	Small, solid, circular raised spot on the surface of the skin less than 0.5 cm in diameter.
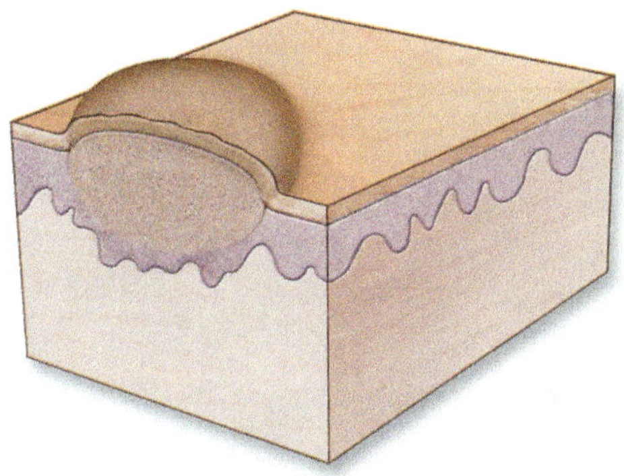 **Figure 3.11** Papule.		
petechiae (peh-TEE-kee-eye)		Pinpoint purple or red spots from minute hemorrhages under the skin.
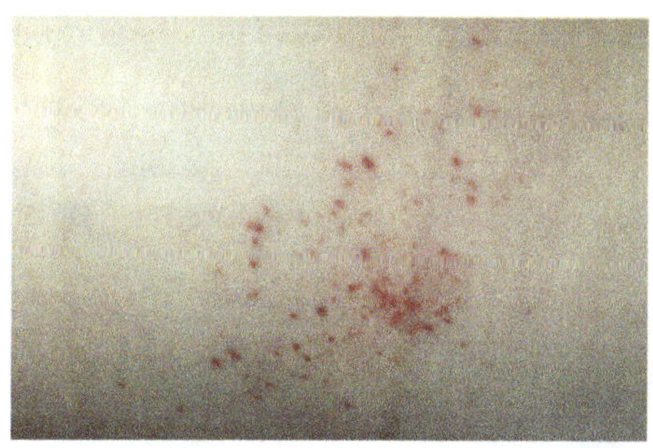 **Figure 3.12** Petechiae, pinpoint skin hemorrhages. *(Custom Medical Stock)*		
photosensitivity (foh-toh-sen-sih-TIH-vih-tee)	phot/o = light	Condition in which the skin reacts abnormally when exposed to light, such as the ultraviolet (UV) rays of the sun.
pruritus (proo-RIGH-tus)		Severe itching.
purpura (PER-pew-rah)		Hemorrhages into the skin due to fragile blood vessels. Commonly seen in older adults.
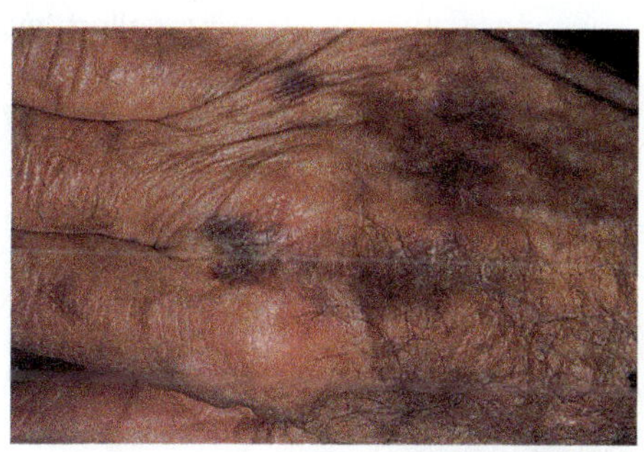 **Figure 3.13** Purpura, hemorrhaging into the skin due to fragile blood vessels. *(Caroll H. Weiss/Camera M.D. Studios)*		**MED TERM TIP** *Purpura* comes from the Latin word for "purple," which refers to the color of these pinpoint hemorrhages.
purulent (PYUR-yoo-lent)		Containing pus or an infection that is producing pus. Pus consists of dead bacteria, white blood cells, and tissue debris.

Pathology *(continued)*

TERM	WORD PARTS	DEFINITION
pustule (PUS-tyool)	-ule = small	Raised spot on the skin containing pus.

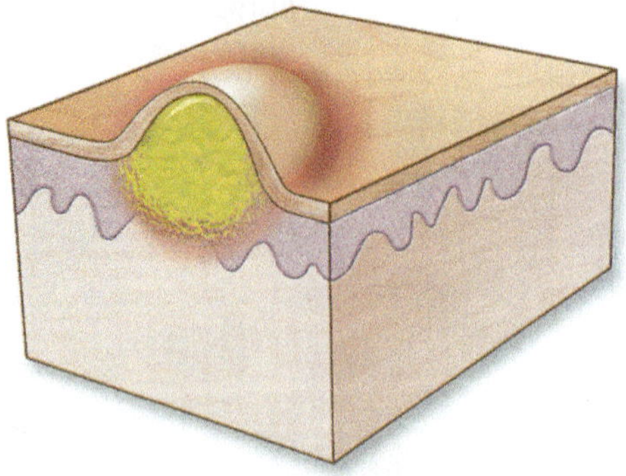

■ **Figure 3.14** Pustule.

TERM	WORD PARTS	DEFINITION
pyoderma (pye-oh-DER-mah)	py/o = pus -derma = skin condition	The presence of pus on or in the layers of skin. A sign of a bacterial infection.
scleroderma (sklair-ah-DER-mah)	scler/o = hard -derma = skin condition	A condition in which the skin has lost its elasticity and become hardened.
seborrhea (seb-or-EE-ah)	seb/o = oil -rrhea = discharge	Oily discharge.
suppurative (SUP-pure-a-tiv)		Containing or producing pus.
ulcer (ULL-ser)		Open sore or lesion in skin or mucous membrane.

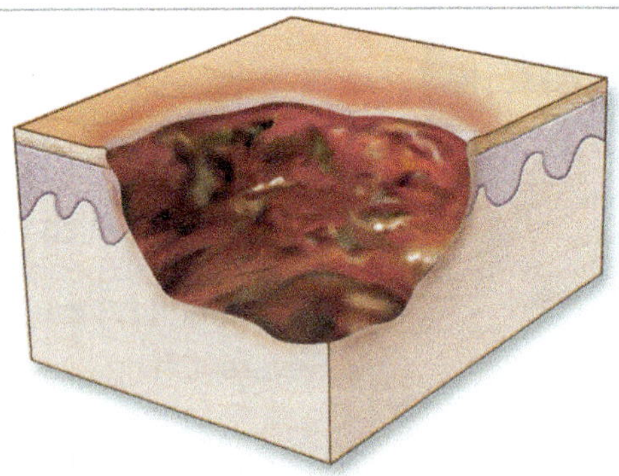

■ **Figure 3.15** Ulcer.

TERM	WORD PARTS	DEFINITION
urticaria (er-tih-KAY-ree-ah)		Also called *hives;* a skin eruption of pale reddish wheals with severe itching. Usually associated with food allergy, stress, or drug reactions.
vesicle (VESS-ikl)	vesic/o = bladder	A blister; small, fluid-filled raised spot on the skin.

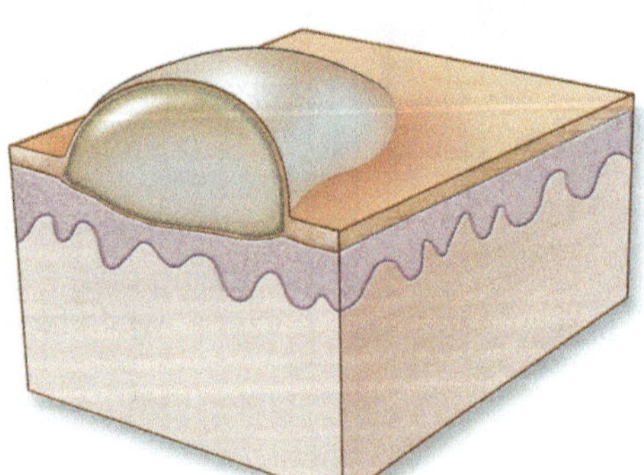

■ **Figure 3.16** Vesicle.

Pathology *(continued)*

TERM	WORD PARTS	DEFINITION
wheal (WEEL) 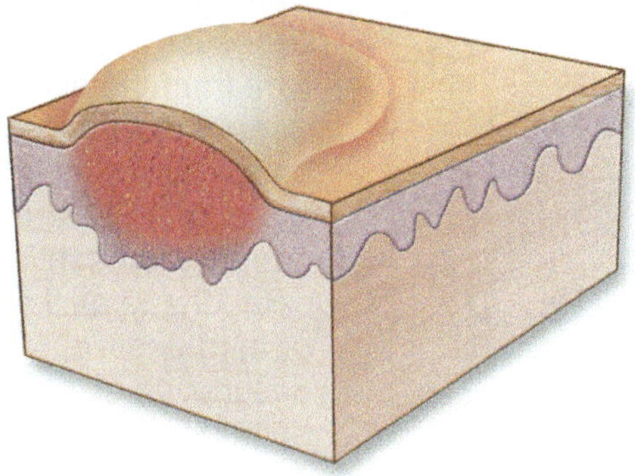 **Figure 3.17** Wheal.		Small, round, swollen area on the skin; typically seen in allergic skin reactions such as *hives* and usually accompanied by urticaria.
xeroderma (zee-roh-DER-mah)	xer/o = dry -derma = skin condition	Condition in which the skin is abnormally dry.
Skin		
abscess (AB-sess)		A collection of pus in the skin.
acne (ACK-nee)		Inflammatory disease of the sebaceous glands and hair follicles resulting in papules and pustules.
acne rosacea (ACK-nee roh-ZAY-she-ah)		Chronic form of acne seen in adults involving redness, tiny pimples, and broken blood vessels, primarily on the nose and cheeks.
acne vulgaris (ACK-nee vul-GAY-ris)		Common form of acne seen in teenagers. Characterized by comedo, papules, and pustules.
albinism (al-BIH-nizm)	albin/o = white -ism = state of	A genetic condition in which the body is unable to make melanin. Characterized by white hair and skin and red pupils due to the lack of pigment. The person with albinism is called an *albino.*
basal cell carcinoma (BCC) (BAY-sal / sell / kar-sin-NOH-ma)	bas/o = the base -al = pertaining to carcin/o = cancer -oma = tumor	Cancerous tumor of the basal cell layer of the epidermis. A frequent type of skin cancer that rarely metastasizes or spreads. These cancers can arise on sun-exposed skin.
Figure 3.18 Basal cell carcinoma, a frequent type of skin cancer that rarely metastasizes. *(Bob Craig/CDC)*	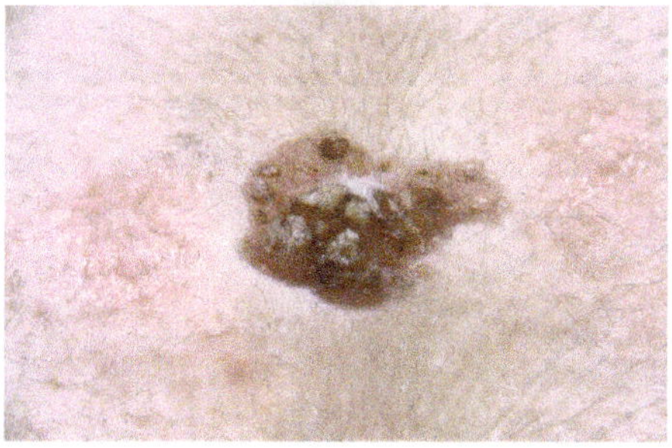	

Pathology *(continued)*

TERM	WORD PARTS	DEFINITION
burn		Damage to the skin that can result from exposure to open fire, electricity, ultraviolet light from the sun, or caustic chemicals. Seriousness depends on the amount of body surface involved and the depth of the burn as determined by the amount of damage to each layer. Skin and burns are categorized as first degree, second degree, or third degree. See Figure 3.19 ■ for a description of the damage associated with each degree of burn. Extent of a burn is estimated using the Rule of Nines (see Figure 3.20 ■).

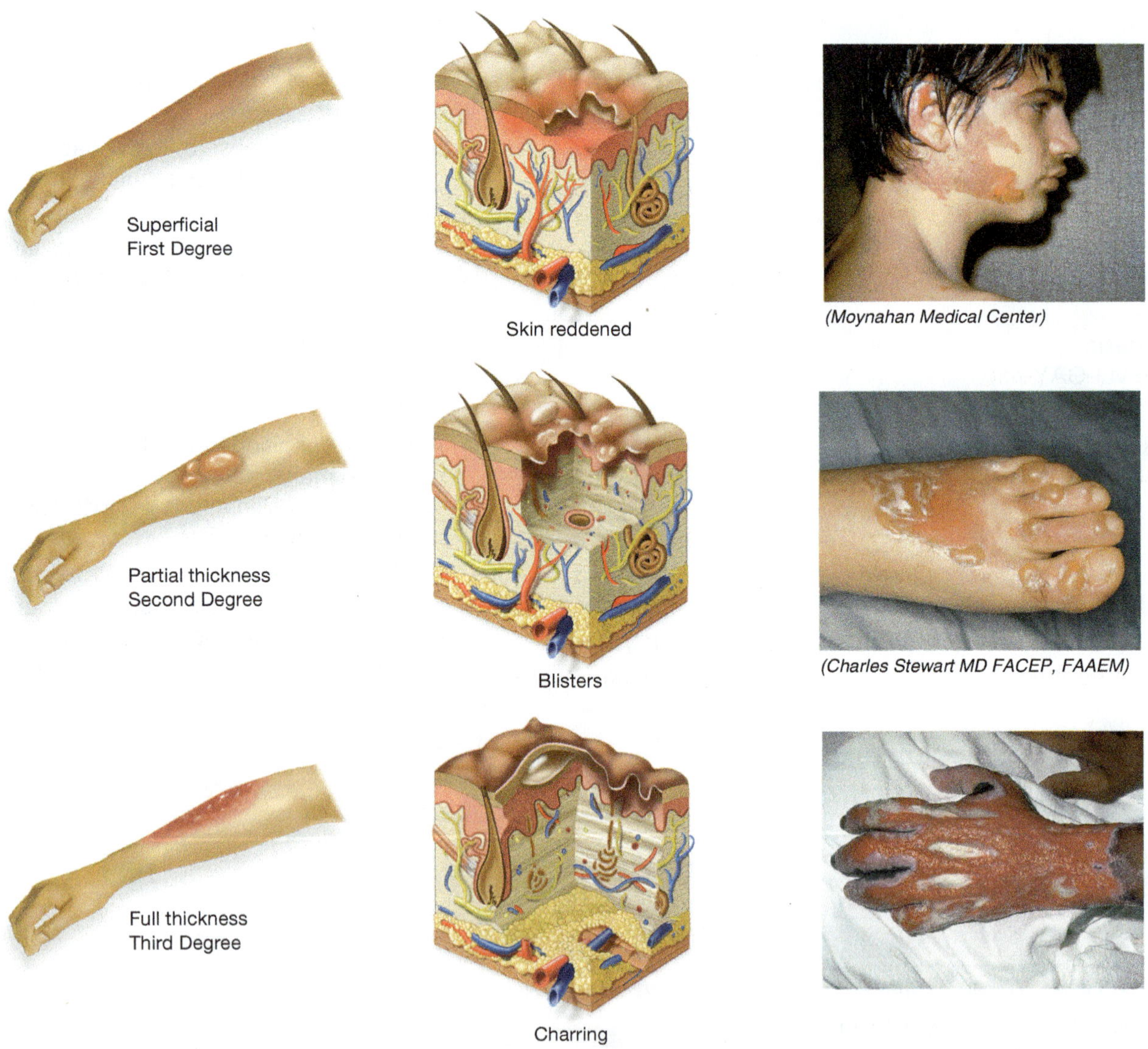

■ **Figure 3.19** Comparison of the level of skin damage as a result of the three different degrees of burns.

Pathology *(continued)*

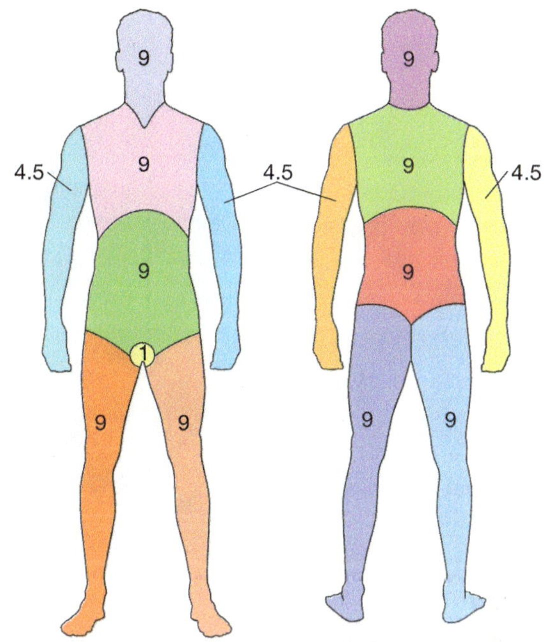

Figure 3.20 Rule of Nines. A method for determining percentage of body burned. Each different-colored section represents a percentage of the body surface. All sections added together will equal 100%.

TERM	WORD PARTS	DEFINITION
cellulitis (sell-you-LYE-tis)	-itis = inflammation	A diffuse, acute infection and inflammation of the connective tissue found in the skin.
cicatrix (SICK-ah-trix)		A scar.
decubitus ulcer (decub) (dee-KYOO-bih-tus)	**MED TERM TIP** *Decubitus* comes from the Latin word *decumbo*, meaning "lying down," which leads to the use of the term for a bedsore or pressure sore.	Open sore caused by pressure over bony prominences cutting off the blood flow to the overlying skin. These can appear in bedridden patients who lie in one position too long and can be difficult to heal. Also called *bedsore* or *pressure sore.*
dermatitis (der-mah-TYE-tis)	dermat/o = skin -itis = inflammation	Inflammation of the skin.
dermatosis (der-mah-TOH-sis)	dermat/o = skin -osis = abnormal condition	A general term indicating the presence of an abnormal skin condition.
dry gangrene (GANG-green)		Late stages of gangrene characterized by the affected area becoming dried, blackened, and shriveled; referred to as *mummified.*
eczema (EK-zeh-mah)		Superficial dermatitis of unknown cause accompanied by redness, vesicles, itching, and crusting.
gangrene (GANG-green)		Tissue necrosis usually due to deficient blood supply.
ichthyosis (ick-thee-OH-sis)	ichthy/o = scaly, dry -osis = abnormal condition	Condition in which the skin becomes dry, scaly, and keratinized.

Pathology *(continued)*

TERM	WORD PARTS	DEFINITION
impetigo (im-peh-TYE-goh)		A highly infectious bacterial infection of the skin with pustules that rupture and become crusted over.

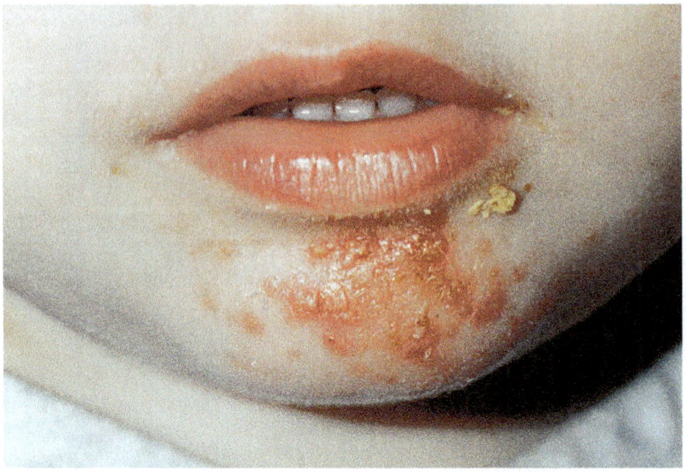

■ **Figure 3.21** Impetigo, a highly contagious bacterial infection. *(Dr. Jason L. Smith)*

TERM	WORD PARTS	DEFINITION
Kaposi's sarcoma (KAP-oh-seez / sar-KOH-mah)	sarc/o = flesh -oma = tumor	Form of skin cancer frequently seen in acquired immunodeficiency syndrome (AIDS) patients. Consists of brownish-purple papules that spread from the skin and metastasize to internal organs.
keloid (KEE-loyd)		Formation of a raised and thickened hypertrophic scar after an injury or surgery.

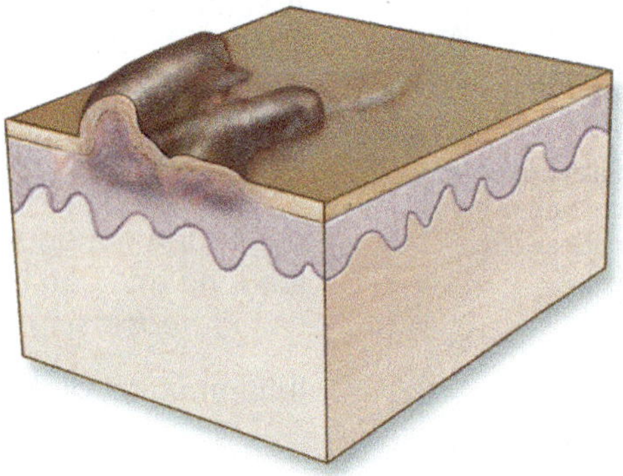

■ **Figure 3.22** Keloid.

TERM	WORD PARTS	DEFINITION
keratosis (kair-ah-TOH-sis)	kerat/o = hard, horny -osis = abnormal condition	Term for any skin condition involving an overgrowth and thickening of the epidermis layer.
laceration		A torn or jagged wound; incorrectly used to describe a cut.
malignant melanoma (MM) (mah-LIG-nant / mel-a-NOH-ma)	melan/o = black -oma = tumor	Dangerous form of skin cancer caused by an uncontrolled growth of melanocytes. May quickly metastasize or spread to internal organs.

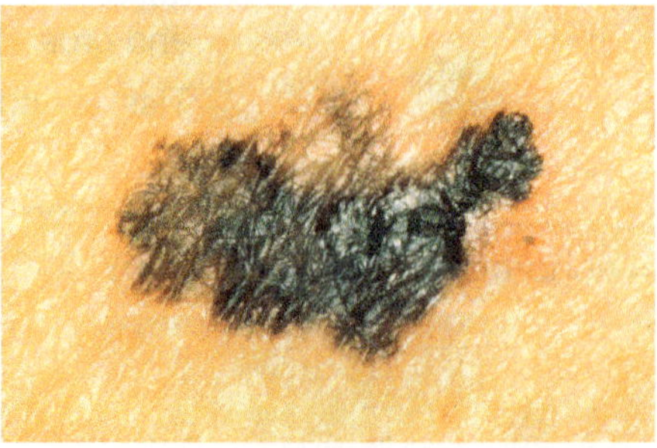

■ **Figure 3.23** Malignant melanoma. This photograph demonstrates the highly characteristic color of this tumor. *(Skin Cancer Foundation/National Cancer Institute)*

Pathology *(continued)*

TERM	WORD PARTS	DEFINITION
pediculosis (peh-dik-you-LOH-sis)	pedicul/o = lice -osis = abnormal condition	Infestation with lice. The eggs laid by the lice are called nits and cling tightly to hair.
psoriasis (soh-RYE-ah-sis)		Chronic inflammatory condition consisting of papules forming "silvery scale" patches with circular borders.

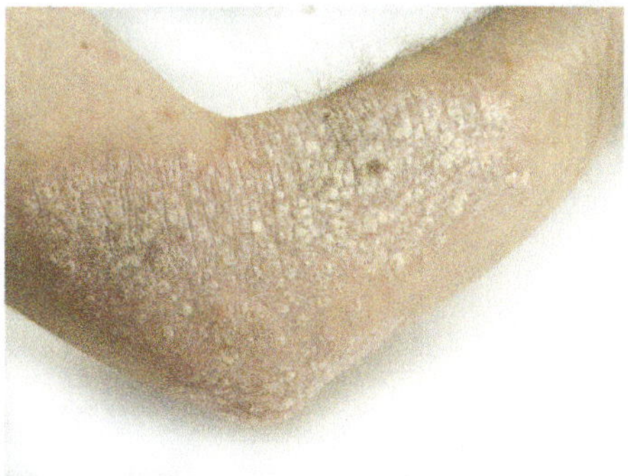

■ **Figure 3.24** Psoriasis. This photograph demonstrates the characteristic white skin patches of this condition. *(kenxro/Shutterstock)*

TERM	WORD PARTS	DEFINITION
rubella (roo-BELL-ah)		Contagious viral skin infection. Commonly called *German measles*.
scabies (SKAY-bees)		Contagious skin disease caused by an egg-laying mite that burrows through the skin and causes redness and intense itching; often seen in children.
sebaceous cyst (see-BAY-shus / SIST)	seb/o = oil	Sac under the skin filled with sebum or oil from a sebaceous gland. This can grow to a large size and may need to be excised.
squamous cell carcinoma (SCC) (SKWAY-mus / sell / kar-sih-NOH-mah)	carcin/o = cancer -oma = tumor	Cancer of the epidermis layer of skin that may invade deeper tissue and metastasize. Often begins as a sore that does not heal.

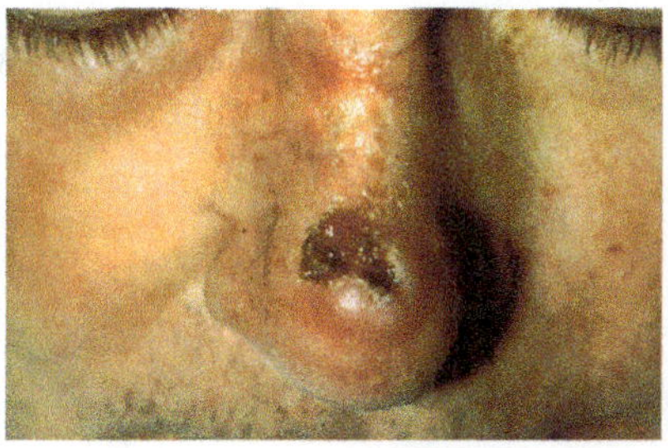

■ **Figure 3.25** Squamous cell carcinoma. *(National Cancer Institute)*

Pathology *(continued)*

TERM	WORD PARTS	DEFINITION
strawberry hemangioma (hee-man-jee-OH-ma)	hem/o = blood angi/o = vessel -oma = tumor	Congenital collection of dilated blood vessels causing a red birthmark that fades a few months after birth.

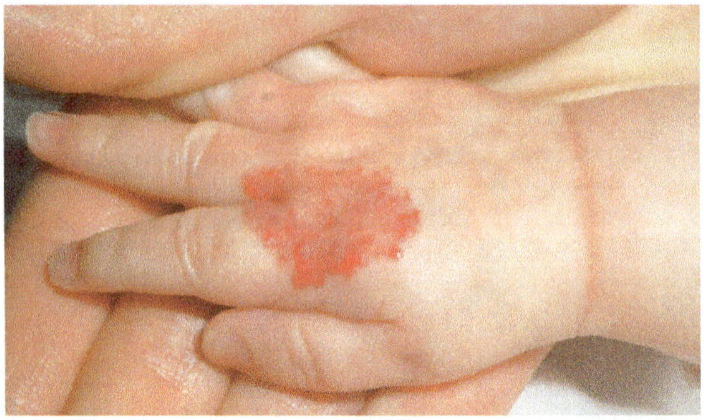

■ **Figure 3.26** Strawberry hemangioma, a birthmark caused by a collection of blood vessels in the skin. *(H.C. Robinson/Science Photo Library/ Photo Researchers)*

TERM	WORD PARTS	DEFINITION
systemic lupus erythematosus (SLE) (sis-TEM-ik / LOO-pus / air-ih-them-ah-TOH-sis)	system/o = system -ic = pertaining to erythr/o = red	Chronic disease of the connective tissue that injures the skin, joints, kidneys, nervous system, and mucous membranes. This is an autoimmune condition meaning that the body's own immune system attacks normal tissue of the body. May produce a characteristic red, scaly butterfly rash across the cheeks and nose.
tinea (TIN-ee-ah)		Fungal skin disease resulting in itching, scaling lesions.
tinea capitis (TIN-ee-ah / CAP-it-is)	*capitis* is the Latin term for the head	Fungal infection of the scalp. Commonly called *ringworm.*
tinea pedis (TIN-ee-ah / PED-is)	*pedis* is the Latin term for the foot	Fungal infection of the foot. Commonly called *athlete's foot.*
varicella (vair-ih-SELL-ah)		Contagious viral skin infection. Commonly called *chickenpox.*

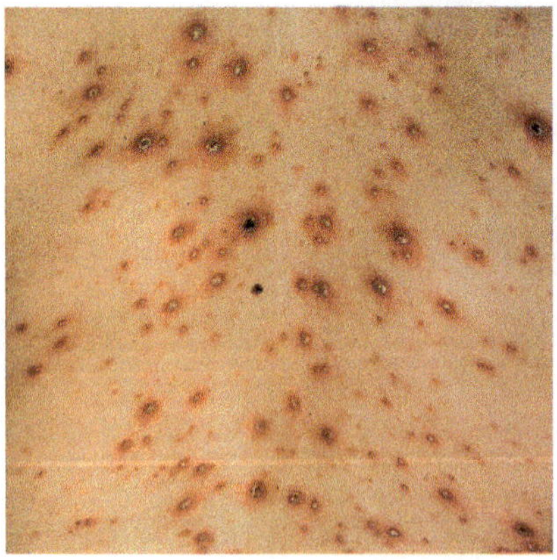

■ **Figure 3.27** Varicella or chickenpox, a viral skin infection. In this photograph, the rash is beginning to form scabs.

TERM	WORD PARTS	DEFINITION
verruca (ver-ROO-kah)		Commonly called *warts;* a benign growth caused by a virus. Has a rough surface that is removed by chemicals and/or laser therapy.

Pathology *(continued)*

TERM	WORD PARTS	DEFINITION
vitiligo (vit-ill-EYE-go)		Disappearance of pigment from the skin in patches, causing a milk-white appearance. Also called *leukoderma.*
wet gangrene (GANG-green)		An area of gangrene that becomes secondarily infected by pus-producing bacteria.
Hair		
alopecia (al-oh-PEE-she-ah)		Absence or loss of hair, especially of the head. Commonly called *baldness.*
carbuncle (CAR-bung-kl)		Furuncle involving several hair follicles.
furuncle (FOO-rung-kl)		Bacterial infection of a hair follicle. Characterized by redness, pain, and swelling. Also called a *boil.*
trichomycosis (trik-oh-my-KOH-sis)	trich/o = hair myc/o = fungus -osis = abnormal condition	Abnormal condition of hair fungus.
Nails		
onychia (oh-NICK-ee-ah)	onych/o = nail -ia = state, condition	Infected nail bed.
onychomycosis (on-ih-koh-my-KOH-sis)	onych/o = nail myc/o = fungus -osis = abnormal condition	Abnormal condition of nail fungus.
onychophagia (on-ih-koh-FAY-jee-ah)	onych/o = nail -phagia = eating	Nail eating (nail biting).
paronychia (pair-oh-NICK-ee-ah)	para- = beside onych/o = nail -ia = state, condition	Infection of the skin fold around a nail.

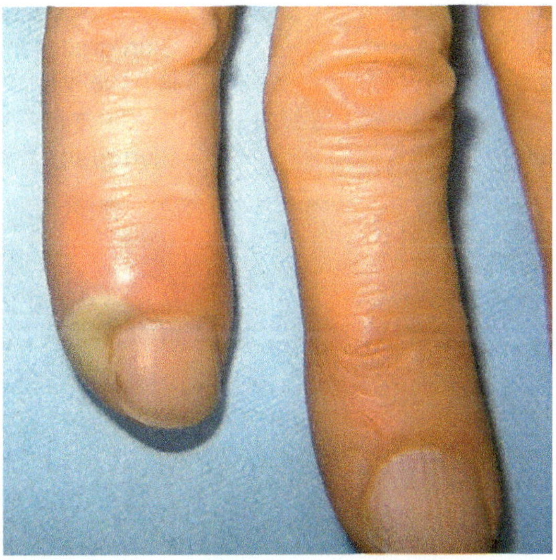

Figure 3.28 Paronychia.
(Local Images Inc.)

Diagnostic Procedures

TERM	WORD PARTS	DEFINITION
Clinical Laboratory Tests		
culture and sensitivity (C&S)		Laboratory test that grows a colony of bacteria removed from an infected area in order to identify the specific infecting bacteria and then determine its sensitivity to a variety of antibiotics.
Biopsy Procedures		
biopsy (BX, bx) (BYE-op-see) MED TERM TIP Word Watch: Be careful when using *bi-* meaning "two" and *bi/o* meaning "life."	bi/o = life -opsy = to view	Piece of tissue removed by syringe and needle, knife, punch, or brush to examine under a microscope. Used to aid in diagnosis.
exfoliative cytology (ex-FOH-lee-ah-tiv / sigh-TALL-oh-jee)	cyt/o = cell -logy = study of	Scraping cells from tissue and then examining them under a microscope.
frozen section (FS)		Thin piece of tissue cut from a frozen specimen for rapid examination under a microscope.
fungal scrapings	-al = pertaining to	Scrapings, taken with a curette or scraper, of tissue from lesions are placed on a growth medium and examined under a microscope to identify fungal growth.

Therapeutic Procedures

TERM	WORD PARTS	DEFINITION
Skin Grafting		
allograft (AL-oh-graft)	allo- = other	Skin graft from one person to another; donor is usually a cadaver. Also called *homograft* (homo = same).
autograft (AW-toh-graft)	auto- = self	Skin graft from a person's own body.

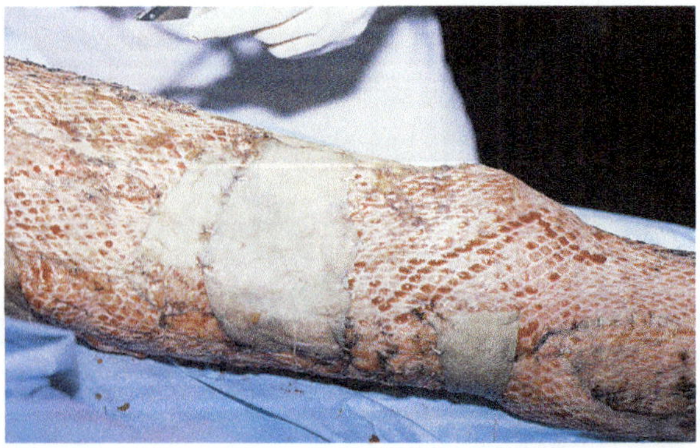

■ **Figure 3.29** A freshly applied autograft. Note that the donor skin has been perforated so that it can be stretched to cover a larger burned area. *(Courtesy of Dr. William Dominic, Community Regional Medical Center)*

TERM	WORD PARTS	DEFINITION
dermatome (DER-mah-tohm)	derm/o = skin -tome = instrument to cut	Instrument for cutting the skin or thin transplants of skin.

Therapeutic Procedures *(continued)*

TERM	WORD PARTS	DEFINITION
dermatoplasty (DER-mah-toh-plas-tee)	dermat/o = skin -plasty = surgical repair	Skin grafting; transplantation of skin.
skin graft (SG)		Transfer of skin from a normal area to cover another site. Used to treat burn victims and after some surgical procedures. Also called *dermatoplasty*.
xenograft (ZEN-oh-graft)	xeno- = strange, foreign	Skin graft from an animal of another species (usually a pig) to a human. Also called *heterograft* (hetero- = other).
Surgical Procedures		
cauterization (kaw-ter-ih-ZAY-shun)		Destruction of tissue by using caustic chemicals, electric currents, heat, or by freezing.
cryosurgery (cry-oh-SER-jer-ee)	cry/o = cold	Use of extreme cold to freeze and destroy tissue.
curettage (koo-REH-tahz)		Removal of superficial skin lesions with a curette (surgical instrument shaped like a spoon) or scraper.
debridement (de-BREED-mint)		Removal of foreign material and dead or damaged tissue from a wound.
electrocautery (ee-leck-troh-KAW-teh-ree)	electr/o = electricity	To destroy tissue with an electric current.
incision and drainage (I&D)	cis/o = to cut	Making an incision to create an opening for the drainage of material such as pus.
onychectomy (on-ee-KECK-toh-mee)	onych/o = nail -ectomy = surgical removal	Removal of a nail.
Plastic Surgery Procedures		
chemabrasion (kee-moh-BRAY-zhun)	chem/o = chemical	Abrasion using chemicals. Also called a *chemical peel*.
dermabrasion (DERM-ah-bray-shun)	derm/o = skin	Abrasion or rubbing using wire brushes or sandpaper. Performed to remove acne scars, tattoos, and scar tissue.
laser therapy		Removal of skin lesions and birthmarks using a laser beam that emits intense heat and power at a close range. The laser converts frequencies of light into one small, powerful beam.
liposuction (LIP-oh-suck-shun)	lip/o = fat	Removal of fat beneath the skin by means of suction.
rhytidectomy (rit-ih-DECK-toh-mee)	rhytid/o = wrinkle -ectomy = surgical removal	Surgical removal of excess skin to eliminate wrinkles. Commonly referred to as a *face lift*.

Pharmacology

CLASSIFICATION	WORD PARTS	ACTION	EXAMPLES
anesthetic (an-es-THET-tic)	an- = without esthesi/o = feeling -ic = pertaining to	Applied to the skin to deaden pain.	lidocaine, Xylocaine; procaine, Novocain
antibiotic (an-tye-bye-AW-tic)	anti- = against bi/o = life -tic = pertaining to	Kill bacteria causing skin infections.	bacitracin/neomycin/polymixinB, Neosporin ointment
antifungal (an-tye-FUNG-all)	anti- = against -al = pertaining to	Kill fungi infecting the skin.	miconazole, Monistat; clotrimazole, Lotrimin
antiparasitic (an-tye-pair-ah-SIT-tic)	anti- = against -ic = pertaining to	Kill mites or lice.	lindane, Kwell; permethrin, Nix
antipruritic (an-tye-proo-RIGH-tik)	anti- = against -ic = pertaining to	Reduce severe itching.	diphenhydramine, Benadryl; camphor/pramoxine/zinc, Caladryl
antiseptic (an-tye-SEP-tic)	anti- = against -tic = pertaining to	Used to kill bacteria in skin cuts and wounds or at a surgical site.	isopropyl alcohol; hydrogen peroxide
corticosteroid cream		Specific type of powerful anti-inflammatory cream.	hydrocortisone, Cortaid; triamcinolone, Kenalog

Abbreviations

BCC	basal cell carcinoma	**MM**	malignant melanoma
BX, bx	biopsy	**SCC**	squamous cell carcinoma
C&S	culture and sensitivity	**SG**	skin graft
decub	decubitus ulcer	**SLE**	systemic lupus erythematosus
Derm, derm	dermatology	**STSG**	split-thickness skin graft
FS	frozen section	**Subc, SubQ**	subcutaneous
I&D	incision and drainage	**UV**	ultraviolet
ID	intradermal		

MED TERM TIP

Word Watch: Be careful when using the abbreviation *ID* meaning "intradermal" and *I&D* meaning "incision and drainage."

Chapter Review

Real-World Applications

Medical Record Analysis

This Dermatology Consultation Report contains 11 medical terms. Underline each term and write it in the list below the report. Then define each term.

Dermatology Consultation Report

Reason for Consultation:	Possible recurrence of basal cell carcinoma, left cheek.
History of Present Illness:	Patient is a 74-year-old male first seen by his regular physician 5 years ago for persistent facial lesions. Biopsies revealed basal cell carcinoma in two lesions, one on the nasal tip and the other on the left cheek. These were successfully excised. The patient noted that the left cheek lesion returned approximately one year ago. Patient reports pruritus and states the lesion is growing larger.
Results of Physical Exam:	Examination revealed a 10 × 14 mm lesion on left cheek 20 mm anterior to the ear. The lesion displays marked erythema and poorly defined borders. The area immediately around the lesion shows depigmentation with vesicles.
Assessment:	Recurrence of basal cell carcinoma.
Recommendations:	Due to the lesion's size, shape, and reoccurrence, deep excision of the carcinoma through the epidermis and dermis layers followed by dermatoplasty is recommended.

	Term	Definition
1	______________	______________________________
2	______________	______________________________
3	______________	______________________________
4	______________	______________________________
5	______________	______________________________
6	______________	______________________________
7	______________	______________________________
8	______________	______________________________
9	______________	______________________________
10	______________	______________________________
11	______________	______________________________

Chart Note Transcription

The chart note below contains 10 phrases that can be reworded with a medical term that you learned in this chapter. Each phrase is identified with an underline. Determine the medical term and write your answers in the spaces provided.

Current Complaint:	A 64-year-old female with an <u>open sore</u> (1) on her right leg is seen by the <u>specialist in treating diseases of the skin.</u> (2)
Past History:	Patient states she first noticed an area of pain, <u>severe itching,</u> (3) and <u>redness of the skin</u> (4) just below her right knee about 6 weeks ago. One week later <u>raised spots containing pus</u> (5) appeared. Patient states the raised spots containing pus ruptured and the open sore appeared.
Signs and Symptoms:	Patient has a deep open sore 5 × 3 cm: It is 4 cm distal to the knee on the lateral aspect of the right leg. It appears to extend into the <u>middle skin layer,</u> (6) and the edges show signs of <u>tissue death.</u> (7) The open sore has a small amount of drainage but there is no odor. A <u>sample of the drainage that was grown in the lab to identify the microorganism and determine the best antibiotic</u> (8) of the drainage revealed *Staphylococcus* bacteria in the open sore.
Diagnosis:	<u>Inflammation of connective tissue in the skin.</u> (9)
Treatment:	<u>Removal of damaged tissue</u> (10) of the open sore followed by application of an antibiotic cream. Patient was instructed to return to the skin disease specialist's office in 2 weeks, or sooner if the open sore does not heal, or if it begins draining pus.

(1) ______________________________

(2) ______________________________

(3) ______________________________

(4) ______________________________

(5) ______________________________

(6) ______________________________

(7) ______________________________

(8) ______________________________

(9) ______________________________

(10) ______________________________

Case Study

Below is a case study presentation of a patient with a condition discussed in this chapter. Read the case study and answer the questions below. Some questions will ask for information not included within this chapter. Use your text, a medical dictionary, or any other reference material you choose to answer these questions.

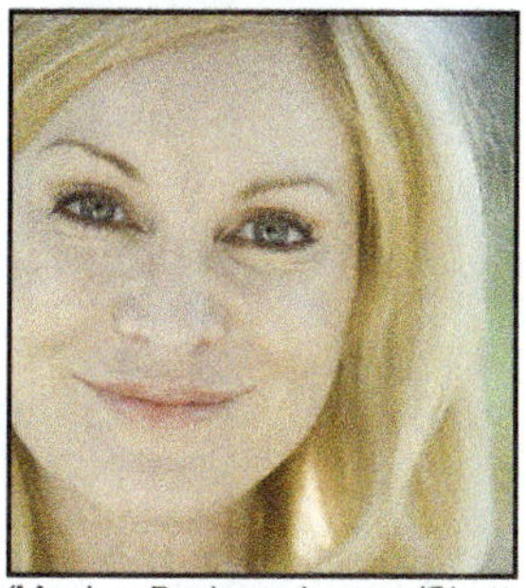
(Monkey Business Images/Shutterstock)

A 40-year-old female is seen in the dermatologist's office, upon the recommendation of her internist, for a workup for suspected SLE. Her presenting symptoms include erythema rash across her cheeks and nose, photosensitivity resulting in raised rash in sun-exposed areas, patches of alopecia, and pain and stiffness in her joints. The dermatologist examines the patient and orders exfoliative cytology and fungal scrapings to rule out other sources of the rash. Her internist had already placed the patient on oral anti-inflammatory medication for joint pain. The dermatologist orders corticosteroid cream for the rash. The patient is advised to use a sunscreen and make a follow-up appointment for results of the biopsy.

1. What pathological condition does the internist think this patient might have? Look this condition up in a reference source, and include a short description of it. SLE is an autoimmune disease. Use a reference source to look up the name of another autoimmune disease.

____

____

2. List and define each of the patient's presenting symptoms in your own words.

____

____

3. What diagnostic tests did the dermatologist perform? Describe it in your own words. Why were they important in helping the dermatologist make a diagnosis?

____

____

4. Each physician initiated a treatment. Describe them in your own words.

____

____

5. What do you think the term "workup" means?

____

____

Practice Exercises

A. Complete the Statement

1. The three layers of skin in order starting with the most superficial layer are ______________________,

______________________, and ______________________.

2. The ______________________ layer is the only living layer of the epidermis.

3. The subcutaneous layer of skin is composed primarily of ______________________.

4. Sensory receptors are located in the ______________________ layer of skin.

5. Nails and hair are composed of a hard protein called ______________________.

6. ______________________ is the pigment that gives skin its color.

7. Another name for the dermis is ______________________.

8. The nail body is connected to underlying tissue by the ______________________.

9. ______________________ glands release their product directly into hair follicles while ______________________ glands release their product into a duct.

10. ______________________ glands are sweat glands found in the underarm and pubic areas.

B. Define the Combining Form

	Definition	Example from Chapter
1. **cry/o**	______________________	______________________
2. **cutane/o**	______________________	______________________
3. **diaphor/o**	______________________	______________________
4. **py/o**	______________________	______________________
5. **cyan/o**	______________________	______________________
6. **ungu/o**	______________________	______________________
7. **lip/o**	______________________	______________________
8. **hidr/o**	______________________	______________________
9. **rhytid/o**	______________________	______________________
10. **seb/o**	______________________	______________________
11. **trich/o**	______________________	______________________
12. **necr/o**	______________________	______________________

C. Describe the Type of Burn

1. first degree ____
2. second degree ____
3. third degree ____

D. Terminology Matching

Match each term to its definition.

1. ________ eczema	a. decubitus ulcer
2. ________ nevus	b. lack of skin pigment
3. ________ lipoma	c. acne commonly seen in adults
4. ________ urticaria	d. hardened skin
5. ________ bedsore	e. redness, vesicles, itching, crusts
6. ________ acne rosacea	f. birthmark
7. ________ acne vulgaris	g. excessive hair growth
8. ________ hirsutism	h. caused by deficient blood supply
9. ________ alopecia	i. fatty tumor
10. ________ gangrene	j. hives
11. ________ scleroderma	k. baldness
12. ________ albinism	l. acne of adolescence

E. Define the Term

1. macule ____
2. papule ____
3. cyst ____
4. fissure ____
5. pustule ____
6. wheal ____
7. vesicle ____
8. ulcer ____
9. nodule ____
10. laceration ____

F. Combining Form Practice

The combining form **dermat/o** refers to the skin. Use it to write a term that means:

1. inflammation of the skin ______________________
2. any abnormal skin condition ______________________
3. an instrument for cutting the skin ______________________
4. specialist in skin ______________________
5. surgical repair of the skin ______________________
6. study of the skin ______________________

The combining form **melan/o** means black. Use it to write a term that means a:

7. black tumor ______________________
8. black cell ______________________

The suffix **-derma** means skin. Use it to write a term that means:

9. scaly skin ______________________
10. white skin ______________________
11. red skin ______________________

The combining form **onych/o** refers to the nail. Use it to write a term that means:

12. softening of the nails ______________________
13. infection around the nail ______________________
14. nail eating (biting) ______________________
15. removal of the nail ______________________

G. Procedure Matching

Match each procedure to its definition.

1.	_______ debridement	a.	surgical removal of wrinkled skin
2.	_______ cauterization	b.	instrument to cut thin slices of skin
3.	_______ chemabrasion	c.	removal of fat with suction
4.	_______ dermatoplasty	d.	use of extreme cold to destroy tissue
5.	_______ liposuction	e.	skin grafting
6.	_______ rhytidectomy	f.	removal of lesions with scraper
7.	_______ curettage	g.	removal of skin with brushes
8.	_______ dermabrasion	h.	removal of damaged skin
9.	_______ dermatome	i.	destruction of tissue with electric current
10.	_______ cryosurgery	j.	chemical peel

H. What's the Abbreviation?

1. frozen section ______________________
2. incision and drainage ______________________
3. intradermal ______________________
4. subcutaneous ______________________
5. ultraviolet ______________________
6. biopsy ______________________

I. What Does it Stand For?

1. C&S ______________________
2. BCC ______________________
3. derm ______________________
4. SG ______________________
5. decub ______________________
6. MM ______________________

J. Fill in the Blank

impetigo	tinea	keloid	exfoliative cytology	xeroderma
petechiae	frozen section	paronychia	scabies	Kaposi's sarcoma

1. The winter climates can cause dry skin. The medical term for this is ______________________.
2. Kim has experienced small pinpoint purplish spots caused by bleeding under the skin. This is called ______________________.
3. Janet has a fungal skin disease. This is called ______________________.
4. A contagious skin disease caused by a mite is ______________________.
5. An infection around the entire nail is called ______________________.
6. A form of skin cancer affecting AIDS patients is called ______________________.
7. Latrivia has a bacterial skin infection that results in pustules crusting and rupturing. It is called ______________________.
8. James's burn scar became a hypertrophic ______________________.
9. For a(n) ______________________ test, cells scraped off the skin are examined under a microscope.
10. During surgery a ______________________ was ordered for a rapid exam of tissue cut from a tumor.

K. Pharmacology Challenge

Fill in the classification for each drug description, then match the brand name.

	Drug Description	Classification		Brand Name
1.	________ kills fungi	____________________	a.	Kwell
2.	________ reduces severe itching	____________________	b.	Cortaid
3.	________ kills mites and lice	____________________	c.	Benadryl
4.	________ powerful anti-inflammatory	____________________	d.	Neosporin
5.	________ deadens pain	____________________	e.	Monistat
6.	________ kills bacteria	____________________	f.	Xylocaine

L. Liquid Conversion

Even after the United States became independent, the people continued to use the English system of measurement. This system had grown naturally for hundreds of years. People used familiar objects and parts of the body, such as "feet," as measuring devices. They measured liquid volume with common household items such as teaspoons, cups, and pails (the word "gallon" comes from an old name for a pail). Although this system could be quite confusing, it is still used in the United States today.

The metric system was developed in France during the French Revolution in the 1790s. The metric system has several advantages over the English system. The metric system was based on a decimal system, which made it much easier to do calculations. The scientific community adopted the metric system almost from its inception. It came to be used by most other nations of the world. The dual systems create problems for Americans.

Liquid measurement seems to be an incomprehensible whirl of drams, milliliters, cups, and tablespoons.

The situation is not helped by the fact that one cubic centimeter (cc) equals one milliliter (ml); they are the same.
Here's a conversion chart to help you out on the trickier volume conversions:

one teaspoon = 5 cc = 5 ml
one tablespoon (tbl) = three teaspoons
one tablespoon = 15 cc = 15 ml
one fluid ounce (U.S. liquid) = 30 cc = 30 ml = 2 tablespoons = 6 teaspoons
one cup = eight fluid ounces = 16 tablespoons
one pint = 2 cups = 16 fluid ounces

Actually, one teaspoon equals 4.928921594 milliliters, but the chart has rounded it off to make things easier. Similarly, one fluid ounce (U.S.) equals 29.573529562 milliliters. Believe it or not, it actually makes a difference. At some point, "rounding off" errors would become serious. However, for the problems below, you can use the easier equivalents.

Example 1

Billy must drink 2,250 cc of water each day. How many pints of water will he drink? Round to the nearest tenth of a pint.
1 pint = 16 oz.
1 oz = 30 cc
16 oz × 30 cc = 480 cc
2,250 cc divided by 480 cc = 4.688 pints
4.7 pints

Example 2

Convert 55 tbsp into an equal volume of cups. Round to the nearest tenth of a cup.
1 cup = 6 tbs
55 divided by 6 = 9.167 cups
9.2 cups

1. A dose of a specific medicine is 1 tbs. How many doses does an 8 oz bottle contain?
2. A bottle of juice contains 2 liters. If 1 liter equals 33.8 fl. oz, how many cc of juice are there in the 2-liter bottle?
3. The humidifier for the nursing station holds 14 pints of water.
   a. How many ounces will completely fill the reservoir?
   b. How many 8-oz bottles will be needed to fill the reservoir?
4. U.S. fluid ounces and British fluid ounces are not the same volume. One British fluid ounce equals only 28.41 milliliters. Why is this evidence that the metric system is easier to use than the English system of measurement?

Choose a level of accuracy appropriate to solve the problem when reporting quantities.

M. Online Learning for Professional Development

Many schools, state agencies, and private companies offer distance-learning courses in the health sciences. These courses are taught over the Internet. Offerings range from single classes that teach a particular skill, to entire programs, such as a Certificate of Leadership for Health Care Professionals. The programs are especially helpful to students who live in rural areas or in regions without access to a wide range of options in health science education.

Before you participate in any online learning program, make sure that the program you are interested in is offered by an accredited organization, so that your class work will be accepted by employers. The Web site of the United States Department of Education keeps a list of accredited institutions.

What might be one benefit and one difficulty of learning leadership skills through a distance-learning class?

N. Career Connection

Research professions related to the Integumentary System and report on the following:

1. Profession description to include job responsibilities
2. Educational requirements
3. Job opportunities
4. Opportunities outside of the hospital setting
5. Salary range
6. Licensure and continuing education requirements

Present your findings to your class.

Labeling Exercise

Image A

Write the labels for this figure on the numbered lines provided.

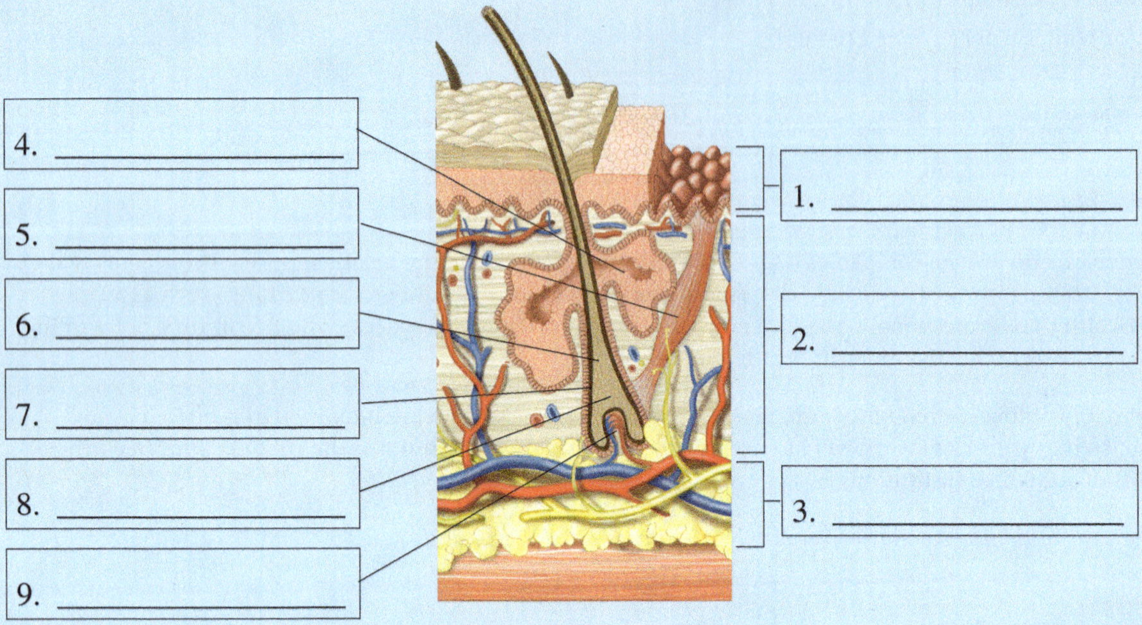

Image B

Write the labels for this figure on the numbered lines provided. companion website

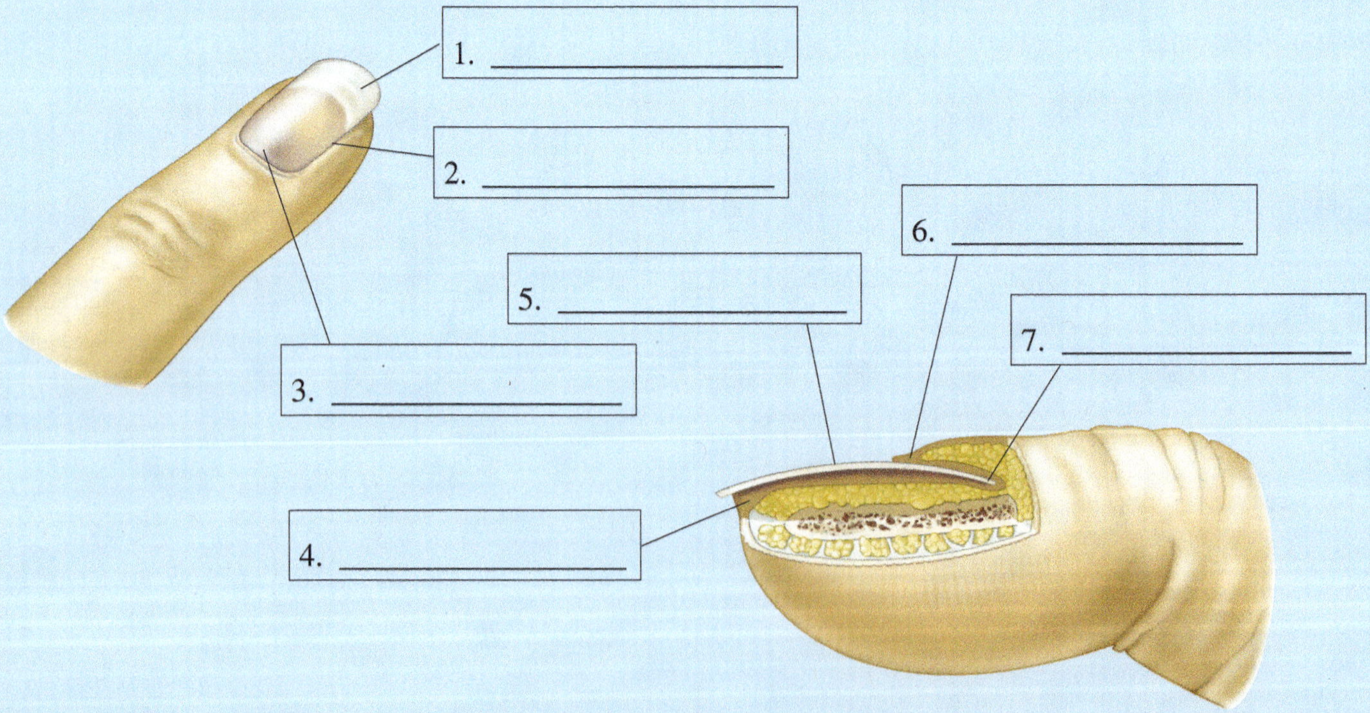

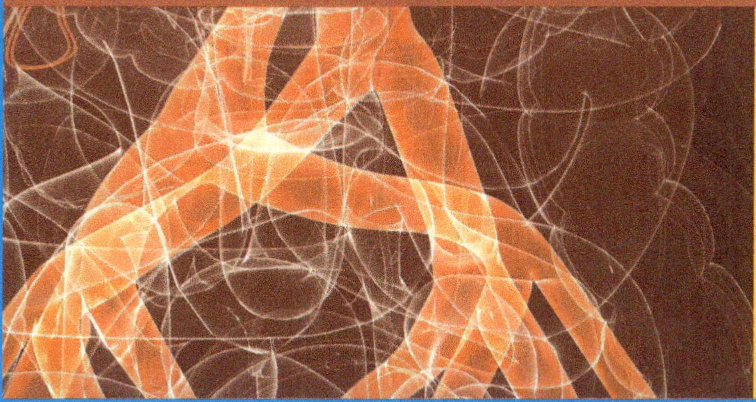

4

MUSCULOSKELETAL SYSTEM

Learning Objectives

Upon completion of this chapter, you will be able to

- Identify and define the combining forms, prefixes, and suffixes introduced in this chapter.
- Correctly spell and pronounce medical terms and major anatomical structures relating to the musculoskeletal system.
- Locate and describe the major organs of the musculoskeletal system and their functions.
- Correctly place bones in either the axial or the appendicular skeleton.
- List and describe the components of a long bone.
- Identify bony projections and depressions.
- Identify the parts of a synovial joint.
- Describe the characteristics of the three types of muscle tissue.
- Use movement terminology correctly.
- Identify and define musculoskeletal system anatomical terms.
- Identify and define selected musculoskeletal system pathology terms.
- Identify and define selected musculoskeletal system diagnostic procedures.
- Identify and define selected musculoskeletal system therapeutic procedures.
- Identify and define selected medications relating to the musculoskeletal system.
- Define selected abbreviations associated with the musculoskeletal system.

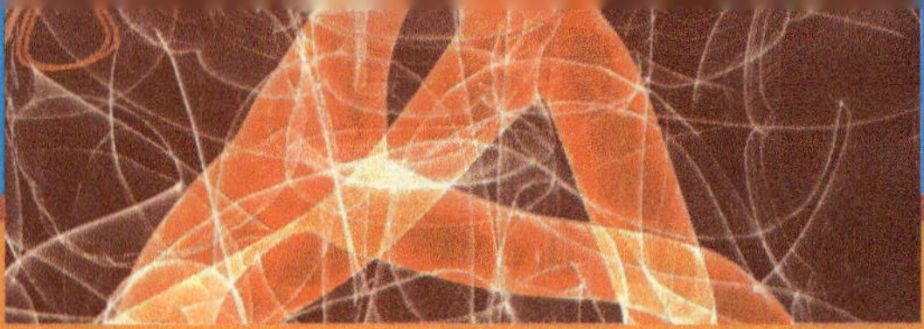

Section I: Skeletal System at a Glance

Function

The skeletal system consists of 206 bones that make up the internal framework of the body, called the skeleton. The skeleton supports the body, protects internal organs, serves as a point of attachment for skeletal muscles for body movement, produces blood cells, and stores minerals.

Structures

Here are the primary structures that comprise the skeletal system.

bones **joints**

Word Parts

Here are the most common word parts (with their meanings) used to build skeletal system terms. For a more comprehensive list, refer to the Terminology section of this chapter.

Combining Forms

Combining Form	Meaning
ankyl/o	stiff joint
arthr/o	joint
articul/o	joint
burs/o	sac
carp/o	wrist
cervic/o	neck
chondr/o	cartilage
clavicul/o	clavicle
coccyg/o	coccyx
cortic/o	outer portion
cost/o	rib
crani/o	skull
femor/o	femur
fibul/o	fibula
humer/o	humerus
ili/o	ilium
ischi/o	ischium
kyph/o	hump
lamin/o	lamina, part of vertebra
lord/o	bent backwards
lumb/o	low back, loin
mandibul/o	mandible
maxill/o	maxilla
medull/o	inner portion
metacarp/o	metacarpals
metatars/o	metatarsals
myel/o	bone marrow, spinal cord
orth/o	straight
oste/o	bone
patell/o	patella
ped/o	child, foot
pelv/o	pelvis
phalang/o	phalanges
pod/o	foot
prosthet/o	addition
pub/o	pubis
radi/o	radius, ray (X-ray)
sacr/o	sacrum
sarc/o	flesh (muscular substance)
scapul/o	scapula
scoli/o	crooked, bent
spin/o	spine
spondyl/o	vertebrae
stern/o	sternum
synovi/o	synovial membrane
synov/o	synovial membrane
tars/o	ankle
thorac/o	chest
tibi/o	tibia
uln/o	ulna
vertebr/o	vertebra

Suffixes

Suffix	Meaning
-blast	immature, embryonic
-clasia	to surgically break
-desis	stabilize, fuse
-listhesis	slipping
-porosis	porous

Skeletal System Illustrated

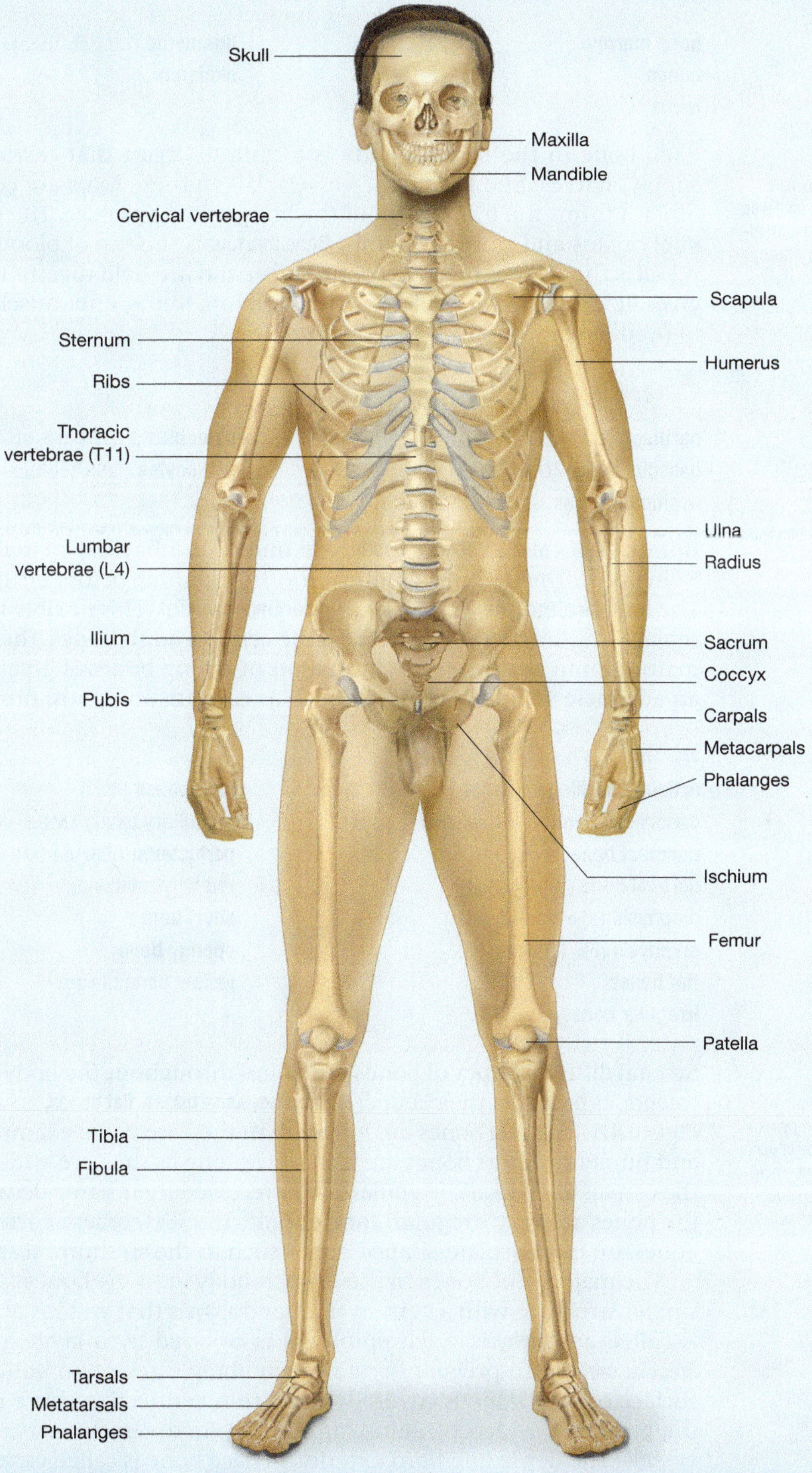

Anatomy and Physiology of the Skeletal System

bone marrow
bones
joints
ligaments (LIG-ah-ments)
skeleton

MED TERM TIP

The term *skeleton*, from the Greek word *skeltos* meaning "dried up," was originally used in reference to a dried-up mummified body, but over time came to be used for bones.

Each bone in the human body is a unique organ that carries its own blood supply, nerves, and lymphatic vessels. When these **bones** are connected to each other it forms the framework of the body called a **skeleton.** The skeleton protects vital organs and stores minerals. **Bone marrow** is the site of blood cell production. A **joint** is the place where two bones meet and are held together by **ligaments.** This gives flexibility to the skeleton. The skeleton, joints, and muscles work together to produce movement.

Bones

cartilage (CAR-tih-lij)
osseous tissue (OSS-ee-us)
ossification (oss-sih-fih-KAY-shun)
osteoblasts (OSS-tee-oh-blasts)
osteocytes (OSS-tee-oh-sights)

Bones, also called **osseous tissue,** are one of the hardest materials in the body. Bones are formed from a gradual process beginning before birth called **ossification.** The fetal skeleton is formed from a **cartilage** model. This flexible tissue is gradually replaced by **osteoblasts,** immature bone cells. In adult bones, the osteoblasts have matured into **osteocytes.** The formation of strong bones is greatly dependent on an adequate supply of minerals such as calcium and phosphorus.

Bone Structure

articular cartilage (ar-TIK-yoo-lar)
cancellous bone (CAN-sell-us)
compact bone
cortical bone (KOR-ti-kal)
diaphysis (dye-AFF-ih-sis)
epiphysis (eh-PIFF-ih-sis)
flat bones
irregular bones
long bones
medullary cavity (MED-you-lair-ee)
periosteum (pair-ee-AH-stee-um)
red bone marrow
short bones
spongy bone
yellow bone marrow

MED TERM TIP

Do not confuse a long bone with a large bone. A long bone is not necessarily a large bone. The bones of your fingers are short in length, but since they are longer than they are wide, they are classified as long bones.

Several different types of bones are found throughout the body and fall into four categories based on their shape: **long bones, short bones, flat bones,** and **irregular bones** (see Figure 4.1 ■). Long bones are longer than they are wide; examples are the femur and humerus. Short bones are roughly as long as they are wide; examples being the carpals and tarsals. Irregular bones received their name because the shapes of the bones are very irregular; for example, the vertebrae are irregular bones. Flat bones are usually plate-shaped bones such as the sternum, scapulae, and pelvis.

The majority of bones in the human body are long bones. These bones have similar structure with a central shaft or **diaphysis** that widens at each end, which is called an **epiphysis.** Each epiphysis is covered by a layer of cartilage called **articular cartilage** to prevent bone from rubbing directly on bone. The remaining surface of each bone is covered with a thin connective tissue membrane called the **periosteum,** which contains numerous blood vessels, nerves, and lymphatic vessels. The dense and hard exterior surface bone is called **cortical** or **compact bone. Cancellous** or **spongy bone** is found inside the bone. As its name indicates, spongy

MED TERM TIP

The term *diaphysis* comes from the Greek term meaning "to grow between."

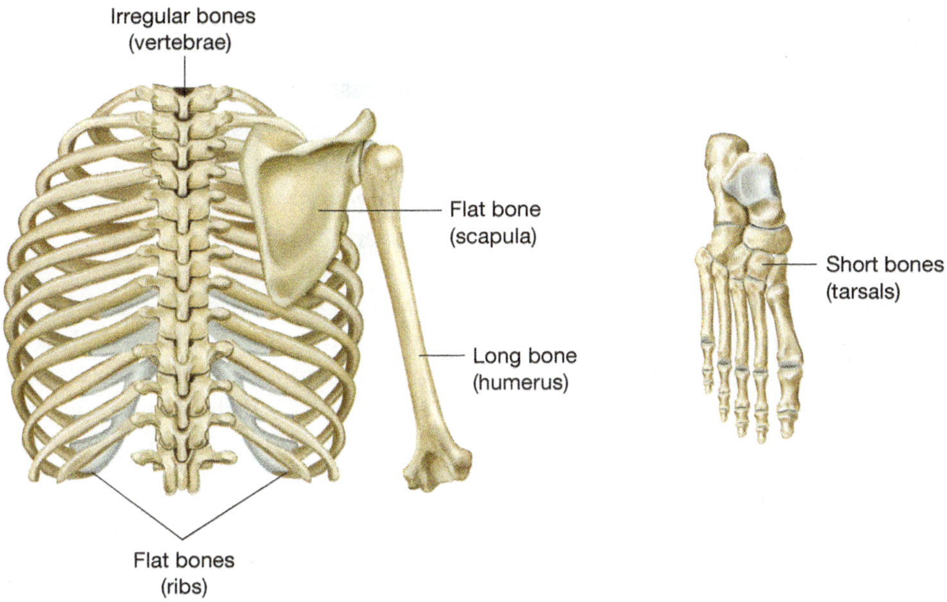

■ **Figure 4.1** Classification of bones by shape.

bone has spaces in it, giving it a spongelike appearance. These spaces contain **red bone marrow,** which manufactures most of the blood cells and is found in some parts of all bones.

The center of the diaphysis contains an open canal called the **medullary cavity.** Early in life this cavity also contains red bone marrow, but as we age the red bone marrow of the medullary cavity gradually converts to **yellow bone marrow,** which consists primarily of fat cells. Figure 4.2 ■ contains an illustration of the structure of long bones.

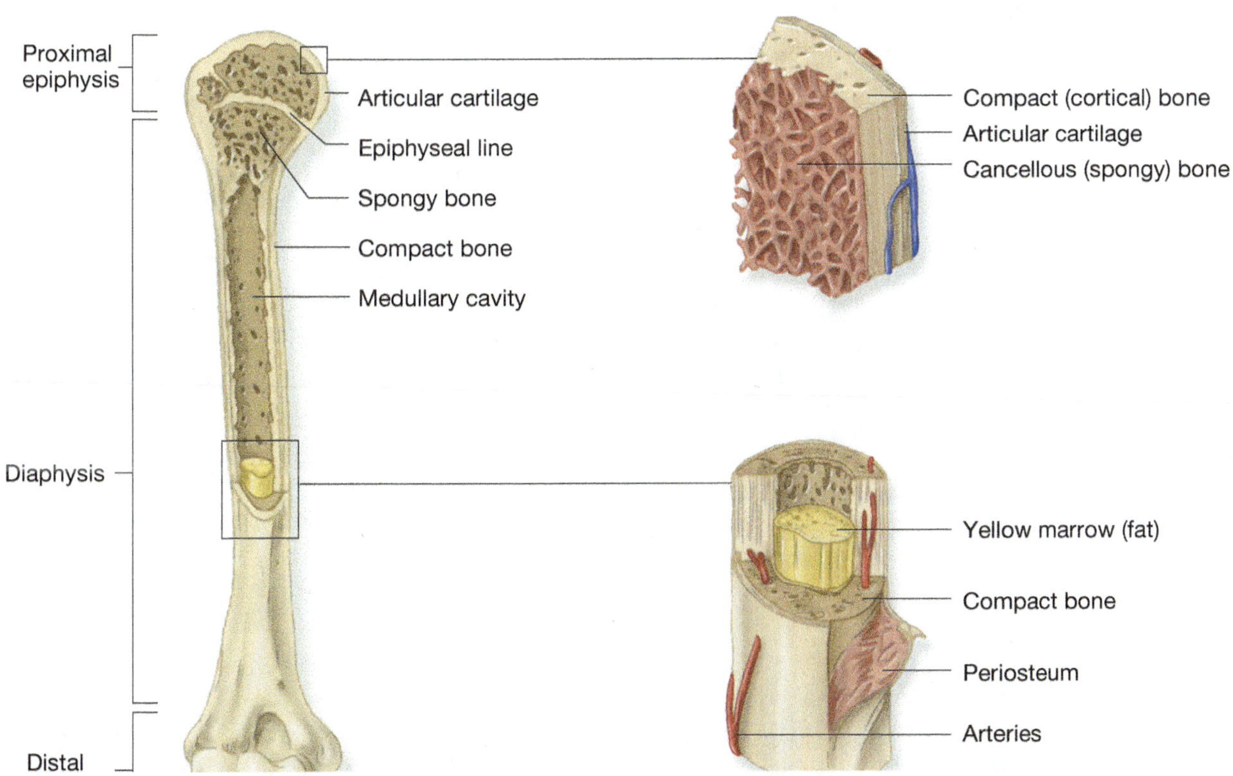

■ **Figure 4.2** Components of a long bone. The entire long bone is on the left side accompanied by a blowup of the proximal epiphysis and a section of the diaphysis.

Bone Projections and Depressions

condyle (KON-dile)
epicondyle (ep-ih-KON-dile)
fissure (FISH-er)
foramen (for-AY-men)
fossa (FOSS-ah)
head
neck
process
sinus (SIGH-nus)
trochanter (tro-KAN-ter)
tubercle (TOO-ber-kl)
tuberosity (too-ber-OSS-ih-tee)

MED TERM TIP

The elbow, commonly referred to as the *funny bone,* is actually a projection of the ulna called the olecranon process.

Bones have many projections and depressions; some are rounded and smooth in order to articulate with another bone in a joint. Others are rough to provide muscles with attachment points. The general term for any bony projection is a **process.** Then there are specific terms to describe the different shapes and locations of various processes. These terms are commonly used on operative reports and in physicians' records for clear identification of areas on the individual bones. Some of the common bony processes include the following:

1. The **head** is a large, smooth, ball-shaped end on a long bone. It may be separated from the body or shaft of the bone by a narrow area called the **neck.**
2. A **condyle** refers to a smooth, rounded portion at the end of a bone.
3. The **epicondyle** is a projection located above or on a condyle.
4. The **trochanter** refers to a large rough process for the attachment of a muscle.
5. A **tubercle** is a small, rough process that provides the attachment for tendons and muscles.
6. The **tuberosity** is a large, rough process that provides the attachment of tendons and muscles.

See Figure 4.3 ■ for an illustration of the processes found on the femur.

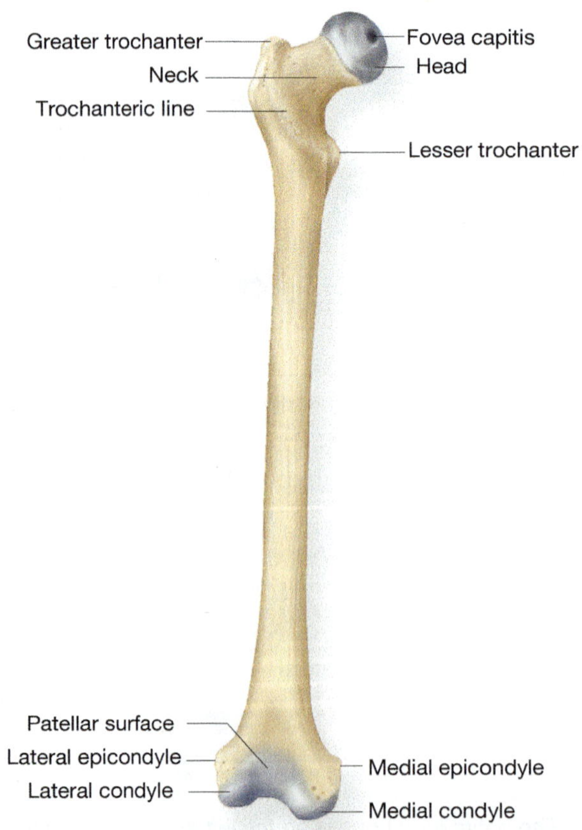

■ **Figure 4.3** Bony processes found on the femur.

Additionally, bones have hollow regions or depressions. The most common are the:

1. **Sinus** is a hollow cavity within a bone.
2. **Foramen** is a smooth, round opening for nerves and blood vessels.
3. **Fossa** consists of a shallow cavity or depression on the surface of a bone.
4. **Fissure** is a slit-type opening.

Skeleton

appendicular skeleton (app-en-DIK-yoo-lar)
axial skeleton (AK-see-al)

The human skeleton has two divisions: the **axial skeleton** and the **appendicular skeleton.** Figures 4.4 and 4.8 illustrate the axial and appendicular skeletons.

MED TERM TIP

Newborn infants have about 300 bones at birth that will fuse into 206 bones as an adult.

Axial Skeleton

cervical vertebrae
coccyx (COCK-six)
cranium (KRAY-nee-um)
ethmoid bone (ETH-moyd)
facial bones
frontal bone
hyoid bone (HIGH-oyd)
intervertebral disc (in-ter-VER-teh-bral)
lacrimal bone (LACK-rim-al)
lumbar vertebrae
mandible (MAN-dih-bl)
maxilla (mack-SIH-lah)
nasal bone
occipital bone (ock-SIP-eh-tal)
palatine bone (PAL-ah-tine)
parietal bone (pah-RYE-eh-tal)
rib cage
sacrum (SAY-crum)
sphenoid bone (SFEE-noyd)
sternum (STER-num)
temporal bone (TEM-por-al)
thoracic vertebrae
vertebral column (VER-teh-bral)
vomer bone (VOH-mer)
zygomatic bone (zeye-go-MAT-ik)

The axial skeleton includes the bones of the head, neck, spine, chest, and trunk of the body (see Figure 4.4 ■). These bones form the central axis for the whole body and protect many of the internal organs such as the brain, lungs, and heart.

The head or skull is divided into two parts consisting of the **cranium** and **facial bones.** These bones surround and protect the brain, eyes, ears, nasal cavity, and oral cavity from injury. The muscles for chewing and moving the head are attached to the cranial bones. The cranium encases the brain and consists of the **frontal, parietal, temporal, ethmoid, sphenoid,** and **occipital bones.** The facial bones surround the mouth, nose, and eyes and include the **mandible, maxilla, zygomatic, vomer, palatine, nasal,** and **lacrimal bones.** The cranial and facial bones are illustrated in Figure 4.5 ■ and described in Table 4.1 ■.

The **hyoid bone** is a single U-shaped bone suspended in the neck between the mandible and larynx. It is a point of attachment for swallowing and speech muscles.

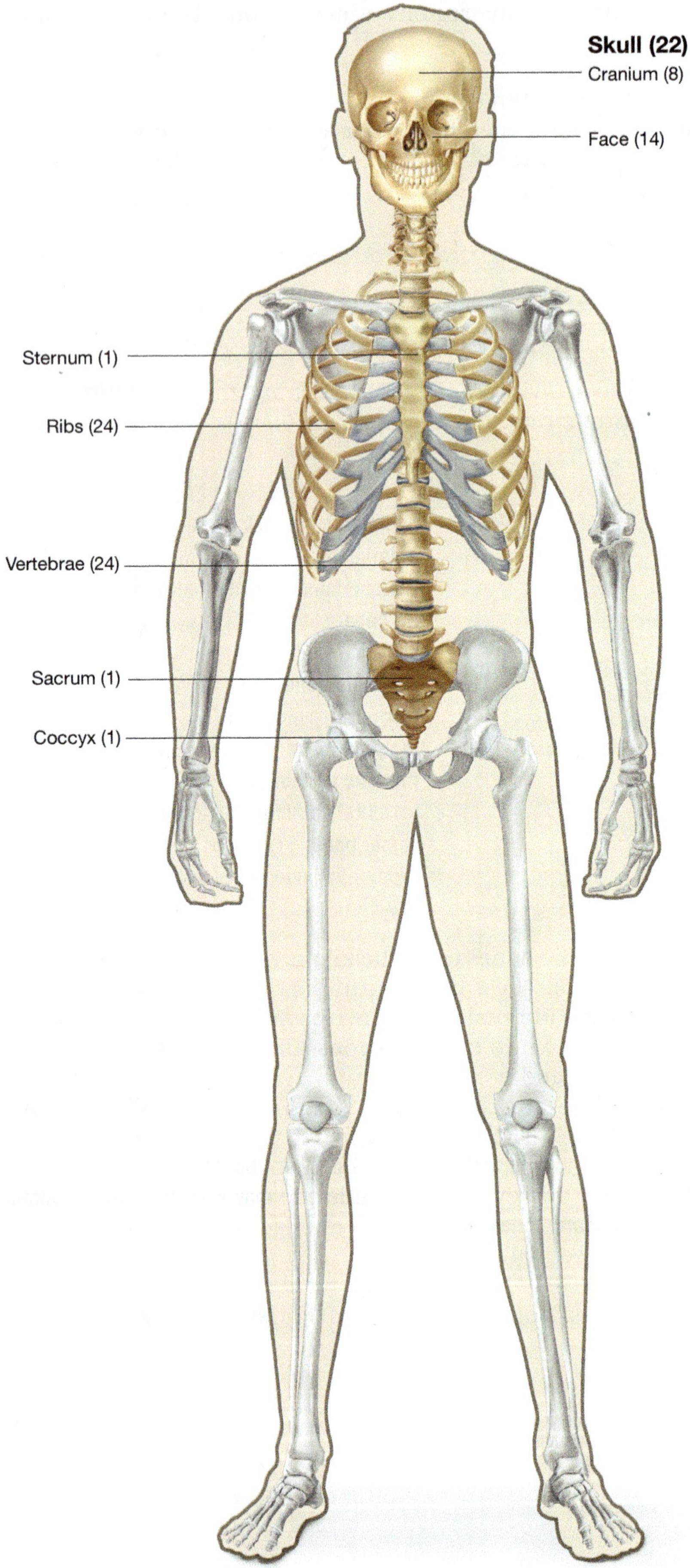

Figure 4.4 Bones of the axial skeleton.

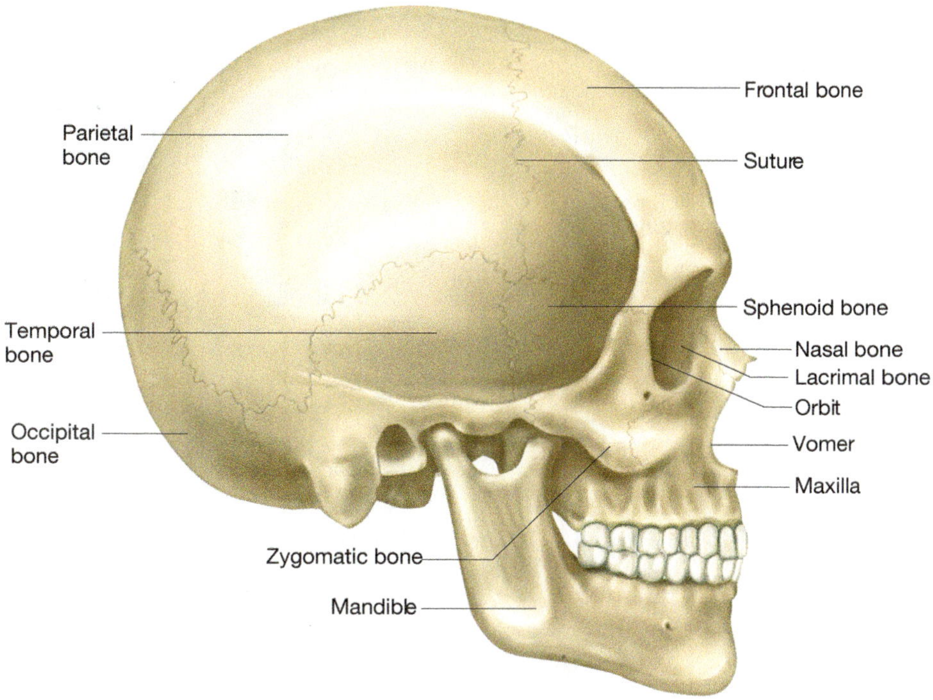

Figure 4.5 Bones of the skull.

Table 4.1 Bones of the Skull

NAME	NUMBER	DESCRIPTION
Cranial Bones		
Frontal bone	1	Forehead
Parietal bone	2	Upper sides of cranium and roof of skull
Occipital bone	1	Back and base of skull
Temporal bone	2	Sides and base of cranium
Sphenoid bone	1	Bat-shaped bone that forms part of the base of the skull, floor, and sides of eye orbit
Ethmoid bone	1	Forms part of eye orbit, nose, and floor of cranium
Facial Bones		
Lacrimal bone	2	Inner corner of each eye
Nasal bone	2	Form part of nasal septum and support bridge of nose
Maxilla	1	Upper jaw
Mandible	1	Lower jawbone; only movable bone of the skull
Zygomatic bone	2	Cheekbones
Vomer bone	1	Base of nasal septum
Palatine bone	1	Hard palate (PAH lat) roof of oral cavity and floor of nasal cavity

The trunk of the body consists of the **vertebral column, sternum,** and **rib cage.** The vertebral or spinal column is divided into five sections: **cervical vertebrae, thoracic vertebrae, lumbar vertebrae, sacrum,** and **coccyx** (see Figure 4.6 ■ and Table 4.2 ■). Located between each pair of vertebrae, from the cervical through the lumbar regions, is an **intervertebral disc.** Each disc is composed of fibrocartilage to provide a cushion between the vertebrae. The rib cage has twelve pairs of ribs attached at the back to the vertebral column. Ten of the pairs are also attached to the sternum in the front (see Figure 4.7 ■). The lowest two pairs are called *floating ribs* and are attached only to the vertebral column. The rib cage serves to provide support for organs, such as the heart and lungs.

MED TERM TIP

The term *coccyx* comes from the Greek word for the cuckoo because the shape of these small bones extending off the sacrum resembles this bird's bill.

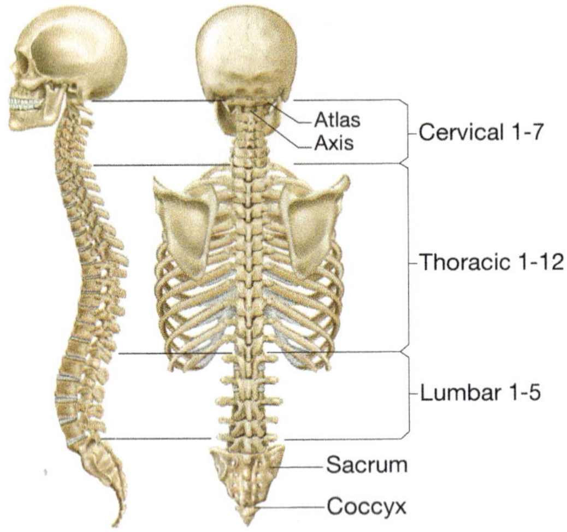

■ **Figure 4.6** Divisions of the vertebral column.

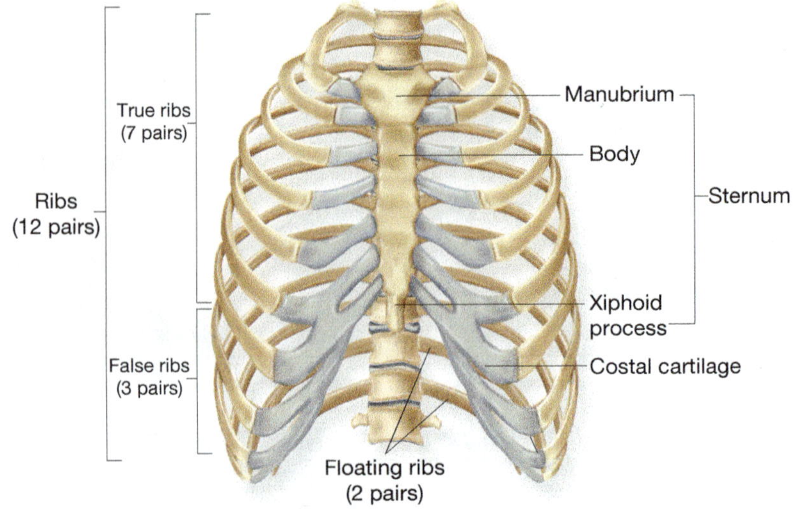

■ **Figure 4.7** The structure of the rib cage.

Table 4.2 Bones of the Vertebral/Spinal Column

NAME	NUMBER	DESCRIPTION
Cervical vertebra	7	Vertebrae in the neck region
Thoracic vertebra	12	Vertebrae in the chest region with ribs attached
Lumbar vertebra	5	Vertebrae in the small of the back, about waist level
Sacrum	1	Five vertebrae that become fused into one triangular-shaped flat bone at the base of the vertebral column
Coccyx	1	Three to five very small vertebrae attached to the sacrum, often become fused

Appendicular Skeleton

carpals (CAR-pals)
clavicle (CLAV-ih-kl)
femur (FEE-mer)
fibula (FIB-yoo-lah)
humerus (HYOO-mer-us)
ilium (ILL-ee-um)
innominate bone (ih-NOM-ih-nayt)
ischium (ISS-kee-um)
lower extremities
metacarpals (met-ah-CAR-pals)
metatarsals (met-ah-TAHR-sals)
os coxae (OSS / KOK-sigh)
patella (pah-TELL-ah)
pectoral girdle
pelvic girdle
phalanges (fah-LAN-jeez)
pubis (PYOO-bis)
radius (RAY-dee-us)
scapula (SKAP-yoo-lah)
tarsals (TAHR-sals)
tibia (TIB-ee-ah)
ulna (UHL-nah)
upper extremities

MED TERM TIP

The term *girdle*, meaning something that encircles or confines, refers to the entire bony structure of the shoulder and the pelvis. If just one bone from these areas is being discussed, like the ilium of the pelvis, it would be named as such. If, however, the entire pelvis is being discussed, it would be called the pelvic girdle.

The appendicular skeleton consists of the **pectoral girdle, upper extremities, pelvic girdle,** and **lower extremities** (see Figure 4.8 ■). These are the bones for our appendages or limbs and along with the muscles attached to them, they are responsible for body movement.

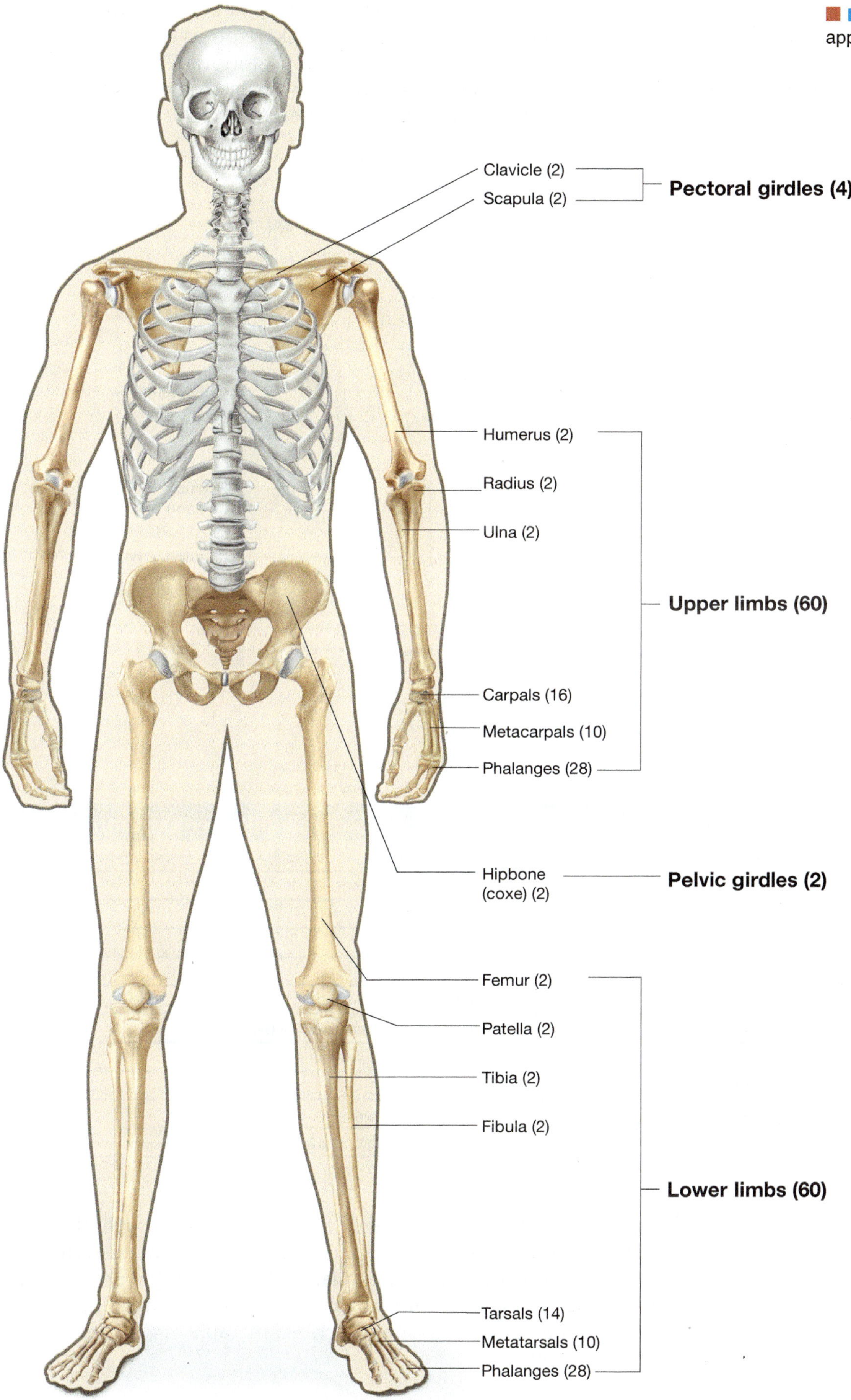

Figure 4.8 Bones of the appendicular skeleton.

The pectoral girdle consists of the **clavicle** and **scapula** bones. It functions to attach the upper extremity, or arm, to the axial skeleton by articulating with the sternum anteriorly and the vertebral column posteriorly. The bones of the upper extremity include the **humerus, ulna, radius, carpals, metacarpals,** and **phalanges.** These bones are illustrated in Figure 4.9 ■ and described in Table 4.3 ■.

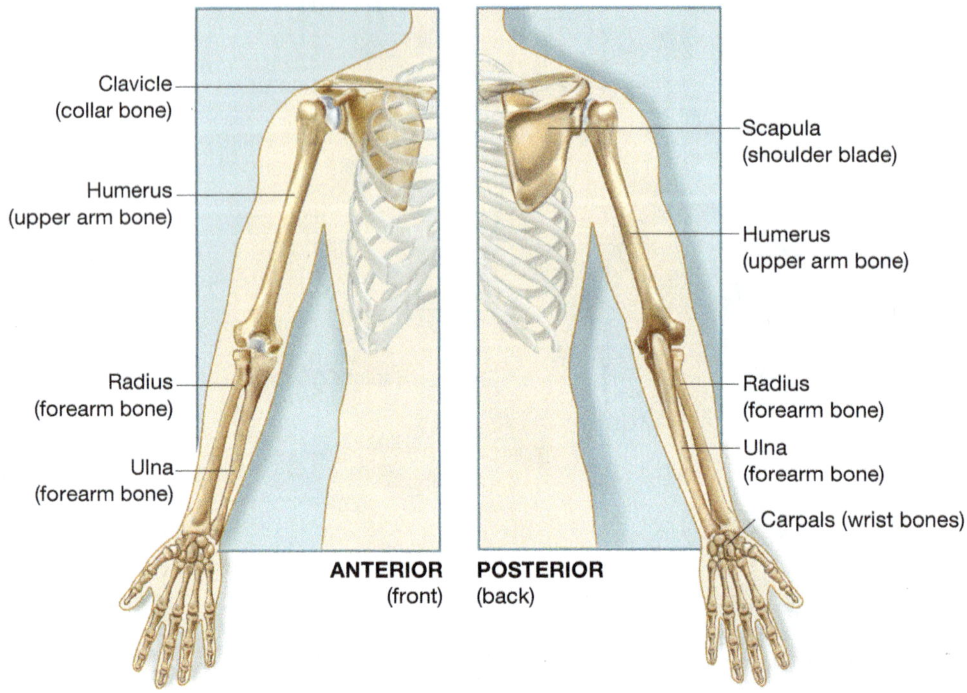

■ **Figure 4.9** Anatomical and common names for the pectoral girdle and upper extremity.

Table 4.3 Bones of the Pectoral Girdle and Upper Extremity

NAME	NUMBER	DESCRIPTION
Pectoral Girdle		
Clavicle	2	Collar bone
Scapula	2	Shoulder blade
Upper Extremity		
Humerus	2	Upper arm bone
Radius	2	Forearm bone on thumb side of lower arm
Ulna	2	Forearm bone on little finger side of lower arm
Carpals	16	Bones of wrist
Metacarpals	10	Bones in palm of hand
Phalanges	28	Finger bones; three in each finger and two in each thumb

The pelvic girdle is called the **os coxae** or the **innominate bone** or hipbone. It contains the **ilium, ischium,** and **pubis.** It articulates with the sacrum posteriorly to attach the lower extremity, or leg, to the axial skeleton. The lower extremity bones include the **femur, patella, tibia, fibula, tarsals, metatarsals,** and phalanges. These bones are illustrated in Figure 4.10 ■ and described in Table 4.4 ■.

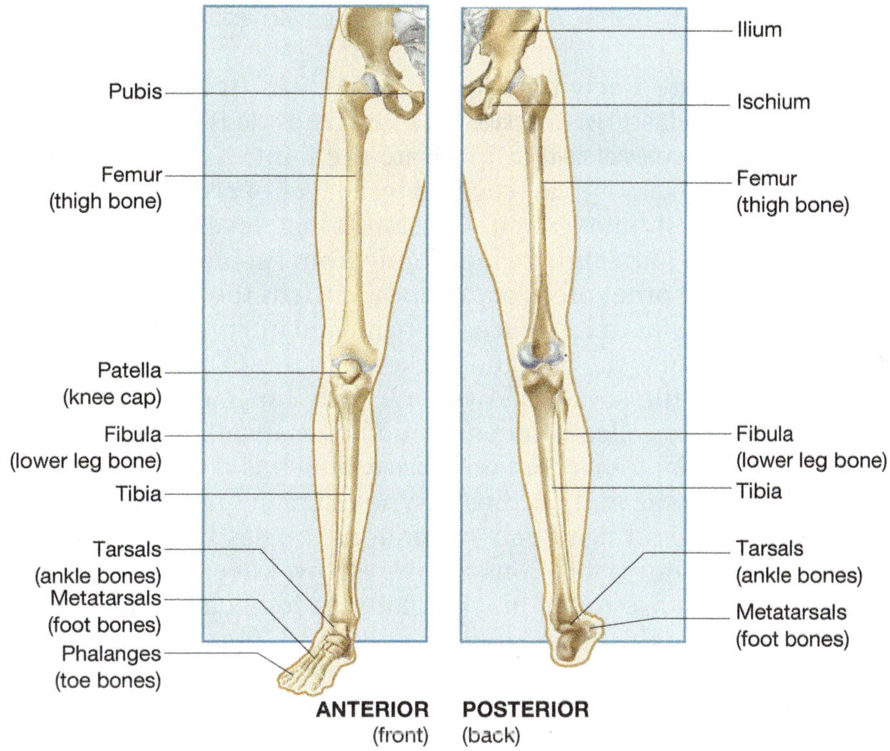

Figure 4.10 Anatomical and common names for the pelvic girdle and lower extremity.

Table 4.4 Bones of the Pelvic Girdle and Lower Extremity

NAME	NUMBER	DESCRIPTION
Pelvic Girdle/Os Coxae		
Ilium	2	Part of the hipbone
Ischium	2	Part of the hipbone
Pubis	2	Part of the hipbone
Lower Extremity		
Femur	2	Upper leg bone; thigh bone
Patella	2	Knee cap
Tibia	2	Shin bone; thicker lower leg bone
Fibula	2	Thinner, long bone in lateral side of lower leg
Tarsals	14	Ankle and heel bones
Metatarsals	10	Forefoot bones
Phalanges	28	Toe bones; three in each toe and two in each great toe

Joints

articulation (ar-tik-yoo-LAY-shun)
bursa (BER-sah)
cartilaginous joints (car-tih-LAJ-ih-nus)
fibrous joints (FYE-bruss)
joint capsule
synovial fluid
synovial joint (sin-OH-vee-al)
synovial membrane

Joints are formed when two or more bones meet. This is also referred to as an **articulation.** There are three types of joints based on the amount of movement allowed between the bones: **synovial joints, cartilaginous joints,** and **fibrous joints** (see Figure 4.11 ■).

Most joints are freely moving synovial joints (see Figure 4.12 ■), which are enclosed by an elastic **joint capsule.** The joint capsule is lined with **synovial membrane,** which secretes **synovial fluid** to lubricate the joint. As noted earlier, the ends of bones in a synovial joint are covered by a layer of articular cartilage. Cartilage is very tough, but still flexible. It withstands high levels of stress to act as a shock absorber for the joint and prevents bone from rubbing against bone. Cartilage is found in several other areas of the body, such as the nasal septum, external ear, eustachian tube, larynx, trachea, bronchi, and intervertebral disks. One example of a synovial joint is the ball-and-socket joint found at the shoulder and hip. The ball rotating in the socket allows for a wide range of motion. Bands of strong connective tissue called ligaments bind bones together at the joint.

Some synovial joints contain a **bursa,** which is a saclike structure composed of connective tissue and lined with synovial membrane. Most commonly found between bones and ligaments or tendons, bursas function to reduce friction. Some common bursa locations are the elbow, knee, and shoulder joints.

Not all joints are freely moving. Fibrous joints allow almost no movement since the ends of the bones are joined by thick fibrous tissue, which may even fuse into solid bone. The sutures of the skull are an example of a fibrous joint. Cartilaginous joints allow for slight movement but hold bones firmly in place by a solid piece of cartilage. An example of this type of joint is the pubic symphysis, the point at which the left and right pubic bones meet in the front of the lower abdomen.

MED TERM TIP

Bursitis is an inflammation of the bursa located between bony prominences such as at the shoulder. Housemaid's knee, a term thought to have originated from the damage to the knees that occurred when maids knelt to scrub floors, is a form of bursitis and carries the medical name *prepatellar bursitis.*

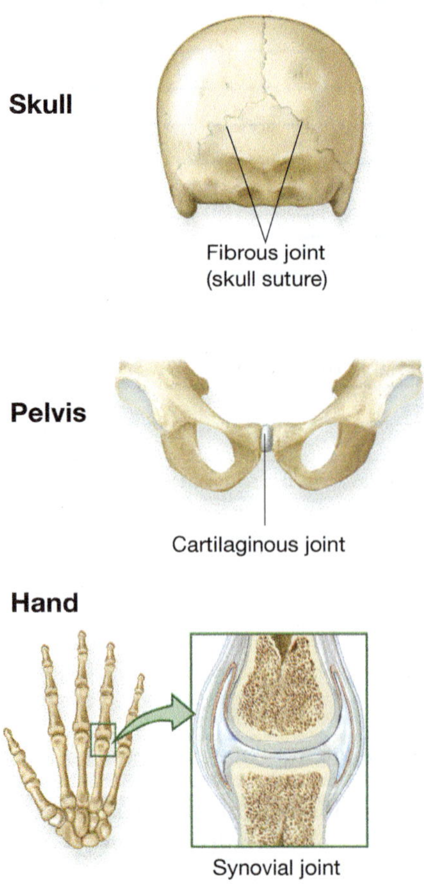

■ **Figure 4.11** Examples of three types of joints found in the body.

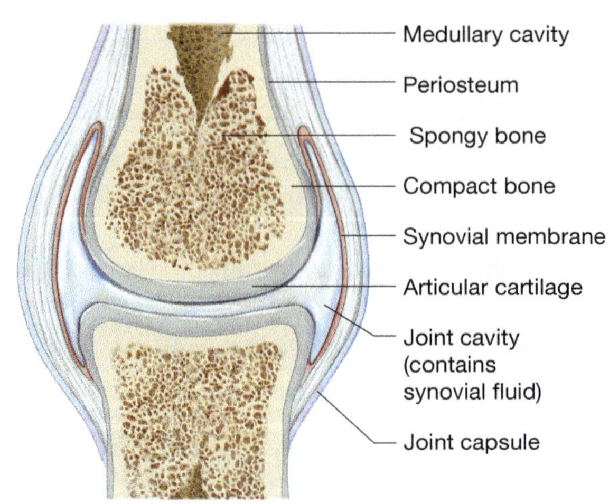

■ **Figure 4.12** Structure of a generalized synovial joint.

Terminology

Word Parts Used to Build Skeletal System Terms

The following lists contain the combining forms, suffixes, and prefixes used to build terms in the remaining sections of this chapter.

Combining Forms

ankyl/o	stiff joint
arthr/o	joint
articul/o	joint
burs/o	bursa
carp/o	carpus
cervic/o	neck
chondr/o	cartilage
clavicul/o	clavicle
coccyg/o	coccyx
cortic/o	outer portion
cost/o	rib
crani/o	skull
cutane/o	skin
erythr/o	red
femor/o	femur
fibul/o	fibula
humer/o	humerus
ili/o	ilium
ischi/o	ischium

kyph/o	hump
lamin/o	lamina, part of vertebra
lord/o	bent backwards
lumb/o	low back
mandibul/o	mandible
maxill/o	maxilla
medull/o	inner portion
metacarp/o	metacarpus
metatars/o	metatarsus
myel/o	bone marrow
orth/o	straight
oste/o	bone
patell/o	patella
path/o	disease
ped/o	child, foot
pelv/o	pelvis
phalang/o	phalanges
pod/o	foot

prosthet/o	addition
pub/o	pubis
radi/o	radius, ray (X-ray)
sacr/o	sacrum
sarc/o	flesh
scapul/o	scapula
scoli/o	crooked, bent
spin/o	spine
spondyl/o	vertebra
stern/o	sternum
synovi/o	synovial membrane
synov/o	synovial membrane
system/o	system
tars/o	tarsus
thorac/o	thorax
tibi/o	tibia
uln/o	ulna
vertebr/o	vertebra

Suffixes

-ac	pertaining to
-al	pertaining to
-algia	pain
-ar	pertaining to
-ary	pertaining to
-centesis	puncture to withdraw fluid
-clasia	surgically break
-desis	fuse
-eal	pertaining to
-ectomy	surgical removal
-genic	producing

-gram	record
-graphy	process of recording
-iatry	medical treatment
-ic	pertaining to
-itis	inflammation
-listhesis	slipping
-logy	study
-malacia	softening
-metry	process of measuring
-oma	tumor
-ory	pertaining to
-osis	abnormal condition

-otomy	cutting into
-ous	pertaining to
-pathy	disease
-plasty	surgical repair
-porosis	porous
-scope	instrument for viewing
-scopy	process of visually examining
-stenosis	narrowing
-tic	pertaining to
-tome	instrument used to cut

Prefixes

anti-	against
bi-	two
ex-	external, outward
inter-	between
intra-	inside
per-	through
sub-	below, under

Anatomical Terms

TERM	WORD PARTS	DEFINITION
articular (ar-TIK-yoo-lar)	articul/o = joint -ar = pertaining to	pertaining to a joint
carpal (CAR-pal)	carp/o = carpus -al = pertaining to	pertaining to the carpus
cervical (CER-vih-kal)	cervic/o = neck -al = pertaining to	pertaining to the neck
clavicular (cla-VIK-yoo-lar)	clavicul/o = clavicle -ar = pertaining to	pertaining to the clavicle
coccygeal (cock-eh-JEE-all)	coccyg/o = coccyx -eal = pertaining to	pertaining to the coccyx
cortical (KOR-ti-kal)	cortic/o = outer portion -al = petaining to	pertaining to the outer portion
costal (COAST-all)	cost/o = rib -al = pertaining to	pertaining to the rib
cranial (KRAY-nee-all)	crani/o = skull -al = pertaining to	pertaining to the skull
femoral (FEM-or-all)	femor/o = femur -al = pertaining to	pertaining to the femur
fibular (FIB-yoo-lar)	fibul/o = fibula -ar = pertaining to	pertaining to the fibula
humeral (HYOO-mer-all)	humer/o = humerus -al = pertaining to	pertaining to the humerus
iliac (ILL-ee-ack)	ili/o = ilium -ac = pertaining to	pertaining to the ilium
intervertebral (in-ter-VER-teh-bral)	inter- = between vertebr/o = vertebra -al = pertaining to	pertaining to between vertebrae
intracranial (in-trah-KRAY-nee-al)	intra- = inside crani/o = skull -al = pertaining to	pertaining to inside the skull
ischial (ISH-ee-all)	ischi/o = ischium -al = pertaining to	pertaining to the ischium
lumbar (LUM-bar)	lumb/o = low back -ar = pertaining to	pertaining to the low back
mandibular (man-DIB-yoo-lar)	mandibul/o = mandible -ar = pertaining to	pertaining to the mandible
maxillary (mack-sih-LAIR-ree)	maxill/o = maxilla -ary = pertaining to	pertaining to the maxilla

Anatomical Terms *(continued)*

TERM	WORD PARTS	DEFINITION
medullary (MED-you-lair-ee)	medull/o = inner portion -ary = pertaining to	pertaining to the inner portion
metacarpal (met-ah-CAR-pal)	metacarp/o = metacarpus -al = pertaining to	pertaining to the metacarpus
metatarsal (met-ah-TAHR-sal)	metatars/o = metatarsus -al = pertaining to	pertaining to the metatarsus
patellar (pa-TELL-ar)	patell/o = patella -ar = pertaining to	pertaining to the patella
pelvic (PEL-vik)	pelv/o = pelvis -ic = pertaining to	pertaining to the pelvis
phalangeal (fay-lan-JEE-all)	phalang/o = phalanges -eal = pertaining to	pertaining to the phalanges
pubic (PYOO-bik)	pub/o = pubis -ic = pertaining to	pertaining to the pubis
radial (RAY-dee-all)	radi/o = radius -al = pertaining to	pertaining to the radius
sacral (SAY-kral)	sacr/o = sacrum -al = pertaining to	pertaining to the sacrum
scapular (SKAP-yoo-lar)	scapul/o = scapula -ar = pertaining to	pertaining to the scapula
sternal (STER-nal)	stern/o = sternum -al = pertaining to	pertaining to the sternum
synovial (sin-OH-vee-al)	synovi/o = synovial membrane -al = pertaining to	pertaining to the synovial membrane
tarsal (TAHR-sal)	tars/o = tarsus -al = pertaining to	pertaining to the tarsus
thoracic (tho-RASS-ik)	thorac/o = thorax -ic = pertaining to	pertaining to the thorax
tibial (TIB-ee-all)	tibi/o = tibia -al = pertaining to	pertaining to the tibia
ulnar (UHL-nar)	uln/o = ulna -ar = pertaining to	pertaining to the ulna

Pathology

TERM	WORD PARTS	DEFINITION
Medical Specialties		
chiropractic (ki-roh-PRAK-tik)	-tic = pertaining to	Healthcare profession concerned with diagnosis and treatment of malalignment conditions of the spine and musculoskeletal system with the intention of affecting the nervous system and improving health. Healthcare professional is a *chiropractor.*

Pathology *(continued)*

TERM	WORD PARTS	DEFINITION
orthopedics (or-thoh-PEE-diks)	orth/o = straight ped/o = child, foot -ic = pertaining to	Branch of medicine specializing in the diagnosis and treatment of conditions of the musculoskeletal system; also called *orthopedic surgery.* Physician is an *orthopedist* or *orthopedic surgeon.* Name derived from straightening (*orth/o*) deformities in children (*ped/o*).
orthotics (or-THOT-iks)	orth/o = straight -tic = pertaining to	Healthcare profession specializing in making orthopedic appliances such as braces and splints. Person skilled in making and adjusting these appliances is an *orthotist.*
podiatry (po-DYE-ah-tree)	pod/o = foot -iatry = medical treatment	Healthcare profession specializing in diagnosis and treatment of disorders of the feet and lower legs. Healthcare professional is a *podiatrist.*
prosthetics (pross-THET-iks)	prosthet/o = addition -ic = pertaining to	Healthcare profession specializing in making artificial body parts. Person skilled in making and adjusting prostheses is a *prosthetist.*
Signs and Symptoms		
arthralgia (ar-THRAL-jee-ah)	arthr/o = joint -algia = pain	joint pain
bursitis (ber-SIGH-tis)	burs/o = bursa -itis = inflammation	inflammation of a bursa
callus (KAL-us)		The mass of bone tissue that forms at a fracture site during its healing.
chondromalacia (kon-droh-mah-LAY-she-ah)	chondr/o = cartilage -malacia = softening	softening of the cartilage
crepitation (krep-ih-TAY-shun)		The noise produced by bones or cartilage rubbing together in conditions such as arthritis. Also called *crepitus.*
ostealgia (oss-tee-AL-jee-ah)	oste/o = bone -algia = pain	bone pain
osteomyelitis (oss-tee-oh-mi-ell-EYE-tis)	oste/o = bone myel/o = bone marrow -itis = inflammation	inflammation of bone and bone marrow
synovitis (sih-no-VI-tis)	synov/o = synovial membrane -itis = inflammation	inflammation of synovial membrane
Fractures		
closed fracture		Fracture in which there is no open skin wound. Also called a *simple fracture.*

Pathology *(continued)*

TERM	WORD PARTS	DEFINITION

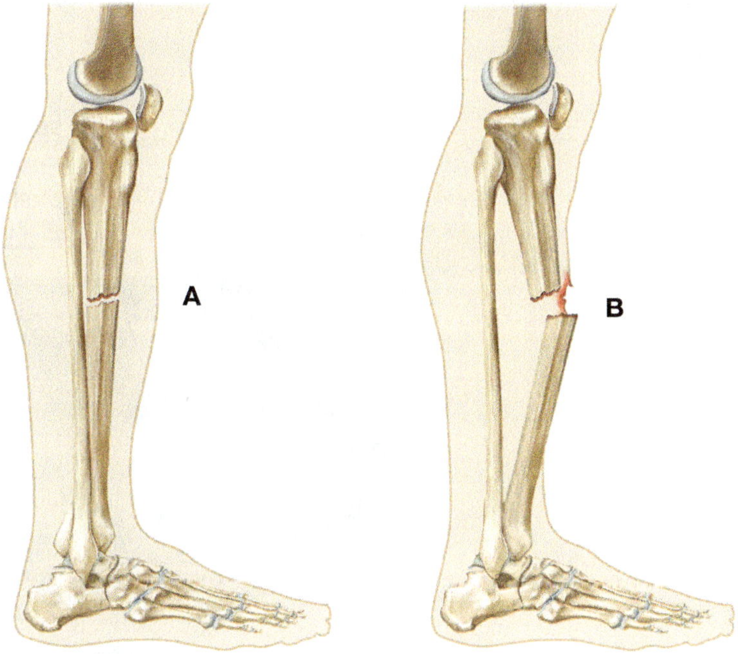

Figure 4.13 (A) Closed (or simple) fracture and (B) open (or compound) fracture.

TERM	WORD PARTS	DEFINITION
Colles' (COL-eez) **fracture**		A common type of wrist fracture.

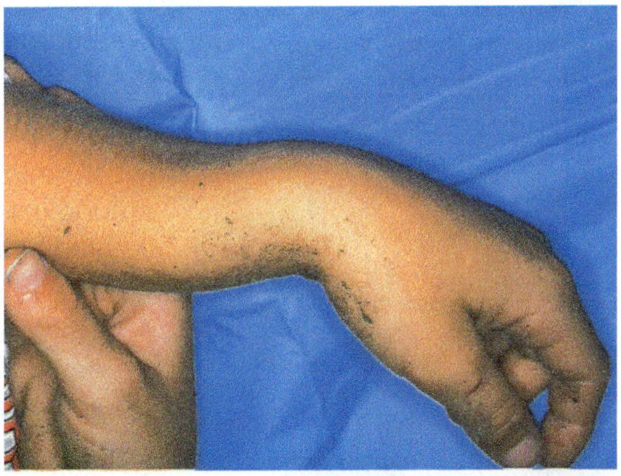

Figure 4.14 Colles' fracture. *(Charles Stewart MD FACEP, FAAEM)*

TERM	WORD PARTS	DEFINITION
comminuted fracture (kom-ih-NYOOT-ed)		Fracture in which the bone is shattered, splintered, or crushed into many small pieces or fragments.
compound fracture		Fracture in which the skin has been broken through to the fracture. Also called an *open fracture* (see Figure 4.13B).
compression fracture		Fracture involving loss of height of a vertebral body. It may be the result of trauma, but in older people, especially women, it may be caused by conditions like osteoporosis.
fracture (FX, Fx)		A broken bone.

Pathology *(continued)*

TERM	WORD PARTS	DEFINITION
greenstick fracture		Fracture in which there is an incomplete break; one side of bone is broken and the other side is bent. This type of fracture is commonly found in children due to their softer and more pliable bone structure.
impacted fracture		Fracture in which bone fragments are pushed into each other.
oblique (oh-BLEEK) fracture ■ **Figure 4.15** X-ray showing oblique fracture of the humerus. *(Charles Stewart MD)*	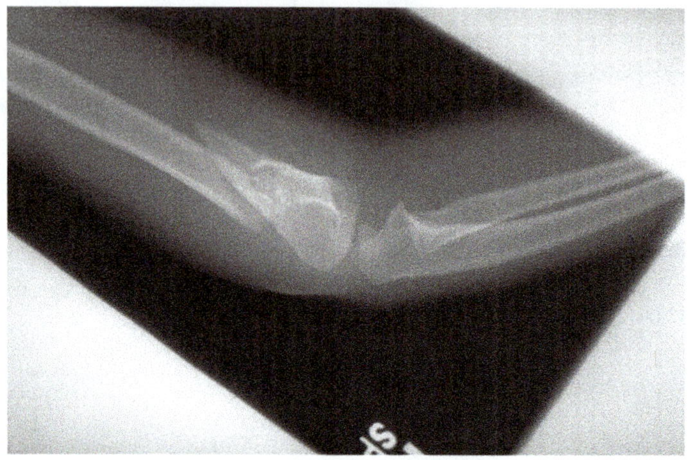	Fracture at an angle to the bone.
pathologic (path-a-LOJ-ik) fracture	path/o = disease -logy = study -ic = pertaining to	Fracture caused by diseased or weakened bone.
spiral fracture		Fracture in which the fracture line spirals around the shaft of the bone. Can be caused by a twisting injury and is often slower to heal than other types of fractures.
stress fracture		A slight fracture caused by repetitive low-impact forces, like running, rather than a single forceful impact.
transverse fracture ■ **Figure 4.16** X-ray showing transverse fracture of radius. *(James Stevenson/Science Photo Library/Photo Researchers, Inc.)*	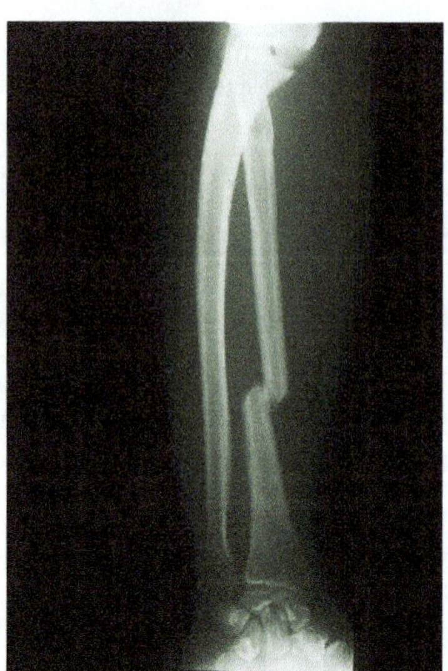	Complete fracture that is straight across the bone at right angles to the long axis of the bone.

Pathology *(continued)*

TERM	WORD PARTS	DEFINITION
Bones		
chondroma (kon-DROH-mah)	chondr/o = cartilage -oma = tumor	A tumor, usually benign, that forms in cartilage.
Ewing's sarcoma (YOO-wings / sar-KOH-mah)	sarc/o = flesh -oma = tumor	Malignant growth found in the shaft of long bones that spreads through the periosteum. Removal is the treatment of choice because this tumor will metastasize or spread to other organs.
exostosis (eck-sos-TOH-sis)	ex- = external, outward oste/o = bone -osis = abnormal condition	A bone spur.
myeloma (my-ah-LOH-mah)	myel/o = bone marrow -oma = tumor	A tumor that forms in bone marrow tissue.
osteochondroma (oss-tee-oh-kon-DROH-mah)	oste/o = bone chondr/o = cartilage -oma = tumor	A tumor, usually benign, that consists of both bone and cartilage tissue.
osteogenic sarcoma (oss-tee-oh-GIN-ik / sark-OH-mah)	oste/o = bone -genic = producing sarc/o = flesh -oma = tumor	The most common type of bone cancer. Usually begins in osteocytes found at the ends of long bones.
osteomalacia (oss-tee-oh-mah-LAY-she-ah)	oste/o = bone -malacia = softening	Softening of the bones caused by a deficiency of calcium. It is thought to be caused by insufficient sunlight and vitamin D in children.
osteopathy (oss-tee-OPP-ah-thee)	oste/o = bone -pathy = disease	A general term for bone disease.
osteoporosis (oss-tee-oh-por-ROH-sis)	oste/o = bone -porosis = porous	Decrease in bone mass producing a thinning and weakening of the bone with resulting fractures. The bone becomes more porous, especially in the spine and pelvis.
Paget's disease (PAH-jets)		A fairly common metabolic disease of the bone from unknown causes. It usually attacks middle-aged and older adults and is characterized by bone destruction and deformity. Named for Sir James Paget, a British surgeon.
rickets (RIK-ets)		Deficiency in calcium and vitamin D found in early childhood that results in bone deformities, especially bowed legs.
Spinal Column		
ankylosing spondylitis (ang-kih-LOH-sing / spon-dih-LYE-tis)	ankyl/o = stiff joint spondyl/o = vertebra -itis = inflammation	Inflammatory spinal condition resembling rheumatoid arthritis and results in gradual stiffening and fusion of the vertebrae. More common in men than women.

Pathology *(continued)*

TERM	WORD PARTS	DEFINITION
herniated nucleus pulposus (HNP) (HER-nee-ated / NOO-klee-us / pull-POH-sus)		Herniation or protrusion of an intervertebral disk; also called *herniated disk* or *ruptured disk.* May require surgery.

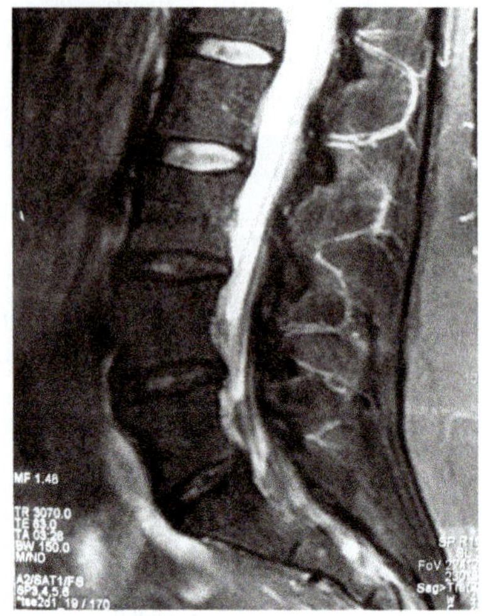

■ **Figure 4.17** Magnetic resonance imaging (MRI) image demonstrating a back herniated disk. *(Michelle Milano/ Shutterstock)*

TERM	WORD PARTS	DEFINITION
kyphosis (ki-FOH-sis)	kyph/o = hump -osis = abnormal condition	Abnormal increase in the outward curvature of the thoracic spine. Also known as *hunchback* or *humpback.* See Figure 4.18 ■ for an illustration of abnormal spine curvatures.

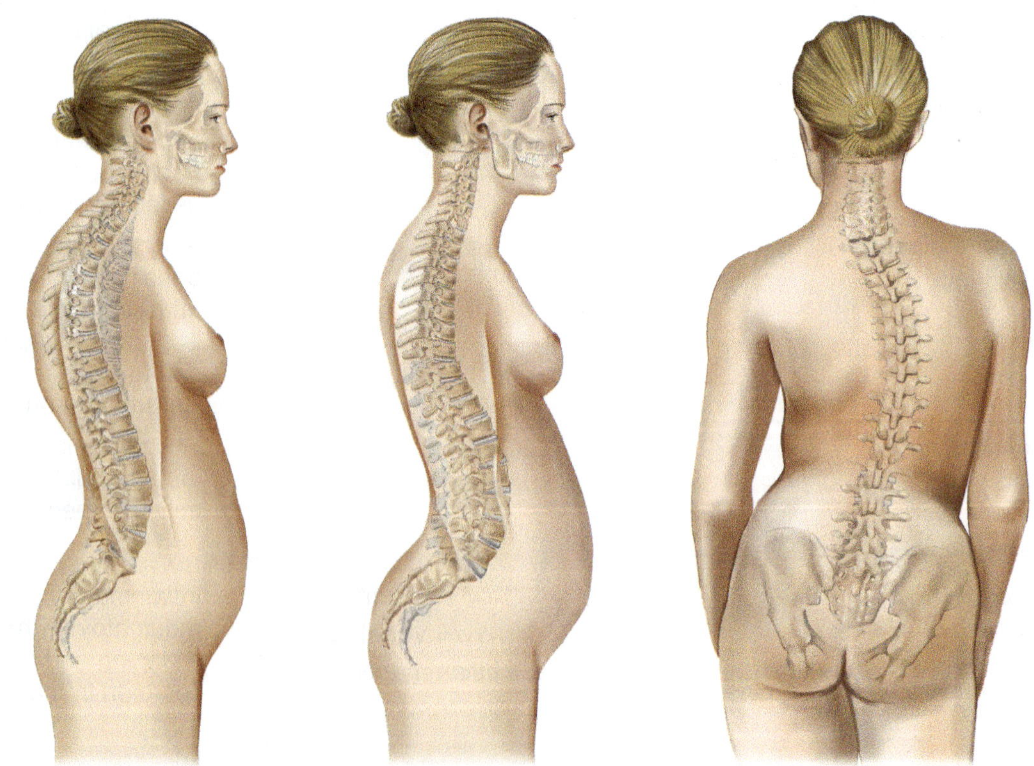

Kyphosis (excessive posterior thoracic curvature - hunchback)

Lordosis (excessive anterior lumbar curvature - swayback)

Scoliosis (lateral curvature)

■ **Figure 4.18** Abnormal spinal curvatures: kyphosis, lordosis, and scoliosis.

Pathology *(continued)*

TERM	WORD PARTS	DEFINITION
lordosis (lor-DOH-sis)	lord/o = bent backwards -osis = abnormal condition	Abnormal increase in the forward curvature of the lumbar spine. Also known as *swayback*. See again Figure 4.18 for an illustration of abnormal spine curvatures.
scoliosis (skoh-lee-OH-sis)	scoli/o = crooked, bent -osis = abnormal condition	Abnormal lateral curvature of the spine. See again Figure 4.18 for an illustration of abnormal spine curvatures.
spina bifida (SPY-nah / BIF-ih-dah)	spin/o = spine bi- = two	Congenital anomaly occurring when a vertebra fails to fully form around the spinal cord.
spinal stenosis (ste-NOH-sis)	spin/o = spine -al = pertaining to	Narrowing of the spinal canal causing pressure on the cord and nerves.
spondylolisthesis (spon-dih-loh-liss-THEE-sis)	spondyl/o = vertebra -listhesis = slipping	The forward sliding of a lumbar vertebra over the vertebra below it.
spondylosis (spon-dih-LOH-sis)	spondyl/o = vertebra -osis = abnormal condition	Specifically refers to ankylosing of the spine, but commonly used in reference to any degenerative condition of the vertebral column.
whiplash		Cervical muscle and ligament sprain or strain as a result of a sudden movement forward and backward of the head and neck. Can occur as a result of a rear-end auto collision.
Joints		
bunion (BUN-yun)		Inflammation of the bursa of the first metatarsophalangeal joint (base of the big toe).
dislocation		Occurs when the bones in a joint are displaced from their normal alignment and the ends of the bones are no longer in contact.
osteoarthritis (OA) (oss-tee-oh-ar-THRY-tis)	oste/o = bone arthr/o = joint -itis = inflammation	Arthritis resulting in degeneration of the bones and joints, especially those bearing weight. Results in bone rubbing against bone.
rheumatoid arthritis (RA) (ROO-mah-toyd / ar-THRY-tis)	arthr/o = joint -itis = inflammation	Chronic form of arthritis with inflammation of the joints, swelling, stiffness, pain, and changes in the cartilage that can result in crippling deformities; considered to be an autoimmune disease.

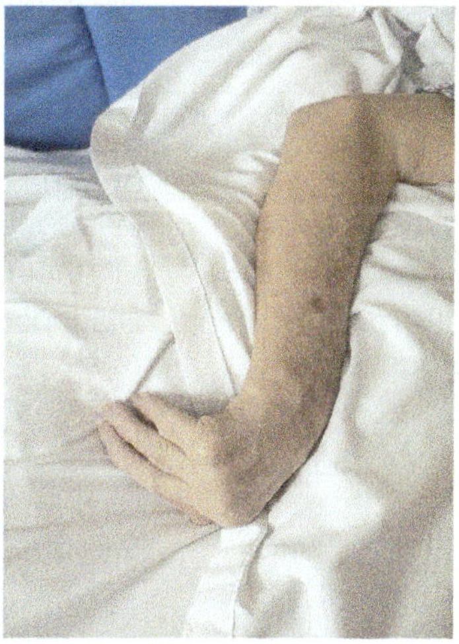

Figure 4.19 Patient with typical rheumatoid arthritis contractures.

Pathology *(continued)*

TERM	WORD PARTS	DEFINITION
sprain		Damage to the ligaments surrounding a joint due to overstretching, but no dislocation of the joint or fracture of the bone.
subluxation (sub-LUCKS-a-shun)	sub- = below, under	An incomplete dislocation, the joint alignment is disrupted, but the ends of the bones remain in contact.
systemic lupus erythematosus (SLE) (sis-TEM-ik / LOOP-us / air-ih-them-ah-TOH-sis)	system/o = system -ic = pertaining to erythr/o = red	Chronic inflammatory autoimmune disease of connective tissue affecting many systems that may include joint pain and arthritis. May be mistaken for rheumatoid arthritis.
talipes (TAL-ih-peez)		Congenital deformity causing misalignment of the ankle joint and foot. Also referred to as a *clubfoot.*

Diagnostic Procedures

TERM	WORD PART	DEFINITION
Diagnostic Imaging		
arthrogram (AR-throh-gram)	arthr/o = joint -gram = record	X-ray record of a joint; usually taken after the joint has been injected by a contrast medium.
arthrography (ar-THROG-rah-fee)	arthr/o = joint -graphy = process of recording	Process of X-raying a joint; usually after injection of a contrast medium into the joint space.
bone scan		Nuclear medicine procedure in which the patient is given a radioactive dye and then scanning equipment is used to visualize bones. It is especially useful in identifying stress fractures, observing progress of treatment for osteomyelitis, and locating cancer metastases to the bone.
dual-energy absorptiometry (DXA) (ab-sorp-she-AHM-eh-tree)	-metry = process of measuring	Measurement of bone density using low-dose X-ray for the purpose of detecting osteoporosis.
myelography (my-eh-LOG-rah-fee)	myel/o = bone marrow -graphy = process of recording	Study of the spinal column after injecting opaque contrast material; particularly useful in identifying herniated nucleus pulposus pinching a spinal nerve.
radiography	radi/o = ray (X-ray) -graphy = process of recording	Diagnostic imaging procedure using X-rays to study the internal structure of the body; especially useful for visualizing bones and joints.
Endoscopic Procedures		
arthroscope (AR-throw-skop)	arthr/o = joint -scope = instrument for viewing	Instrument used to view inside a joint.

Diagnostic Procedures *(continued)*

TERM	WORD PART	DEFINITION
arthroscopy (ar-THROS-koh-pee)	arthr/o = joint -scopy = process of visually examining	Examination of the interior of a joint by entering the joint with an *arthroscope.* The arthroscope contains a small television camera that allows the physician to view the interior of the joint on a monitor during the procedure. Some joint conditions can be repaired during arthroscopy.

Therapeutic Procedures

TERM	WORD PART	DEFINITION
Medical Treatments		
arthrocentesis (ar-thro-sen-TEE-sis)	arthr/o = joint -centesis = puncture to withdraw fluid	Involves the insertion of a needle into the joint cavity in order to remove or aspirate fluid. May be done to remove excess fluid from a joint or to obtain fluid for examination.
orthotic (or-THOT-ik)	orth/o = straight -tic = pertaining to	Orthopedic appliance, such as a brace or splint, used to prevent or correct deformities.
prosthesis (pross-THEE-sis)	prosthet/o = addition	Artificial device used as a substitute for a body part that is either congenitally missing or absent as a result of accident or disease. An example would be an artificial leg.
Surgical Procedures		
amputation (am-pew-TAY-shun)		Partial or complete removal of a limb for a variety of reasons, including tumors, gangrene, intractable pain, crushing injury, or uncontrollable infection.
arthroclasia (ar-throh-KLAY-see-ah)	arthr/o = joint -clasia = surgically break	To forcibly break loose a fused joint while the patient is under anesthetic. Fusion is usually caused by the buildup of scar tissue or adhesions.
arthrodesis (ar-throh-DEE-sis)	arthr/o = joint -desis = fuse	Procedure to stabilize a joint by fusing the bones together.
arthroscopic surgery (ar-throh-SKOP-ic)	arthr/o = joint -scopy = process of visually examining -ic = pertaining to	Performing a surgical procedure while using an arthroscope to view the internal structure, such as a joint.
arthrotomy (ar-THROT-oh-mee)	arthr/o = joint -otomy = cutting into	Surgical procedure that cuts into a joint capsule.
bone graft		Piece of bone taken from the patient used to take the place of a removed bone or a bony defect at another site.
bunionectomy (bun-yun-ECK-toh-mee)	-ectomy = surgical removal	Removal of the bursa at the joint of the great toe.

Therapeutic Procedures *(continued)*

TERM	WORD PART	DEFINITION
bursectomy (ber-SEK-toh-mee)	burs/o = bursa -ectomy = surgical removal	Surgical removal of a bursa.
chondrectomy (kon-DREK-toh-mee)	chondr/o = cartilage -ectomy = surgical removal	Surgical removal of cartilage.
chondroplasty (KON-droh-plas-tee)	chondr/o = cartilage -plasty = surgical repair	Surgical repair of cartilage.
craniotomy (kray-nee-OTT-oh-mee)	chondr/o = cartilage -otomy = cutting into	Surgical procedure that cuts into the skull.
laminectomy (lam-ih-NEK-toh-mee)	lamin/o = lamina, part of vertebra -ectomy = surgical removal	Removal of the vertebral posterior arch to correct severe back problems and pain caused by compression of a spinal nerve.
osteoclasia (oss-tee-oh-KLAY-see-ah)	oste/o = bone -clasia = surgically break	Surgical procedure involving the intentional breaking of a bone to correct a deformity.
osteotome (OSS-tee-oh-tohm)	oste/o = bone -tome = instrument used to cut	Instrument used to cut bone.
osteotomy (oss-tee-OTT-ah-me)	oste/o = bone -otomy = cutting into	Surgical procedure that cuts into a bone.
percutaneous diskectomy (per-kyou-TAY-nee-us / disk-EK-toh-mee)	per- = through cutane/o = skin -ous = pertaining to -ectomy = surgical removal	A thin catheter tube is inserted into the intervertebral disk through the skin and the herniated or ruptured disk material is sucked out or a laser is used to vaporize it.
spinal fusion	spin/o = spine -al = pertaining to	Surgical immobilization of adjacent vertebrae. This may be done for several reasons, including correction for a herniated disk.
synovectomy (sih-no-VEK-toh-mee)	synov/o = synovial membrane -ectomy = surgical removal	Surgical removal of the synovial membrane.
total hip arthroplasty (THA) (ar-thro-PLAS-tee)	arthr/o = joint -plasty = surgical repair	Surgical reconstruction of a hip by implanting a prosthetic or artificial hip joint. Also called *total hip replacement (THR).*

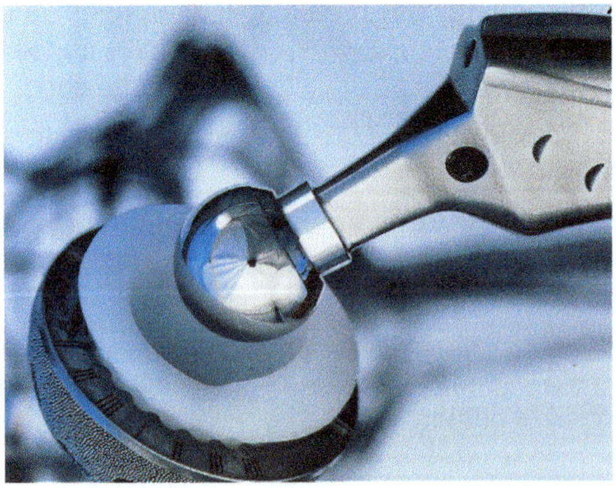

Figure 4.20 Prosthetic hip joint. *(Lawrence Livermore National Library/Science Photo Library/Photo Researchers, Inc.)*

TERM	WORD PART	DEFINITION
total knee arthroplasty (TKA) (ar-thro-PLAS-tee)	arthr/o = joint -plasty = surgical repair	Surgical reconstruction of a knee joint by implanting a prosthetic knee joint. Also called *total knee replacement (TKR).*

Therapeutic Procedures *(continued)*

TERM	WORD PART	DEFINITION
Fracture Care		
cast		Application of a solid material to immobilize an extremity or portion of the body as a result of a fracture, dislocation, or severe injury. It may be made of plaster of Paris or fiberglass.
fixation		Procedure to stabilize a fractured bone while it heals. *External fixation* includes casts, splints, and pins inserted through the skin. *Internal fixation* includes pins, plates, rods, screws, and wires that are applied during an *open reduction.*
reduction		Correcting a fracture by realigning the bone fragments. *Closed reduction* is doing this manipulation without entering the body. *Open reduction* is the process of making a surgical incision at the site of the fracture to do the reduction. This is necessary when bony fragments need to be removed or *internal fixation* such as plates or pins are required.
traction		Applying a pulling force on a fractured or dislocated limb or the vertebral column in order to restore normal alignment.

Pharmacology

CLASSIFICATION	WORD PARTS	ACTION	EXAMPLES
bone reabsorption inhibitors		Conditions that result in weak and fragile bones, such as osteoporosis and Paget's disease, are improved by medications that reduce the reabsorption of bones.	alendronate, Fosamax; ibandronate, Boniva
calcium supplements and vitamin D therapy		Maintaining high blood levels of calcium in association with vitamin D helps maintain bone density; used to treat osteomalacia, osteoporosis, and rickets.	calcium carbonate, Oystercal, Tums; calcium citrate, Cal-Citrate, Citracal
corticosteroids	cortic/o = outer portion	A hormone produced by the adrenal cortex that has very strong anti-inflammatory properties. It is particularly useful in treating rheumatoid arthritis.	prednisone; methylprednisolone, Medrol; dexamethasone, Decadron
nonsteroidal anti-inflammatory drugs (NSAIDs)	-al = pertaining to anti- = against -ory = pertaining to	A large group of drugs that provide mild pain relief and anti-inflammatory benefits for conditions such as arthritis.	ibuprofen, Advil, Motrin; naproxen, Aleve, Naprosyn; salicylates, Aspirin

Abbreviations

AE	above elbow
AK	above knee
BDT	bone density testing
BE	below elbow
BK	below knee
BMD	bone mineral density
C1, C2, etc.	first cervical vertebra, second cervical vertebra, etc.
Ca	calcium
DJD	degenerative joint disease
DXA	dual-energy absorptiometry
FX, Fx	fracture
HNP	herniated nucleus pulposus
JRA	juvenile rheumatoid arthritis
L1, L2, etc.	first lumbar vertebra, second lumbar vertebra, etc.
LE	lower extremity
LLE	left lower extremity
LUE	left upper extremity
NSAID	nonsteroidal anti-inflammatory drug
OA	osteoarthritis
ORIF	open reduction–internal fixation
Orth, ortho	orthopedics
RA	rheumatoid arthritis
RLE	right lower extremity
RUE	right upper extremity
SLE	systemic lupus erythematosus
T1, T2, etc.	first thoracic vertebra, second thoracic vertebra, etc.
THA	total hip arthroplasty
THR	total hip replacement
TKA	total knee arthroplasty
TKR	total knee replacement
UE	upper extremity

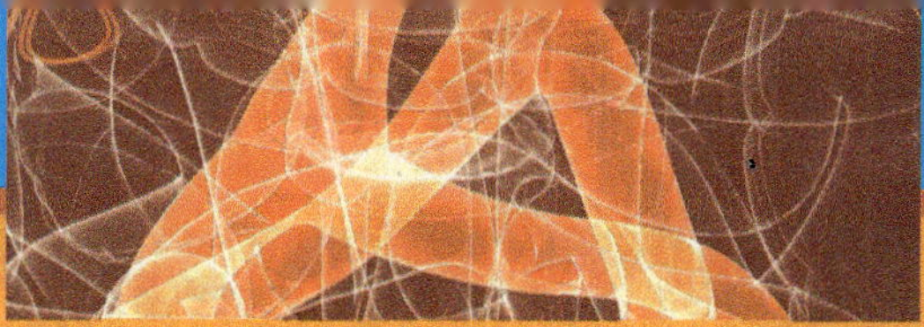

Section II: Muscular System at a Glance

Function

Muscles are bundles, sheets, or rings of tissue that produce movement by contracting and pulling on the structures to which they are attached.

Structures

Here is the primary structure that comprises the muscular system.
muscles

Word Parts

Here are the most common word parts (with their meanings) used to build muscular system terms. For a more comprehensive list, refer to the Terminology section of this chapter.

Combining Forms

duct/o	to bring
extens/o	to stretch out
fasci/o	fibrous band
fibr/o	fibers
flex/o	to bend
kinesi/o	movement
muscul/o	muscle
my/o	muscle
myocardi/o	heart muscle
myos/o	muscle
plant/o	sole of foot
rotat/o	to revolve
ten/o	tendon
tend/o	tendon
tendin/o	tendon
vers/o	to turn

Suffixes

-asthenia	weakness
-ion	action, condition
-kinesia	movement
-tonia	tone

Prefixes

ab-	away from
ad-	toward
circum-	around
e-	outward, without
in-	inward, without

Muscular System Illustrated

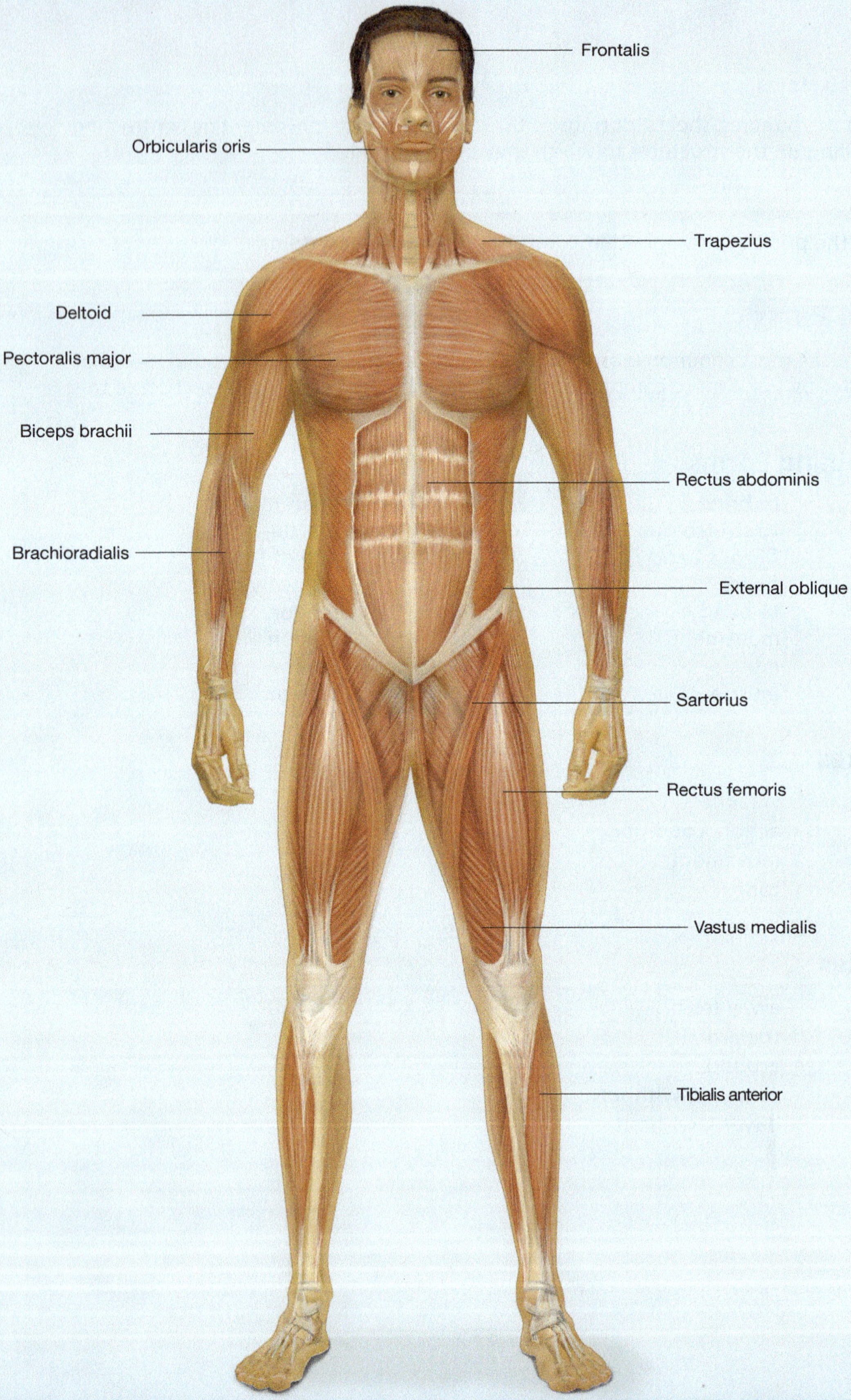

Anatomy and Physiology of the Muscular System

muscle tissue fibers
muscles

Muscles are bundles of parallel **muscle tissue fibers.** As these fibers contract (shorten in length) they produce movement of or within the body. The movement may take the form of bringing two bones closer together, pushing food through the digestive system, or pumping blood through blood vessels. In addition to producing movement, muscles also hold the body erect and generate heat.

MED TERM TIP

The term *muscle* is the diminutive form of the Latin word *mus* or "little mouse." This is thought to describe how the skin ripples when a muscle contracts, like a little mouse running.

Types of Muscles

cardiac muscle
involuntary muscles
skeletal muscle
smooth muscle
voluntary muscles

The three types of muscle tissue are **skeletal muscle, smooth muscle,** and **cardiac muscle** (see Figure 4.21 ■). Muscle tissue may be either voluntary or involuntary. **Voluntary muscles** are those muscles for which a person consciously chooses to contract and for how long and how hard to contract them. The skeletal muscles of the arm and leg are examples of this type of muscle. **Involuntary muscles** are the muscles under the control of the subconscious regions of the brain. The smooth muscles found in internal organs and cardiac muscles are examples of involuntary muscle tissue.

MED TERM TIP

Combining Latin and Greek roots will help form terms related to conditions of the muscular system.

Condition:	fibromyalgia
Latin:	fibro (fibrous tissue)
Greek:	myo (muscle) algia (pain)

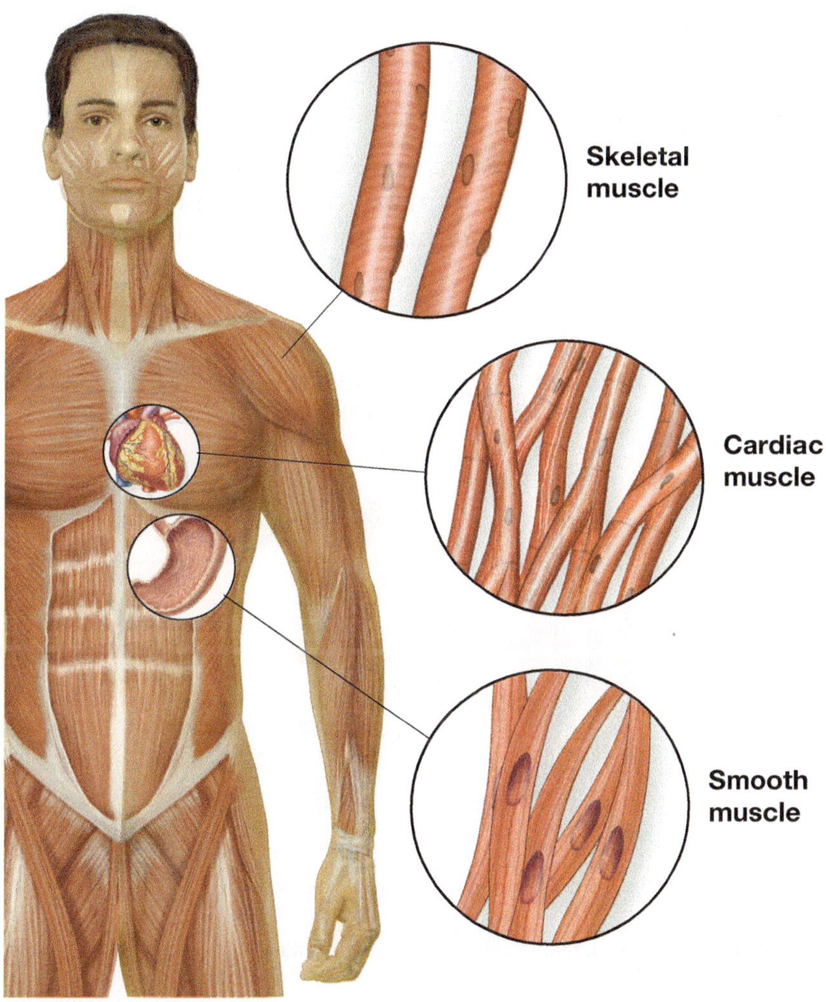

■ **Figure 4.21** The three types of muscles: skeletal, smooth, and cardiac.

Skeletal Muscle

fascia (FASH-ee-ah)
motor neurons
myoneural junction (MY-oh-NOO-rall)
striated muscles (stry-a-ted)
tendon (TEN-dun)

MED TERM TIP

The human body has more than 400 skeletal muscles, which account for almost 50% of the body weight.

A skeletal muscle is directly or indirectly attached to a bone and produces voluntary movement of the skeleton. It is also referred to as a **striated muscle** because of its striped appearance under the microscope (see Figure 4.22 ■). Each muscle is wrapped in layers of fibrous connective tissue called **fascia.** The fascia tapers at each end of a skeletal muscle to form a very strong **tendon.** The tendon then inserts into the periosteum covering a bone to anchor the muscle to the bone. Skeletal muscles are stimulated by **motor neurons** of the nervous system. The point at which the motor nerve contacts a muscle fiber is called the **myoneural junction.**

Smooth Muscle

visceral muscle (vis-she-ral)

Smooth muscle tissue is found in association with internal organs. For this reason, it is also referred to as **visceral muscle.** The name smooth muscle refers to the muscle's microscopic appearance; it lacks the striations of skeletal muscle (see again Figure 4.22). Smooth muscle is found in the walls of the hollow organs, such as the stomach, tube-shaped organs, such as the respiratory airways, and blood vessels. It is responsible for the involuntary muscle action associated with movement of the internal organs, such as churning food, constricting a blood vessel, and uterine contractions.

Cardiac Muscle

myocardium (my-oh-CAR-dee-um)

Cardiac muscle, or **myocardium,** makes up the wall of the heart (see again Figure 4.22). With each involuntary contraction the heart squeezes to pump blood out of its chambers and through the blood vessels.

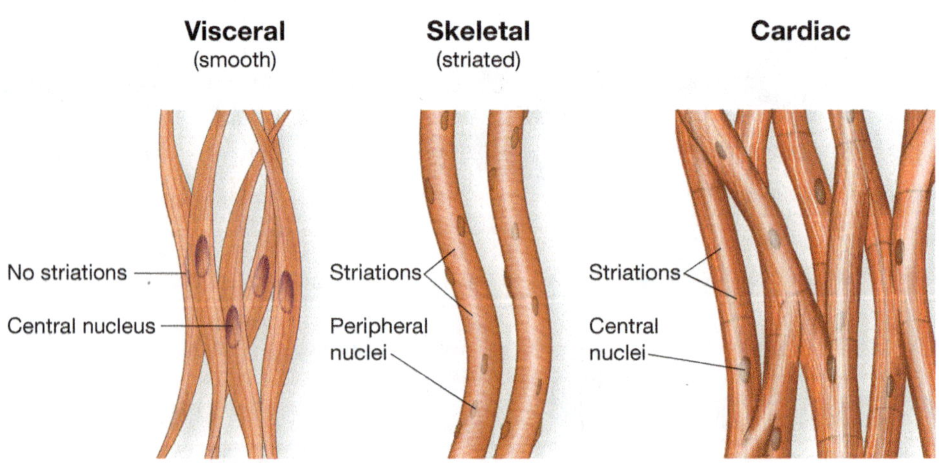

	Visceral	Skeletal	Cardiac
Contracts	Slowly	Rapidly	Rapidly
Found	Viscera, blood vessels	Trunk, extremities, head and neck	Heart
Control	Involuntary	Voluntary	Involuntary

■ **Figure 4.22** Characteristics of the three types of muscles.

Naming Skeletal Muscles

biceps (BYE-seps)
extensor carpi
external oblique
flexor carpi
gluteus maximus (GLOO-tee-us / MACKS-ih-mus)
rectus abdominis (REK-tus / ab-DOM-ih-nis)
sternocleidomastoid (STER-noh-KLY-doh-MASS-toid)

The name of a muscle often reflects its location, origin and insertion, size, action, fiber direction, or number of attachment points, as illustrated by the following examples:

- **Location:** the term **rectus abdominis** means straight (rectus) abdominal muscle.
- **Origin and insertion:** the **sternocleidomastoid** is named for its two origins (stern/o for sternum and cleid/o for clavicle) and single insertion (mastoid process).
- **Size:** when gluteus, meaning rump area, is combined with maximus, meaning large, we have the term **gluteus maximus.**
- **Action:** the **flexor carpi** and **extensor carpi** muscles are named as such because they produce flexion and extension at the wrist.
- **Fiber direction:** the **external oblique** muscle is an abdominal muscle whose fibers run at an oblique angle.
- **Number of attachment points:** the term *bi,* meaning two, can form the medical term **biceps,** which refers to the muscle in the upper arm that has two heads or connecting points.

Skeletal Muscle Actions

action
antagonistic pairs
insertion
origin

Skeletal muscles are attached to two different bones and overlap a joint. When a muscle contracts, the two bones move, but not usually equally. The less movable of the two bones is considered to be the starting point of the muscle and is called the **origin.** The more movable bone is considered to be where the muscle ends and is called the **insertion.** The type of movement a muscle produces is called its **action.** Muscles are often arranged around joints in **antagonistic pairs,** meaning that they produce opposite actions. For example, one muscle will bend a joint while its antagonist is responsible for straightening the joint. Some common terminology for muscle actions are described in Table 4.5 ■.

Table 4.5 Muscle Actions Grouped by Antagonistic Pairs

ACTION	WORD PARTS	DESCRIPTION
abduction (ab-DUCK-shun)	ab- = away from duct/o = to bring -ion = action, condition	Movement away from midline of the body (see Figure 4.23 ■)
adduction (ah-DUCK-shun)	ad- = toward duct/o = to bring -ion = action, condition	Movement toward midline of the body (see again Figure 4.23)
flexion (FLEK-shun)	flex/o = to bend -ion = action, condition	Act of bending or being bent (see Figure 4.24 ■)
extension (eks-TEN-shun)	extens/o = to stretch out -ion = action, condition	Movement that brings limb into or toward a straight condition (see again Figure 4.24)
dorsiflexion (dor-see-FLEK-shun)	dors/o = back of body flex/o = to bend -ion = action, condition	Backward bending, as of hand or foot (see Figure 4.25A ■)
plantar flexion (PLAN-tar / FLEK-shun)	plant/o = sole of foot -ar = pertaining to flex/o = to bend -ion = action, condition	Bending sole of foot; pointing toes downward (see Figure 4.25B ■)

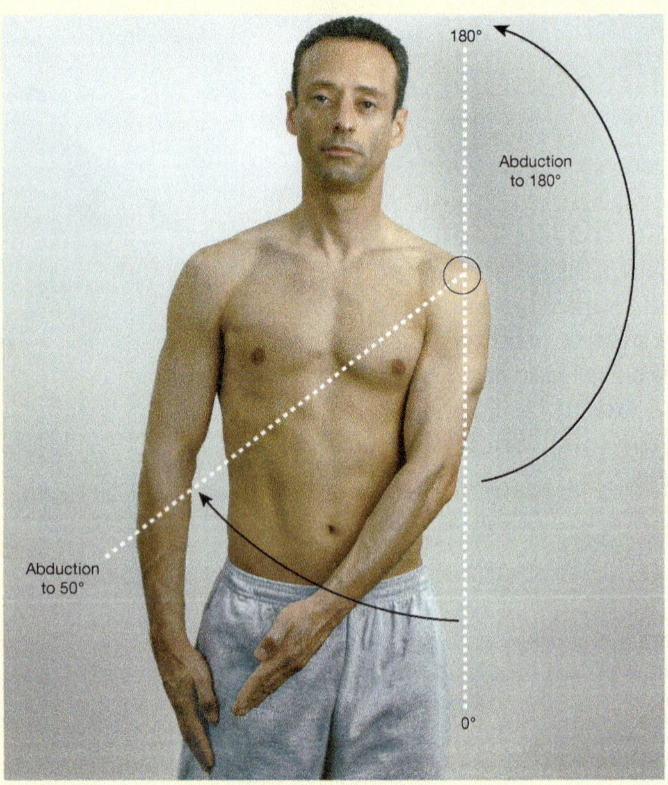

■ **Figure 4.23** Abduction and adduction of the shoulder joint.

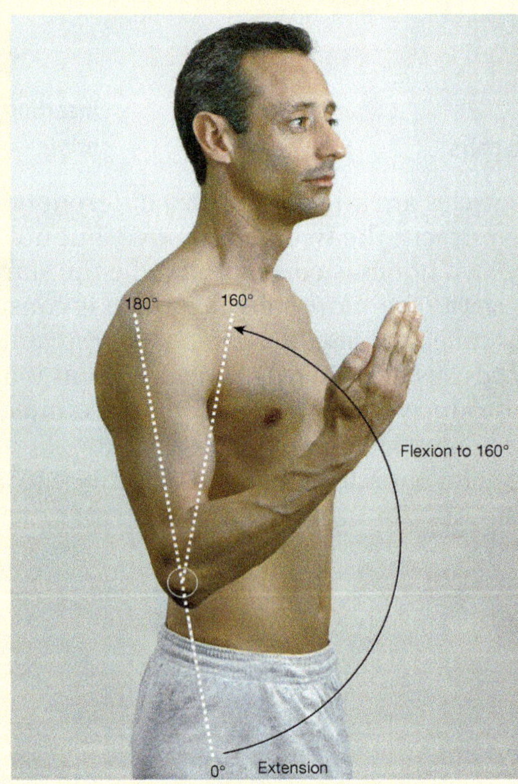

■ **Figure 4.24** Flexion and extension of the elbow joint.

Table 4.5	Muscle Actions Grouped by Antagonistic Pairs (continued)	
ACTION	**WORD PARTS**	**DESCRIPTION**
eversion (ee-VER-zhun)	e- = outward, without vers/o = to turn -ion = action, condition	Turning outward (see Figure 4.26 ■)
inversion (in-VER-zhun)	in- = inward, without vers/o = to turn -ion = action, condition	Turning inward (see again Figure 4.26)

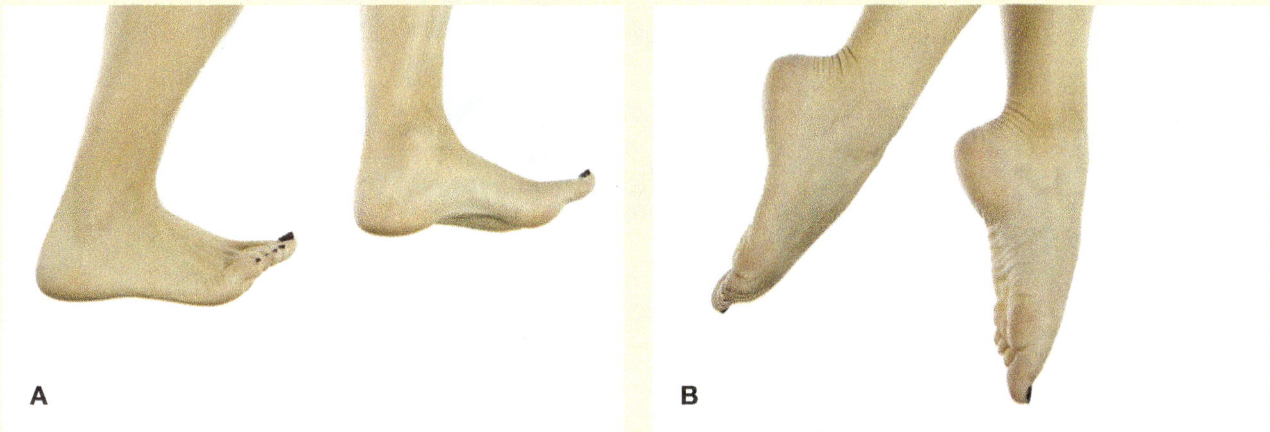

■ **Figure 4.25** Dorsiflexion (A) and plantar flexion (B) of the ankle joint. *(Poulsons Photography/Shutterstock)*

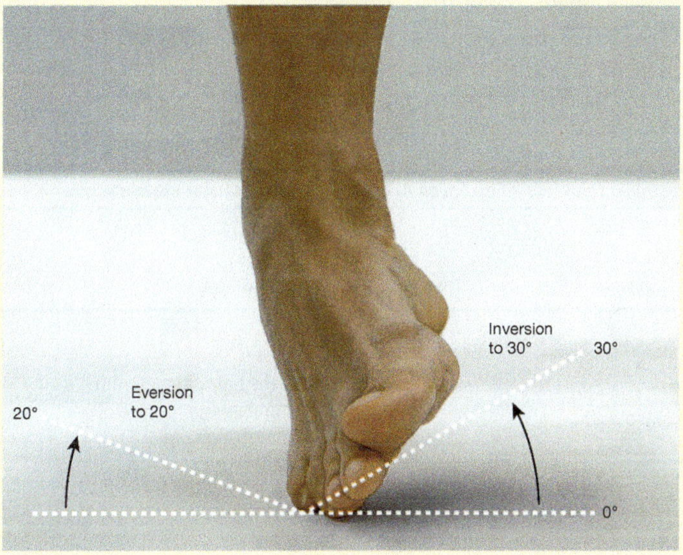

■ **Figure 4.26** Eversion and inversion of the foot.

(Continued)

Table 4.5 Muscle Actions Grouped by Antagonistic Pairs (continued)

ACTION	WORD PARTS	DESCRIPTION
pronation (proh-NAY-shun)		To turn downward or backward as with the hand or foot (see Figure 4.27)
supination (soo-pin-NAY-shun)		Turning the palm or foot upward (see again Figure 4.27)
elevation		To raise a body part, as in shrugging the shoulders
depression		A downward movement, as in dropping the shoulders
The circular actions described below are an exception to the antagonistic pair arrangement.		
circumduction (sir-kum-DUCK-shun)	circum- = around duct/o = to bring -ion = action, condition	Movement in a circular direction from a central point as if drawing a large, imaginary circle in the air
opposition	**MED TERM TIP** Primates are the only animals with opposable thumbs.	Moving thumb away from palm; the ability to move the thumb into contact with the other fingers
rotation	rotat/o = to revolve -ion = action, condition	Moving around a central axis

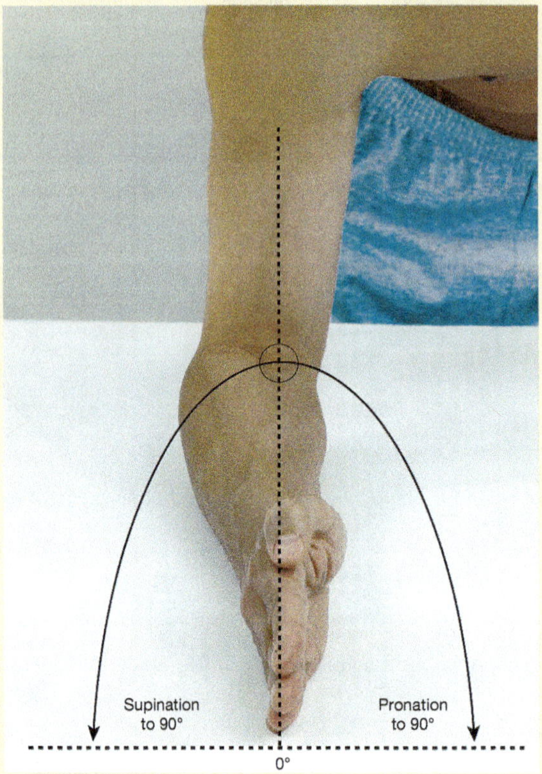

Figure 4.27 Pronation and supination of the forearm.

Terminology

Word Parts Used to Build Muscular System Terms

The following lists contain the combining forms, suffixes, and prefixes used to build terms in the remaining sections of this chapter.

Combining Forms

bi/o	life
carp/o	wrist
electr/o	electricity
fasci/o	fibrous band
fibr/o	fibers
kinesi/o	movement
later/o	side
muscul/o	muscle
my/o	muscle
myocardi/o	heart muscle
myos/o	muscle
ten/o	tendon
tend/o	tendon
tendin/o	tendon

Suffixes

-al	pertaining to
-algia	pain
-ar	pertaining to
-asthenia	weakness
-desis	fuse
-dynia	pain
-gram	record
-graphy	process of recording
-itis	inflammation
-kinesia	movement
-logy	study of
-opsy	view of
-otomy	cutting into
-ous	pertaining to
-pathy	disease
-plasty	surgical repair
-rrhaphy	suture
-rrhexis	rupture
-tonia	tone
-trophy	development

Prefixes

a-	without
brady-	slow
dys-	abnormal, difficult, painful
epi-	over
hyper-	excessive
hypo-	insufficient
poly-	many
pseudo-	false

Anatomical Terms

TERM	WORD PARTS	DEFINITION
fascial (FAS-ee-all)	fasci/o = fibrous band -al = pertaining to	pertaining to fascia
muscular (MUSS-kew-lar)	muscul/o = muscle -ar = pertaining to	pertaining to muscles
myocardial (my-oh-CAR-dee-al)	myocardi/o = heart muscle -al = pertaining to	pertaining to heart muscle
skeletal (SKEL-eh-tal)	-al = pertaining to	pertaining to the skeleton
tendinous (TEN-din-us)	tendin/o = tendon -ous = pertaining to	pertaining to tendons

Pathology

TERM	WORD PARTS	DEFINITION
Medical Specialties		
kinesiology (kih-NEE-see-oh-loh-jee)	kinesi/o = movement -logy = study of	The science that studies movement, how it is produced, and the muscles involved.
Signs and Symptoms		
adhesion		Scar tissue forming in the fascia surrounding a muscle, making it difficult to stretch the muscle.
atonia	a- = without -tonia = tone	The lack of muscle tone.
atrophy (AT-rah-fee)	a- = without -trophy = development	Poor muscle development as a result of muscle disease, nervous system disease, or lack of use; commonly referred to as *muscle wasting*.
bradykinesia (brad-ee-kih-NEE-see-ah)	brady- = slow -kinesia = movement	Having slow movements.
contracture (kon-TRACK-chur)		Abnormal shortening of muscle fibers, tendons, or fascia, making it difficult to stretch the muscle.
dyskinesia (dis-kih-NEE-see-ah)	dys- = difficult, painful -kinesia = movement	Having difficult or painful movement.
dystonia	dys- = abnormal -tonia = tone	Having abnormal muscle tone.
hyperkinesia (high-per-kih-NEE-see-ah)	hyper- = excessive -kinesia = movement	Having an excessive amount of movement.
hypertonia	hyper- = excessive -tonia = tone	Having excessive muscle tone.
hypertrophy (high-PER-troh-fee)	hyper- = excessive -trophy = development	Increase in muscle bulk as a result of use, as with lifting weights.
hypokinesia (HI-poh-kih-NEE-see-ah)	hypo- = insufficient -kinesia = movement	Having an insufficient amount of movement.
hypotonia	hypo- = insufficient -tonia = tone	Having insufficient muscle tone.
intermittent claudication (klaw-dih-KAY-shun)		Attacks of severe pain and lameness caused by ischemia of the muscles, typically the calf muscles; brought on by walking even very short distances.
myalgia (my-AL-jee-ah)	my/o = muscle -algia = pain	Muscle pain.
myasthenia (my-ass-THEE-nee-ah)	my/o = muscle -asthenia = weakness	Muscle weakness.
myotonia	my/o = muscle -tonia = tone	Muscle tone.
spasm		Sudden, involuntary, strong muscle contraction.

Pathology *(continued)*

TERM	WORD PARTS	DEFINITION
tenodynia (ten-oh-DIN-ee-ah)	ten/o = tendon -dynia = pain	Tendon pain.
Muscles		
fasciitis (fas-ee-EYE-tis)	fasci/o = fibrous band -itis = inflammation	Inflammation of fascia.
fibromyalgia (figh-broh-my-AL-jee-ah)	fibr/o = fibers my/o = muscle -algia = pain	Condition with widespread aching and pain in the muscles and soft tissue.
lateral epicondylitis (ep-ih-kon-dih-LYE-tis)	later/o = side -al = pertaining to epi- = over -itis = inflammation	Inflammation of the muscle attachment to the lateral epicondyle of the elbow. Often caused by strongly gripping. Commonly called *tennis elbow.*
muscular dystrophy (MD) (MUSS-kew-ler / DIS-troh-fee)	muscul/o = muscle -ar = pertaining to dys- = abnormal -trophy = development	Inherited disease causing a progressive muscle degeneration, weakness, and atrophy.
myopathy (my-OPP-ah-thee)	my/o = muscle -pathy = disease	A general term for muscle disease.
myorrhexis (my-oh-REK-sis)	my/o = muscle -rrhexis = rupture	Tearing a muscle.
polymyositis (pol-ee-my-oh-SIGH-tis)	poly- = many myos/o = muscle -itis = inflammation	The simultaneous inflammation of two or more muscles.
pseudohypertrophic muscular dystrophy (soo-doh-HIGH-per-troh-fic)	pseudo- = false hyper- = excessive -trophy = development muscul/o = muscle -ar = pertaining to dys- = abnormal -trophy = development	A type of inherited muscular dystrophy in which the muscle tissue is gradually replaced by fatty tissue, making the muscle look strong. Also called *Duchenne's muscular dystrophy.*
torticollis (tore-tih-KOLL-iss)		Severe neck spasms pulling the head to one side. Commonly called *wryneck* or a *crick in the neck.*
Tendons, Muscles, and/or Ligaments		
carpal tunnel syndrome (CTS)	carp/o = wrist -al = pertaining to	Repetitive motion disorder with pain caused by compression of the finger flexor tendons and median nerve as they pass through the carpal tunnel of the wrist.
ganglion cyst (GANG-lee-on)		Cyst that forms on tendon sheath, usually on hand, wrist, or ankle.
repetitive motion disorder		Group of chronic disorders involving the tendon, muscle, joint, and nerve damage, resulting from the tissue being subjected to pressure, vibration, or repetitive movements for prolonged periods.

Pathology *(continued)*

TERM	WORD PARTS	DEFINITION
rotator cuff injury		The rotator cuff consists of the joint capsule of the shoulder joint reinforced by the tendons from several shoulder muscles. The high degree of flexibility at the shoulder joint puts the rotator cuff at risk for strain and tearing.
strain		Damage to the muscle, tendons, or ligaments due to overuse or overstretching.
tendinitis (ten-dih-NIGH-tis)	tendin/o = tendon -itis = inflammation	Inflammation of a tendon.

Diagnostic Procedures

TERM	WORD PARTS	DEFINITION
Clinical Laboratory Test		
creatine phosphokinase (CPK) (KREE-ah-teen / foss-foe-KYE-nase)		Muscle enzyme found in skeletal muscle and cardiac muscle. Blood levels become elevated in disorders such as heart attack, muscular dystrophy, and other skeletal muscle pathologies.
Additional Diagnostic Procedures		
deep tendon reflexes (DTR)		Muscle contraction in response to a stretch caused by striking the muscle tendon with a reflex hammer. Test used to determine if muscles are responding properly.
electromyogram (EMG) (ee-lek-troh-MY-oh-gram)	electr/o = electricity my/o = muscle -gram = record	The hardcopy record produced by electromyography.
electromyography (EMG) (ee-lek-troh-my-OG-rah-fee)	electr/o = electricity my/o = muscle -graphy = process of recording	Study and record of the strength and quality of muscle contractions as a result of electrical stimulation.
muscle biopsy (BYE-op-see)	bi/o = life -opsy = view of	Removal of muscle tissue for pathological examination.

Therapeutic Procedures

TERM	WORD PARTS	DEFINITION
Surgical Procedures		
carpal tunnel release	carp/o = wrist -al = pertaining to	Surgical cutting of the ligament in the wrist to relieve nerve pressure caused by carpal tunnel syndrome, which can result from repetitive motion such as typing.
fasciotomy (fas-ee-OT-oh-mee)	fasci/o = fibrous band -otomy = cutting into	A surgical procedure that cuts into fascia.

Therapeutic Procedures *(continued)*

TERM	WORD PARTS	DEFINITION
myoplasty (MY-oh-plas-tee)	my/o = muscle -plasty = surgical repair	A surgical procedure to repair a muscle.
myorrhaphy (MY-or-ah-fee)	my/o = muscle -rrhaphy = suture	To suture a muscle.
tendoplasty (TEN-doh-plas-tee)	tend/o = tendon -plasty = surgical repair	A surgical procedure to repair a tendon.
tendotomy (tend-OT-oh-mee)	tend/o = tendon -otomy = cutting into	A surgical procedure that cuts into a tendon.
tenodesis (ten-oh-DEE-sis)	ten/o = tendon -desis = fuse	Surgical procedure to stabilize a joint by anchoring down the tendons of the muscles that move the joint.
tenoplasty (TEN-oh-plas-tee)	ten/o = tendon -plasty = surgical repair	A surgical procedure to repair a tendon.
tenorrhaphy (tah-NOR-ah-fee)	ten/o = tendon -rrhaphy = suture	To suture a tendon.

Pharmacology

CLASSIFICATION	WORD PARTS	ACTION	EXAMPLES
skeletal muscle relaxants	-al = pertaining to	Medication to relax skeletal muscles in order to reduce muscle spasms. Also called *antispasmodics.*	cyclobenzaprine, Flexeril; carisoprodol, Soma

Abbreviations

CTS	carpal tunnel syndrome	**EMG**	electromyogram
CPK	creatine phosphokinase	**IM**	intramuscular
DTR	deep tendon reflex	**MD**	muscular dystrophy

Chapter Review

Real-World Applications

Medical Record Analysis

This Discharge Summary contains 10 medical terms. Underline each term and write it in the list below the report. Then define each term.

Discharge Summary

Admitting Diagnosis:	Osteoarthritis bilateral knees.
Final Diagnosis:	Osteoarthritis bilateral knees with right TKA
History of Present Illness:	Patient is a 68-year-old male. He reports he has experienced occasional knee pain and swelling since he injured his knees playing football in high school. These symptoms became worse while he was in his 50s and working on a concrete surface. The right knee has always been more painful than the left. He saw his orthopedic surgeon six months ago because of constant knee pain and swelling severe enough to interfere with sleep and all activities. He required a cane to walk. CT scan indicated severe bilateral osteoarthritis. He is admitted to the hospital at this time for TKR right knee.
Summary of Hospital Course:	Patient tolerated the surgical procedure well. He began intensive physical therapy for lower extremity ROM and strengthening exercises and gait training with a walker. He received occupational therapy instruction in ADLs, especially dressing and personal care. He was able to transfer himself out of bed by the third post-op day and was able to ambulate 150 ft with a walker and dress himself on the fifth post-op day.
Discharge Plans:	Patient was discharged home with his wife one week post-op. He will continue rehabilitation as an outpatient. Return to office for post-op checkup in one week.

	Term	Definition
1	______	______
2	______	______
3	______	______
4	______	______
5	______	______
6	______	______
7	______	______
8	______	______
9	______	______
10	______	______

Chart Note Transcription

The chart note below contains 11 phrases that can be reworded with a medical term that you learned in this chapter. Each phrase is identified with an underline. Determine the medical term and write your answers in the space provided.

Current Complaint:	An 82-year-old female was transported to the Emergency Room via ambulance with severe left hip pain following a fall on the ice.
Past History:	Patient suffered a wrist broken bone (1) 2 years earlier that required immobilization by solid material. (2) Following this broken bone, (3) her physician who specializes in treatment of bone conditions (4) diagnosed her with moderate porous bones (5) on the basis of a computer-assisted X-ray. (6)
Signs and Symptoms:	Patient reported severe left hip pain, rating it as 8 on a scale of 1 to 10. She held her hip in a bent position (7) and could not tolerate movement toward a straight position. (8) X-rays of the left hip and leg were taken.
Diagnosis:	Shattered broken bone (9) in the neck of the left thigh bone. (10)
Treatment:	Implantation of an artificial hip joint (11) on the left.

1. ______________________________
2. ______________________________
3. ______________________________
4. ______________________________
5. ______________________________
6. ______________________________
7. ______________________________
8. ______________________________
9. ______________________________
10. ______________________________
11. ______________________________

Case Study

Below is a case study presentation of a patient with a condition covered by this chapter. Read the case study and answer the questions below. Some questions will ask for information not included within this chapter. Use your text, a medical dictionary, or any other reference material you choose to answer these questions.

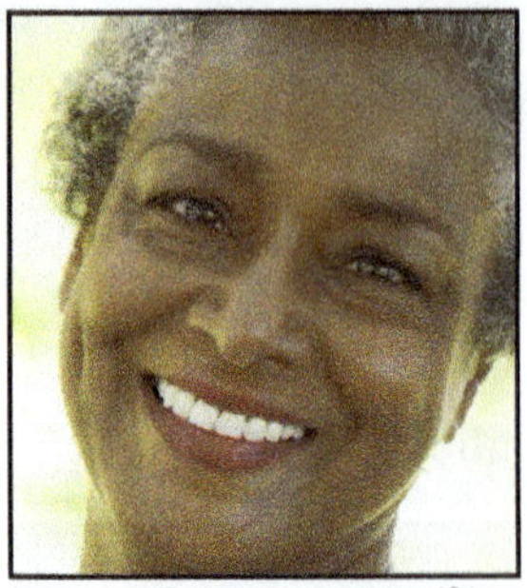
(Monkey Business Images/Shutterstock)

Mary Pearl, age 60, has come into the physician's office complaining of swelling, stiffness, and arthralgia, especially in her elbows, wrists, and hands. A bone scan revealed acute inflammation in multiple joints with damaged articular cartilage and an erythrocyte sedimentation rate blood test indicated a significant level of acute inflammation in the body. A diagnosis of acute episode of rheumatoid arthritis was made. The physician ordered nonsteroidal anti-inflammatory medication and physical therapy. The therapist initiated a treatment program of hydrotherapy and AROM exercises.

1. What pathological condition does this patient have? Look this condition up in a reference source and include a short description of it.

   ____

   ____

2. What type of long-term damage may occur in a patient with rheumatoid arthritis?

   ____

   ____

3. Describe the other major type of arthritis mentioned in your textbook.

   ____

   ____

4. What two diagnostic procedures did the physician order? Describe them in your own words. What were the results?

   ____

   ____

5. What treatments were ordered? Explain what the physical therapy procedures involve.

   ____

   ____

6. This patient is experiencing an acute episode. Explain what this phrase means and contrast it with chronic.

   ____

   ____

Practice Exercises

A. Complete the Statement

1. The two divisions of the human skeleton are the ______________________ and ______________________.
2. Another name for visceral muscle is ______________________ muscle.
3. The five functions of the skeletal system are to ______________________, ______________________, ______________________, ______________________, and ______________________.
4. Nerves contact skeletal muscle fibers at the ______________________ junction.
5. ______________________ bones are roughly as long as they are wide.
6. The membrane covering bones is called the ______________________.
7. A Colles' fracture occurs in the ______________________.
8. Another name for spongy bone is ______________________ bone.
9. ______________________ joints are the most common joints in the body.
10. The three types of muscle are ______________________, ______________________, and ______________________.
11. A ______________________ is a smooth, round opening in bones.
12. The ______________________ is the shaft of a long bone.

B. Adjective Form Practice

Give the adjective form for the following bones.

1. femur ______________________
2. sternum ______________________
3. clavicle ______________________
4. coccyx ______________________
5. maxilla ______________________
6. tibia ______________________
7. patella ______________________
8. phalanges ______________________
9. humerus ______________________
10. pubis ______________________

C. Combining Form Practice

The combining form **oste/o** refers to bone. Use it to write a term that means:

1. bone cell __________
2. embryonic bone cell __________
3. porous bone __________
4. disease of the bone __________
5. cutting into a bone __________
6. instrument to cut bone __________
7. inflammation of the bone and bone marrow __________
8. softening of the bones __________
9. tumor composed of both bone and cartilage __________

The combining form **my/o** refers to muscle. Use it to write a term that means:

10. muscle disease __________
11. surgical repair of muscle __________
12. suture of muscle __________
13. record of muscle electricity __________
14. muscle weakness __________

The combining form **ten/o** refers to tendons. Use it to write a term that means:

15. tendon pain __________
16. tendon suture __________

The combining form **arthr/o** refers to the joints. Use it to write a term that means:

17. surgical fusion of a joint __________
18. surgical repair of a joint __________
19. cutting into a joint __________
20. inflammation of a joint __________
21. puncture to withdraw fluid from a joint __________
22. pain in the joints __________

The combining form **chondr/o** refers to cartilage. Use it to write a term that means:

23. cartilage removal ______________________________

24. cartilage tumor ______________________________

25. cartilage softening ______________________________

D. Name That Suffix

	Suffix	Example from Chapter
1. fuse	______________	______________
2. weakness	______________	______________
3. slipping	______________	______________
4. to surgically break	______________	______________
5. movement	______________	______________
6. porous	______________	______________

E. Spinal Column Practice

Name the five regions of the spinal column and indicate the number of bones in each area.

	Name	Number of Bones
1.	______________	______________
2.	______________	______________
3.	______________	______________
4.	______________	______________
5.	______________	______________

F. Prefix and Suffix Practice

Circle the prefix and/or suffix. Place a *P* for prefix or an *S* for suffix over these word parts then, define the term.

1. arthroscopy ______________________________

2. intervertebral ______________________________

3. chondromalacia ______________________________

4. diskectomy ______________________________

5. intracranial ______________________________

6. subscapular ______________________________

G. Define the Combining Form

	Definition	Example from Chapter
1. **lamin/o**	______	______
2. **ankyl/o**	______	______
3. **chondr/o**	______	______
4. **spondyl/o**	______	______
5. **my/o**	______	______
6. **orth/o**	______	______
7. **kyph/o**	______	______
8. **tend/o**	______	______
9. **myel/o**	______	______
10. **articul/o**	______	______

H. What's the Abbreviation?

1. intramuscular ______
2. total knee replacement ______
3. herniated nucleus pulposus ______
4. deep tendon reflex ______
5. upper extremity ______
6. fifth lumbar vertebra ______
7. bone density testing ______
8. above the knee ______
9. fracture ______
10. nonsteroidal anti-inflammatory drug ______

I. Define the Term

1. orthopedics ______
2. chiropractic ______
3. podiatry ______
4. orthotics ______
5. prosthetics ______

J. Terminology Matching

Match each term to its definition.

1. ________ abduction
2. ________ rotation
3. ________ plantar flexion
4. ________ extension
5. ________ dorsiflexion
6. ________ flexion
7. ________ adduction
8. ________ opposition

a. backward bending of the foot
b. bending the foot to point toes toward the ground
c. straightening motion
d. motion around a central axis
e. motion away from the body
f. moving the thumb away from the palm
g. motion toward the body
h. bending motion

K. Fill in the Blank

carpal tunnel syndrome	rickets	lateral epicondylitis	systemic lupus erythematosus
scoliosis	osteogenic sarcoma	pseudohypertrophic muscular dystrophy	
herniated nucleus pulposus	osteoporosis		
	spondylolisthesis		

1. Mrs. Lewis, age 84, broke her hip. Her physician will be running tests for what potential ailment? ________________
2. Jamie, age 6 months, is being given orange juice and vitamin supplements to avoid what condition? ________________
3. George has severe elbow pain after playing tennis four days in a row. He may have ________________.
4. Marshall's doctor told him that he had a ruptured disk. The medical term for this is ________________.
5. Mr. Jefferson's physician has discovered a tumor at the end of his femur. He has been admitted to the hospital for a biopsy to rule out what type of bone cancer? ________________
6. The school nurse has asked Janelle to bend over so that she may examine her back to see if she is developing a lateral curve. What is the nurse looking for? ________________
7. Gerald has experienced a gradual loss of muscle strength over the past 5 years even though his muscles look large and healthy. The doctors believe he has an inherited muscle disease. What is that disease? ________________
8. Roberta has suddenly developed arthritis in her hands and knees. Rheumatoid arthritis had been ruled out, but what other auto-immune disease might Roberta have? ________________
9. Mark's X-ray demonstrated forward sliding of a lumbar vertebra; the radiologist diagnosed ________________.
10. The orthopedist determined that Marcia's repetitive wrist movements at work caused her to develop ________________.

L. Fracture Type Matching

Match each fracture type to its definition.

1.	________ comminuted	a.	fracture line is at an angle
2.	________ greenstick	b.	fracture line curves around the bone
3.	________ compound	c.	bone is splintered or crushed
4.	________ simple	d.	bone is pressed into itself
5.	________ impacted	e.	fracture line is straight across bone
6.	________ transverse	f.	skin has been broken
7.	________ oblique	g.	no open wound
8.	________ spiral	h.	bone only partially broken

M. Name That Anatomical Name

1. knee cap ____
2. ankle bones ____
3. collar bone ____
4. thigh bone ____
5. toe bones ____
6. wrist bones ____
7. shin bone ____
8. shoulder blade ____
9. finger bones ____

N. What Does it Stand For?

1. DJD ____
2. EMG ____
3. C1 ____
4. T6 ____
5. IM ____
6. DTR ____
7. JRA ____

8. LLE ______________________________

9. ortho ______________________________

10. CTS ______________________________

O. Define the Term

1. chondroplasty ______________________________

2. bradykinesia ______________________________

3. osteoporosis ______________________________

4. lordosis ______________________________

5. atrophy ______________________________

6. myeloma ______________________________

7. prosthesis ______________________________

8. craniotomy ______________________________

9. arthrocentesis ______________________________

10. bursitis ______________________________

P. Pharmacology Challenge

Fill in the classification for each drug description, then match the brand name.

	Drug Description	Classification		Brand Name
1.	________ Treats mild pain and anti-inflammatory	________	a.	Flexeril
2.	________ Hormone with anti-inflammatory properties	________	b.	Aleve
3.	________ Reduces muscle spasms	________	c.	Fosamax
4.	________ Treats conditions of weakened bones	________	d.	Oystercal
5.	________ Maintains blood calcium levels	________	e.	Medrol

Q. Professionalism

Professional standards needed by health workers include a model of excellent care and service. Professionalism brings together soft skills: work ethic, character, relationships, teamwork, communication, honesty, cultural competence, personal image, personal health, and wellness. Working with a partner, create a poster or presentation on how to demonstrate professionalism in the workplace.

Labeling Exercise

Image A

Write the labels for this figure on the numbered lines provided.

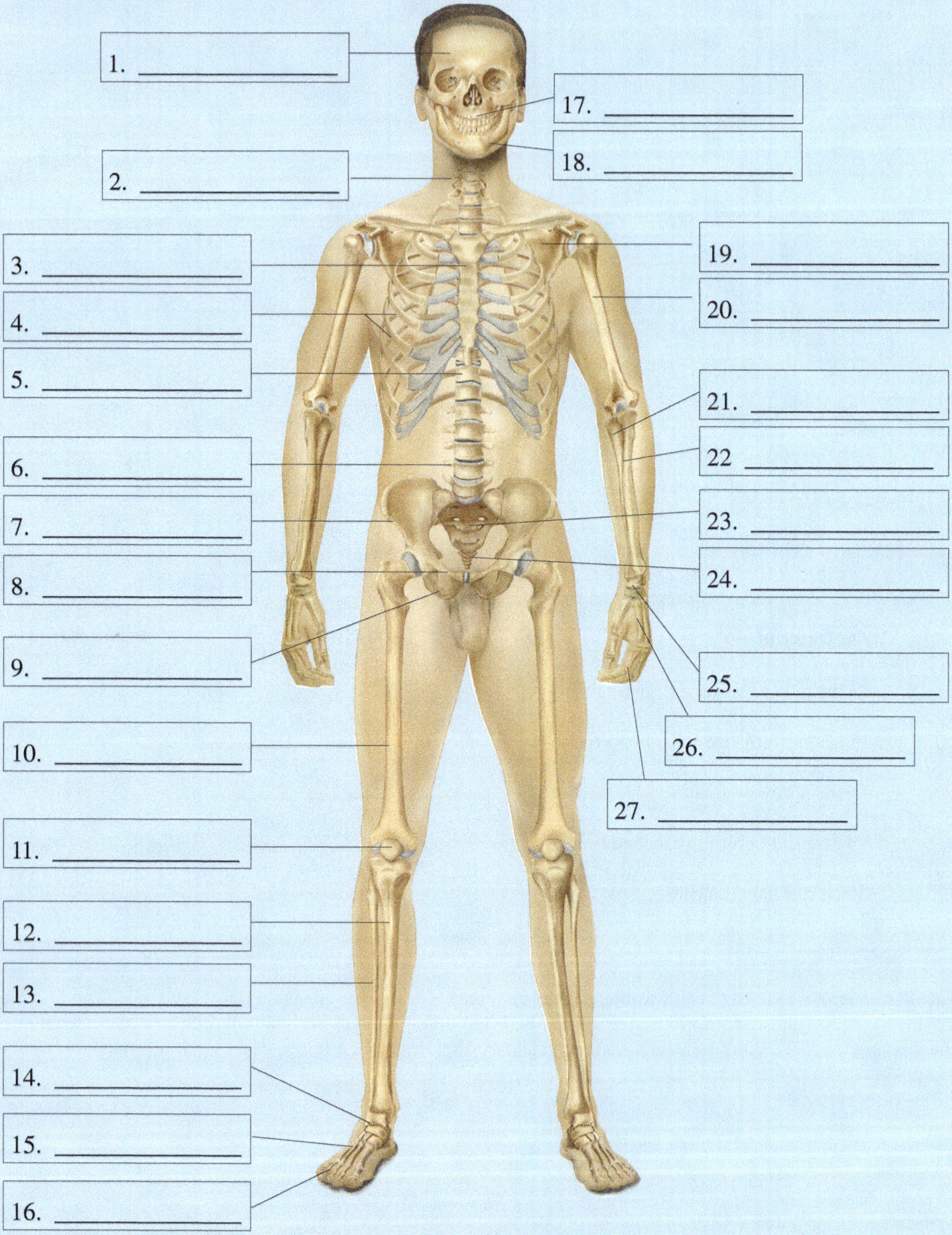

Image B

Write the labels for this figure on the numbered lines provided.

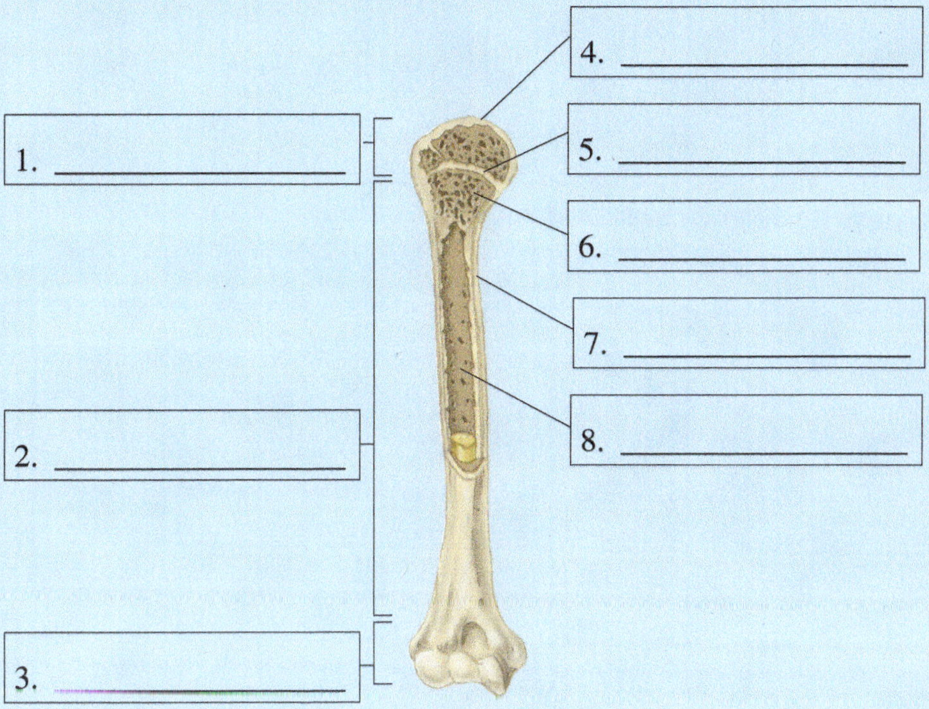

Image C

Write the labels for this figure on the numbered lines provided.

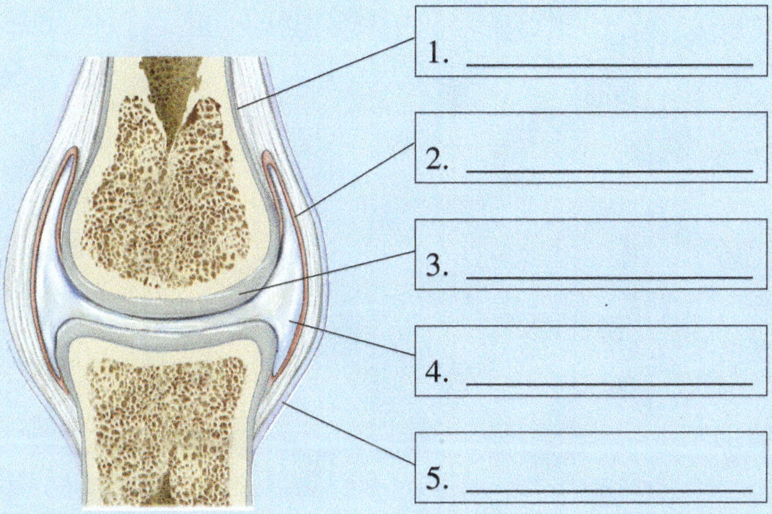

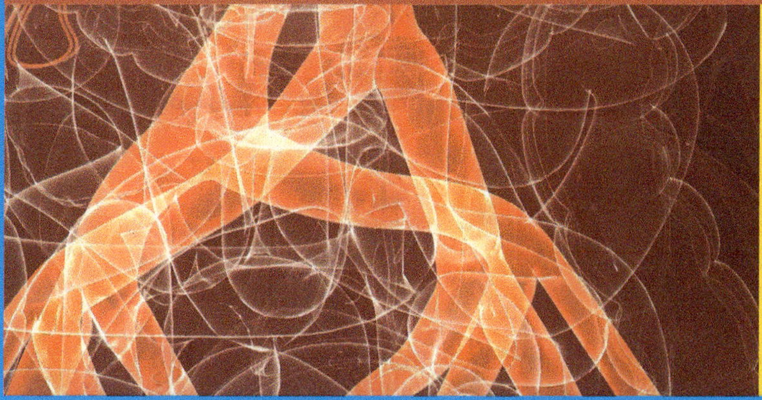

5

CARDIOVASCULAR SYSTEM

Learning Objectives

Upon completion of this chapter, you will be able to

- Identify and define the combining forms and suffixes introduced in this chapter.
- Correctly spell and pronounce medical terms and major anatomical structures relating to the cardiovascular system.
- Describe the major organs of the cardiovascular system and their functions.
- Describe the anatomy of the heart.
- Describe the flow of blood through the heart.
- Explain how the electrical conduction system controls the heartbeat.
- List and describe the characteristics of the three types of blood vessels.
- Define pulse and blood pressure.
- Identify and define cardiovascular system anatomical terms.
- Identify and define selected cardiovascular system pathology terms.
- Identify and define selected cardiovascular system diagnostic procedures.
- Identify and define selected cardiovascular system therapeutic procedures.
- Identify and define selected medications relating to the cardiovascular system.
- Define selected abbreviations associated with the cardiovascular system.

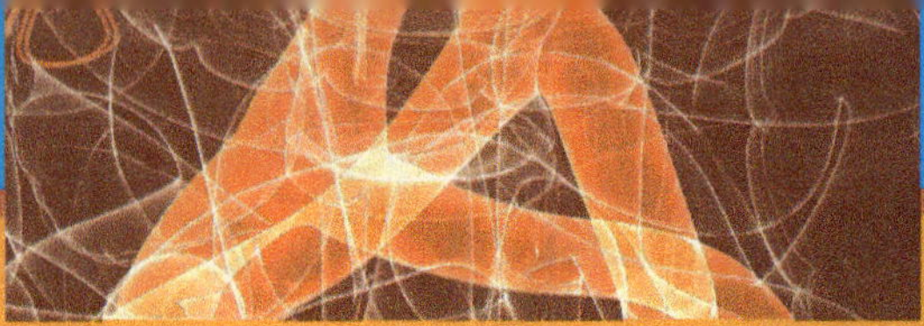

Cardiovascular System at a Glance

Function

The cardiovascular system consists of the pump and vessels that distribute blood to all areas of the body. This system allows for the delivery of needed substances to the cells of the body as well as for the removal of wastes.

Structures

Here are the primary structures that comprise the cardiovascular system.

blood vessels
- **arteries**
- **capillaries**
- **veins**

heart

Word Parts

Here are the most common word parts (with their meanings) used to build cardiovascular system terms. For a more comprehensive list, refer to the Terminology section of this chapter.

Combining Forms

angi/o	vessel
aort/o	aorta
arteri/o	artery
ather/o	fatty substance
atri/o	atrium
cardi/o	heart
coron/o	heart
corpor/o	body
embol/o	plug
isch/o	to hold back
myocardi/o	heart muscle
pect/o	chest
phleb/o	vein
sphygm/o	pulse
steth/o	chest
thromb/o	clot
valv/o	valve
valvul/o	valve
varic/o	dilated vein
vascul/o	blood vessel
vas/o	vessel, duct
ven/o	vein
ventricul/o	ventricle

Suffixes

-manometer	instrument to measure pressure
-ole	small
-tension	pressure
-tonic	pertaining to tone
-ule	small

Cardiovascular System Illustrated

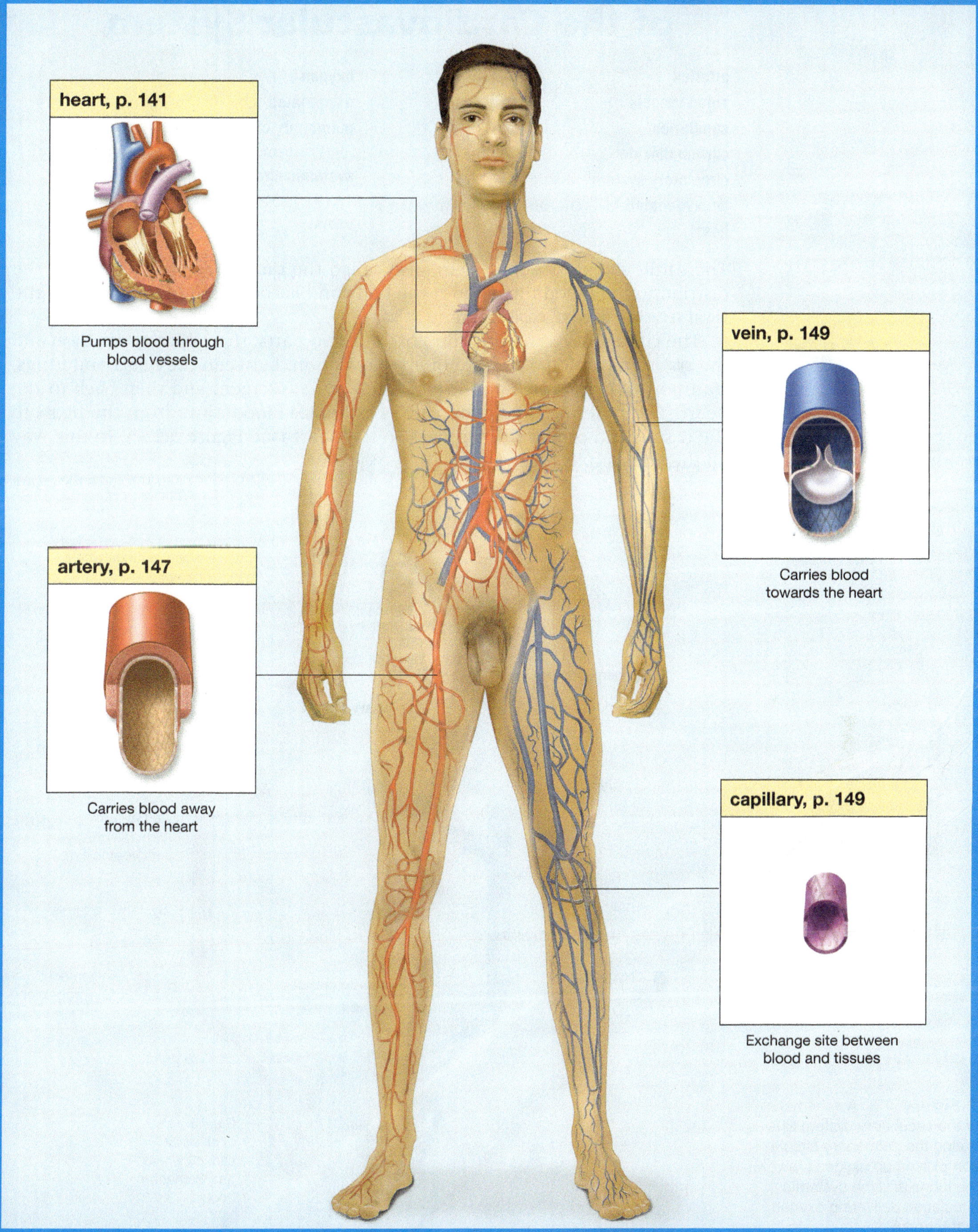

Anatomy and Physiology of the Cardiovascular System

arteries
blood vessels
capillaries
carbon dioxide
circulatory system
deoxygenated (dee-OK-sih-jen-ay-ted)
heart
oxygen
oxygenated (OK-sih-jen-ay-ted)
pulmonary circulation (PULL-mon-air-ee / ser-kew-LAY-shun)
systemic circulation (sis-TEM-ik / ser-kew-LAY-shun)
veins

The cardiovascular (CV) system, also called the **circulatory system,** maintains the distribution of blood throughout the body and is composed of the **heart** and the **blood vessels—arteries, capillaries,** and **veins.**

The circulatory system is composed of two parts: the **pulmonary circulation** and the **systemic circulation.** The pulmonary circulation, between the heart and lungs, transports **deoxygenated** blood to the lungs to get oxygen, and then back to the heart. The systemic circulation carries **oxygenated** blood away from the heart to the tissues and cells, and then back to the heart (see Figure 5.1 ■). In this way all the body's cells receive blood and oxygen.

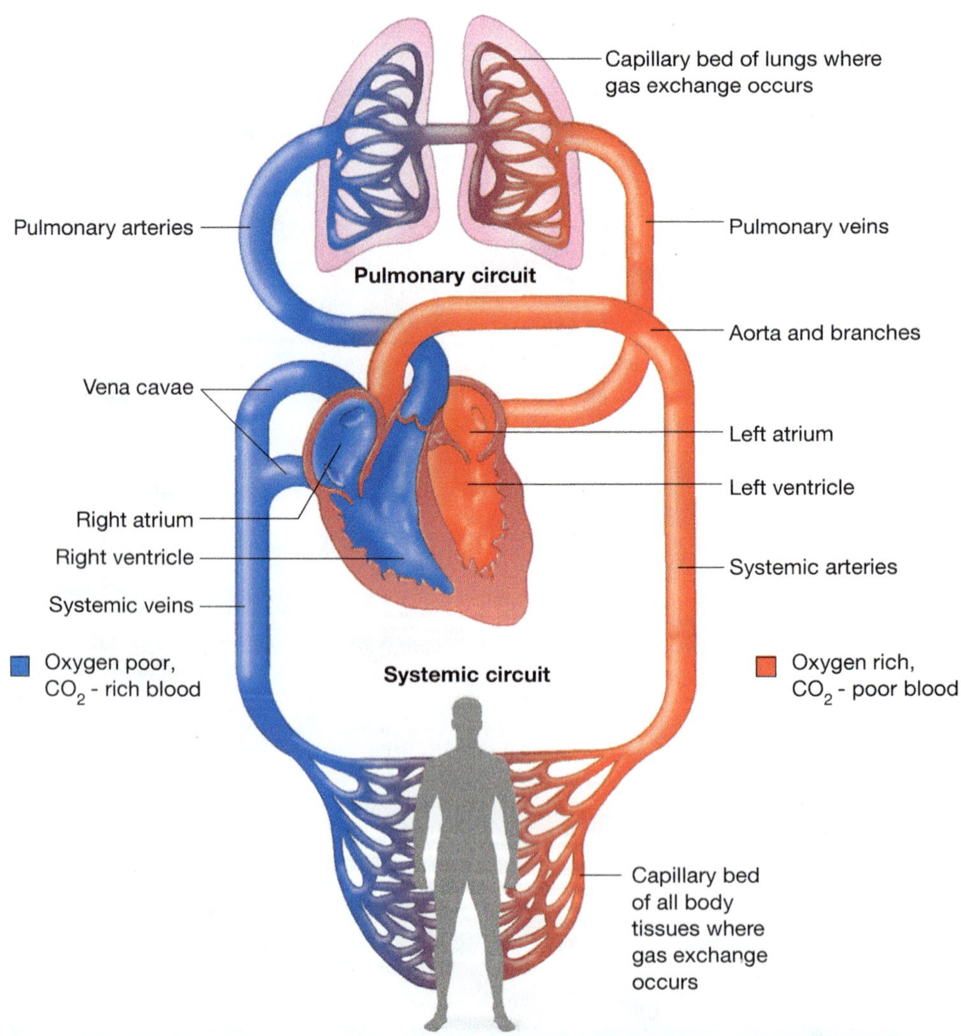

■ **Figure 5.1** A schematic of the circulatory system illustrating the pulmonary circulation picking up oxygen from the lungs and the systemic circulation delivering oxygen to the body.

In addition to distributing **oxygen** and other nutrients, such as glucose and amino acids, the cardiovascular system also collects the waste products from the body's cells. **Carbon dioxide** and other waste products produced by metabolic reaction are transported by the cardiovascular system to the lungs, liver, and kidneys where they are eliminated from the body.

MED TERM TIP

Many terms that were initiated in Greek were modified for use in Latin which does not have a "k" in their alphabet. The Latin terms replace the k with a "c". When using terms common to the cardiovascular system for example the original root term kardia was modified to *cardia.* commonly used in heart related words and word parts today.

Heart

apex (AY-peks)
cardiac muscle (CAR-dee-ak)

The heart is a muscular pump made up of **cardiac muscle** fibers that could be considered a muscle rather than an organ. It has four chambers, or cavities, and beats an average of 60–100 beats per minute (bpm) or about 100,000 times in one day. Each time the cardiac muscle contracts, blood is ejected from the heart and pushed throughout the body within the blood vessels.

The heart is located in the mediastinum in the center of the chest cavity; however, it is not exactly centered; more of the heart is on the left side of the mediastinum than the right (see Figure 5.2 ■). At about the size of a fist and shaped like an upside-down pear, the heart lies directly behind the sternum. The tip of the heart at the lower edge is called the **apex**.

MED TERM TIP

Your heart is approximately the size of your clenched fist and pumps 4,000 gallons of blood each day. It will beat at least three billion times during your lifetime.

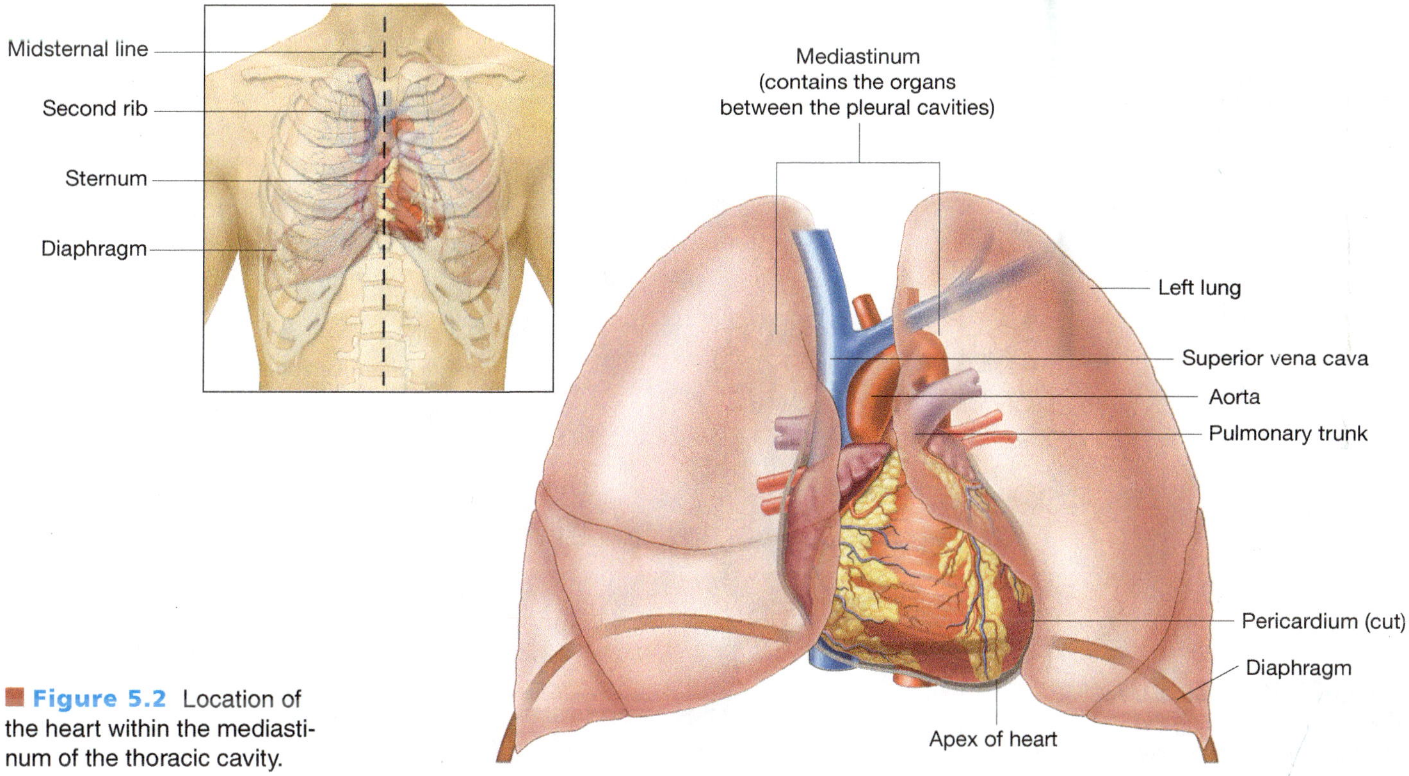

■ **Figure 5.2** Location of the heart within the mediastinum of the thoracic cavity.

Heart Layers

endocardium (en-doh-CAR-dee-um)
epicardium (ep-ih-CAR-dee-um)
myocardium (my-oh-CAR-dee-um)
parietal pericardium (pah-RYE-eh-tal / pair-ih-CAR-dee-um)
pericardium (pair-ih-CAR-dee-um)
visceral pericardium (VISS-er-al / pair-ih-CAR-dee-um)

The wall of the heart is quite thick and composed of three layers (see Figure 5.3 ■):

1. The **endocardium** is the inner layer of the heart lining the heart chambers. It is a very smooth, thin layer that serves to reduce friction as the blood passes through the heart chambers.
2. The **myocardium** is the thick, muscular middle layer of the heart. Contraction of this muscle layer develops the pressure required to pump blood through the blood vessels.
3. The **epicardium** is the outer layer of the heart. The heart is enclosed within a double-layered pleural sac, called the **pericardium.** The epicardium is the **visceral pericardium,** or inner layer of the sac. The outer layer of the sac is the **parietal pericardium.** Fluid between the two layers of the sac reduces friction as the heart beats.

MED TERM TIP

These layers become important when studying the disease conditions affecting the heart. For instance, when the prefix *endo-* is added to *carditis,* forming *endocarditis,* we know that the inflammation is within the "inner layer of the heart." In discussing the muscular action of the heart, the prefix *myo-,* meaning "muscle," is added to *cardium* to form the word *myocardium.* The diagnosis *myocardial infarction* (MI), or heart attack, means that the patient has an infarct or "dead tissue in the muscle of the heart." The prefix *peri-,* meaning "around," when added to the word *cardium* refers to the sac "surrounding the heart." Therefore, *pericarditis* is an "inflammation of the outer sac of the heart."

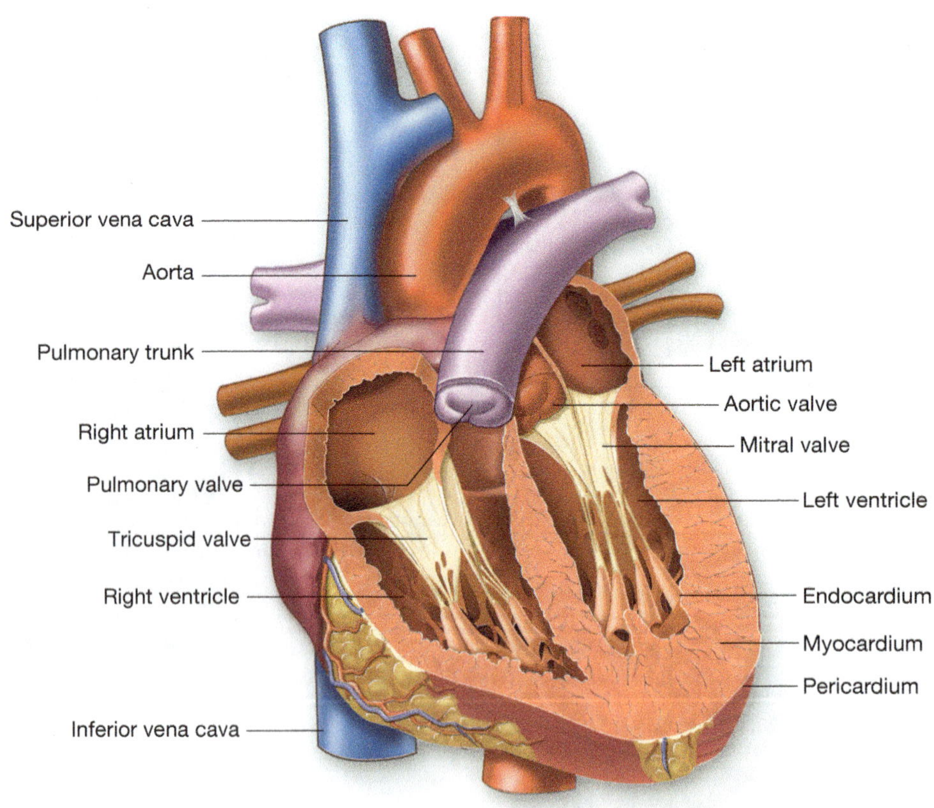

■ **Figure 5.3** Internal view of the heart illustrating the heart chambers, heart layers, and major blood vessels associated with the heart.

Heart Chambers

atria (AY-tree-ah)

interatrial septum (in-ter-AY-tree-al / SEP-tum)

interventricular septum (in-ter-ven-TRIK-yoo-lar / SEP-tum)

ventricles (VEN-trik-lz)

The heart is divided into four chambers or cavities (see Figures 5.3 and 5.4). There are two **atria,** or upper chambers, and two **ventricles,** or lower chambers. These chambers are divided into right and left sides by walls called the **interatrial septum** and the **interventricular septum.** The atria are the receiving chambers of the heart. Blood returning to the heart via veins first collects in the atria. The ventricles are the pumping chambers. They have a much thicker myocardium and their contraction ejects blood out of the heart and into the great arteries.

MED TERM TIP

The term *ventricle* comes from the Latin term *venter,* which means "little belly." Although it originally referred to the abdomen and then the stomach, it came to stand for any hollow region inside an organ.

Heart Valves

aortic valve (ay-OR-tik)

atrioventricular valve (ay-tree-oh-ven-TRIK-yoo-lar)

bicuspid valve (bye-CUSS-pid)

cusps

mitral valve (MY-tral)

pulmonary valve (PULL-mon-air-ee)

semilunar valve (sem-ih-LOO-nar)

tricuspid valve (try-CUSS-pid)

Four valves act as restraining gates to control the direction of blood flow. They are situated at the entrances and exits to the ventricles (see Figure 5.4 ■). Properly functioning valves allow blood to flow only in the forward direction by blocking it from returning to the previous chamber.

The four valves are as follows:

1. **Tricuspid valve:** an **atrioventricular valve** (AV), meaning that it controls the opening between the right atrium and the right ventricle. Once the blood enters the right ventricle, it cannot go back up into the atrium again. The prefix *tri-,* meaning three, indicates that this valve has three leaflets or **cusps.**
2. **Pulmonary valve:** a **semilunar valve.** The prefix *semi-,* meaning half, and the term **lunar,** meaning moon, indicate that this valve looks like a half moon. Located between the right ventricle and the pulmonary artery, this valve prevents blood that has been ejected into the pulmonary artery from returning to the right ventricle as it relaxes.
3. **Mitral valve:** also called the **bicuspid valve,** indicating that it has two cusps. Blood flows through this atrioventricular valve to the left ventricle and cannot go back up into the left atrium.
4. **Aortic valve:** a semilunar valve located between the left ventricle and the aorta. Blood leaves the left ventricle through this valve and cannot return to the left ventricle.

MED TERM TIP

The heart makes two distinct sounds referred to as "lub-dupp." These sounds are produced by the forceful snapping shut of the heart valves. *Lub* is the closing of the atrioventricular valves. *Dupp* is the closing of the semilunar valves.

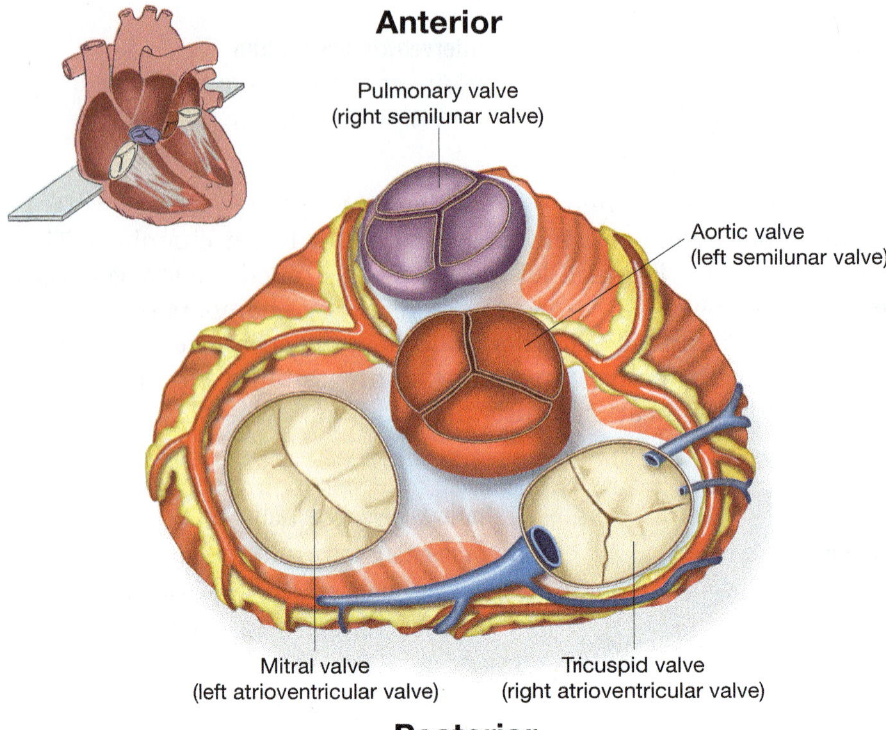

■ **Figure 5.4** Superior view of heart valves illustrating position, size, and shape of each valve.

Blood Flow Through the Heart

aorta (ay-OR-tah)
diastole (dye-ASS-toe-lee)
inferior vena cava (VEE-nah / KAY-vah)
pulmonary artery (PULL-mon-air-ee)
pulmonary veins
superior vena cava
systole (SIS-toe-lee)

The flow of blood through the heart is very orderly (see Figure 5.5 ■). It progresses through the heart to the lungs, where it receives oxygen; then goes back to the heart; and then out to the body tissues and parts. The normal process of blood flow is:

1. Deoxygenated blood from all the tissues in the body enters a relaxed right atrium via two large veins called the **superior vena cava** and **inferior vena cava.**
2. The right atrium contracts and blood flows through the tricuspid valve into the relaxed right ventricle.
3. The right ventricle then contracts and blood is pumped through the pulmonary valve into the **pulmonary artery,** which carries it to the lungs for oxygenation.
4. The left atrium receives blood returning to the heart after being oxygenated by the lungs. This blood enters the relaxed left atrium from the four **pulmonary veins.**
5. The left atrium contracts and blood flows through the mitral valve into the relaxed left ventricle.
6. When the left ventricle contracts, the blood is pumped through the aortic valve and into the **aorta,** the largest artery in the body. The aorta carries blood to all parts of the body.

It can be seen that the heart chambers alternate between relaxing in order to fill and contracting to push blood forward. The period of time a chamber is relaxed is **diastole.** The contraction phase is **systole.**

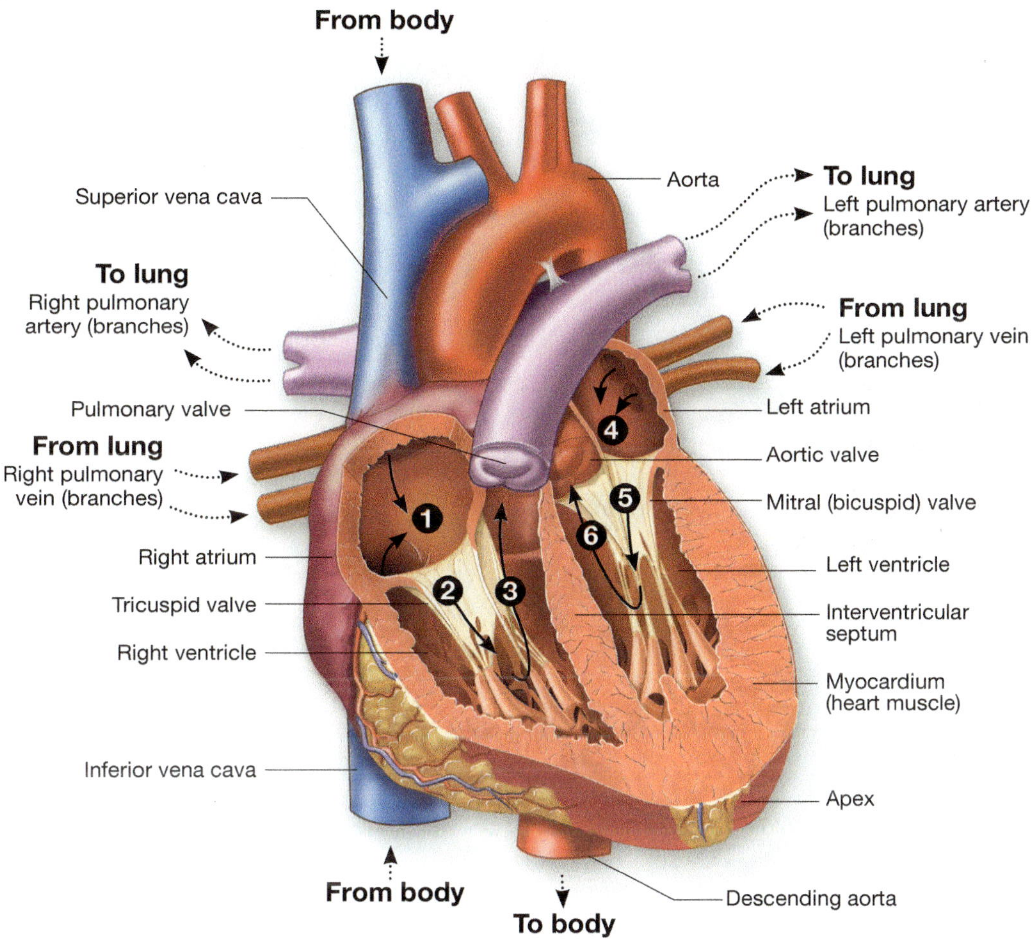

■ **Figure 5.5** The path of blood flow through the chambers of the left and right side of the heart, including the veins delivering blood to the heart and arteries receiving blood ejected from the heart.

Conduction System of the Heart

atrioventricular bundle
atrioventricular node
autonomic nervous system (aw-toh-NOM-ik / NER-vus / SIS-tem)
bundle branches
bundle of His
pacemaker
Purkinje fibers (per-KIN-gee)
sinoatrial node (sigh-noh-AY-tree-al)

The heart rate is regulated by the **autonomic nervous system;** therefore, we have no voluntary control over the beating of our heart. Special tissue within the heart is responsible for conducting an electrical impulse stimulating the different chambers to contract in the correct order.

The path that the impulses travel is as follows (see Figure 5.6 ■):

1. The **sinoatrial (SA) node,** or **pacemaker,** is where the electrical impulses begin. From the sinoatrial node a wave of electricity travels through the atria, causing them to contract, or go into systole.
2. The **atrioventricular node** is stimulated.
3. This node transfers the stimulation wave to the **atrioventricular bundle** (formerly called **bundle of His**).
4. The electrical signal next travels down the **bundle branches** within the interventricular septum.
5. The **Purkinje fibers** out in the ventricular myocardium are stimulated, resulting in ventricular systole.

■ **Figure 5.6** The conduction system of the heart; traces the path of the electrical impulse that stimulates the heart chambers to contract in the correct sequence.

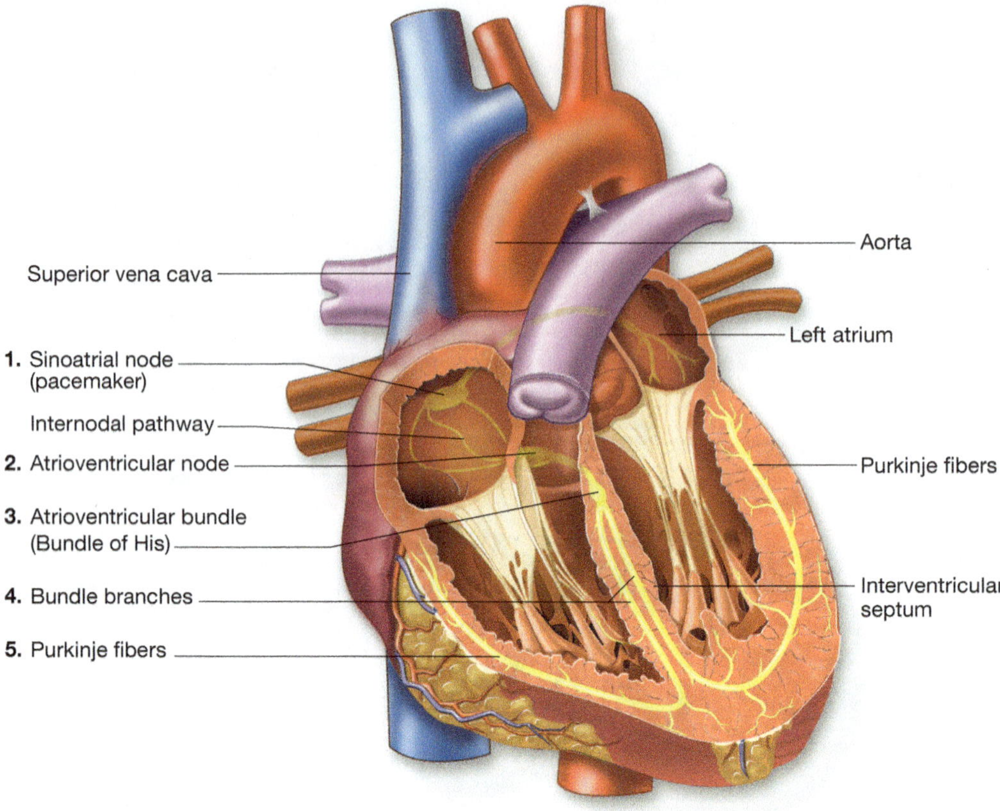

■ **Figure 5.7** An electrocardiogram (EKG) wave, a record of the electrical signal as it moves through the conduction system of the heart. This signal stimulates the chambers of the heart to contract and relax in the proper sequence.

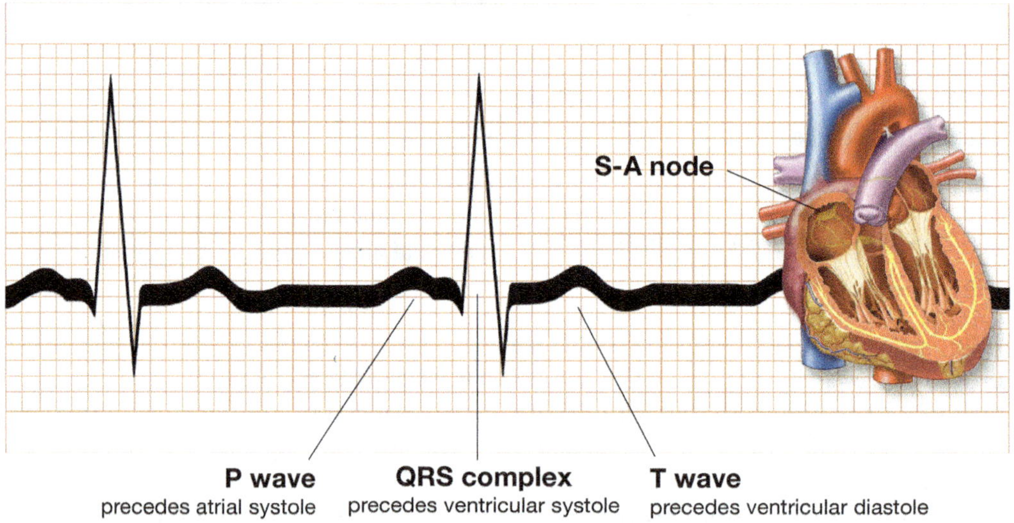

MED TERM TIP

The electrocardiogram, referred to as an EKG or ECG, is a measurement of the electrical activity of the heart (see Figure 5.7 ■). This can give the physician information about the health of the heart, especially the myocardium.

Blood Vessels

lumen (LOO-men)

There are three types of blood vessels: arteries, capillaries, and veins (see Figure 5.8 ■). These are the pipes that circulate blood throughout the body. The **lumen** is the channel within these vessels through which blood flows.

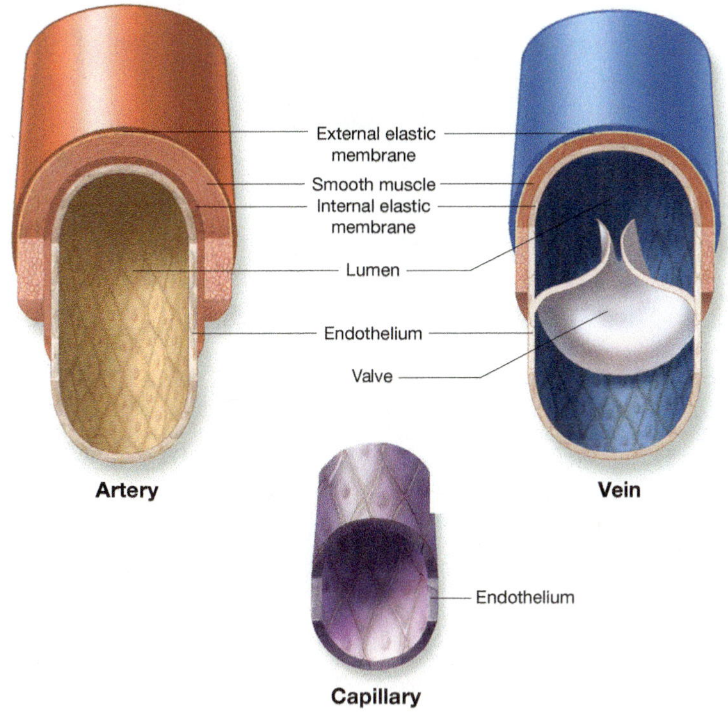

■ **Figure 5.8** Comparative structure of arteries, capillaries, and veins.

Arteries

arterioles (ar-TEE-ree-ohlz)

coronary arteries (KOR-ah-nair-ee / AR-te-reez)

The arteries are the large, thick-walled vessels that carry the blood away from the heart. The walls of arteries contain a thick layer of smooth muscle that can contract or relax to change the size of the arterial lumen. The pulmonary artery carries deoxygenated blood from the right ventricle to the lungs. The largest artery, the aorta, begins from the left ventricle of the heart and carries oxygenated blood to all the body systems. The **coronary arteries** then branch from the aorta and provide blood to the myocardium (see Figure 5.9 ■). As they travel through the body, the arteries branch into progressively smaller sized arteries. The smallest of the arteries, called **arterioles,** deliver blood to the capillaries. Figure 5.10 ■ illustrates the major systemic arteries.

MED TERM TIP

The term *coronary,* from the Latin word for crown, describes how the great vessels encircle the heart as they emerge from the top of the heart.

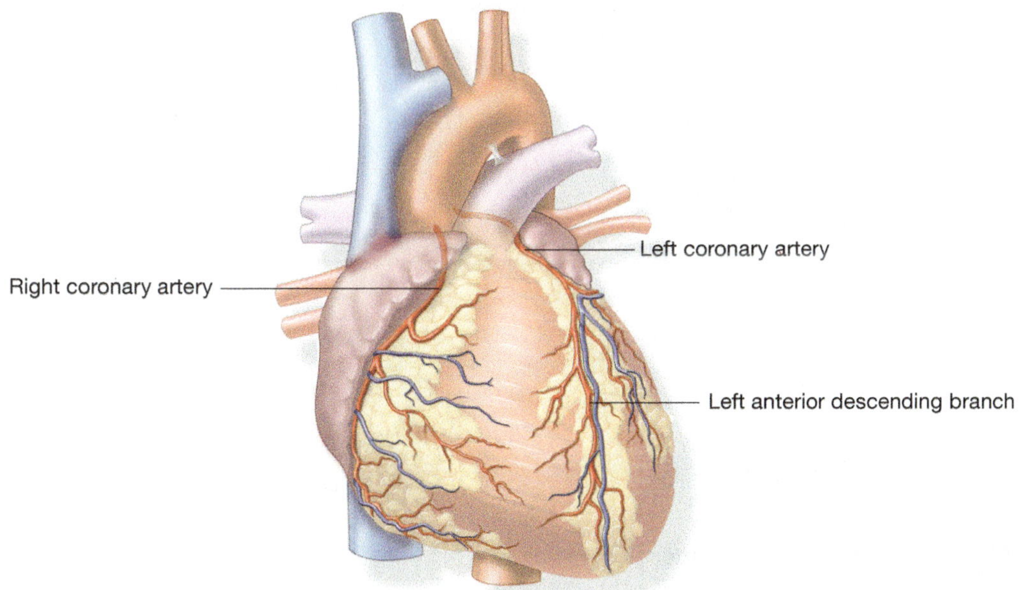

■ **Figure 5.9** The coronary arteries.

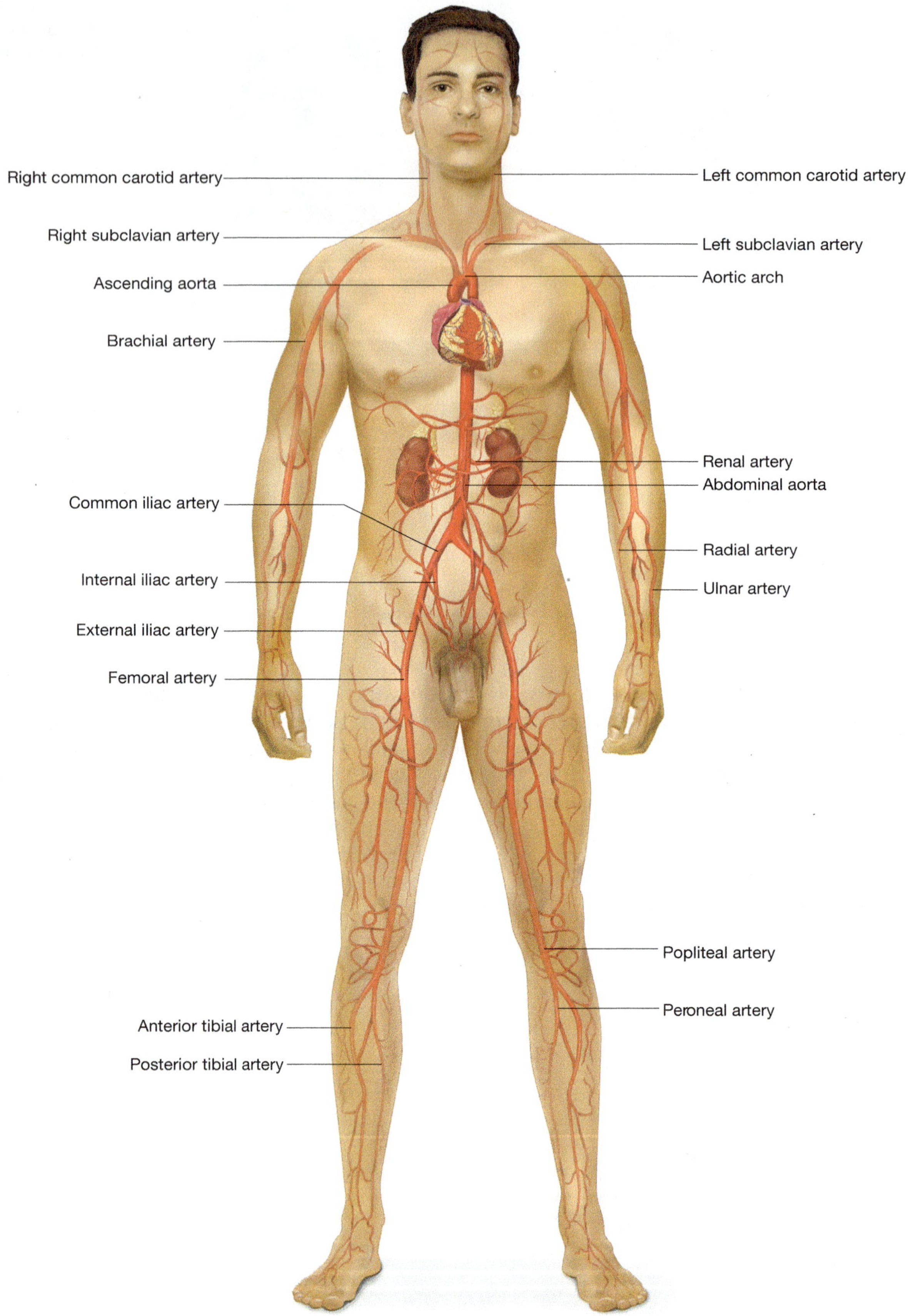

Figure 5.10 The major arteries of the body.

Capillaries

capillary bed

Capillaries are a network of tiny blood vessels referred to as a **capillary bed.** Arterial blood flows into a capillary bed, and venous blood flows back out. Capillaries are very thin walled, allowing for the diffusion of the oxygen and nutrients from the blood into the body tissues (see Figure 5.8). Likewise, carbon dioxide and waste products are able to diffuse out of the body tissues and into the bloodstream to be carried away. Since the capillaries are so small in diameter, the blood will not flow as quickly through them as it does through the arteries and veins. This means that the blood has time for an exchange of nutrients, oxygen, and waste material to take place. As blood exits a capillary bed, it returns to the heart through a vein.

Veins

venules (VEN-yools)

The veins carry blood back to the heart (see Figure 5.8). Blood leaving capillaries first enters small **venules,** which then merge into larger veins. Veins have much thinner walls than arteries, causing them to collapse easily. The veins also have valves that allow the blood to move only toward the heart. These valves prevent blood from backflowing, ensuring that blood always flows toward the heart. The two large veins that enter the heart are the superior vena cava, which carries blood from the upper body, and the inferior vena cava, which carries blood from the lower body. Blood pressure in the veins is much lower than in the arteries. Muscular action against the veins and skeletal muscle contractions help in the movement of blood. Figure 5.11 ■ illustrates the major systemic veins.

Pulse and Blood Pressure

blood pressure (BP)
diastolic pressure (dye-ah-STOL-ik)
pulse
systolic pressure (sis-TOL-ik)

Blood pressure (BP) is a measurement of the force exerted by blood against the wall of a blood vessel. During ventricular systole, blood is under a lot of pressure from the ventricular contraction, giving the highest blood pressure reading—the **systolic pressure.** The **pulse** felt at the wrist or throat is the surge of blood caused by the heart contraction. This is why pulse rate is normally equal to heart rate. During ventricular diastole, blood is not being pushed by the heart at all and the blood pressure reading drops to its lowest point—the **diastolic pressure.** Therefore, to see the full range of what is occurring with blood pressure, both numbers are required. Blood pressure is also affected by several other characteristics of the blood and the blood vessels. These include the elasticity of the arteries, the diameter of the blood vessels, the viscosity of the blood, the volume of blood flowing through the vessels, and the amount of resistance to blood flow.

MED TERM TIP

The instrument used to measure blood pressure is called a *sphygmomanometer.* The combining form *sphygm/o* means "pulse" and the suffix *-manometer* means "instrument to measure pressure." A blood pressure reading is reported as two numbers, for example, 120/80. The 120 is the systolic pressure and the 80 is the diastolic pressure. There is no one "normal" blood pressure number. The normal blood pressure for an adult is a systolic pressure less than 120 and diastolic pressure less than 80.

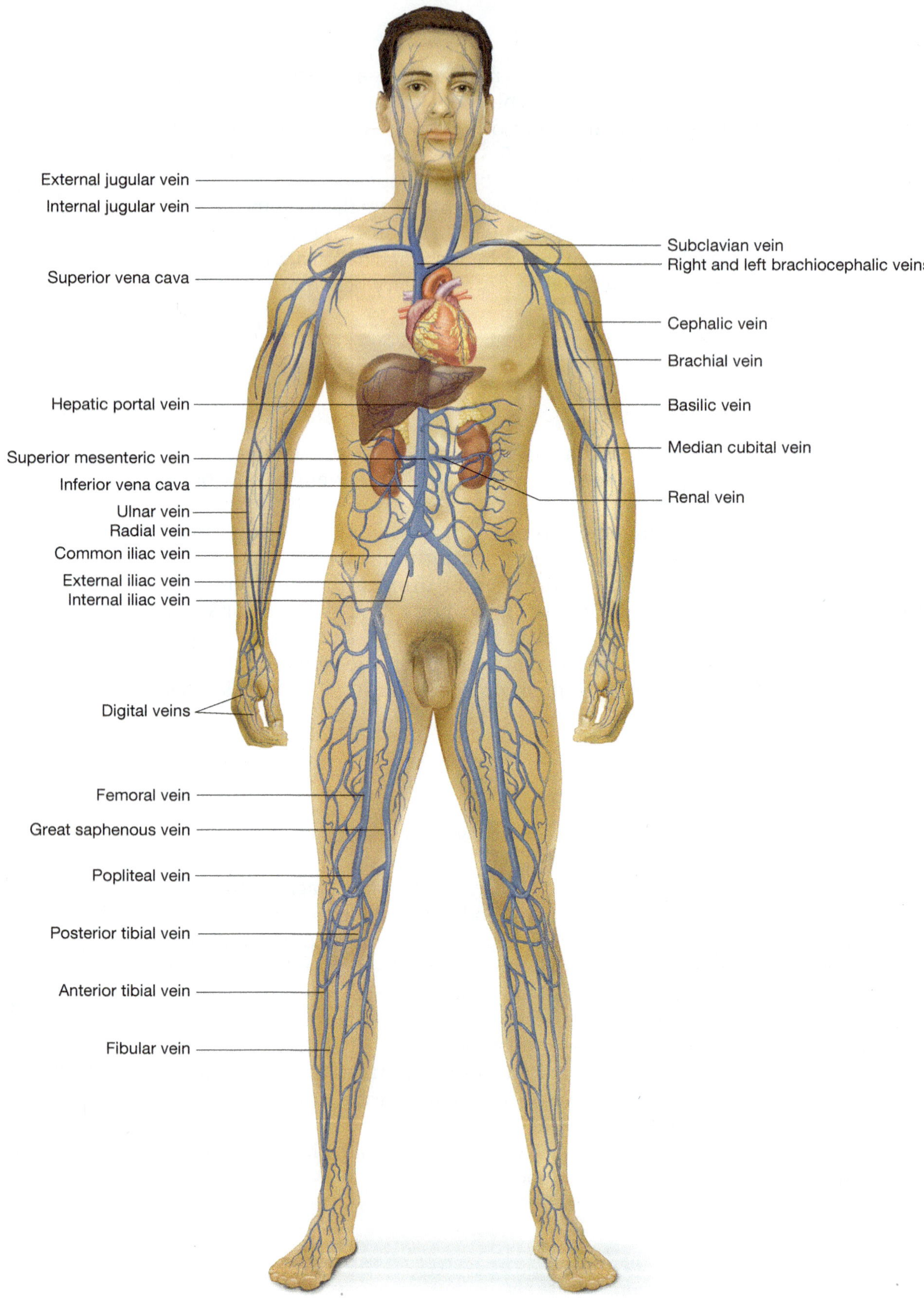

Figure 5.11 The major veins of the body.

Terminology

Word Parts Used to Build Cardiovascular System Terms

The following lists contain the combining forms, suffixes, and prefixes used to build terms in the remaining sections of this chapter.

Combining Forms

aort/o	aorta
angi/o	vessel
arteri/o	artery
ather/o	fatty substance
atri/o	atrium
cardi/o	heart
coron/o	heart
corpor/o	body
cutane/o	skin
duct/o	to bring
electr/o	electricity

embol/o	plug
hem/o	blood
isch/o	to hold back
lip/o	fat
my/o	muscle
myocardi/o	heart muscle
orth/o	straight
pector/o	chest
phleb/o	vein
pulmon/o	lung
sept/o	a wall

son/o	sound
sphygm/o	pulse
steth/o	chest
thromb/o	clot
valv/o	valve
valvul/o	valve
varic/o	dilated vein
vas/o	vessel
vascul/o	blood vessel
ven/o	vein
ventricul/o	ventricle

Suffixes

-ac	pertaining to
-al	pertaining to
-ar	pertaining to
-ary	pertaining to
-eal	pertaining to
-ectomy	surgical removal
-gram	record
-graphy	process of recording
-ia	condition
-ic	pertaining to
-itis	inflammation

-logy	study of
-lytic	destruction
-manometer	instrument to measure pressure
-megaly	enlarged
-ole	small
-oma	growth
-ose	pertaining to
-ous	pertaining to
-pathy	disease
-plasty	surgical repair

-rrhexis	rupture
-sclerosis	hardening
-scope	instrument for viewing
-spasm	involuntary muscle contraction
-stenosis	narrowing
-tension	pressure
-tic	pertaining to
-tonic	pertaining to tone
-ule	small

Prefixes

a-	without
anti-	against
brady-	slow
de-	without
endo-	inner
extra-	outside of

hyper-	excessive
hypo-	insufficient
inter-	between
intra-	within
per-	through
peri-	around

poly-	many
tachy-	fast
tetra-	four
trans-	across
ultra-	beyond

Anatomical Terms

TERM	WORD PARTS	DEFINITION
aortic (ay-OR-tik)	aort/o = aorta -ic = pertaining to	Pertaining to the aorta
arterial (ar-TEE-ree-al)	arteri/o = artery -al = pertaining to	Pertaining to an artery
arteriole (ar-TEE-ree-ohl)	arteri/o = artery -ole = small	A small (narrow in diameter) artery
atrial (AY-tree-al)	atri/o = atrium -al = pertaining to	Pertaining to the atrium
cardiac (CAR-dee-ak)	cardi/o = heart -ac = pertaining to	Pertaining to the heart
coronary (KOR-ah-nair-ee)	coron/o = heart -ary = pertaining to	Pertaining to the heart
interatrial (in-ter-AY-tree-al)	inter- = between atri/o = atrium -al = pertaining to	Pertaining to between the atria
interventricular (in-ter-ven-TRIK-yoo-lar)	inter- = between ventricul/o = ventricle -ar = pertaining to	Pertaining to between the ventricles
myocardial (my-oh-CAR-dee-al)	myocardi/o = heart muscle -al = pertaining to	Pertaining to heart muscle
valvular (VAL-view-lar)	valvul/o = valve -ar = pertaining to	Pertaining to a valve
vascular (VAS-kwee-lar)	vascul/o = blood vessel -ar = pertaining to	Pertaining to a blood vessel
venous (VEE-nus)	ven/o = vein -ous = pertaining to	Pertaining to a vein
ventricular (ven-TRIK-yoo-lar)	ventricul/o = ventricle -ar = pertaining to	Pertaining to a ventricle
venule (VEN-yool)	ven/o = vein -ule = small	A small (narrow in diameter) vein

Pathology

TERM	WORD PARTS	DEFINITION
Medical Specialties		
cardiology (car-dee-ALL-oh-jee)	cardi/o = heart -logy = study of	The branch of medicine involving diagnosis and treatment of conditions and diseases of the cardiovascular system. Physician is a *cardiologist.*
cardiovascular technician	cardi/o = heart vascul/o = blood vessel -ar = pertaining to	Healthcare professional trained to perform a variety of diagnostic and therapeutic procedures including electrocardiography, echocardiography, and exercise stress tests.

Pathology *(continued)*

TERM	WORD PARTS	DEFINITION
Signs and Symptoms		
angiitis (an-jee-EYE-tis)	angi/o = vessel -itis = inflammation	Inflammation of a vessel.
angiospasm (AN-jee-oh-spazm)	angi/o = vessel -spasm = involuntary muscle contraction	An involuntary muscle contraction of the smooth muscle in the wall of a vessel; narrows the vessel.
angiostenosis (an-jee-oh-sten-OH-sis)	angi/o = vessel -stenosis = narrowing	The narrowing of a vessel.
bradycardia (brad-ee-CAR-dee-ah)	brady- = slow cardi/o = heart -ia = condition	The condition of having a slow heart rate; typically less than 60 beats/minute; highly trained aerobic persons may normally have a slow heart rate.
embolus (EM-boh-lus)	embol/o = plug	The obstruction of a blood vessel by a blood clot that has broken off from a thrombus somewhere else in the body and traveled to the point of obstruction. If it occurs in a coronary artery, it may result in a myocardial infarction.

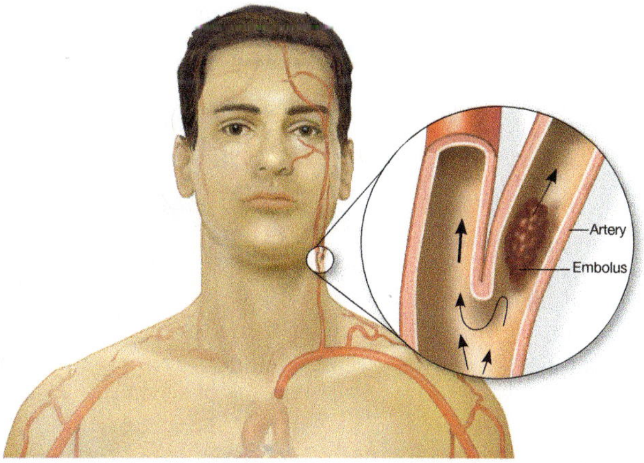

Figure 5.12 Illustration of an embolus floating in an artery. The embolus will become lodged in a blood vessel that is smaller than it is, resulting in occlusion of that artery.

TERM	WORD PARTS	DEFINITION
infarct (IN-farkt)		An area of tissue within an organ or part that undergoes necrosis (death) following the loss of its blood supply.
ischemia (is-KEYH-mee-ah)	isch/o = to hold back hem/o = blood -ia = condition	The localized and temporary deficiency of blood supply due to an obstruction to the circulation.
murmur (MUR-mur)		A sound, in addition to the normal heart sounds, arising from blood flowing through the heart. This extra sound may or may not indicate a heart abnormality.
orthostatic hypotension (or-thoh-STAT-ik)	orth/o = straight hypo- = insufficient -tension = pressure	The sudden drop in blood pressure a person experiences when standing straight up suddenly.
palpitations (pal-pih-TAY-shunz)		Pounding, racing heartbeats.

Pathology *(continued)*

TERM	WORD PARTS	DEFINITION
plaque (plak)		A yellow, fatty deposit of lipids in an artery that is the hallmark of atherosclerosis. Also called an *atheroma.*
regurgitation (re-ger-gih-TAY-shun)		To flow backwards. In the cardiovascular system this refers to the backflow of blood through a valve.
tachycardia (tak-ee-CAR-dee-ah)	tachy- = fast cardi/o = heart -ia = condition	The condition of having a fast heart rate; typically more than 100 beats/minute while at rest.
thrombus (THROM-bus)	thromb/o = clot	A blood clot forming within a blood vessel. May partially or completely occlude the blood vessel.

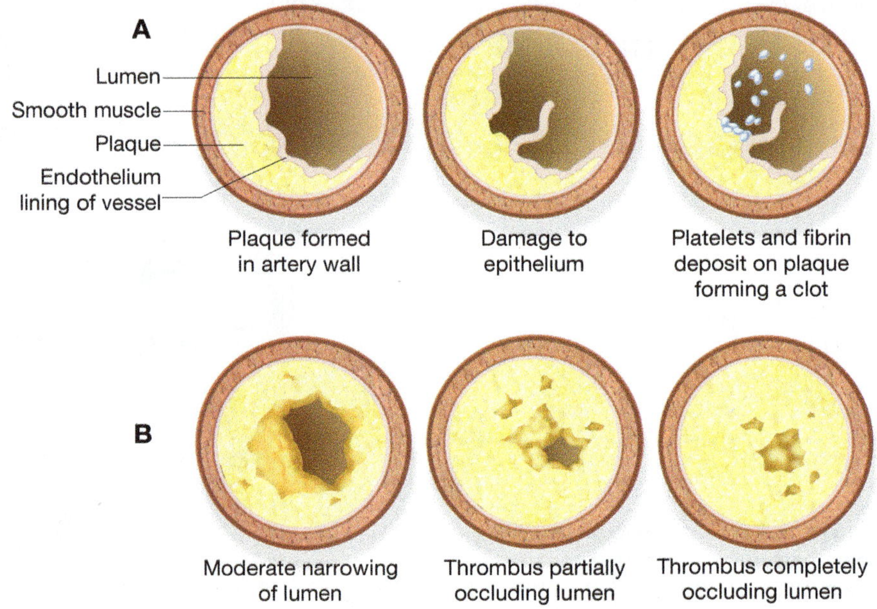

Figure 5.13 Development of an atherosclerotic plaque that progressively narrows the lumen of an artery to the point that a thrombus fully occludes the lumen.

Heart

TERM	WORD PARTS	DEFINITION
angina pectoris (an-JYE-nah / PECK-tor-is)	pector/o = chest	Condition in which there is severe pain with a sensation of constriction around the heart. Caused by a deficiency of oxygen to the heart muscle.
arrhythmia (ah-RITH-mee-ah)	a- = without -ia = condition	Irregularity in the heartbeat or action. Comes in many different forms; some are not serious, while others are life-threatening.
bundle branch block (BBB)		Occurs when the electrical impulse is blocked from traveling down the bundle of His or bundle branches. Results in the ventricles beating at a different rate than the atria. Also called a *heart block.*
cardiac arrest	cardi/o = heart -ac = pertaining to	Complete stopping of heart activity.
cardiomegaly (car-dee-oh-MEG-ah-lee)	cardi/o = heart -megaly = enlarged	An enlarged heart.

Pathology *(continued)*

TERM	WORD PARTS	DEFINITION
cardiomyopathy (car-dee-oh-my-OP-ah-thee)	cardi/o = heart my/o = muscle -pathy = disease	General term for a disease of the myocardium. Can be caused by alcohol abuse, parasites, viral infection, and congestive heart failure. One of the most common reasons a patient may require a heart transplant.
congenital septal defect (CSD)	sept/o = a wall -al = pertaining to	A hole, present at birth, in the septum between two heart chambers; results in a mixture of oxygenated and deoxygenated blood. There can be an *atrial septal defect* (ASD) and a *ventricular septal defect* (VSD).
congestive heart failure (CHF) (kon-JESS-tiv)		Pathological condition of the heart in which there is a reduced outflow of blood from the left side of the heart because the left ventricle myocardium has become too weak to efficiently pump blood. Results in weakness, breathlessness, and edema.
coronary artery disease (CAD) (KOR-ah-nair-ee)	coron/o = heart -ary = pertaining to	Insufficient blood supply to the heart muscle due to an obstruction of one or more coronary arteries. May be caused by atherosclerosis and may cause angina pectoris and myocardial infarction.

MED TERM TIP

All types of cardiovascular disease have been the number one killer of Americans since the 19th century. This disease kills more people annually than the next six causes of death combined.

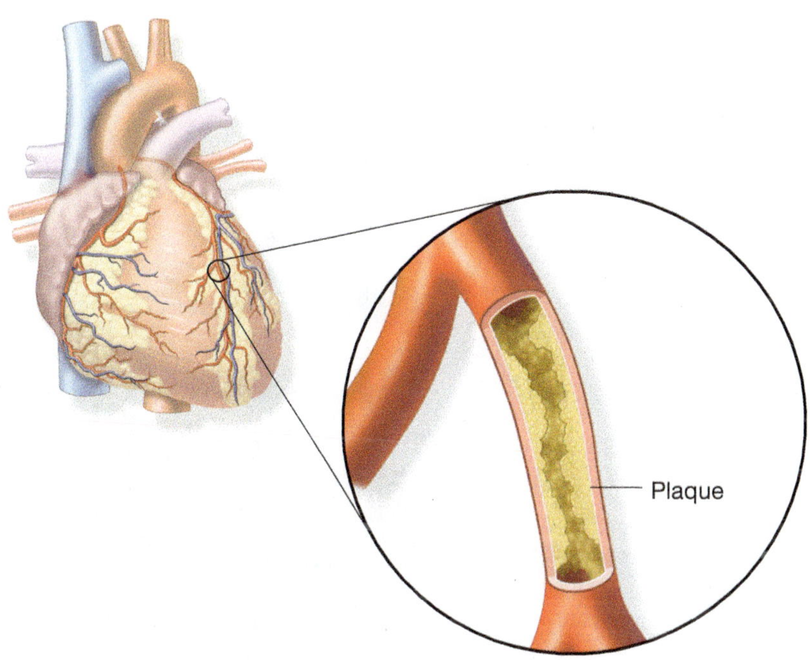

Figure 5.14 Formation of an atherosclerotic plaque within a coronary artery; may lead to coronary artery disease, angina pectoris, and myocardial infarction.

TERM	WORD PARTS	DEFINITION
endocarditis (en-doh-car-DYE-tis)	endo- = inner cardi/o = heart -itis = inflammation	Inflammation of the lining membranes of the heart. May be due to bacteria or to an abnormal immunological response. In bacterial endocarditis, the mass of bacteria that forms is referred to as *vegetation.*

Pathology *(continued)*

TERM	WORD PARTS	DEFINITION
fibrillation (fih-brill-AY-shun)		An extremely serious arrhythmia characterized by an abnormal quivering or contraction of heart fibers. When this occurs in the ventricles, cardiac arrest and death can occur. Emergency equipment to defibrillate, or convert the heart to a normal beat, is necessary.
flutter		An arrhythmia in which the atria beat too rapidly, but in a regular pattern.
heart valve prolapse (PROH-laps)		Condition in which the cusps or flaps of the heart valve are too loose and fail to shut tightly, allowing blood to flow backward through the valve when the heart chamber contracts. Most commonly occurs in the mitral valve, but may affect any of the heart valves.
heart valve stenosis (steh-NOH-sis)	-stenosis = narrowing	The cusps or flaps of the heart valve are too stiff. Therefore, they are unable to open fully, making it difficult for blood to flow through, or shut tightly, allowing blood to flow backward. This condition may affect any of the heart valves.
myocardial infarction (MI) (my-oh-CAR-dee-al / in-FARC-shun)	myocardi/o = heart muscle -al = pertaining to	Condition caused by the partial or complete occlusion or closing of one or more of the coronary arteries. Symptoms include a squeezing pain or heavy pressure in the middle of the chest (angina pectoris). A delay in treatment could result in death. Also referred to as a *heart attack.*

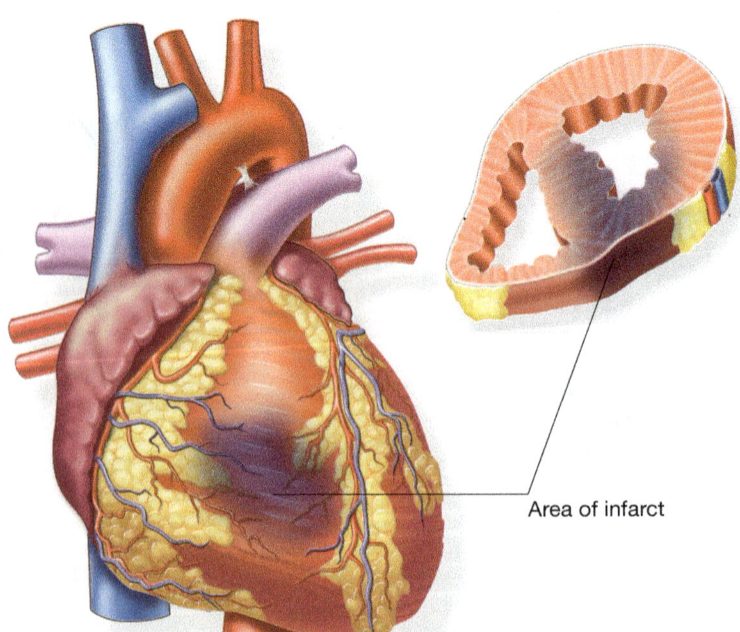

Figure 5.15 External and cross-sectional view of an infarct caused by a myocardial infarction.

Pathology *(continued)*

TERM	WORD PARTS	DEFINITION
myocarditis (my-oh-car-DYE-tis)	myocardi/o = heart muscle -itis = inflammation	Inflammation of the muscle layer of the heart wall.
pericarditis (pair-ih-car-DYE-tis)	peri- = around cardi/o = heart -itis = inflammation	Inflammation of the pericardial sac around the heart.
tetralogy of Fallot (teh-TRALL-oh-jee / fal-LOH)	tetra- = four -logy = study of	Combination of four congenital anomalies: pulmonary stenosis, an interventricular septal defect, improper placement of the aorta, and hypertrophy of the right ventricle. Needs immediate surgery to correct.
valvulitis (val-view-LYE-tis)	valvul/o = valve -itis = inflammation	The inflammation of a heart valve.
Blood Vessels		
aneurysm (AN-yoo-rizm)		Weakness in the wall of an artery resulting in localized widening of the artery. Although an aneurysm may develop in any artery, common sites include the aorta in the abdomen and the cerebral arteries in the brain.

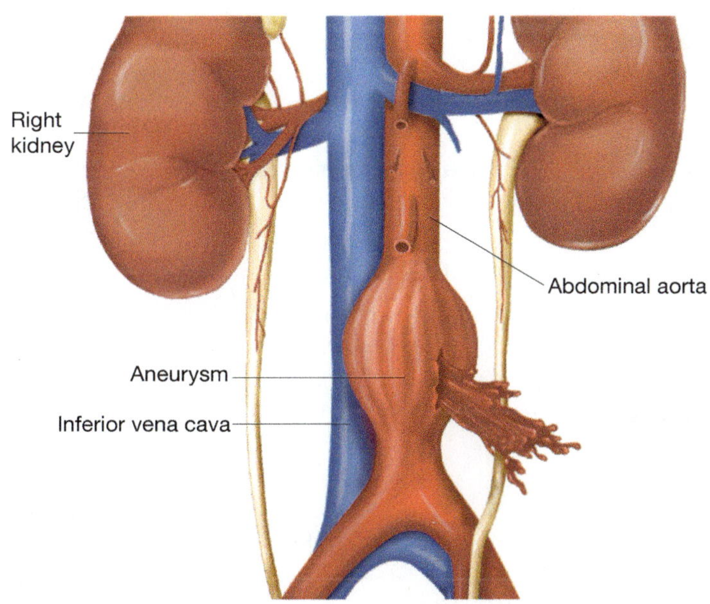

■ **Figure 5.16** Illustration of a large aneurysm in the abdominal aorta that has ruptured.

TERM	WORD PARTS	DEFINITION
arteriorrhexis (ar-tee-ree-oh-REK-sis)	arteri/o = artery -rrhexis = rupture	A ruptured artery; may occur if an aneurysm ruptures an arterial wall.
arteriosclerosis (ar-tee-ree-oh-skleh-ROH-sis)	arteri/o = artery -sclerosis = hardening	Thickening, hardening, and loss of elasticity of the walls of the arteries. Most often due to atherosclerosis.
atheroma (ath-er-OH-mah)	ather/o = fatty substance -oma = growth	A deposit of fatty substance in the wall of an artery that bulges into and narrows the lumen of the artery; a characteristic of atherosclerosis. Also called a *plaque*.

Pathology *(continued)*

TERM	WORD PARTS	DEFINITION
atherosclerosis (ath-er-oh-skleh-ROH-sis)	ather/o = fatty substance -sclerosis = hardening	The most common form of arteriosclerosis. Caused by the formation of yellowish plaques of cholesterol on the inner walls of arteries (see again Figures 5.13 & 5.14).
coarctation of the aorta (CoA) (koh-ark-TAY-shun)		Severe congenital narrowing of the aorta.
hemorrhoid (HIM-oh-royd)	hem/o = blood	Varicose veins in the anal region.
hypertension (HTN) (high-per-TEN-shun)	hyper- = excessive -tension = pressure	Blood pressure above the normal range. *Essential* or *primary hypertension* occurs directly from cardiovascular disease. *Secondary hypertension* refers to high blood pressure resulting from another disease such as kidney disease.
hypotension (high-poh-TEN-shun)	hypo- = insufficient -tension = pressure	Decrease in blood pressure. Can occur in shock, infection, cancer, anemia, or as death approaches.
patent ductus arteriosus (PDA) (PAY-tent / DUCK-tus / ar-tee-ree-OH-sis)	duct/o = to bring arteri/o = artery	Congenital heart anomaly in which the fetal connection between the pulmonary artery and the aorta fails to close at birth. This condition may be treated with medication and resolve with time. However, in some cases surgery is required.
peripheral vascular disease (PVD)	-al = pertaining to vascul/o = blood vessel -ar = pertaining to	Any abnormal condition affecting blood vessels outside the heart. Symptoms may include pain, pallor, numbness, and loss of circulation and pulses.
phlebitis (fleh-BYE-tis)	phleb/o = vein -itis = inflammation	The inflammation of a vein.
polyarteritis (pol-ee-ar-ter-EYE-tis)	poly- = many arteri/o = artery -itis = inflammation	Inflammation of several arteries.
Raynaud's phenomenon (ray-NOZ)		Periodic ischemic attacks affecting the extremities of the body, especially the fingers, toes, ears, and nose. The affected extremities become cyanotic and very painful. These attacks are brought on by arterial constriction due to extreme cold or emotional stress.
thrombophlebitis (throm-boh-fleh-BYE-tis)	thromb/o = clot phleb/o = vein -itis = inflammation	Inflammation of a vein resulting in the formation of blood clots within the vein.
varicose veins (VAIR-ih-kohs)	varic/o = dilated vein -ose = pertaining to	Swollen and distended veins, usually in the legs.

Diagnostic Procedures

TERM	WORD PARTS	DEFINITION
Medical Procedures		
auscultation (oss-kul-TAY-shun)		Process of listening to the sounds within the body by using a stethoscope.
sphygmomanometer (sfig-moh-mah-NOM-eh-ter)	sphygm/o = pulse -manometer = instrument to measure pressure	Instrument for measuring blood pressure. Also referred to as a *blood pressure cuff.*

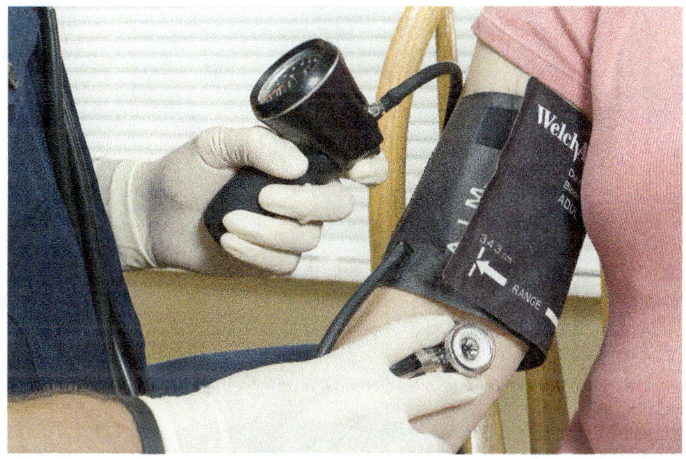

Figure 5.17 Using a sphygmomanometer to measure blood pressure.

TERM	WORD PARTS	DEFINITION
stethoscope (STETH-oh-scope)	steth/o = chest -scope = instrument for viewing	Instrument for listening to body sounds (auscultation), such as the chest, heart, or intestines.
Clinical Laboratory Tests		
cardiac enzymes (CAR-dee-ak / EN-zyms)	cardi/o = heart -ac = pertaining to	Blood test to determine the level of enzymes specific to heart muscles in the blood. An increase in the enzymes may indicate heart muscle damage such as a myocardial infarction. These enzymes include creatine phosphokinase (CPK), lactate dehydrogenase (LDH), and glutamic oxaloacetic transaminase (GOT).
serum lipoprotein level (SEE-rum / lip-oh-PROH-teen)	lip/o = fat	Blood test to measure the amount of cholesterol and triglycerides in the blood. An indicator of atherosclerosis risk.
Diagnostic Imaging		
angiogram (AN-jee-oh-gram)	angi/o = vessel -gram = record	X-ray record of a vessel taken during angiography.
angiography (an-jee-OG-rah-fee)	angi/o = vessel -graphy = process of recording	X-rays taken after the injection of an opaque material into a blood vessel. Can be performed on the aorta as an aortic angiography, on the heart as angiocardiography, and on the brain as a cerebral angiography.
cardiac scan	cardi/o = heart -ac = pertaining to	Patient is given radioactive thallium intravenously and then scanning equipment is used to visualize the heart. It is especially useful in determining myocardial damage.

Diagnostic Procedures *(continued)*

TERM	WORD PARTS	DEFINITION
Doppler ultrasonography (DOP-ler / ul-trah-son-OG-rah-fee)	ultra- = beyond son/o = sound -graphy = process of recording	Measurement of sound-wave echoes as they bounce off tissues and organs to produce an image. In this system, used to measure velocity of blood moving through blood vessels to look for blood clots or deep vein thromboses.
echocardiography (ek-oh-car-dee-OG-rah-fee)	cardi/o = artery -graphy = process of recording	Noninvasive diagnostic method using ultrasound to visualize internal cardiac structures. Cardiac valve activity can be evaluated using this method.
Cardiac Function Tests		
catheter (KATH-eh-ter)		Flexible tube inserted into the body for the purpose of moving fluids into or out of the body. In the cardiovascular system a catheter is used to place dye into blood vessels so they may be visualized on x-rays.
cardiac catheterization (CAR-dee-ak / cath-eh-ter-ih-ZAY-shun)	cardi/o = heart -ac = pertaining to	Passage of a thin tube catheter through a blood vessel leading to the heart. Done to detect abnormalities, to collect cardiac blood samples, and to determine the blood pressure within the heart.
electrocardiogram (ee-lek-tro-CAR-dee-oh-gram)	electr/o = electricity cardi/o = heart -gram = record	Hard copy record produced by electrocardiography.
electrocardiography (ECG, EKG) (ee-lek-troh-car-dee-OG-rah-fee)	electr/o = electricity cardi/o = heart -graphy = process of recording	Process of recording the electrical activity of the heart. Useful in the diagnosis of abnormal cardiac rhythm and heart muscle (myocardium) damage.
Holter monitor		Portable ECG monitor worn by a patient for a period of a few hours to a few days to assess the heart and pulse activity as the person goes through the activities of daily living. Used to assess a patient who experiences chest pain and unusual heart activity during exercise and normal activities.
stress testing		Method for evaluating cardiovascular fitness. The patient is placed on a treadmill or a bicycle and then subjected to steadily increasing levels of work. An EKG and oxygen levels are taken while the patient exercises. The test is stopped if abnormalities occur on the EKG. Also called an *exercise test* or a *treadmill test*.

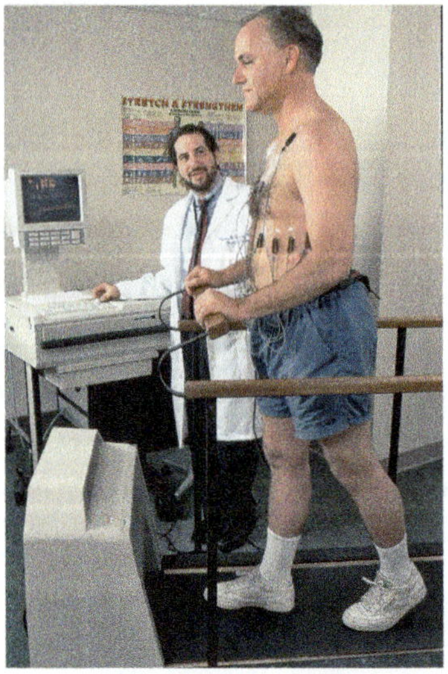

Figure 5.18 Man undergoing a stress test on a treadmill while physician monitors his condition. *(Jonathan Nourok/PhotoEdit Inc.)*

Therapeutic Procedures

TERM	WORD PARTS	DEFINITION
Medical Procedures		
cardiopulmonary resuscitation (CPR) (car-dee-oh-PULL-mon-air-ee / ree-suss-ih-TAY-shun)	cardi/o = heart pulmon/o = lung -ary = pertaining to	Procedure to restore cardiac output and oxygenated air to the lungs for a person in cardiac arrest. A combination of chest compressions (to push blood out of the heart) and artificial respiration (to blow air into the lungs) performed by one or two CPR-trained rescuers.
defibrillation (dee-fib-rih-LAY-shun)	de- = without	Procedure that converts serious irregular heartbeats, such as fibrillation, by giving electric shocks to the heart using an instrument called a defibrillator. Also called *cardioversion.* Automated external defibrillators (AED) are portable devices that automatically detect life-threatening arrhythmias and deliver the appropriate electrical shock. They are designed to be used by nonmedical personnel and are found in public places such as shopping malls and schools.

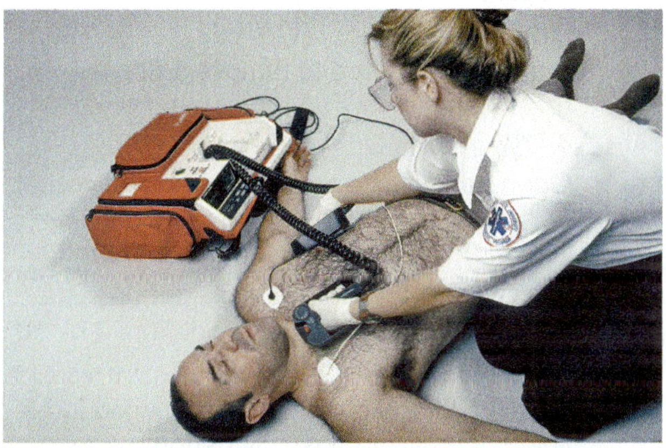

Figure 5.19 An emergency medical technician positions defibrillator paddles on the chest of a supine male patient.

TERM	WORD PARTS	DEFINITION
extracorporeal circulation (ECC) (EX-tra-core-poor-EE-al)	extra- = outside of corpor/o = body -eal = pertaining to	During open-heart surgery, the routing of blood to a heart-lung machine so it can be oxygenated and pumped to the rest of the body.
implantable cardioverter-defibrillator (ICD) (CAR-dee-oh-ver-ter / de-FIB-rih-lay-tor)	cardi/o = heart de- = without	Device implanted in the heart that delivers an electrical shock to restore a normal heart rhythm. Particularly useful for persons who experience ventricular fibrillation.
pacemaker implantation		Electrical device that substitutes for the natural pacemaker of the heart. It controls the beating of the heart by a series of rhythmic electrical impulses. An external pacemaker has the electrodes on the outside of the body. An internal pacemaker has the electrodes surgically implanted within the chest wall.

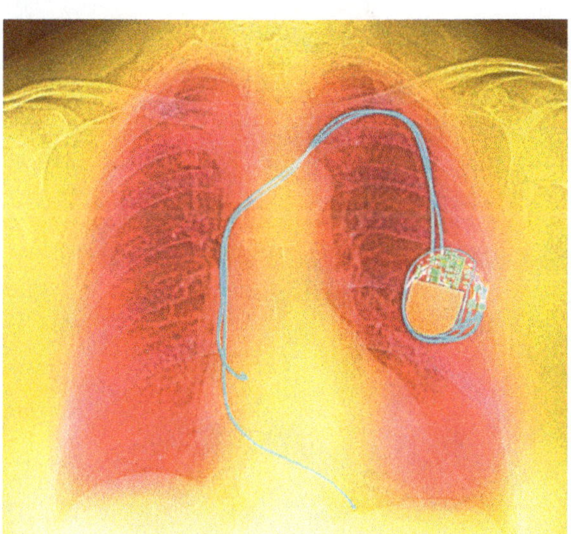

Figure 5.20 Color enhanced X-ray showing a pacemaker implanted in the left side of the chest and the electrode wires running to the heart muscle. *(UHB Trust/Getty Images)*

Therapeutic Procedures *(continued)*

TERM	WORD PARTS	DEFINITION
thrombolytic therapy (throm-boh-LIT-ik / THAIR-ah-pee)	thromb/o = clot -lytic = destruction	Process in which drugs, such as streptokinase (SK) or tissue-type plasminogen activator (tPA), are injected into a blood vessel to dissolve clots and restore blood flow.
Surgical Procedures		
aneurysmectomy (an-yoo-riz-MEK-toh-mee)	-ectomy = surgical removal	Surgical removal of the sac of an aneurysm.
arterial anastomosis (ar-TEE-ree-all / ah-nas-toe-MOE-sis)	arteri/o = artery -al = pertaining to	Surgical joining together of two arteries. Performed if an artery is severed or if a damaged section of an artery is removed.
atherectomy (ath-er-EK-toh-mee)	ather/o = fatty substance -ectomy = surgical removal	Surgical procedure to remove a deposit of fatty substance, an atheroma, from an artery.
coronary artery bypass graft (CABG) (KOR-ah-nair-ee)	coron/o = heart -ary = pertaining to	Open-heart surgery in which a blood vessel from another location in the body (often a leg vein) is grafted to route blood around a blocked coronary artery.
embolectomy (em-boh-LEK-toh-mee)	embol/o = plug -ectomy = surgical removal	Removal of an embolus or clot from a blood vessel.
endarterectomy (end-ar-teh-REK-toh-mee)	endo- = inner arteri/o = artery -ectomy = surgical removal	Removal of the diseased or damaged inner lining of an artery. Usually performed to remove atherosclerotic plaques.
heart transplantation		Replacement of a diseased or malfunctioning heart with a donor's heart.
intracoronary artery stent (in-trah-KOR-ah-nair-ee / AR-ter-ee)	intra- = within coron/o = heart -ary = pertaining to	Placement of a stent within a coronary artery to treat coronary ischemia due to atherosclerosis.

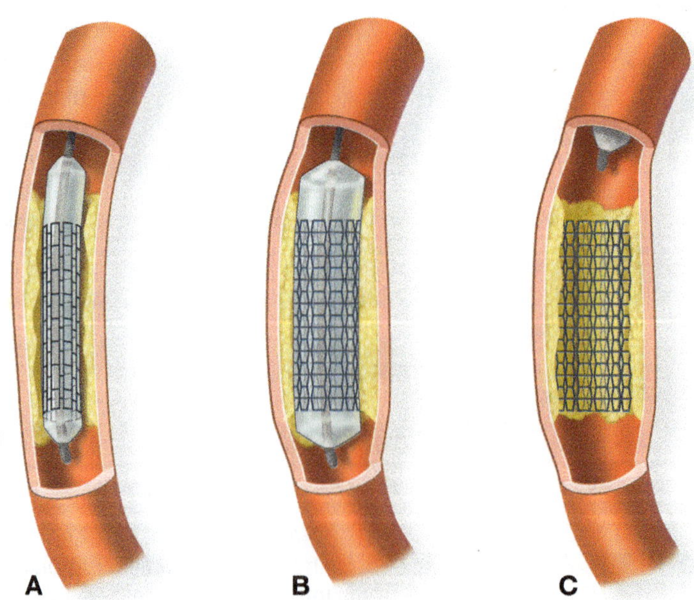

Figure 5.21 The process of placing a stent in a blood vessel. (A) A catheter is used to place a collapsed stent next to an atherosclerotic plaque; (B) stent is expanded; (C) catheter is removed, leaving the expanded stent behind.

Therapeutic Procedures *(continued)*

TERM	WORD PARTS	DEFINITION
ligation and stripping (lye-GAY-shun)		Surgical treatment for varicose veins. The damaged vein is tied off (ligation) and removed (stripping).
percutaneous transluminal coronary angioplasty (PTCA) (per-kyoo-TAY-nee-us / trans-LOO-mih-nal / KOR-ah-nair-ee / AN-jee-oh-plas-tee)	per- = through cutane/o = skin -ous = pertaining to trans- = across -al = pertaining to angi/o = vessel -plasty = surgical repair	Method for treating localized coronary artery narrowing. A balloon catheter is inserted through the skin into the coronary artery and inflated to dilate the narrow blood vessel.
stent		Stainless steel tube placed within a blood vessel or a duct to widen the lumen (see again Figure 5.21).
valve replacement		Removal of a diseased heart valve and replacement with an artificial valve.
valvoplasty (VAL-voh-plas-tee)	valv/o = valve -plasty = surgical repair	Surgical procedure to repair a heart valve.

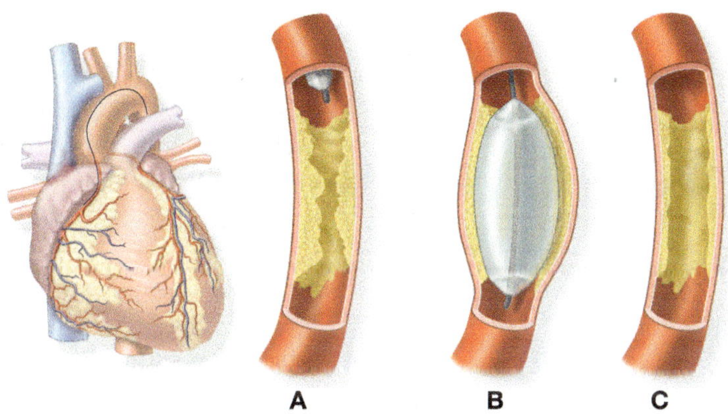

Figure 5.22 Balloon angioplasty: (A) deflated balloon catheter is approaching an atherosclerotic plaque; (B) plaque is compressed by inflated balloon; (C) plaque remains compressed after balloon catheter is removed.

Pharmacology

CLASSIFICATION	WORD PARTS	ACTION	EXAMPLES
ACE inhibitor drugs		Produce vasodilation and decrease blood pressure.	benazepril, Lotensin; catopril, Capoten
antiarrhythmic (an-tye-a-RHYTH-mik)	anti- = against a- = without -ic = pertaining to	Reduces or prevents cardiac arrhythmias.	flecainide, Tambocor; ibutilide, Corvert
anticoagulant (an-tye-koh-AG-you-lant)	anti- = against	Prevents blood clot formation.	heparin; warfarin, Coumadin
antilipidemic (an-tye-lip-ih-DEM-ik)	anti- = against lip/o = fat -ic = pertaining to	Reduces amount of cholesterol and lipids in the bloodstream; treats hyperlipidemia.	atorvastatin, Lipitor; simvastatin, Zocor
antiplatelet agents	anti- = against	Inhibits the ability of platelets to clump together as part of a blood clot.	clopidogrel, Plavix; aspirin; ticlopidine, Ticlid

Pharmacology *(continued)*

CLASSIFICATION	WORD PARTS	ACTION	EXAMPLES
beta-blocker drugs		Treats hypertension and angina pectoris by lowering the heart rate.	metoprolol, Lopressor; propranolol, Inderal
calcium channel blocker drugs		Treats hypertension, angina pectoris, and congestive heart failure by causing the heart to beat less forcefully and less often.	diltiazem, Cardizem; nifedipine, Procardia
cardiotonic (card-ee-oh-TAHN-ik)	cardi/o = heart -tonic = pertaining to tone	Increases the force of cardiac muscle contraction; treats congestive heart failure.	digoxin, Lanoxin
diuretic (dye-you-RET-ik)	-tic = pertaining to	Increases urine production by the kidneys, which works to reduce plasma and therefore blood volume, resulting in lower blood pressure.	furosemide, Lasix
thrombolytic (throm-boh-LIT-ik)	thromb/o = clot -lytic = destruction	Dissolves existing blood clots.	tissue plasminogen activator (tPA); alteplase, Activase
vasoconstrictor (vaz-oh-kon-STRICK-tor)	vas/o = vessel	Contracts smooth muscle in walls of blood vessels; raises blood pressure.	metaraminol, Aramine
vasodilator (vaz-oh-DYE-late-or)	vas/o = vessel	Relaxes the smooth muscle in the walls of arteries, thereby increasing diameter of the blood vessel. Used for two main purposes: increasing circulation to an ischemic area; reducing blood pressure.	nitroglycerine, Nitro-Dur; isoxsuprine, Vasodilan

Abbreviations

AED	automated external defibrillator
AF	atrial fibrillation
AMI	acute myocardial infarction
AS	arteriosclerosis
ASD	atrial septal defect
ASHD	arteriosclerotic heart disease
AV, A-V	atrioventricular
BBB	bundle branch block (L for left; R for right)
BP	blood pressure
bpm	beats per minute
CABG	coronary artery bypass graft
CAD	coronary artery disease
cath	catheterization
CC	cardiac catheterization, chief complaint
CCU	coronary care unit
CHF	congestive heart failure
CoA	coarctation of the aorta
CP	chest pain
CPR	cardiopulmonary resuscitation
CSD	congenital septal defect
CV	cardiovascular
DVT	deep vein thrombosis
ECC	extracorporeal circulation
ECG, EKG	electrocardiogram
ECHO	echocardiogram
GOT	glutamic oxaloacetic transaminase
HTN	hypertension
ICD	implantable cardioverter-defibrillator
ICU	intensive care unit
IV	intravenous

Abbreviations *(continued)*

LVAD	left ventricular assist device
LVH	left ventricular hypertrophy
MI	myocardial infarction, mitral insufficiency
mm Hg	millimeters of mercury
MR	mitral regurgitation
MS	mitral stenosis
MVP	mitral valve prolapse
P	pulse
PAC	premature atrial contraction
PDA	patent ductus arteriosus
PTCA	percutaneous transluminal coronary angioplasty
PVC	premature ventricular contraction
S1	first heart sound
S2	second heart sound
SA, S-A	sinoatrial
SK	streptokinase
tPA	tissue-type plasminogen activator
V fib	ventricular fibrillation
VSD	ventricular septal defect
VT	ventricular tachycardia

MED TERM TIP

Word Watch: Be careful using the abbreviation *MS*, which can mean either "mitral stenosis" or "multiple sclerosis."

Chapter Review

Real-World Applications

Medical Record Analysis

This Discharge Summary contains 12 medical terms. Underline each term and write it in the list below the report. Then define each term.

PEARSON GENERAL HOSPITAL

5500 University Avenue, Metropolis, TX
Phone: (211) 594-4000 • Fax: (211) 594-4001

Medical Consultation Osteology
Date 6/1/2013
Patient Jorge Johnson
Patient complaint: Sever pain in the right ankle with any movement of lower limb.

Discharge Summary

Admitting Diagnosis:	Difficulty breathing, hypertension, tachycardia
Final Diagnosis:	CHF secondary to mitral valve prolapse
History of Present Illness:	Patient was brought to the Emergency Room by her family because of difficulty breathing and palpitations. Patient reports that she has experienced these symptoms for the past 6 months, but this episode is more severe than any previous. Upon admission in the ER, heart rate was 120 beats per minute and blood pressure was 180/110. The results of an EKG and cardiac enzyme blood tests were normal. She was admitted for a complete workup for tachycardia and hypertension.
Summary of Hospital Course:	Patient underwent a full battery of diagnostic tests. A prolapsed mitral valve was observed by echocardiography. A stress test had to be stopped early due to onset of severe difficulty in breathing. Angiocardiography failed to demonstrate significant CAD. Blood pressure and tachycardia were controlled with medications. At discharge, HR was 88 beats per minute and blood pressure was 165/98.
Discharge Plans:	There was no evidence of a myocardial infarction or significant CAD. Patient was placed on a low-salt and low-cholesterol diet. She received instructions on beginning a carefully graded exercise program. She is to continue her medications. If symptoms are not controlled by these measures, a mitral valve replacement will be considered.

	Term	Definition
1	______________	______________________________
2	______________	______________________________
3	______________	______________________________
4	______________	______________________________
5	______________	______________________________
6	______________	______________________________
7	______________	______________________________
8	______________	______________________________
9	______________	______________________________
10	______________	______________________________
11	______________	______________________________
12	______________	______________________________

Chart Note Transcription

The chart note below contains 11 phrases that can be reworded with a medical term that you learned in this chapter. Each phrase is identified with an underline. Determine the medical term and write your answers in the space provided.

Current Complaint:	A 56-year-old male was admitted to the Cardiac Care Unit from the Emergency Room with left arm pain, severe pain around the heart, ❶ an abnormally slow heartbeat, ❷ nausea, and vomiting.
Past History:	Patient reports no heart problems prior to this episode. He has taken medication for high blood pressure ❸ for the past 5 years. His family history is significant for a father and brother who both died in their 50s from death of heart muscle. ❹
Signs and Symptoms:	Patient reports severe pain around the heart that radiates into his left jaw and arm. A record of the heart's electrical activity ❺ and a blood test to determine the amount of heart damage ❻ were abnormal.
Diagnosis:	An acute death of heart muscle ❹ resulting from insufficient blood flow to heart muscle due to obstruction of coronary artery. ❼
Treatment:	First, provide supportive care during the acute phase. Second, evaluate heart damage by passing a thin tube through a blood vessel into the heart to detect abnormalities ❽ and evaluate heart fitness by having patient exercise on a treadmill. ❾ Finally, perform surgical intervention by either inflating a balloon catheter to dilate a narrow vessel ❿ or by open heart surgery to create a shunt around a blocked vessel. ⓫

❶ ____________________

❷ ____________________

❸ ____________________

❹ ____________________

❺ ____________________

❻ ____________________

❼ ____________________

❽ ____________________

❾ ____________________

❿ ____________________

⓫ ____________________

Case Study

Below is a case study presentation of a patient with a condition covered by this chapter. Read the case study and answer the questions below. Some questions will ask for information not included within this chapter. Use your text, a medical dictionary, or any other reference material you choose to answer these questions.

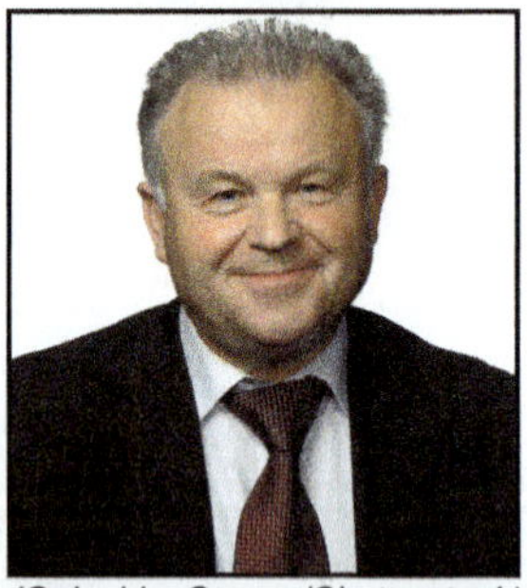

(Galushko Sergey/Shutterstock)

Mr. Thomas is a 62-year-old man who has been diagnosed with an acute myocardial infarction with the following symptoms and history. His chief complaint is a persistent, crushing chest pain that radiates to his left arm, jaw, neck, and shoulder blade. He describes the pain, which he has had for the past 12 hours, as a "squeezing" sensation around his heart. He has also suffered nausea, dyspnea, and diaphoresis. He has a low-grade temperature and his blood pressure is within a normal range at 130/82. He states that he smokes two packs of cigarettes a day, is overweight by 50 pounds, and has a family history of hypertension and coronary artery disease. He leads a relatively sedentary lifestyle.

1. What is the common name for Mr. Thomas's acute condition? Look this condition up in a reference source and include a short description of it.

____

____

2. What do you think the phrase "chief complaint" means?

____

____

3. What is the medical term for this patient's chief complaint? Define this term.

____

____

4. List and define each of the patient's additional symptoms in your own words. (These terms appear in other chapters of the book or use a medical dictionary.)

____

____

5. Using your text as a resource, name and describe three diagnostic tests that may be performed to determine the extent of the patient's heart damage.

____

____

6. What risk factors for developing heart disease does Mr. Thomas have? What changes should he make?

____

____

Practice Exercises

A. Complete the Statement

1. The study of the heart is called ______________________.
2. The three layers of the heart are ______________________, ______________________, and ______________________.
3. The impulse for the heartbeat (the pacemaker) originates in the ______________________.
4. Arteries carry blood ______________________ the heart.
5. The four heart valves are ______________________, ______________________, ______________________, and ______________________.
6. The ______________________ are the receiving chambers of the heart and the ______________________ are the pumping chambers.
7. The ______________________ circulation carries blood to and from the lungs.
8. The pointed tip of the heart is called the ______________________.
9. The ______________________ divides the heart into left and right halves.
10. ______________________ is the contraction phase of the heartbeat and ______________________ is the relaxation phase.

B. Combining Form Practice

The combining form **cardi/o** refers to the heart. Use it to write a term that means:

1. pertaining to the heart ______________________
2. disease of the heart muscle ______________________
3. enlargement of the heart ______________________
4. abnormally fast heart rate ______________________
5. abnormally slow heart rate ______________________
6. record of heart electricity ______________________

The combining form **angi/o** refers to the vessel. Use it to write a term that means:

7. vessel narrowing ______________________
8. vessel inflammation ______________________
9. involuntary muscle contraction of a vessel ______________________

The combining form **arteri/o** refers to the artery. Use it to write a term that means:

10. pertaining to an artery ______________________
11. hardening of an artery ______________________
12. small artery ______________________

C. Prefix Practice

Add the appropriate prefix to **-carditis** to form the term that matches each definition.

1. inflammation of the inner lining of the heart ______________________
2. inflammation of the outer layer of the heart ______________________
3. inflammation of the muscle of the heart ______________________

D. Define the Combining Form

	Definition	Example from Chapter
1. **cardi/o**	______________	______________
2. **valvul/o**	______________	______________
3. **steth/o**	______________	______________
4. **arteri/o**	______________	______________
5. **phleb/o**	______________	______________
6. **angi/o**	______________	______________
7. **ventricul/o**	______________	______________
8. **thromb/o**	______________	______________
9. **atri/o**	______________	______________
10. **ather/o**	______________	______________

E. Name That Term

1. pertaining to a vein ______________________
2. study of the heart ______________________
3. record of a vein ______________________
4. process of recording electrical activity of the heart ______________________
5. high blood pressure ______________________
6. low blood pressure ______________________
7. surgical repair of valve ______________________
8. pertaining to between ventricles ______________________
9. removal of fatty substance ______________________
10. narrowing of the arteries ______________________

F. Name That Suffix

	Suffix	Example from Chapter
1. pressure	______	______
2. abnormal narrowing	______	______
3. instrument to measure pressure	______	______
4. small	______	______
5. hardening	______	______

G. Terminology Matching

Match each term to its definition.

1.	_______ arrhythmia	a. swollen, distended veins
2.	_______ thrombus	b. inflammation of vein
3.	_______ bradycardia	c. serious congenital anomaly
4.	_______ murmur	d. slow heart rate
5.	_______ phlebitis	e. insertion of thin tubing
6.	_______ hypotension	f. irregular heartbeat
7.	_______ varicose vein	g. an abnormal heart sound
8.	_______ tetralogy of Fallot	h. clot in blood vessel
9.	_______ catheterization	i. low blood pressure
10.	_______ sphygmomanometer	j. blood pressure cuff

H. What Does it Stand For?

1. BP ______
2. CHF ______
3. MI ______
4. CCU ______
5. PVC ______
6. CPR ______
7. CAD ______
8. CP ______
9. EKG ______
10. S1 ______

I. What's the Abbreviation?

1. mitral valve prolapse ______________________________
2. ventricular septal defect ______________________________
3. percutaneous transluminal coronary angioplasty ______________________________
4. ventricular fibrillation ______________________________
5. deep vein thrombosis ______________________________
6. lactate dehydrogenase ______________________________
7. coarctation of the aorta ______________________________
8. tissue-type plasminogen activator ______________________________
9. cardiovascular ______________________________
10. extracorporeal circulation ______________________________

J. Procedure Matching

Match each procedure to its definition.

1. _______ cardiac enzymes	a. visualizes heart after patient is given radioactive thallium
2. _______ Doppler ultrasound	b. uses ultrasound to visualize heart beating
3. _______ Holter monitor	c. blood test that indicates heart muscle damage
4. _______ cardiac scan	d. uses treadmill to evaluate cardiac fitness
5. _______ stress testing	e. removes varicose veins
6. _______ echocardiography	f. clot-dissolving drugs
7. _______ extracorporeal circulation	g. measures velocity of blood moving through blood vessels
8. _______ ligation and stripping	h. balloon angioplasty
9. _______ thrombolytic therapy	i. use of a heart-lung machine
10. _______ PTAC	j. portable EKG monitor

K. Define the Term

1. catheter ______________________________
2. infarct ______________________________
3. thrombus ______________________________
4. palpitation ______________________________
5. regurgitation ______________________________

6. aneurysm ______________________________

7. cardiac arrest ______________________________

8. fibrillation ______________________________

9. myocardial infarction ______________________________

10. hemorrhoid ______________________________

L. Fill in the Blank

angiography	murmur	varicose veins	echocardiogram
pacemaker	CHF	defibrillation	angina pectoris
Holter monitor	hypertension	MI	CCU

1. Tiffany was born with a congenital condition resulting in an abnormal heart sound called a(n) ____________.
2. Joseph suffered an arrhythmia resulting in cardiac arrest. The emergency team used an instrument to give electric shocks to the heart to create a normal heart rhythm. This procedure is called ____________.
3. Marguerite has been placed on a low-sodium diet and medication to bring her blood pressure down to a normal range. She suffers from ____________.
4. Tony has had an artificial device called a(n) ____________ inserted to control the beating of his heart by producing rhythmic electrical impulses.
5. Derrick's physician determined that he had ____________ after examining his legs and finding swollen, tortuous veins.
6. Laura has persistent chest pains that require medication. The term for the pain is ____________.
7. La Tonya will be admitted to what hospital unit after surgery to correct her heart condition? ____________
8. Stephen is going to have a coronary artery bypass graft to correct the blockage in his coronary arteries. He recently suffered a heart attack as a result of this occlusion. His attack is called a(n) ____________.
9. Stephen's physician scheduled a(n) ____________, an X-ray to determine the extent of his blood vessel damage.
10. A patient scheduled to have a diagnostic procedure that uses ultrasound to produce an image of the heart valves is going to have a(n) ____________.
11. Eric must wear a device for 24 hours that will keep track of his heart activity as he performs his normal daily routine. This device is called a(n) ____________.
12. Lydia is 82 years old and is suffering from a heart condition that causes weakness, edema, and breathlessness. Her heart failure is the cause of her lung congestion. This condition is called ____________.

M. Pharmacology Challenge

Fill in the classification for each drug description, then match the brand name.

	Drug Description	Classification		Brand Name
1.	_______ prevents arrhythmia	____________________	a.	tPA
2.	_______ reduces cholesterol	____________________	b.	Coumadin
3.	_______ increases force of heart contraction	____________________	c.	Cardizem
4.	_______ increases urine production	____________________	d.	Nitro-Dur
5.	_______ prevents blood clots	____________________	e.	Tambocor
6.	_______ dissolves blood clots	____________________	f.	Lanoxin
7.	_______ relaxes smooth muscle in artery wall	____________________	g.	Lipitor
8.	_______ cause heart to beat less forcefully	____________________	h.	Lasix

N. Career Connection

Research professions related to the Cardiovascular System and report on the following:

1. Profession description to include job responsibilities
2. Educational requirements
3. Job opportunities
4. Opportunities outside of the hospital setting
5. Salary range
6. Licensure and continuing education requirements

Present your findings to your class.

O. Communication

The health care worker should understand that there are many factors in communication. A knowledge of these techniques will increase your skills in communicating with co-workers and patients/clients. With this knowledge, you will be able to do a better job and to make good observations about your patients.

List three effective skills to remember when communicating with a child, a peer, and an older person. List the skills in order of importance, and then evaluate and analyze how each communication skill contributes to maintaining a healthy relationship at each stage of the life span.

P. EKG Graph Paper Speed

ECG/EKG graph paper can be run through the EKG machine at different speeds. The standard speed is 25 mm per second. However, faster speeds are sometimes used.

Each small block of EKG paper equals 1 square mm. At a standard paper speed of 25 mm per second, one small block of EKG paper equals 1/25th of a second or 0.04.

If five small blocks equal one large block, how many seconds are represented by one large block?

5 blocks × 0.04 seconds = 0.20 seconds

If one large block equals 0.20 seconds, how many large blocks equal one second?

1 large block = 0.20 seconds

1 second divided by 0.20 seconds = 5

5 × 1 large block = 5 large blocks

Example 1

A sample EKG reading takes 5 ½ minutes. How many large blocks of graph paper would that take up 25 mm per second? How many small blocks?

5.5 minutes = 330 seconds
330 seconds × 5 blocks/second = 1,650 large blocks
1 large block = 5 small blocks
1,650 large blocks = 8,250 small blocks

How many small blocks would be used in an EKG procedure at 25 mm per second for the following times?

a. 50 seconds
b. 1.5 minutes

If an EKG reads at 25 mm per second, how long were the following procedures?

a. 998 large blocks
b. 50,000 small blocks

Why would it matter if the EKG paper speed were 25mm per second or 50 mm per second? Fluently add, subtract, multiply, and divide multi-digit decimals to determine the solution to a problem similar to the examples given.

Labeling Exercise

Image A

Write the labels for this figure on the numbered lines provided.

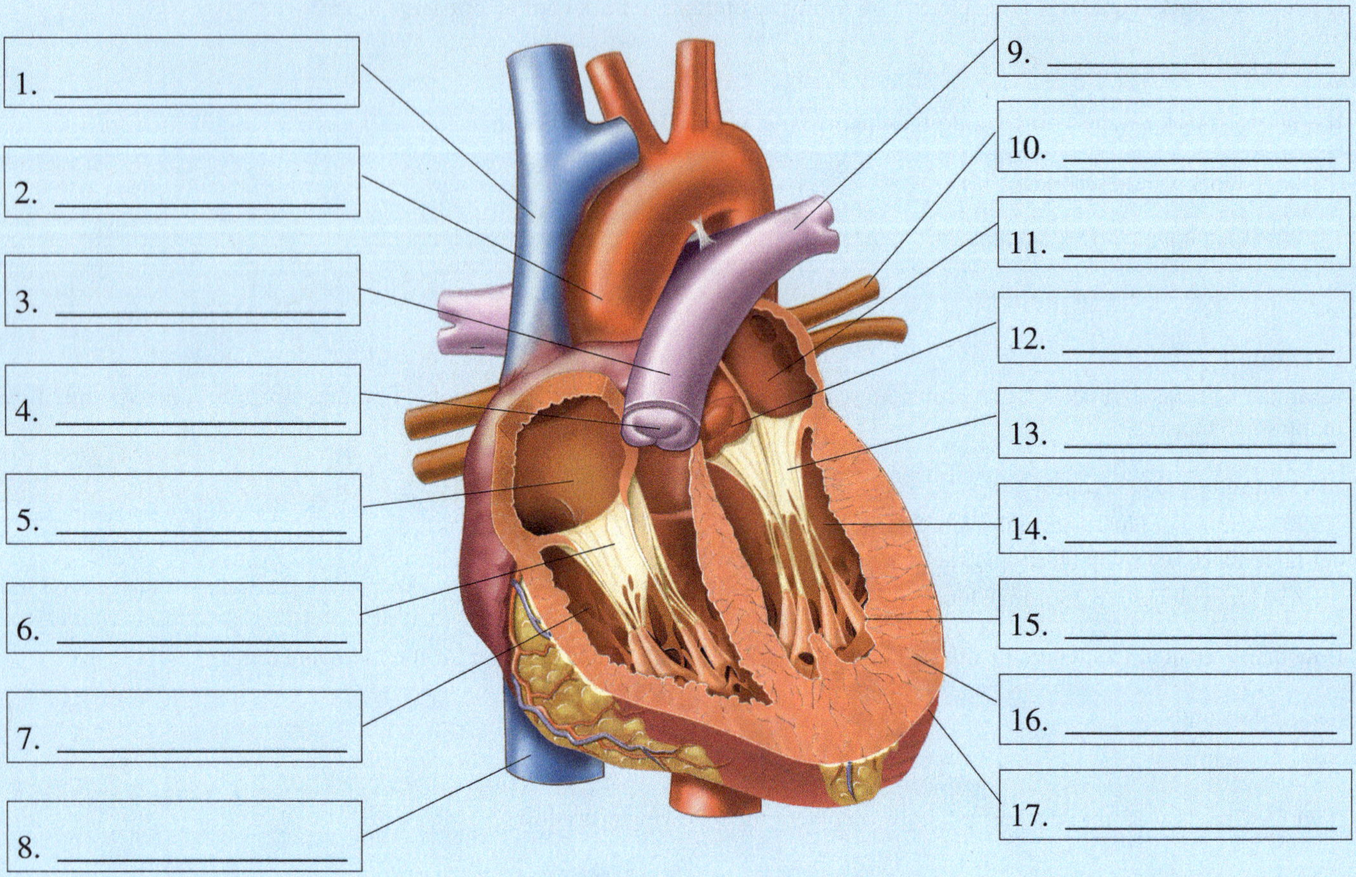

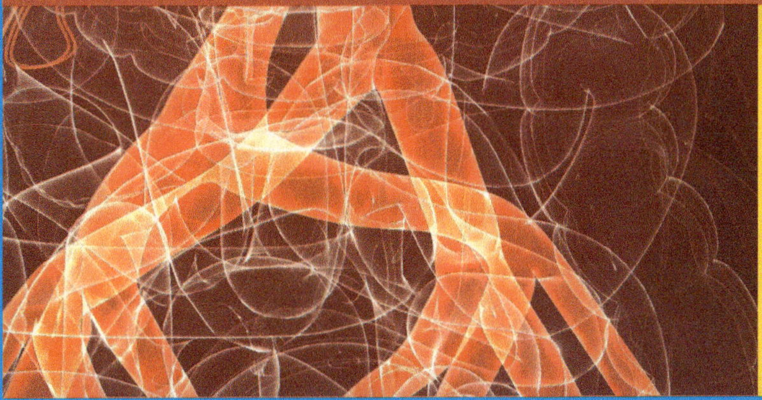

6

BLOOD AND THE LYMPHATIC AND IMMUNE SYSTEMS

Learning Objectives

Upon completion of this chapter, you will be able to

- Recognize the combining forms and suffixes introduced in this chapter.
- Gain the ability to pronounce medical terms and major anatomical structures.
- List the major components, structures, and organs of the blood and lymphatic and immune systems and their functions.
- Describe the blood typing systems.
- Discuss immunity, the immune response, and standard precautions.
- Identify and define blood and lymphatic and immune system anatomical terms.
- Identify and define selected blood and lymphatic and immune system pathology terms.
- Identify and define selected blood and lymphatic and immune system diagnostic procedures.
- Identify and define selected blood and lymphatic and immune system therapeutic procedures.
- Identify and define selected medications associated with blood and the lymphatic and immune systems.
- Define selected abbreviations associated with blood and the lymphatic and immune systems.

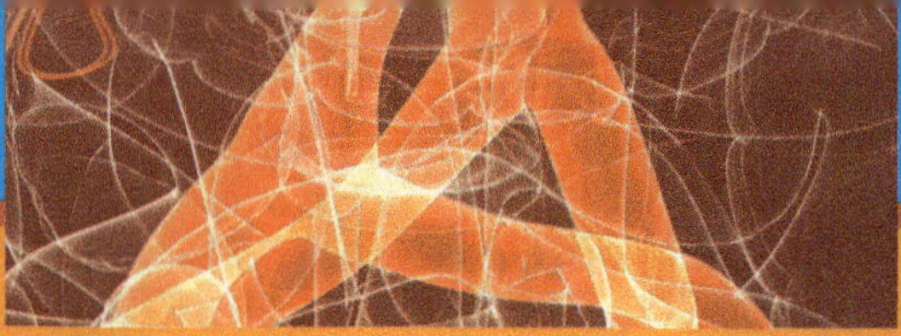

Section I: Blood at a Glance

Function

Blood transports gases, nutrients, and wastes to all areas of the body either attached to red blood cells or dissolved in the plasma. White blood cells fight infection and disease, and platelets initiate the blood clotting process.

Structures

Here are the primary components that comprise blood.

formed elements
- **erythrocytes**
- **leukocytes**
- **platelets**

plasma

Word Parts

Here are the most common word parts (with their meanings) used to build blood terms. For a more comprehensive list, refer to the Terminology section of this chapter.

Combining Forms

agglutin/o	clumping	**hem/o**	blood
bas/o	base	**hemat/o**	blood
chrom/o	color	**leuk/o**	white
coagul/o	clotting	**lymph/o**	lymph
cyt/o	cell	**morph/o**	shape
eosin/o	rosy red	**neutr/o**	neutral
erythr/o	red	**phag/o**	eat, swallow
fibrin/o	fibers, fibrous	**sanguin/o**	blood
fus/o	pouring	**septic/o**	infection
granul/o	granules	**thromb/o**	clot

Suffixes

-apheresis	removal, carry away
-crit	separation of
-cytosis	more than the normal number of cells
-emia	blood condition
-globin	protein
-penia	abnormal decrease, too few
-phil	attracted to
-poiesis	formation
-stasis	standing still

Blood Illustrated

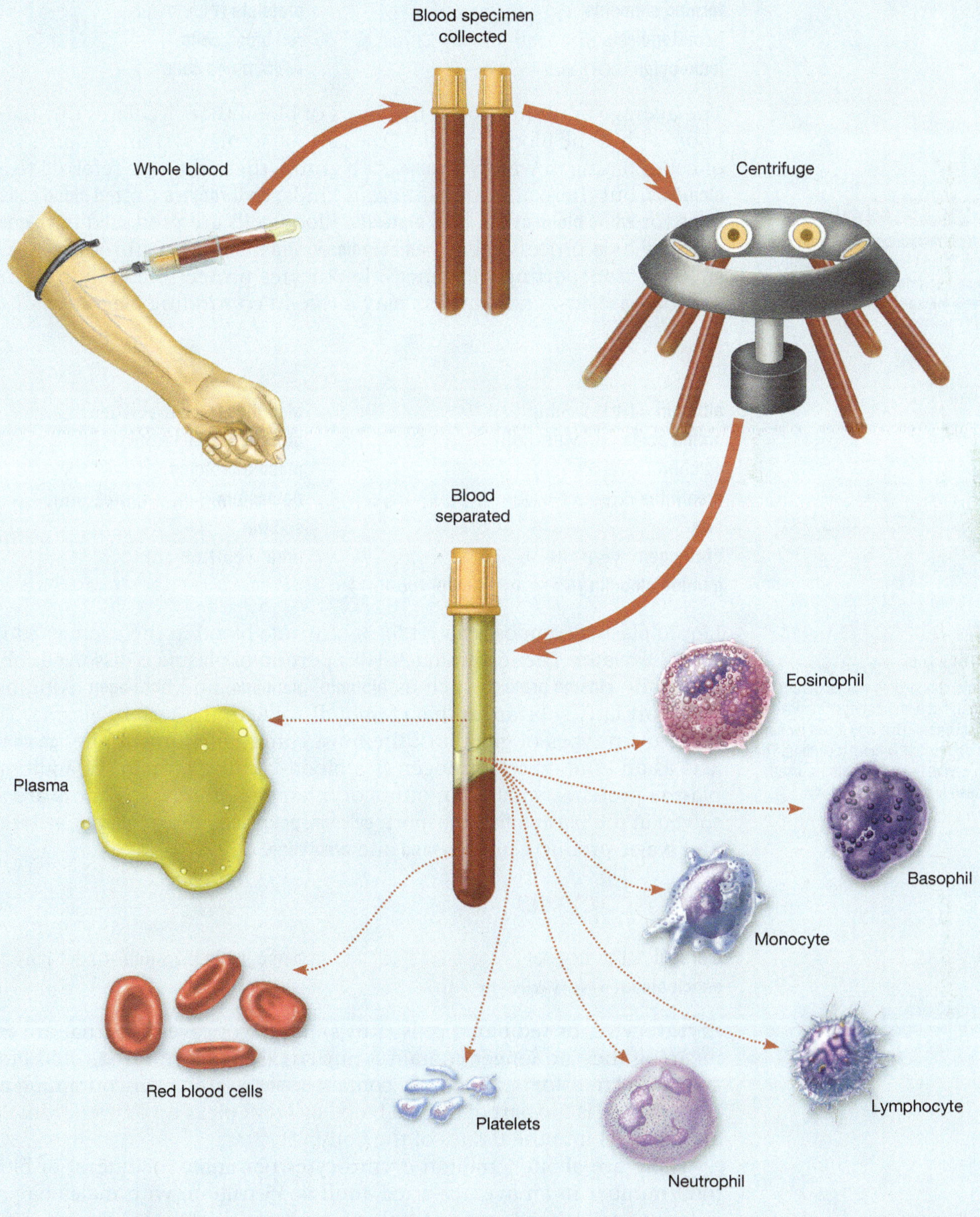

Anatomy and Physiology of Blood

erythrocytes (eh-RITH-roh-sights)
formed elements
hematopoiesis (hee-mah-toh-poy-EE-sis)
leukocytes (LOO-koh-sights)
plasma (PLAZ-mah)
platelets (PLAYT-lets)
red blood cells
white blood cells

The average adult has about five liters of blood that circulates throughout the body within the blood vessels of the cardiovascular system. Blood is a mixture of cells floating in watery **plasma.** As a group, these cells are referred to as **formed elements,** but there are three different kinds: **erythrocytes** (or **red blood cells**), **leukocytes** (or **white blood cells**), and **platelets.** Blood cells are produced in the red bone marrow by a process called **hematopoiesis.** Plasma and erythrocytes are responsible for transporting substances, leukocytes protect the body from invading microorganisms, and platelets play a role in controlling bleeding.

MED TERM TIP

The term *hematopoiesis* literally means "blood formation" by combining hemat/o (meaning blood) with -poiesis (meaning formation).

Plasma

albumin (al-BEW-min)
amino acids (ah-MEE-noh)
calcium (KAL-see-um)
creatinine (kree-AT-in-in)
fats
fibrinogen (fye-BRIN-oh-jen)
gamma globulin (GAM-ah / GLOB-yoo-lin)
globulins (GLOB-yew-lenz)
glucose (GLOO-kohs)
plasma proteins
potassium (poh-TASS-ee-um)
sodium
urea (yoo-REE-ah)

Liquid plasma composes about 55% of whole blood in the average adult and is 90–92% water. The remaining 8–10% portion of plasma is dissolved substances, especially **plasma proteins** such as **albumin, globulins,** and **fibrinogen.** Albumin helps transport fatty substances that cannot dissolve in the watery plasma. There are three main types of globulins; the most commonly known one, **gamma globulin,** acts as an antibody. Fibrinogen is a blood-clotting protein. In addition to the plasma proteins, smaller amounts of other important substances are also dissolved in the plasma for transport: **calcium, potassium, sodium, glucose, amino acids, fats,** and waste products such as **urea** and **creatinine.**

MED TERM TIP

Word Watch: *Plasma* and *serum* are not interchangeable words. Serum is plasma, but with fibrinogen removed or inactivated. This way it can be handled and tested without it clotting. The term *serum* is also sometimes used to mean antiserum or antitoxin.

Erythrocytes

bilirubin (bil-ly-ROO-bin)
enucleated (ee-NEW-klee-ate-ed)
hemoglobin (hee-moh-GLOH-bin)

Erythrocytes, or red blood cells (RBCs), are biconcave disks that are **enucleated,** meaning they no longer contain a nucleus (see Figure 6.1 ■). Red blood cells appear red in color because they contain **hemoglobin,** an iron-containing pigment. Hemoglobin is the part of the red blood cell that picks up oxygen from the lungs and delivers it to the tissues of the body.

There are about 5 million erythrocytes per cubic millimeter of blood. The total number in an average-sized adult is 35 trillion, with males having more red blood cells than females. Erythrocytes have an average lifespan of 120 days,

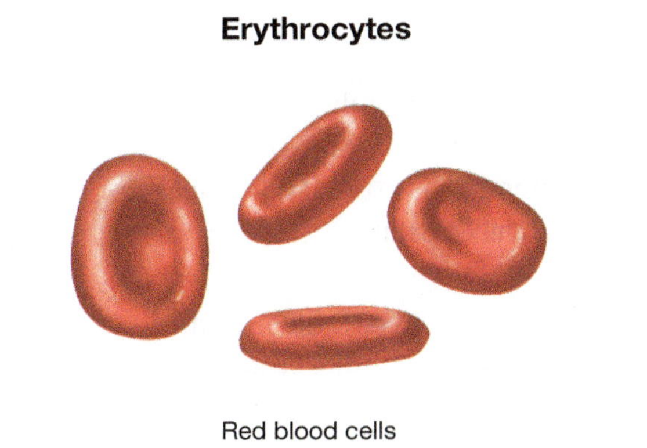

■ **Figure 6.1** The biconcave disk shape of erythrocytes (red blood cells).

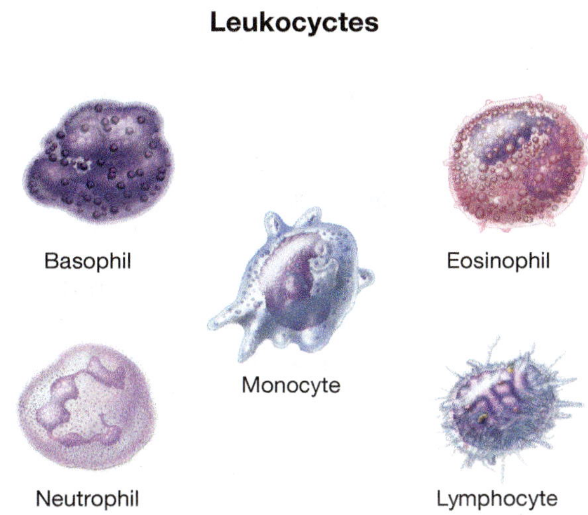

■ **Figure 6.2** The five different types of leukocytes (white blood cells).

and then the spleen removes the worn-out and damaged ones from circulation. Much of the red blood cell, such as the iron, can be reused, but one portion, **bilirubin,** is a waste product disposed of by the liver.

> **MED TERM TIP**
> Your body makes about 2 million erythrocytes every second. Of course, it must then destroy 2 million every second to maintain a relatively constant 30 trillion red blood cells.

Leukocytes

agranulocytes (ah-GRAN-yew-loh-sights)
granulocytes (GRAN-yew-loh-sights)
pathogens (PATH-oh-ginz)

Leukocytes, also referred to as white blood cells (WBCs), provide protection against the invasion of **pathogens** such as bacteria, viruses, and other foreign material. In general, white blood cells have a spherical shape with a large nucleus, and there are about 8,000 per cubic millimeter of blood (see Figure 6.2 ■). There are five different types of white blood cells, each with its own strategy for protecting the body. The five can be subdivided into two categories: **granulocytes** (with granules in the cytoplasm) and **agranulocytes** (without granules in the cytoplasm). The name and function of each type is presented in Table 6.1 ■.

> **MED TERM TIP**
> A *phagocyte* is a cell that has the ability to ingest (phag/o = eat; -cyte = cell) and digest bacteria and other foreign particles. This process, *phagocytosis,* is critical for the control of bacteria within the body.

Table 6.1 Leukocyte Classification

LEUKOCYTE	FUNCTION
Granulocytes	
Basophils (basos) (BAY-soh-fillz)	Release histamine and heparin to damaged tissues
Eosinophils (eosins) (ee-oh-SIN-oh-fillz)	Destroy parasites and increase during allergic reactions
Neutrophils (NOO-troh-fillz)	Engulfs foreign and damaged cells (phagocytosis); most numerous of the leukocytes
Agranulocytes	
Monocytes (monos) (MON-oh-sights)	Engulfs foreign and damaged cells (phagocytosis)
Lymphocytes (lymphs) (LIM-foh-sights)	Plays several different roles in immune response

Platelets

agglutinate (ah-GLOO-tih-nayt)
fibrin (FYE-brin)
hemostasis (hee-moh-STAY-sis)
prothrombin (proh-THROM-bin)
thrombin (THROM-bin)
thrombocyte (THROM-boh-sight)
thromboplastin (throm-boh-PLAS-tin)

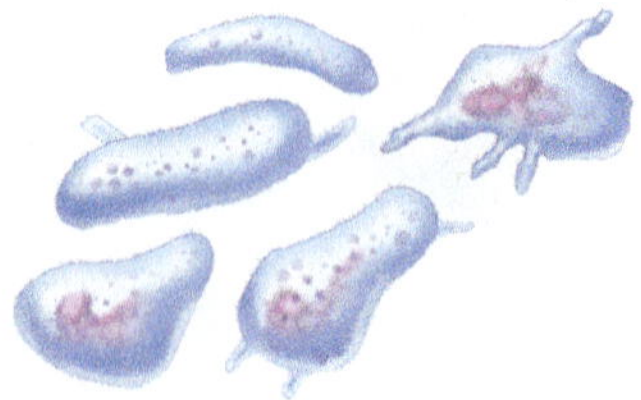

■ **Figure 6.3** Platelet structure.

MED TERM TIP

You can find a clue to the meaning of many terms associated with platelets because they contain word parts:

- fibrinogen: fibrin/o = fibers + -gen = that which produces
- hemostasis: hem/o = blood + -stasis = standing still
- agglutinate: agglutin/o = clumping
- prothrombin: pro- = before + thromb/o = clot
- thromboplastin: thromb/o = clot + -plastin = formation

Platelet, the modern term for **thrombocyte,** refers to the smallest of all the formed blood elements. Platelets are not whole cells, but rather are formed when the cytoplasm of a large precursor cell shatters into small plate-like fragments (see Figure 6.3 ■). There are between 200,000 and 300,000 per cubic millimeter in the body.

Platelets play a critical part in the blood-clotting process or **hemostasis.** They **agglutinate** or clump together into small clusters when a blood vessel is cut or damaged. Platelets also release a substance called **thromboplastin,** which, in the presence of calcium, reacts with **prothrombin** (a clotting protein in the blood) to form **thrombin.** Then thrombin, in turn, works to convert fibrinogen to **fibrin,** which eventually becomes the meshlike blood clot.

Blood Typing

ABO system
blood typing
Rh factor

Each person's blood is different due to the presence of antigens or markers on the surface of erythrocytes. Before a person receives a blood transfusion, it is important to do **blood typing.** This laboratory test determines if the donated blood is compatible with the recipient's blood. There are many different subgroups of blood markers, but the two most important ones are the **ABO system** and **Rh factor.**

ABO System

type A
type AB
type B
type O
universal donor
universal recipient

In the ABO blood system there are two possible red blood cell markers, A and B. A marker is one method by which cells identify themselves. A person with an A marker is said to have **type A** blood. Type A blood produces anti-B antibodies that will attack type B blood. The presence of a B marker gives **type B** blood and anti-A antibodies (that will attack type A blood). If both markers are present, the blood is **type AB** and does not contain any antibodies. Therefore, type AB blood will not attack any other blood type. The absence of either an A or a B marker results in **type O** blood, which contains both anti-A and anti-B antibodies. Type O blood will attack all other blood types (A, B, and AB). For further information on antibodies, refer to the lymphatic section later in this chapter.

Because type O blood does not have either marker A or B, it will not react with anti-A or anti-B antibodies. For this reason, a person with type O blood is referred to as a **universal donor.** In extreme cases, type O blood may be given to a person with any of the other blood types. Similarly, type AB blood is the **universal recipient.** A person with type AB blood has no antibodies against the other blood types and, therefore, in extreme cases, can receive any type of blood.

Rh Factor

Rh-negative **Rh-positive**

Rh factor is not as difficult to understand as the ABO system. A person with the Rh factor on his or her red blood cells is said to be **Rh-positive** (Rh+). Since this person has the factor, he or she will not make anti-Rh antibodies. A person without the Rh factor is **Rh-negative** (Rh–) and will produce anti-Rh antibodies. Therefore, an Rh+ person may receive both an Rh+ and an Rh– transfusion, but an Rh– person can receive only Rh– blood.

Terminology

Word Parts Used to Build Blood Terms

The following lists contain the combining forms, suffixes, and prefixes used to build terms in the remaining sections of this chapter.

Combining Forms

bas/o	base
chrom/o	color
coagul/o	clotting
cyt/o	cell
eosin/o	rosy red
erythr/o	red
fibrin/o	fibers

fus/o	pouring
granul/o	granules
hem/o	blood
hemat/o	blood
leuk/o	white
lip/o	fat
lymph/o	lymph

morph/o	shape
neutr/o	neutral
phleb/o	vein
sanguin/o	blood
septic/o	infection
thromb/o	clot

Suffixes

-apheresis	removal, carry away
-crit	separation of
-cyte	cell
-cytosis	more than the normal number of cells
-emia	blood condition
-globin	protein

-ia	condition
-ic	pertaining to
-ion	action
-logy	study of
-lytic	destruction
-oma	swelling
-otomy	cutting into

-ous	pertaining to
-penia	too few
-phil	attracted to
-plastic	pertaining to development
-rrhage	abnormal flow
-rrhagic	pertaining to abnormal flow

Prefixes

a-	without
an-	without
anti-	against
auto-	self

dys-	abnormal
homo-	same
hyper-	excessive
hypo-	insufficient

mono-	one
pan-	all
poly-	many
trans-	across

Anatomical Terms

TERM	WORD PARTS	DEFINITION
agranulocyte (ah-GRAN-yew-loh-sight)	a- = without granul/o = granules -cyte = cell	A leukocyte without granules in its cytoplasm; monocytes and lymphocytes.
basophil (BAY-soh-fill)	bas/o = base -phil = attracted to	A granulocytic leukocyte that attracts a basic pH stain.
eosinophil (ee-oh-SIN-oh-fill)	eosin/o = rosy red -phil = attracted to	A granulocytic leukocyte that attracts a rosy red stain.
erythrocyte (eh-RITH-roh-sight)	erythr/o = red -cyte = cell	A red blood cell.
fibrinous (fye-brin-us)	fibrin/o = fibers -ous = pertaining to	Pertaining to fibers.
granulocyte (GRAN-yew-loh-sight)	granul/o = granules -cyte = cell	A leukocyte with granules in its cytoplasm; basophils, eosinophils, neutrophils.
hematic (hee-MAT-ik)	hemat/o = blood -ic = pertaining to	Pertaining to blood.
leukocyte (LOO-koh-sight)	leuk/o = white -cyte = cell	A white blood cell.
lymphocyte (LIM-foh-sight)	lymph/o = lymph -cyte = cell	An agranulocytic leukocyte formed in lymphatic tissue.
monocyte (MON-oh-sight)	mono- = one -cyte = cell	An agranulocytic leukocyte with a single, large nucleus.
neutrophil (NOO-troh-fill)	neutr/o = neutral -phil = attracted to	A granulocytic leukocyte that attracts a neutral pH stain.
sanguinous (SANG-gwih-nus)	sanguin/o = blood -ous = pertaining to	Pertaining to blood.
thrombocyte (THROM-boh-sight)	thromb/o = clot -cyte = cell	A clotting cell; a platelet.

Pathology

TERM	WORD PARTS	DEFINITION
Medical Specialties		
hematology (hee-mah-TALL-oh-jee)	hemat/o = blood -logy = study of	The branch of medicine specializing in treatment of diseases and conditions of the blood. Physician is a *hematologist.*
Signs and Symptoms		
blood clot		The hard collection of fibrin, blood cells, and tissue debris that is the end result of hemostasis or the blood-clotting process (see Figure 6.4 ■).

Pathology *(continued)*

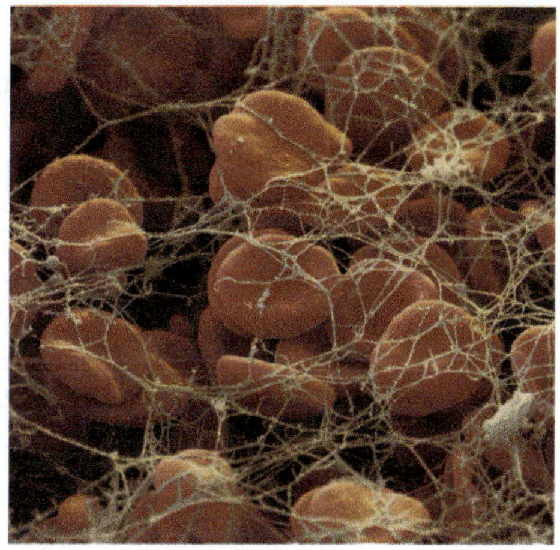

Figure 6.4 Electronmicrograph showing a blood clot composed of fibrin, red blood cells, and tissue debris. *(Eye of Science/Photo Researchers, Inc.)*

TERM	WORD PARTS	DEFINITION
coagulate (koh-ag-YOO-late)	coagul/o = clotting	To convert from a liquid to a gel or solid, as in blood coagulation.
dyscrasia (dis-CRAZ-ee-ah)	dys- = abnormal -ia = condition	A general term indicating the presence of a disease affecting blood.
hematoma (hee-mah-TOH-mah)	hemat/o = blood -oma = swelling	The collection of blood under the skin as the result of blood escaping into the tissue from damaged blood vessels. Commonly referred to as a *bruise.*
hemorrhage (HEM-er-rij)	hem/o = blood -rrhage = abnormal flow	Rapid flow of blood.
Blood		
hemophilia (hee-moh-FILL-ee-ah)	hem/o = blood -phil = attracted to -ia = condition	Hereditary blood disease in which blood-clotting time is prolonged due to a lack of one vital clotting factor. It is transmitted by a sex-linked trait from females to males, appearing almost exclusively in males.
hyperlipidemia (HYE-per-lip-id-ee-mee-ah)	hyper- = excessive lip/o = fat -emia = blood condition	Condition of having too high a level of lipids such as cholesterol in the bloodstream. A risk factor for developing atherosclerosis and coronary artery disease.
pancytopenia (pan-sigh-toe-PEN-ee-ah)	pan- = all cyt/o = cell -penia = too few	Having too few of all cells.
septicemia (sep-tih-SEE-mee-ah)	septic/o = infection -emia = blood condition	Having bacteria or their toxins in the bloodstream. *Sepsis* is a term that means putrefaction or infection. Commonly referred to as *blood poisoning.*

MED TERM TIP

Word Watch: The term *hematoma* is confusing. Its simple translation is "blood tumor." However, it is used to refer to blood that has leaked out of a blood vessel and has pooled in the tissues causing swelling.

Pathology *(continued)*

TERM	WORD PARTS	DEFINITION
Erythrocytes		
anemia (an-NEE-mee-ah)	an- = without -emia = blood condition	A large group of conditions characterized by a reduction in the number of red blood cells or the amount of hemoglobin in the blood; results in less oxygen reaching the tissues.
aplastic anemia (a-PLAS-tik / an-NEE-mee-ah)	a- = without -plastic = pertaining to development an- = without -emia = blood condition	Severe form of anemia that develops as a consequence of loss of functioning red bone marrow. Results in a decrease in the number of all the formed elements. Treatment may eventually require a bone marrow transplant.
erythrocytosis (ee-RITH-row-sigh-toe-sis)	erythr/o = red -cytosis = more than normal number of cells	The condition of having too many red blood cells.
erythropenia (ee-RITH-row-pen-ee-ah)	erythr/o = red -penia = too few	The condition of having too few red blood cells.
hemolytic anemia (hee-moh-LIT-ik / an-NEE-mee-ah)	hem/o = blood -lytic = destruction an- = without -emia = blood condition	An anemia that develops as the result of the destruction of erythrocytes.
hemolytic reaction (hee-moh-LIT-ik)	hem/o = blood -lytic = destruction	The destruction of a patient's erythrocytes that occurs when receiving a transfusion of an incompatible blood type. Also called a *transfusion reaction.*
hypochromic anemia (hi-poe-CHROME-ik / an-NEE-mee-ah)	hypo- = insufficient chrom/o = color -ic = pertaining to an- = without -emia = blood condition	Anemia resulting from having insufficient hemoglobin in the erythrocytes. Named because the hemoglobin molecule is responsible for the dark red color of the erythrocytes.
iron-deficiency anemia	an- = without -emia = blood condition	Anemia resulting from not having sufficient iron to manufacture hemoglobin.
pernicious anemia (PA) (per-NISH-us / an-NEE-mee-ah)	an- = without -emia = blood condition	Anemia associated with insufficient absorption of vitamin B_{12} by the digestive system. Vitamin B_{12} is necessary for erythrocyte production.
polycythemia vera (pol-ee-sigh-THEE-mee-ah / VAIR-rah)	poly- = many cyt/o = cell hem/o = blood -ia = condition	Production of too many red blood cells by the bone marrow. Blood becomes too thick to easily flow through the blood vessels.
sickle cell anemia	an- = without -emia = blood condition	A genetic disorder in which erythrocytes take on an abnormal curved or "sickle" shape. These cells are fragile and are easily damaged, leading to a hemolytic anemia (see Figure 6.5 ■).

Pathology *(continued)*

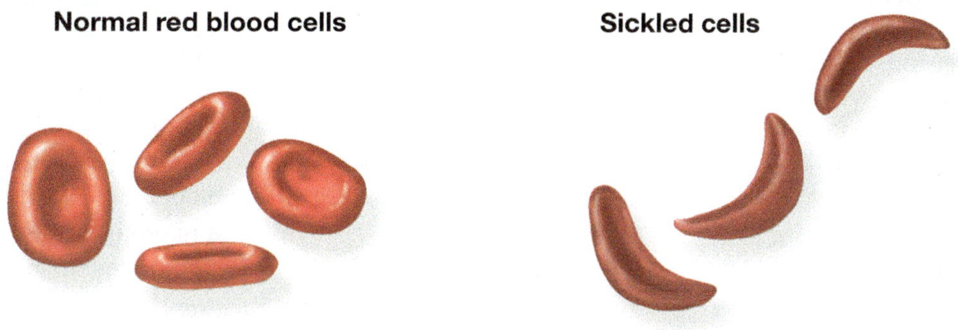

■ **Figure 6.5** Comparison of normal-shaped erythrocytes and the abnormal sickle shape noted in patients with sickle cell anemia.

TERM	WORD PARTS	DEFINITION
thalassemia (thal-ah-SEE-mee-ah)	-emia = blood condition	A genetic disorder in which the body is unable to make functioning hemoglobin, resulting in anemia.
Leukocytes		
leukemia (loo-KEE-mee-ah)	leuk/o = white -emia = blood condition	Cancer of the white blood cell–forming red bone marrow resulting in a large number of abnormal and immature white blood cells circulating in the blood.
leukocytosis (LOO-koh-sigh-toh-sis)	leuk/o = white -cytosis = more than normal number of cells	The condition of having too many white blood cells.
leukopenia (LOO-koh-pen-ee-ah)	leuk/o = white -penia = too few	The condition of having too few white blood cells.
Platelets		
thrombocytosis (throm-boh-sigh-TOH-sis)	thromb/o = clot -cytosis = more than normal number of cells	The condition of having too many platelets.
thrombopenia (THROM-boh-pen-ee-ah)	thromb/o = clot -penia = too few	The condition of having too few platelets.

Diagnostic Procedures

TERM	WORD PARTS	DEFINITION
Clinical Laboratory Tests		
blood culture and sensitivity (C&S)		Sample of blood is incubated in the laboratory to check for bacterial growth. If bacteria are present, they are identified and tested to determine which antibiotics they are sensitive to.
complete blood count (CBC)		Combination of blood tests including red blood cell count (RBC), white blood cell count (WBC), hemoglobin (Hgb), hematocrit (Hct), white blood cell differential, and platelet count.

Diagnostic Procedures *(continued)*

TERM	WORD PARTS	DEFINITION
erythrocyte sedimentation rate (ESR, sed rate) (eh-RITH-roh-sight / sed-ih-men-TAY-shun)	erythr/o = red -cyte = cell	Blood test to determine the rate at which mature red blood cells settle out of the blood after the addition of an anticoagulant. This is an indicator of the presence of an inflammatory disease.
hematocrit (HCT, Hct, crit) (hee-MAT-oh-krit)	hemat/o = blood -crit = separation of	Blood test to measure the volume of red blood cells (erythrocytes) within the total volume of blood.
hemoglobin (Hgb, hb, HGB) (hee-moh-GLOH-bin)	hem/o = blood -globin = protein	A blood test to measure the amount of hemoglobin present in a given volume of blood.
platelet count (PLAYT-let)		Blood test to determine the number of platelets in a given volume of blood.
prothrombin time (pro-time, PT) (proh-THROM-bin)	thromb/o = clot	A measure of the blood's coagulation abilities by measuring how long it takes for a clot to form after prothrombin has been activated.
red blood cell count (RBC)		Blood test to determine the number of erythrocytes in a volume of blood. A decrease in red blood cells may indicate anemia; an increase may indicate polycythemia.
red blood cell morphology	morph/o = shape -logy = study of	Examination of a specimen of blood for abnormalities in the shape (morphology) of the erythrocytes. Used to determine diseases like sickle cell anemia.
sequential multiple analyzer computer (SMAC)		Machine for doing multiple blood chemistry tests automatically.
white blood cell count (WBC)		Blood test to measure the number of leukocytes in a volume of blood. An increase may indicate the presence of infection or a disease such as leukemia. A decrease in white blood cells may be caused by radiation therapy or chemotherapy.
white blood cell differential (diff) (diff-er-EN-shal)		Blood test to determine the number of each variety of leukocytes.
Medical Procedures		
bone marrow aspiration (as-pih-RAY-shun)		Sample of bone marrow is removed by aspiration with a needle and examined for diseases such as leukemia or aplastic anemia.
phlebotomy (fleh-BOT-oh-me)	phleb/o = vein -otomy = cutting into	Incision into a vein in order to remove blood for a diagnostic test. Also called *venipuncture*.

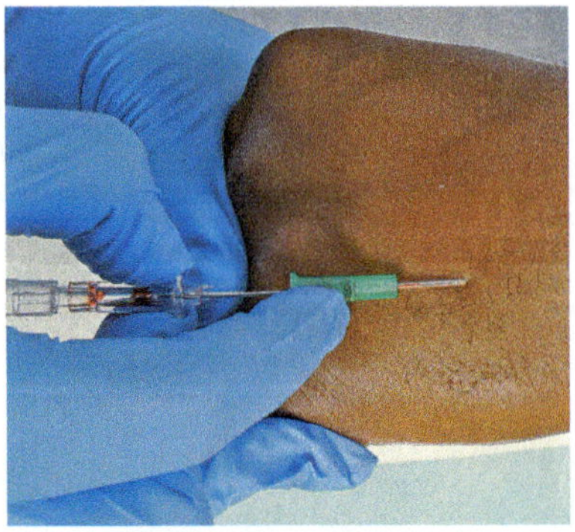

Figure 6.6 Phlebotomist using a needle to withdraw blood.

Therapeutic Procedures

TERM	WORD PARTS	DEFINITION
Medical Procedures		
autologous transfusion (aw-TALL-oh-gus / trans-FYOO-zhun)	auto- = self	Procedure for collecting and storing a patient's own blood several weeks prior to the actual need. It can then be used to replace blood lost during a surgical procedure.
blood transfusion (trans-FYOO-zhun)	trans- = across fus/o = pouring -ion = action	Artificial transfer of blood into the bloodstream.
bone marrow transplant (BMT)		Patient receives red bone marrow from a donor after the patient's own bone marrow has been destroyed by radiation or chemotherapy.
homologous transfusion (hoh-MALL-oh-gus / trans-FYOO-zhun)	homo- = same	Replacement of blood by transfusion of blood received from another person.
packed red cells		A transfusion in which most of the plasma, leukocytes, and platelets have been removed, leaving on erythrocytes.
plasmapheresis (plaz-mah-fah-REE-sis)	-apheresis = removal, carry away	Method of removing plasma from the body without depleting the formed elements. Whole blood is removed and the cells and plasma are separated. The cells are returned to the patient along with a donor plasma transfusion.
whole blood		Refers to the mixture of both plasma and formed elements.

MED TERM TIP

Before a patient receives a blood transfusion, the laboratory performs a **type and cross-match**. This test first double-checks the blood type of both the donor's and recipient's blood. Then a cross-match is performed. This process mixed together small samples of both bloods and observes the mixture for adverse reactions.

Pharmacology

CLASSIFICATION	WORD PARTS	ACTION	EXAMPLES
anticoagulant (an-tih-koh-AG-yoo-lant)	anti- = against coagul/o = clotting	Substance that prevents blood clot formation. Commonly referred to as *blood thinners*.	heparin, HepLock; warfarin, Coumadin
antihemorrhagic (an-tih-hem-er-RAJ-ik)	anti- = against hem/o = blood -rrhagic = pertaining to abnormal flow	Substance that prevents or stops hemorrhaging; a *hemostatic agent.*	aminocaproic acid, Amicar; vitamin K
antiplatelet agents (an-tih-PLATE-let)	anti- = against	Substance that interferes with the action of platelets. Prolongs bleeding time. Used to prevent heart attacks and strokes.	clopidogrel, Plavix; ticlopidine, Ticlid

Pharmacology *(continued)*

CLASSIFICATION	WORD PARTS	ACTION	EXAMPLES
hematinic (hee-mah-TIN-ik)	hemat/o = blood -ic = pertaining to	Substance that increases the number of erythrocytes or the amount of hemoglobin in the blood.	epoetin alfa, Procrit; darbepoetin alfa, Aranesp
thrombolytic (throm-boh-LIT-ik)	thromb/o = clot -lytic = destruction	Term meaning able to dissolve existing blood clots.	alteplase, Activase; streptokinase, Streptase

Abbreviations

ALL	acute lymphocytic leukemia
AML	acute myelogenous leukemia
basos	basophils
BMT	bone marrow transplant
CBC	complete blood count
CLL	chronic lymphocytic leukemia
CML	chronic myelogenous leukemia
diff	differential
eosins, eos	eosinophils
ESR, SR, sed rate	erythrocyte sedimentation rate
HCT, Hct, crit	hematocrit
Hgb, Hb, HGB	hemoglobin
lymphs	lymphocytes
monos	monocytes
PA	pernicious anemia
PCV	packed cell volume
PMN, polys	polymorphonuclear neutrophil
PT, pro-time	prothrombin time
RBC	red blood cell
Rh+	Rh-positive
Rh–	Rh-negative
segs	segmented neutrophils
SMAC	sequential multiple analyzer computer
WBC	white blood cell

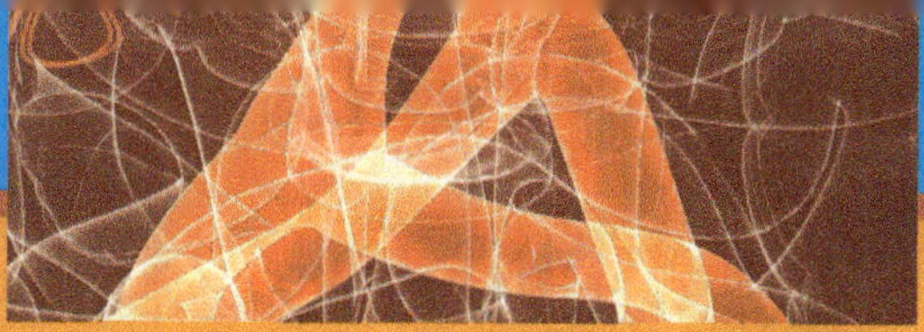

Section II: The Lymphatic and Immune Systems at a Glance

Function

The lymphatic system consists of a network of lymph vessels that pick up excess tissue fluid, cleanse it, and return it to the circulatory system. It also picks up fats that have been absorbed by the digestive system. The immune system fights disease and infections.

Structures

Here are the primary structures that comprise the lymphatic and immune system.

lymph nodes
lymphatic vessels
spleen
thymus gland
tonsils

Word Parts

Here are the most common word parts (with their meanings) used to build lymphatic and immune system terms. For a more comprehensive list, refer to the Terminology section of this chapter.

Combining Forms

adenoid/o	adenoids
axill/o	axilla, underarm
immun/o	protection
inguin/o	groin region
lymph/o	lymph
lymphaden/o	lymph node
lymphangi/o	lymph vessel
nucle/o	nucleus
path/o	disease
splen/o	spleen
thym/o	thymus gland
tonsill/o	tonsils
tox/o	poison

Suffixes

-edema	swelling
-globulin	protein

The Lymphatic and Immune Systems Illustrated

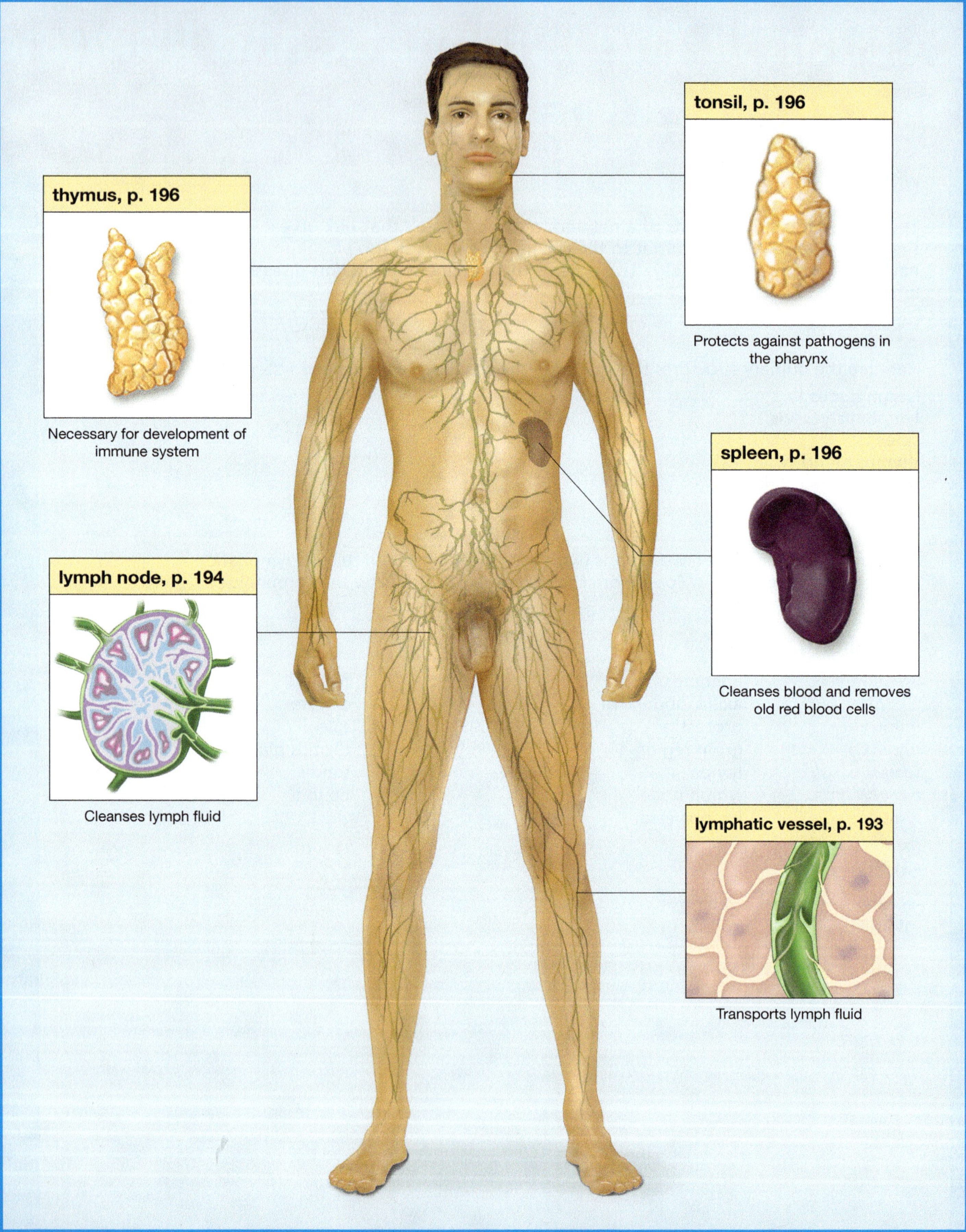

Anatomy and Physiology of the Lymphatic and Immune Systems

lacteals (lack-TEE-als)
lymph (LIMF)
lymph nodes
lymphatic vessels (lim-FAT-ik)
spleen
thymus gland (THIGH-mus)
tonsils (TON-sulls)

The lymphatic system consists of a network of **lymphatic vessels, lymph nodes,** the **spleen,** the **thymus gland,** and the **tonsils.** These organs perform several quite diverse functions for the body. First, they collect excess tissue fluid throughout the body and return it to the circulatory system. The fluid, once inside a lymphatic vessel, is referred to as **lymph.** Lymph vessels located around the small intestines, called **lacteals,** are able to pick up absorbed fats for transport. Additionally, the lymphatic system works with the immune system to form the groups of cells, tissues, organs, and molecules that serve as the body's primary defense against the invasion of pathogens. These systems work together defending the body against foreign invaders and substances, as well as removing our own cells that have become diseased.

Lymphatic Vessels

lymphatic capillaries (CAP-ih-lair-eez)
lymphatic ducts
right lymphatic duct
thoracic duct
valves

The lymphatic vessels form an extensive network of ducts throughout the entire body. However, unlike the circulatory system, these vessels are not in a closed loop. Instead, they serve as one-way pipes conducting lymph from the tissues toward the thoracic cavity (see Figure 6.7 ■). These vessels begin as very small

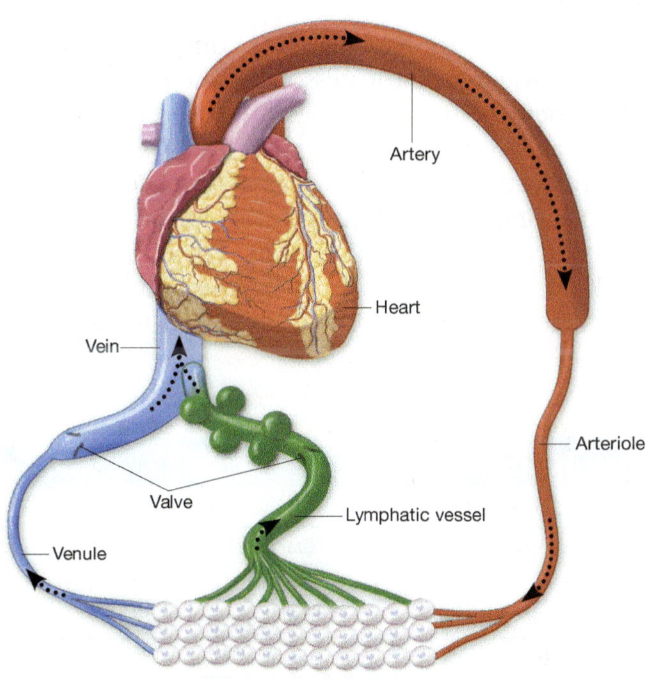

■ **Figure 6.7** Lymphatic vessels (green) pick up excess tissue fluid, purify it in lymph nodes, and return it to the circulatory system.

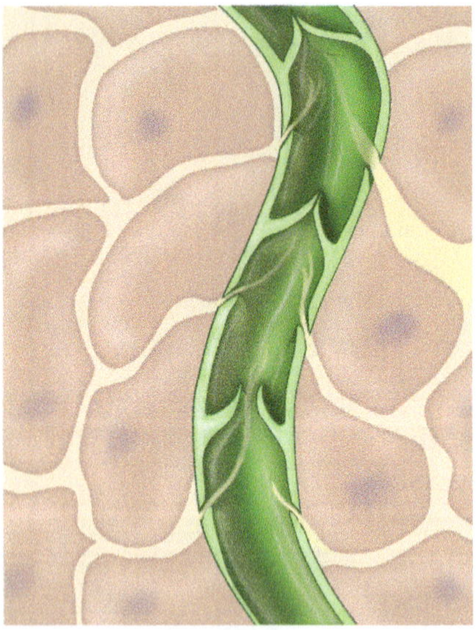
A

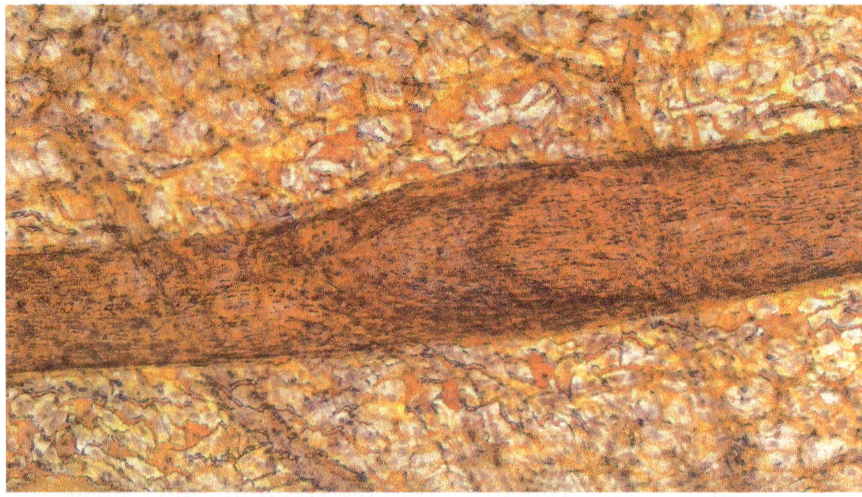
B

■ **Figure 6.8** (A) Lymphatic vessel with valves within tissue cells; (B) photomicrograph of lymphatic vessel with valve clearly visible. *(Michael Abbey/Photo Researchers, Inc.)*

lymphatic capillaries in the tissues. Excessive tissue fluid enters these capillaries to begin the trip back to the circulatory system. The capillaries merge into larger lymphatic vessels. This is a very low pressure system, so these vessels have **valves** along their length to ensure that lymph can only move forward toward the thoracic cavity (see Figure 6.8 ■). These vessels finally drain into one of two large **lymphatic ducts,** the **right lymphatic duct** or the **thoracic duct.** The smaller right lymphatic duct drains the right arm and the right side of the head, neck, and chest. This duct empties lymph into the right subclavian vein. The larger thoracic duct drains lymph from the rest of the body and empties into the left subclavian vein (see Figure 6.9 ■).

MED TERM TIP

The term *capillary* is also used to describe the minute blood vessels within the circulatory system. This is one of several general medical terms, such as valves, cilia, and hair, that are used in several systems.

Lymph Nodes

lymph glands

Lymph nodes are small organs composed of lymphatic tissue located along the route of the lymphatic vessels. These nodes, also referred to as **lymph glands,** house lymphocytes and antibodies and therefore work to remove pathogens and cell debris as lymph passes through them on its way back to the thoracic cavity (see Figure 6.10 ■). Lymph nodes also serve to trap and destroy cells from cancerous tumors. Although found throughout the body, lymph nodes are particularly concentrated in several regions. For example, lymph nodes concentrated in the neck region drain lymph from the head. See again Figure 6.9 and Table 6.2 ■ for a description of some of the most important sites for lymph nodes.

MED TERM TIP

In surgical procedures to remove a malignancy from an organ, such as a breast, the adjacent lymph nodes are also tested for cancer. If cancerous cells are found in the tested lymph nodes, the disease is said to have spread or *metastasized.* Tumor cells may then spread to other parts of the body by means of the lymphatic system.

Table 6.2 Sites for Lymph Nodes

NAME	LOCATION	FUNCTION
axillary (AK-sih-lair-ee)	armpits	Drain arms and shoulder region; cancer cells from breasts may be present
cervical (SER-vih-kal)	neck	Drain head and neck; may be enlarged during upper respiratory infections
inguinal (ING-gwih-nal)	groin	Drain legs and lower pelvis
mediastinal (mee-dee-ass-TYE-nal)	chest	Drain chest cavity

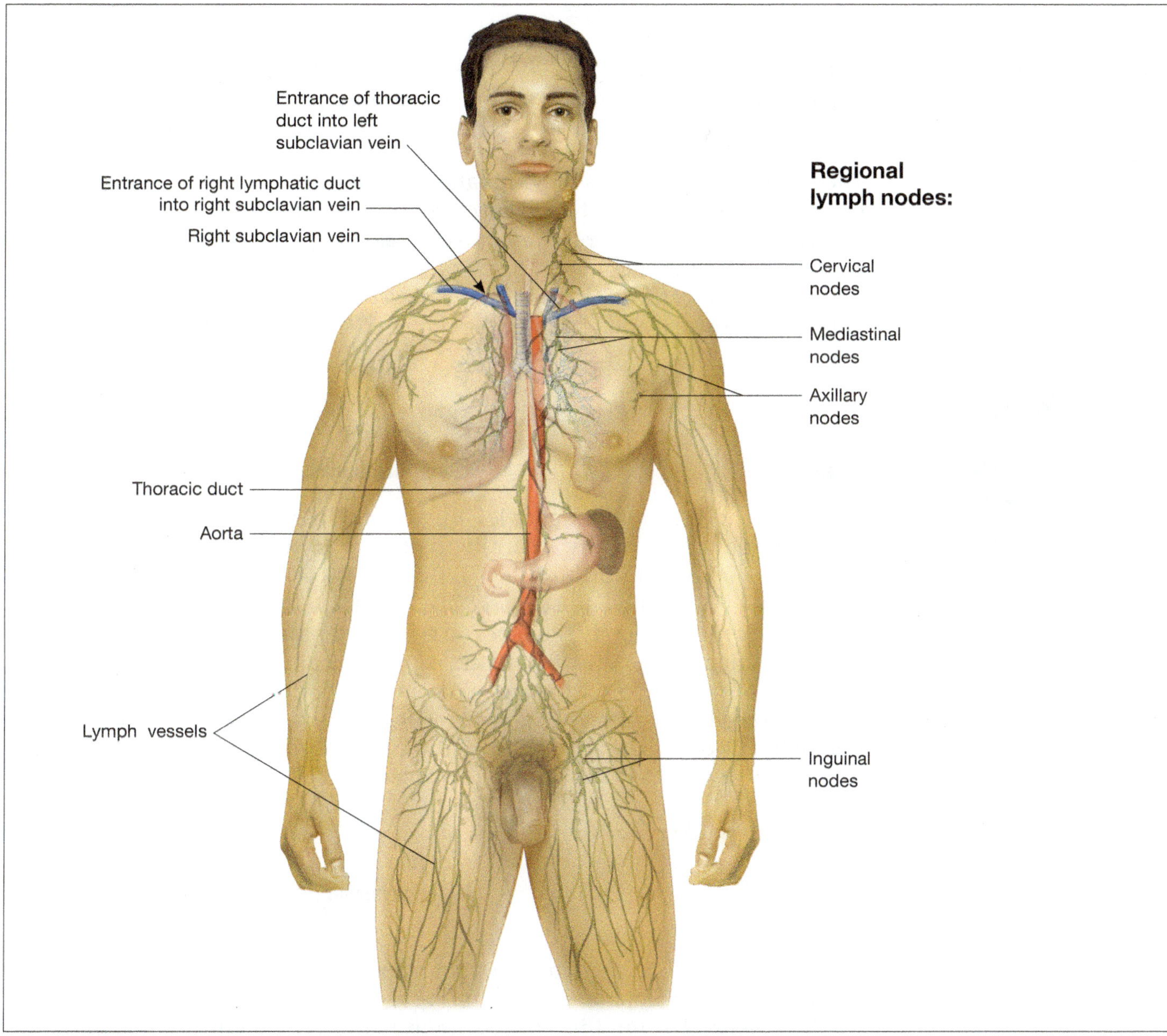

Figure 6.9 Location of lymph vessels, lymphatic ducts, and areas of lymph node concentrations.

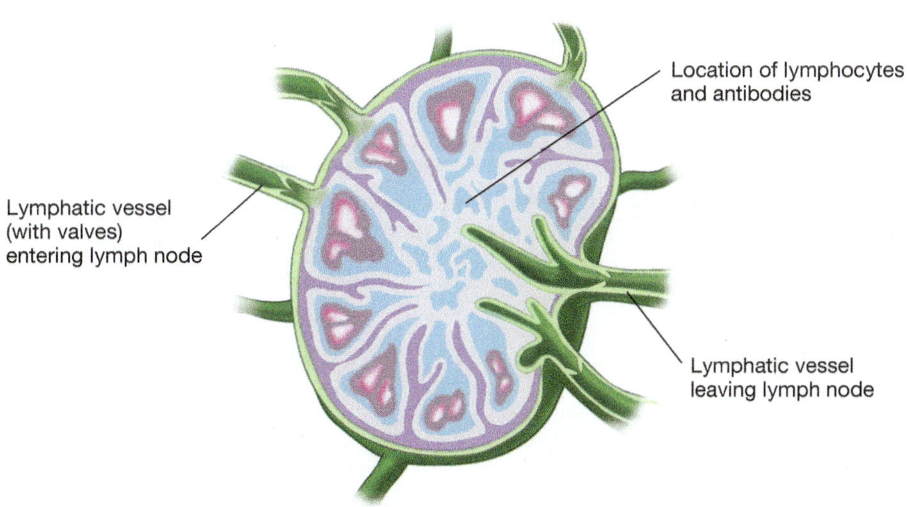

Figure 6.10 Structure of a lymph node.

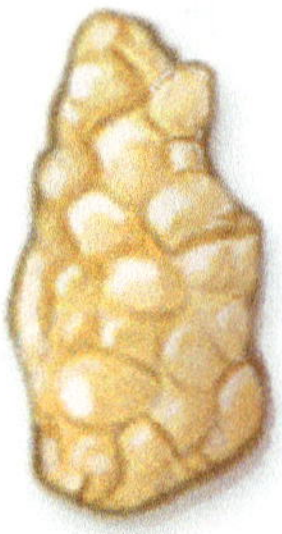

■ **Figure 6.11** Shape of a tonsil.

Tonsils

adenoids (ADD-eh-noydz)
lingual tonsils (LING-gwal)
palatine tonsils (PAL-ah-tyne)
pharyngeal tonsils (fair-IN-jee-al)
pharynx (FAIR-inks)

The tonsils are collections of lymphatic tissue located on each side of the throat or **pharynx** (see Figure 6.11 ■). There are three sets of tonsils: **palatine tonsils, pharyngeal tonsils** (commonly referred to as the **adenoids**), and **lingual tonsils.** All tonsils contain a large number of leukocytes and act as filters to protect the body from the invasion of pathogens through the digestive or respiratory systems. Tonsils are not vital organs and can safely be removed if they become a continuous site of infection.

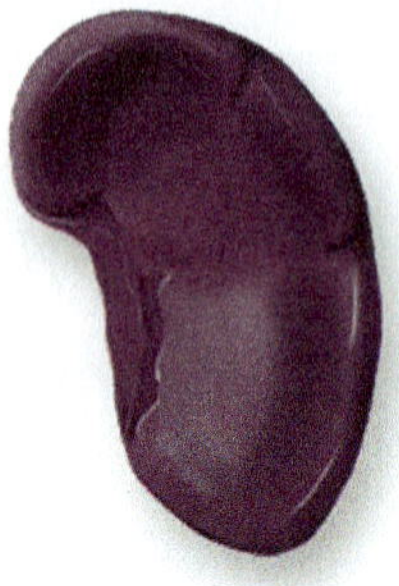

■ **Figure 6.12** Shape of the spleen.

Spleen

blood sinuses
macrophages (MACK-roh-fayj-ez)

The spleen, located in the upper left quadrant of the abdomen, consists of lymphatic tissue that is highly infiltrated with blood vessels (see Figure 6.12 ■). These vessels spread out into slow-moving **blood sinuses.** The spleen filters out and destroys old red blood cells, recycles the iron, and also stores some of the blood supply for the body. Phagocytic **macrophages** line the blood sinuses in the spleen to engulf and remove pathogens. Because the blood is moving through the organ slowly, the macrophages have time to carefully identify pathogens and worn-out red blood cells. The spleen is also not a vital organ and can be removed due to injury or disease. However, without the spleen, a person's susceptibility to a bloodstream infection may be increased.

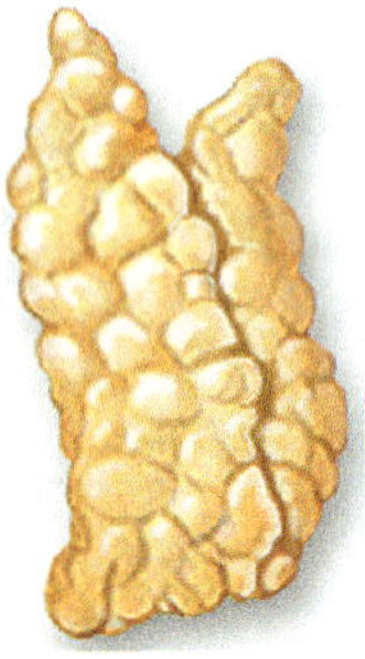

■ **Figure 6.13** Shape of the thymus gland.

Thymus Gland

T cells
T lymphocytes
thymosin (thigh-MOH-sin)

The thymus gland, located in the upper portion of the mediastinum, is essential for the proper development of the immune system (see Figure 6.13 ■). It assists the body with the immune function and the development of antibodies. This organ's hormone, **thymosin,** changes lymphocytes to **T lymphocytes** (simply called **T cells**), which play an important role in the immune response. The thymus is active in the unborn child and throughout childhood until adolescence, when it begins to shrink in size.

Immunity

acquired immunity
active acquired immunity
bacteria (bak-TEE-ree-ah)
cancerous tumors
fungi (FUN-jee)
immune response
immunity (im-YOO-nih-tee)
immunizations (im-yoo-nih-ZAY-shuns)
natural immunity
passive acquired immunity
protozoans (proh-toh-ZOH-anz)
toxins
vaccinations (vak-sih-NAY-shuns)
viruses

Immunity is the body's ability to defend itself against pathogens, such as **bacteria, viruses, fungi, protozoans, toxins,** and **cancerous tumors.** Immunity comes in two forms: **natural immunity** and **acquired immunity.** Natural immunity, also called *innate immunity,* is not specific to a particular disease and does not require prior exposure to the pathogenic agent. A good example of natural immunity is the macrophage. These leukocytes are present throughout all the tissues of the body, but are concentrated in areas of high exposure to invading bacteria, like the lungs and digestive system. They are very active phagocytic cells, ingesting and digesting any pathogen they encounter (see Figure 6.14 ■).

Acquired immunity is the body's response to a specific pathogen and may be established either passively or actively. **Passive acquired immunity** results when a person receives protective substances produced by another human or animal. This may take the form of maternal antibodies crossing the placenta to a baby or an antitoxin or gamma globulin injection. **Active acquired immunity** develops following direct exposure to the pathogenic agent. The agent stimulates the body's **immune response,** a series of different mechanisms all geared to neutralize the agent. For example, a person typically can catch chickenpox only once because once the body has successfully fought the virus, it will be able to more quickly recognize and kill it in the future. **Immunizations** or **vaccinations** are special types of active acquired immunity. Instead of actually being exposed to the infectious agent and having the disease, a person is exposed to a modified or weakened pathogen that is still capable of stimulating the immune response but not actually causing the disease.

Immune Response

antibody (AN-tih-bod-ee)
antibody-mediated immunity
antigen–antibody complex
antigens (AN-tih-jens)
B cells
B lymphocytes
cell-mediated immunity
cellular immunity
cytotoxic (sigh-toh-TOK-sik)
humoral immunity (HYOO-mor-al)
natural killer (NK) **cells**

Disease-causing agents are recognized as being foreign because they display proteins that are different from a person's own natural proteins. Those foreign proteins, called **antigens,** stimulate the immune response. The immune response consists of two distinct and different processes: **humoral immunity** (also called **antibody-mediated immunity**) and **cellular immunity** (also called **cell-mediated immunity**).

MED TERM TIP

The term *humoral* comes from the Latin word for "liquid." It is the old-fashioned term to refer to the fluids of the body.

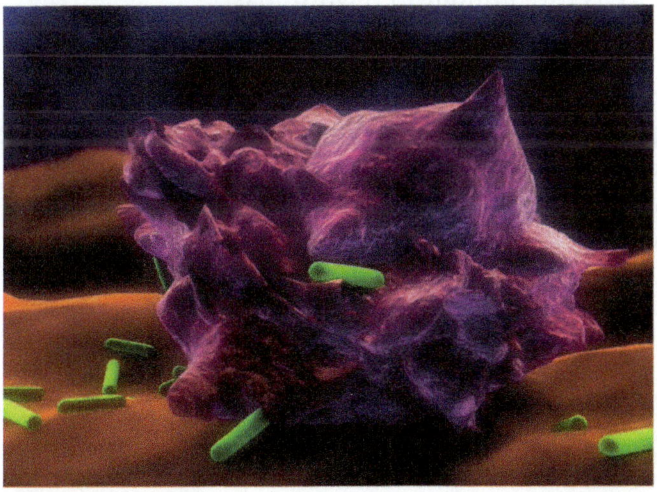

■ **Figure 6.14** Enhanced photomicrograph showing a macrophage (purple) attacking bacillus *Escherichia coli* (green). *(Sebastian Kaulitzki/Shutterstock)*

Humoral immunity refers to the production of **B lymphocytes,** also called **B cells,** which respond to antigens by producing a protective protein, an **antibody.** Antibodies combine with the antigen to form an **antigen–antibody complex.** This complex either targets the foreign substance for phagocytosis or prevents the infectious agent from damaging healthy cells.

Cellular immunity involves the production of T cells and **natural killer** (NK) **cells.** These defense cells are **cytotoxic,** meaning that they physically attack and destroy pathogenic cells.

MED TERM TIP

Analyzing the word parts that make up the term *cytotoxic* gives you a quick idea of this cell's function.

- cyt/o = cell
- tox/o = poison
- -ic = pertaining to

Standard Precautions

cross-infection
nosocomial infection (no-so-KOH-mee-all)
Occupational Safety and Health Administration (OSHA)
reinfection
self-inoculation

Hospitals and other healthcare settings contain a large number of infective pathogens. Patients and healthcare workers are exposed to each other's pathogens and sometimes become infected. An infection acquired in this manner, as a result of hospital exposure, is referred to as a **nosocomial infection.** Nosocomial infections can spread in several ways. **Cross-infection** occurs when a person, either a patient or healthcare worker, acquires a pathogen from another patient or healthcare worker. **Reinfection** takes place when a patient becomes infected again with the same pathogen that originally brought him or her to the hospital. **Self-inoculation** occurs when a person becomes infected in a different part of the body by a pathogen from another part of his or her own body—such as intestinal bacteria spreading to the urethra.

With the appearance of the hepatitis B virus (HBV) in the mid-1960s and the human immunodeficiency virus (HIV) in the mid-1980s, the fight against spreading infections took on even greater significance. In 1987 the **Occupational Safety and Health Administration** (OSHA) issued mandatory guidelines to ensure that all employees at risk of exposure to body fluids are provided with personal protective equipment. These guidelines state that all human blood, tissue, and body fluids must be treated as if they were infected with HIV, HBV, or other bloodborne pathogens. These guidelines were expanded in 1992 and 1996 to encourage the fight against not just bloodborne pathogens, but all nosocomial infections spread by contact with blood, mucous membranes, nonintact skin, and all body fluids (including amniotic fluid, vaginal secretions, pleural fluid, cerebrospinal fluid, peritoneal fluid, pericardial fluid, and semen). These guidelines are commonly referred to as the Standard Precautions:

MED TERM TIP

The simple act of thoroughly washing your hands is the most effective method of preventing the spread of infectious diseases.

1. Wash hands before putting on and after removing gloves and before and after working with each patient or patient equipment.
2. Wear gloves when in contact with any body fluid, mucous membrane, or nonintact skin or if you have chapped hands, a rash, or open sores.
3. Wear a nonpermeable gown or apron during procedures that are likely to expose you to any body fluid, mucous membrane, or nonintact skin.
4. Wear a mask and protective equipment or a face shield when patients are coughing often or if body fluid droplets or splashes are likely.
5. Wear a facemask and eyewear that seal close to the face during procedures that cause body tissues to be vaporized.
6. Remove for proper cleaning any shared equipment—such as a thermometer, stethoscope, or blood pressure cuff—that has come into contact with body fluids, mucous membrane, or nonintact skin.

Terminology

Word Parts Used to Build Lymphatic and Immune System Terms

The following lists contain the combining forms, suffixes, and prefixes used to build terms in the remaining sections of this chapter.

Combining Forms

adenoid/o	adenoids
axill/o	axilla, underarm
cortic/o	outer region, cortex
immun/o	protection
inguin/o	groin
lymph/o	lymph
lymphaden/o	lymph node
lymphangi/o	lymph vessel
nucle/o	nucleus
path/o	disease
pneumon/o	lung
sarc/o	flesh
splen/o	spleen
thym/o	thymus gland
tonsill/o	tonsils

Suffixes

-al	pertaining to
-ar	pertaining to
-ary	pertaining to
-atic	pertaining to
-ectomy	surgical removal
-edema	swelling
-genic	producing
-globulin	protein
-gram	record
-graphy	process of recording
-ia	condition
-iasis	abnormal condition
-ic	pertaining to
-itis	inflammation
-logy	study of
-megaly	enlarged
-oma	tumor
-osis	abnormal condition
-pathy	disease
-therapy	treatment

Prefixes

anti-	against
auto-	self
mono-	one

Anatomical Terms

TERM	WORD PARTS	DEFINITION
axillary (AK-sih-lair-ee)	axill/o = axilla, underarm -ary = pertaining to	Pertaining to the underarm region.
immunoglobulins (im-yoo-noh-GLOB-yoo-linz)	immun/o = protection -globulin = protein	Antibodies secreted by the B cells. All antibodies are immunoglobulins and assist in protecting the body and its surfaces from the invasion of bacteria. For example, the immunoglobulin IgA in colostrum, the first milk from the mother, helps to protect the newborn from infection.
inguinal (ING-gwih-nal)	inguin/o = groin -al = pertaining to	Pertaining to the groin region.
lymphangial (lim-FAN-gee-al)	lymphangi/o = lymph vessel -al = pertaining to	Pertaining to lymph vessels.

Anatomical Terms *(continued)*

TERM	WORD PARTS	DEFINITION
lymphatic (lim-FAT-ik)	lymph/o = lymph -atic = pertaining to	Pertaining to lymph.
splenic (SPLEN-ik)	splen/o = spleen -ic = pertaining to	Pertaining to the spleen.
thymic (THIGH-mik)	thym/o = thymus gland -ic = pertaining to	Pertaining to the thymus gland.
tonsillar (ton-sih-lar)	tonsill/o = tonsils -ar = pertaining to	Pertaining to the tonsils.

Pathology

TERM	WORD PARTS	DEFINITION
Medical Specialties		
allergist (AL-er-jist)		A physician who specializes in testing for and treating allergies.
immunology (im-yoo-NALL-oh-jee)	immun/o = protection -logy = study of	A branch of medicine concerned with diagnosis and treatment of infectious diseases and other disorders of the immune system. Physician is an *immunologist.*
pathology (path-OL-oh-gee)	path/o = disease -logy = study of	A branch of medicine concerned with determining the underlying causes and development of diseases. Physician is an *immunologist.*
Signs and Symptoms		
hives		Appearance of wheals as part of an allergic reaction.
inflammation (in-flah-MA-shun)		The tissues' response to injury from pathogens or physical agents. Characterized by redness, pain, swelling, and feeling hot to touch.

MED TERM TIP

Word Watch: The terms *inflammation* and *inflammatory* are spelled with two *m*'s, while *inflame* and *inflamed* each have only one *m*. These may be the most commonly misspelled terms by medical terminology students.

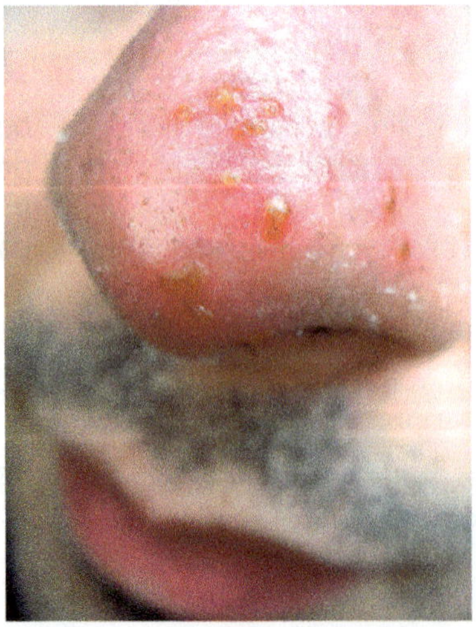

Figure 6.15 Inflammation as illustrated by cellulitis of the nose. Note that the area is red and swollen. It is also painful and hot to touch.

Pathology *(continued)*

TERM	WORD PARTS	DEFINITION
lymphedema (limf-eh-DEE-mah)	lymph/o = lymph -edema = swelling	Edema appearing in the extremities due to an obstruction of the lymph flow through the lymphatic vessels.
pathogenic (path-oh-JEN-ik)	path/o = disease -genic = producing	An adjective term to describe something—such as bacteria, viruses, or toxins—that produce disease.
splenomegaly (splee-noh-MEG-ah-lee)	splen/o = spleen -megaly = enlarged	An enlarged spleen.
urticaria (er-tih-KAY-ree-ah)		Severe itching associated with hives, usually linked to food allergy, stress, or drug reactions.
Allergic Reactions		
allergy (AL-er-jee)		Hypersensitivity to a common substance in the environment or to a medication. The substance causing the allergic reaction is called an *allergen.*
anaphylactic shock (an-ah-fih-LAK-tik)		Life-threatening condition resulting from a severe allergic reaction. Examples of instances that may trigger this reaction include bee stings, medications, or the ingestion of foods. Circulatory and respiratory problems occur, including respiratory distress, hypotension, edema, tachycardia, and convulsions. Also called **anaphylaxis.**
Lymphatic System		
adenoiditis (add-eh-noyd-EYE-tis)	adenoid/o = adenoids -itis = inflammation	Inflammation of the adenoids.
autoimmune disease	auto- = self	A disease resulting from the body's immune system attacking its own cells as if they were pathogens. Examples include systemic lupus erythematosus, rheumatoid arthritis, and multiple sclerosis.
elephantiasis (el-eh-fan-TYE-ah-sis)	-iasis = abnormal condition	Inflammation, obstruction, and destruction of the lymph vessels resulting in enlarged tissues due to edema.
Hodgkin's disease (HD) (HOJ-kins)		Also called *Hodgkin's lymphoma.* Cancer of the lymphatic cells found in concentration in the lymph nodes. Named after Thomas Hodgkin, a British physician, who first described it.
lymphadenitis (lim-fad-en-EYE-tis)	lymphaden/o = lymph node -itis = inflammation	Inflammation of the lymph nodes. Referred to as *swollen glands.*
lymphadenopathy (lim-fad-eh-NOP-ah-thee)	lymphaden/o = lymph node -pathy = disease	A general term for lymph node diseases.
lymphangioma (lim-fan-jee-OH-mah)	lymphangi/o = lymph vessel -oma = tumor	A tumor in a lymphatic vessel.

Pathology *(continued)*

TERM	WORD PARTS	DEFINITION
lymphoma (lim-FOH-mah)	lymph/o = lymph -oma = tumor	A tumor in lymphatic tissue.
mononucleosis (mono) (mon-oh-nook-lee-OH-sis)	mono- = one nucle/o = nucleus -osis = abnormal condition	Acute infectious disease with a large number of abnormal mononuclear lymphocytes. Caused by the Epstein–Barr virus. Abnormal liver function may occur.
non-Hodgkin's lymphoma (NHL)	lymph/o = lymph -oma = tumor	Cancer of the lymphatic tissues other than Hodgkin's lymphoma.

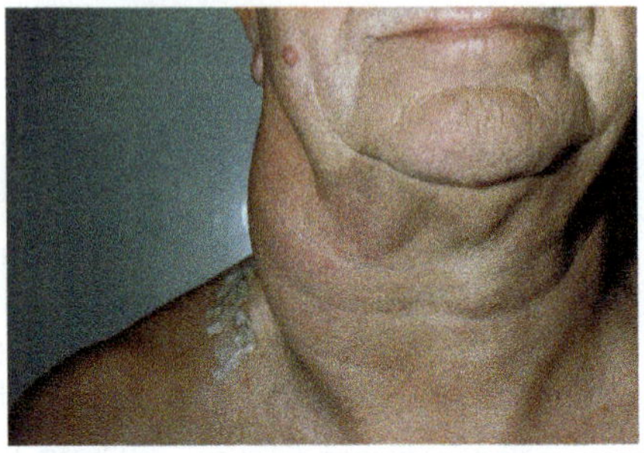

■ **Figure 6.16** Photo of the neck of a patient with non-Hodgkin's lymphoma showing the swelling associated with enlarged lymph nodes.

TERM	WORD PARTS	DEFINITION
thymoma (thigh-MOH-mah)	thym/o = thymus gland -oma = tumor	A tumor of the thymus gland.
tonsillitis (ton-sil-EYE-tis)	tonsill/o = tonsils -itis = inflammation	Inflammation of the tonsils.
Immune System		
acquired immunodeficiency syndrome (AIDS) (ac-quired / im-you-noh-dee-FIH-shen-see / SIN-drohm)	immun/o = protection	Disease involving a defect in the cell-mediated immunity system. A syndrome of opportunistic infections occurring in the final stages of infection with the human immunodeficiency virus (HIV). This virus attacks T4 lymphocytes and destroys them, reducing the person's ability to fight infection.
AIDS-related complex (ARC)		Early stage of AIDS. There is a positive test for the virus, but only mild symptoms of weight loss, fatigue, skin rash, and anorexia.
graft versus host disease (GVHD)		Serious complication of bone marrow transplant (graft). Immune cells from the donor bone marrow attack the recipient's (host's) tissues.
human immunodeficiency virus (HIV) (im-yoo-noh-dee-FIH-shen-see)	immun/o = protection	Virus that causes AIDS; also known as a **retrovirus**.

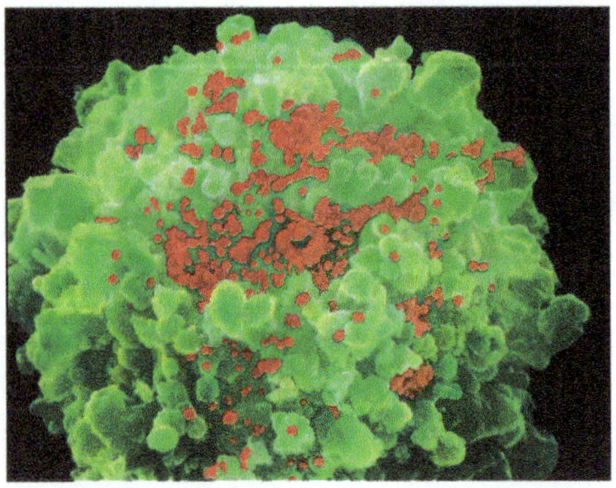

■ **Figure 6.17** Color-enhanced scanning electron micrograph of HIV virus (red) infecting T-helper cells (green). *(National Institute for Biological Standards and Control (U.K.)/Science Photo Library/Photo Researchers, Inc.)*

Pathology *(continued)*

TERM	WORD PARTS	DEFINITION
immunocompromised (im-you-noh-KOM-pro-mized)	immun/o = protection	Having an immune system that is unable to respond properly to pathogens. Also called *immunodeficiency disorder.*
Kaposi's sarcoma (KS) (KAP-oh-seez / sar-KOH-mah)	sarc/o = flesh -oma = tumor	Form of skin cancer frequently seen in patients with AIDS. It consists of brownish-purple papules that spread from the skin and metastasize to internal organs. Named for Moritz Kaposi, an Austrian dermatologist.
opportunistic infections		Infectious diseases associated with patients who have compromised immune systems and therefore a lowered resistance to infections and parasites. May be the result of HIV infection.
pneumocystis pneumonia (PCP) (noo-moh-SIS-tis / new-MOH-nee-ah)	pneumon/o = lung -ia = condition	Pneumonia common in patients with weakened immune systems, such as AIDS patients, caused by the *Pneumocystis jiroveci* fungus.
sarcoidosis (sar-koyd-OH-sis)	-osis = abnormal condition	Disease of unknown cause that forms fibrous lesions commonly appearing in the lymph nodes, liver, skin, lungs, spleen, eyes, and small bones of the hands and feet.
severe combined immunodeficiency syndrome (SCIDS)	immun/o = protection	Disease seen in children born with a nonfunctioning immune system. Often these children are forced to live in sealed sterile rooms.

Diagnostic Procedures

TERM	WORD PARTS	DEFINITION
Clinical Laboratory Tests		
enzyme-linked immunosorbent assay (ELISA) (EN-zym / LINK'T / im-yoo-noh-sor-bent / ASS-say)	immun/o = protection	Blood test for an antibody to the HIV virus. A positive test means that the person has been exposed to the virus. There may be a false-positive reading, and then the Western blot test would be used to verify the results.
Western blot		Test used as a backup to the ELISA blood test to detect the presence of the antibody to HIV (AIDS virus) in the blood.
Diagnostic Imaging		
lymphangiogram (lim-FAN-jee-oh-gram)	lymphangi/o = lymph vessel -gram = record	X-ray record of the lymphatic vessels produced by lymphangiography.
lymphangiography (lim-FAN-jee-oh-graf-ee)	lymphangi/o = lymph vessel -graphy = process of recording	X-ray taken of the lymph vessels after the injection of dye into the foot. The lymph flow through the chest is traced.

Diagnostic Procedures *(continued)*

TERM	WORD PARTS	DEFINITION
Additional Diagnostic Procedures		
Monospot		Blood test for infectious mononucleosis.
scratch test		Form of allergy testing in which the body is exposed to an allergen through a light scratch on the skin.

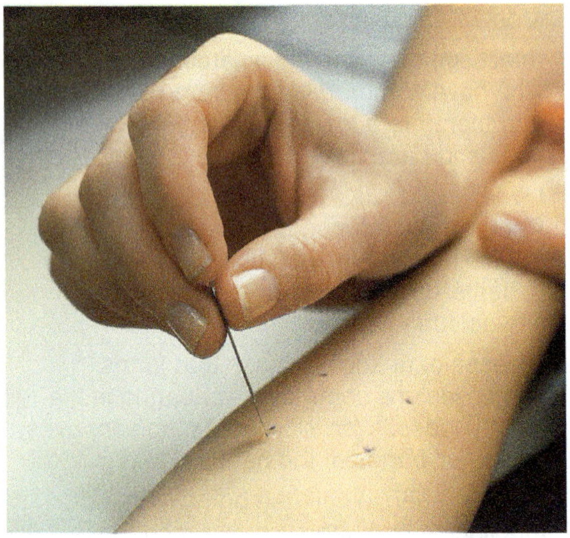

A

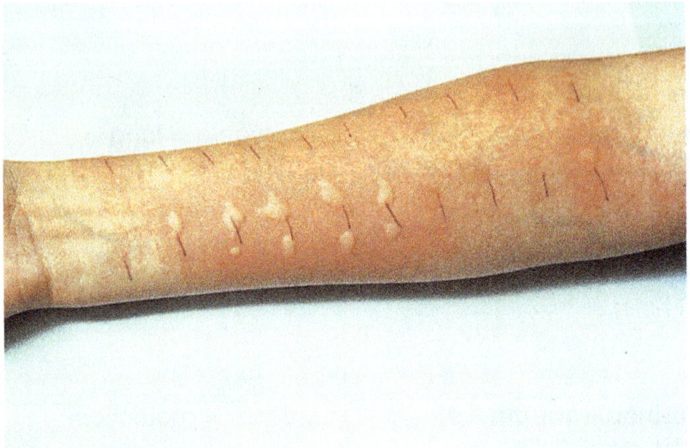

B

■ **Figure 6.18** (A) Scratch test; patient is exposed to allergens through a light scratch on the skin; (B) Positive scratch test results. Inflammation indicates person is allergic to that substance. *(A. James King-Holmes/ Science Photo Library/Photo Researchers, Inc. B. SUI/Photo Researchers, Inc.)*

Therapeutic Procedures

TERM	WORD PARTS	DEFINITION
Medical Procedures		
immunotherapy (IM-yoo-noh-thair-ah-pee)	immun/o = protection -therapy = treatment	Giving a patient an injection of immunoglobulins or antibodies in order to treat a disease. The antibodies may be produced by another person or animal, for example, antivenom for snake bites. More recent developments include treatments to boost the activity of the immune system, especially to treat cancer and AIDS.
vaccination (vak-sih-NAY-shun)		Exposure to a weakened pathogen that stimulates the immune response and antibody production in order to confer protection against the full-blown disease. Also called *immunization.*

Therapeutic Procedures *(continued)*

TERM	WORD PARTS	DEFINITION
Surgical Procedures		
adenoidectomy (add-eh-noyd-EK-toh-mee)	adenoid/o = adenoids -ectomy = surgical removal	Surgical removal of the adenoids.
lymphadenectomy (lim-fad-eh-NEK-toh-mee)	lymphaden/o = lymph node -ectomy = surgical removal	Removal of a lymph node. This is usually done to test for malignancy.
splenectomy (splee-NEK-toh-mee)	splen/o = spleen -ectomy = surgical removal	Surgical removal of the spleen.
thymectomy (thigh-MEK-toh-mee)	thym/o = thymus gland -ectomy = surgical removal	Surgical removal of the thymus gland.
tonsillectomy (ton-sih-LEK-toh-mee)	tonsill/o = tonsils -ectomy = surgical removal	Surgical removal of the tonsils.

Pharmacology

CLASSIFICATION		ACTION	EXAMPLES
antihistamine (an-tih-HIST-ah-meen)	anti- = against	Blocks the effects of histamine released by the body during an allergic reaction.	cetirizine, Zyrtec; diphenhydramine, Benadryl
corticosteroids (core-tih-koh-STARE-royds)	cortic/o = outer region, cortex	A hormone produced by the adrenal cortex that has very strong anti-inflammatory properties. Particularly useful in treating autoimmune diseases.	prednisone; methylprednisolone, Solu-Medrol
immunosuppressants (im-yoo-noh-sue-PRESS-antz)	immun/o = protection	Blocks certain actions of the immune system. Required to prevent rejection of a transplanted organ.	mycophenolate mofetil, CellCept; cyclosporine, Neoral
protease inhibitor drugs (PROH-tee-ace)		Inhibits protease, an enzyme viruses need to reproduce.	indinavir, Crixivan; saquinavir, Fortovase
reverse transcriptase inhibitor drugs (trans-KRIP-tays)		Inhibits reverse transcriptase, an enzyme needed by viruses to reproduce.	lamivudine, Epivir; zidovudine, Retrovir

Abbreviations

AIDS	acquired immunodeficiency syndrome	**KS**	Kaposi's sarcoma
ARC	AIDS-related complex	**mono**	mononucleosis
ELISA	enzyme-linked immunosorbent assay	**NHL**	non-Hodgkin's lymphoma
GVHD	graft versus host disease	**NK**	natural killer cells
HD	Hodgkin's disease	**PCP**	pneumocystis pneumonia
HIV	human immunodeficiency virus	**SCIDS**	severe combined immunodeficiency syndrome
Ig	immunoglobulins (IgA, IgD, IgE, IgG, IgM)		

Chapter Review

Real-World Applications

Medical Record Analysis

This Discharge Summary contains 11 medical terms. Underline each term and write it in the list below the report. Then define each term. Note: Some terms are defined in other chapters; use your glossary-index to locate and define these terms.

Discharge Summary

Admitting Diagnosis:	Splenomegaly, weight loss, diarrhea, fatigue, chronic cough
Final Diagnosis:	Non-Hodgkin's lymphoma of spleen; splenectomy
History of Present Illness:	Patient is a 36-year-old businessman who was first seen in the office with complaints of feeling generally "run down," intermittent diarrhea, weight loss, and, more recently, a dry cough. He states he has been aware of these symptoms for approximately six months. Monospot and ELISA are both negative. In spite of a 35-pound weight loss, he has abdominal swelling and splenomegaly was detected. He was admitted to the hospital for further evaluation and treatment.
Summary of Hospital Course:	Full-body MRI confirmed splenomegaly and located a 3-cm encapsulated tumor in the spleen. Biopsies taken from the splenic tumor confirmed the diagnosis of non-Hodgkin's lymphoma. The patient underwent splenectomy for removal of the tumor.
Discharge Plans:	Patient was discharged home following recovery from the splenectomy. The abdominal swelling and diarrhea were resolved, but the dry cough persisted. He was referred to an oncologist for evaluation and surveillance for metastases.

	Term	Definition
1	______	______
2	______	______
3	______	______
4	______	______
5	______	______
6	______	______
7	______	______
8	______	______
9	______	______
10	______	______
11	______	______

Chart Note Transcription

The chart note below contains 10 phrases that can be reworded with a medical term that you learned in this chapter. Each phrase is identified with an underline. Determine the medical term and write your answers in the space provided.

Current Complaint: Patient is a 22-year-old female referred to the specialist in treating blood disorders ❶ by her internist. Her complaints include fatigue, weight loss, and easy bruising.

Past History: Patient had normal childhood diseases. She is a college student and was feeling well until symptoms gradually appeared starting approximately 3 months ago.

Signs and Symptoms: An immunoassay test for HIV exposure ❷ was normal. The measure of the blood's coagulation abilities ❸ indicated that the blood took too long to form a clot. A blood test to count all the blood cells ❹ reported too few red blood cells ❺ and too few clotting cells. ❻ There were too many white blood cells, ❼ but they were immature and abnormal. A sample of bone marrow obtained for microscopic examination ❽ found an excessive number of immature white blood cells.

Diagnosis: Cancer of the white blood cell–forming bone marrow. ❾

Treatment: Aggressive chemotherapy for the cancer of the white blood cell–forming bone marrow ❾ and replacement blood from another person ❿ to replace the erythrocytes and platelets.

❶ ____________________

❷ ____________________

❸ ____________________

❹ ____________________

❺ ____________________

❻ ____________________

❼ ____________________

❽ ____________________

❾ ____________________

❿ ____________________

Case Study

Below is a case study presentation of a patient with a condition covered in this chapter. Read the case study and answer the questions below. Some questions will ask for information not included within this chapter. Use your text, a medical dictionary, or any other reference material you choose to answer these questions.

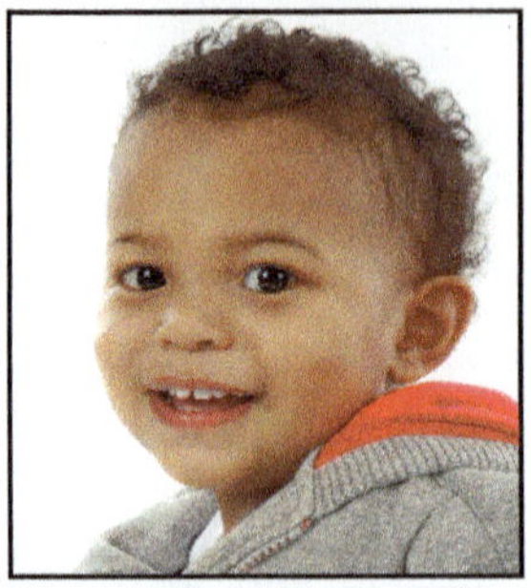

(Flashon Studio/Shutterstock)

A 2-year-old boy is being seen by a hematologist. The child's symptoms include the sudden onset of high fevers, thrombopenia, epistaxis, gingival bleeding, petechiae, and ecchymoses after minor traumas. The physician has ordered a bone marrow aspiration to confirm the clinical diagnosis of acute lymphocytic leukemia. If the diagnosis is positive, the child will be placed immediately on intensive chemotherapy. The physician has informed the parents that treatment produces remission in 90% of children with ALL, especially those between the ages of 2 and 8.

1. What pathological condition does the hematologist suspect? Look this condition up in a reference source and include a short description of it.

____

____

2. List and define each of the patient's presenting symptoms in your own words.

____

____

3. What diagnostic test did the physician perform? Describe it in your own words.

____

____

4. Explain the phrase "clinical diagnosis" in your own words.

____

____

5. If the suspected diagnosis is correct, explain the treatment that will begin.

____

____

6. What do you think the term "remission" means?

____

____

Practice Exercises

A. Complete the Statement

1. The study of the blood is called ______________________.
2. The organs of the lymphatic system other than lymphatic vessels and lymph nodes are the ______________________, ______________________, and ______________________.
3. The two lymph ducts are the ______________________ and ______________________.
4. The primary concentrations of lymph nodes are the ______________________, ______________________, ______________________, and ______________________ regions.
5. The process whereby cells ingest and destroy bacteria within the body is ______________________.
6. The formed elements of blood are the ______________________, ______________________, and ______________________.
7. The fluid portion of blood is called ______________________.
8. ______________________ immunity develops following direct exposure to a pathogen.
9. Humoral immunity is also referred to as ______________________ immunity.
10. The medical term for blood clotting is ______________________.

B. Suffix Practice

Use the following suffixes to create medical terms for the following definitions.

-penia	-globin	-cytosis	-cyte	–globulin

1. too few white (cells) ______________________
2. too few red (cells) ______________________
3. too few clotting (cells) ______________________
4. too few of all cells ______________________
5. increase in white cells ______________________
6. increase in red cells ______________________
7. increase in clotting cells ______________________
8. blood protein ______________________
9. immunity protein ______________________
10. red cell ______________________
11. white cell ______________________
12. lymph cell ______________________

C. Combining Form Practice

The combining form **splen/o** refers to the spleen. Use it to write a term that means:

1. enlargement of the spleen ______
2. surgical removal of the spleen ______
3. cutting into the spleen ______

The combining form **lymph/o** refers to the lymph. Use it to write a term that means:

4. lymph cells ______
5. tumor of the lymph system ______

The combining form **lymphaden/o** refers to the lymph nodes. Use it to write a term that means:

6. disease of a lymph gland ______
7. tumor of a lymph gland ______
8. inflammation of a lymph gland ______

The combining form **immun/o** refers to the immune system. Use it to write a term that means:

9. specialist in the study of the immune system ______
10. immune protein ______
11. study of the immune system ______

The combining form **hemat/o** refers to blood. Use it to write a term that means:

12. relating to the blood ______
13. blood tumor or mass ______
14. blood formation ______

The combining form **hem/o** refers to blood. Use it to write a term that means:

15. blood destruction ______
16. blood protein ______

D. What Does it Stand For?

1. basos ______
2. CBC ______
3. Hgb ______
4. PT ______
5. GVHD ______

6. RBC ______________________________

7. PCV ______________________________

8. ESR ______________________________

9. diff ______________________________

10. lymphs ______________________________

E. Terminology Matching

Match each term to its definition.

1. ______ thalassemia	a.	fluid portion of blood
2. ______ lacteals	b.	disease in which blood does not clot
3. ______ A, B, AB, O	c.	conditions with reduced number of RBCs
4. ______ plasma	d.	mass of blood
5. ______ dyscrasia	e.	blood type
6. ______ hematoma	f.	blood-clotting protein
7. ______ anemia	g.	type of anemia
8. ______ serum	h.	general term for blood disorders
9. ______ hemophilia	i.	lymph vessels around intestine
10. ______ fibrinogen	j.	plasma with inactivated fibrinogen

F. What's the Abbreviation?

1. acquired immunodeficiency syndrome ______________________________

2. AIDS-related complex ______________________________

3. human immunodeficiency virus ______________________________

4. acute lymphocytic leukemia ______________________________

5. bone marrow transplant ______________________________

6. mononucleosis ______________________________

7. Kaposi's sarcoma ______________________________

8. eosinophils ______________________________

9. immunoglobulin ______________________________

10. severe combined immunodeficiency syndrome ______________________________

G. Define the Combining Form

	Combining Form	Example from Chapter
1. lymph node	_______________	_______________
2. clot	_______________	_______________
3. blood	_______________	_______________
4. tonsil	_______________	_______________
5. poison	_______________	_______________
6. eat/swallow	_______________	_______________
7. lymph vessel	_______________	_______________
8. disease	_______________	_______________
9. spleen	_______________	_______________
10. lymph	_______________	_______________

H. Fill in the Blank

Kaposi's sarcoma	mononucleosis	Hodgkin's disease	aplastic
polycythemia vera	anaphylactic shock	AIDS	pernicious
pneumocystis	HIV		

1. The condition characterized by the production of too many red blood cells is called _______________.
2. The Epstein–Barr virus is thought to be responsible for what infectious disease? _______________.
3. A life-threatening allergic reaction is _______________.
4. The virus responsible for causing AIDS is _______________.
5. A cancer that is seen frequently in AIDS patients is _______________.
6. An ELISA is used to test for _______________.
7. Malignant tumors concentrate in lymph nodes with this disease: _______________.
8. A type of pneumonia seen in AIDS patients is _______________ pneumonia.
9. _______________ anemia is a severe form of anemia caused by nonfunctioning red bone marrow.
10. _______________ anemia is the result of a vitamin B_{12} deficiency.

I. Terminology Matching

Match each term to its definition.

1. ________ allergy
2. ________ nosocomial
3. ________ phagocytosis
4. ________ hives
5. ________ antibody
6. ________ antigen
7. ________ Hodgkin's disease
8. ________ sarcoidosis
9. ________ vaccination
10. ________ ELISA

a. seen in an allergic reaction
b. substance that stimulates antibody formation
c. a hypersensitivity reaction
d. engulfing
e. protective blood protein
f. a type of cancer
g. autoimmune disease
h. infection acquired in the hospital
i. blood test for AIDS
j. immunization

J. Pharmacology Challenge

Fill in the classification for each drug description, then match the brand name.

	Drug Description	Classification	Brand Name
1.	________ inhibits enzyme needed for viral reproduction	____________________	a. HepLock
2.	________ prevents blood clot formation	____________________	b. Activase
3.	________ stops bleeding	____________________	c. Solu-Medrol
4.	________ blocks effects of histamine	____________________	d. Amicar
5.	________ prevents rejection of a transplanted organ	____________________	e. Epivir
6.	________ dissolves existing blood clots	____________________	f. CellCept
7.	________ increases number of erythrocytes	____________________	g. Procrit
8.	________ strong anti-inflammatory properties	____________________	h. Zyrtec
9.	________ interferes with action of platelets	____________________	i. Plavix

K. Terminology Matching

Match each term to its definition.

1. ________ culture and sensitivity
2. ________ hematocrit
3. ________ complete blood count
4. ________ erythrocyte sedimentation rate
5. ________ prothrombin time
6. ________ white cell differential
7. ________ red cell morphology

a. measure of blood's clotting ability
b. counts number of each type of blood cell
c. examines cells for abnormal shape
d. checks blood for bacterial growth and best antibiotic to use
e. determines number of each type of white blood cell
f. measures percent of whole blood that is red blood cells
g. an indicator of the presence of an inflammatory condition

L. Career Pathways

Select one of the career pathways. Use the Internet and various Web search engines to research the pathway. Once you are done with your research, write a brief report on what you have learned, including required skills, certification, licensure, and academic requirements. If you have e-mail access, send an e-mail to your instructor with the report as an attachment. Remember to follow guidelines for writing a professional e-mail.

M. Professional Organizations

Career-ready individuals seek new methods, practices, and ideas from a variety of sources that they can apply to their own workplace. A professional organization is one such resource. Joining a professional organization provides you with opportunities to learn more about your industry, strengthen your job skills, achieve accreditation or certification in your field, and expand your network of personal contacts. To an employer, it shows that you are motivated to look beyond the workplace to find new and innovative ideas that can help you and your organization be more productive.

One way that a professional organization helps its members is by distributing information about the industry through Web sites, newsletters, or magazines. Working in teams of three or four, select a health care career and create a two-page publication for a professional organization that would serve it. Use the Internet to research current trends, policies, or events affecting the industry. Be sure to gather information on the organization's accreditation and certification procedures, if applicable, and how they prepare members to achieve the credentials necessary for certification and/or licensure in their field. Give the publication a suitable name, and write three or four articles that the members would find useful. Include correct medical terminology and cite all sources used in your research applying conventional citation methods. Share your article with a peer. Provide feedback and suggestions to each other; then revise your document as necessary. When your project is complete, print it to share with the class.

Labeling Exercise

Image A

Write the labels for this figure on the numbered lines provided.

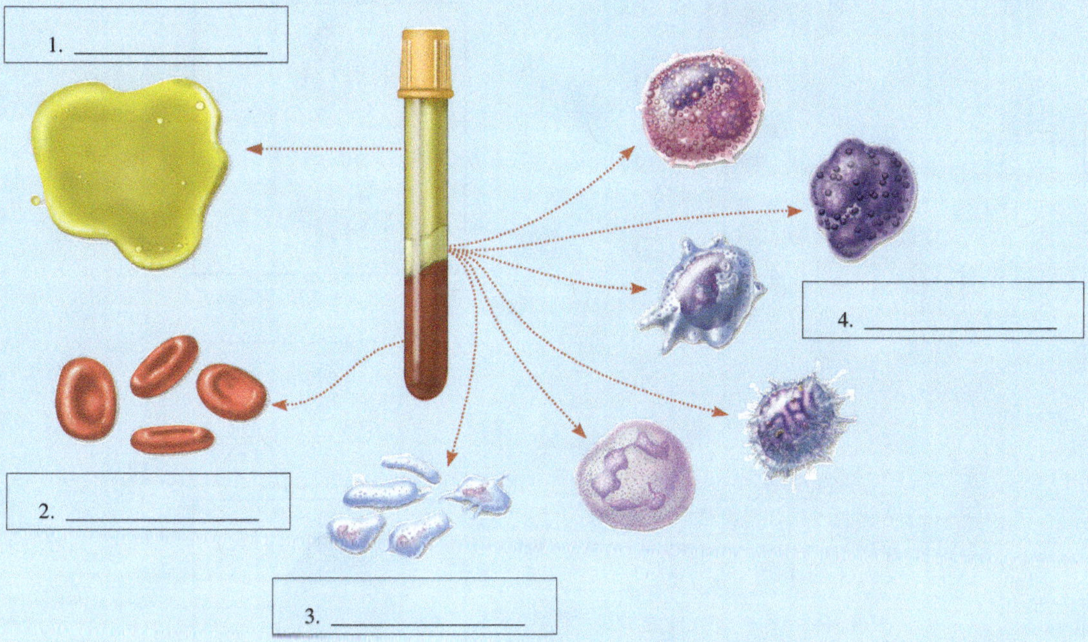

Image B

Write the labels for this figure on the numbered lines provided.

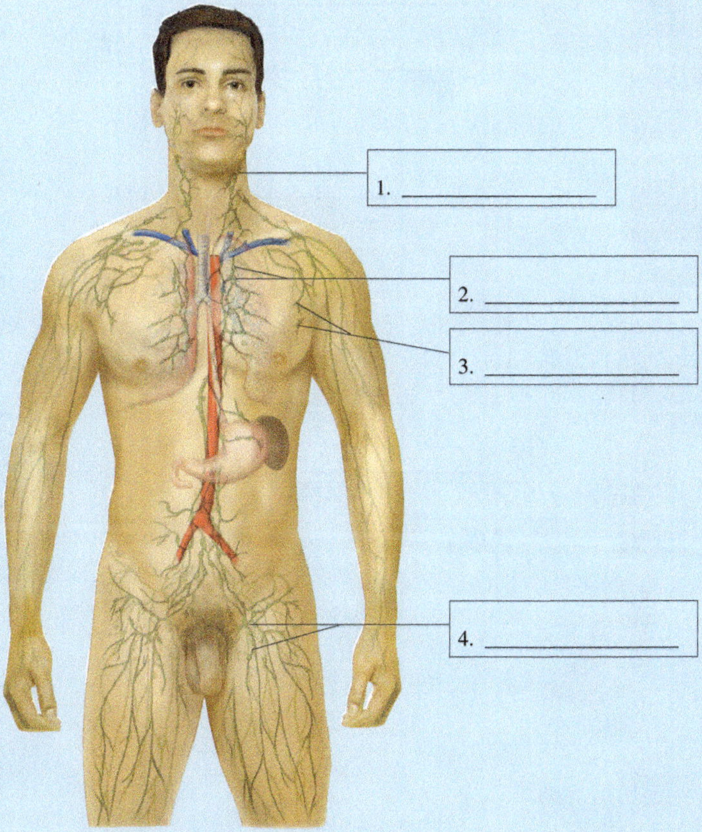

Image C

Write the labels for this figure on the numbered lines provided.

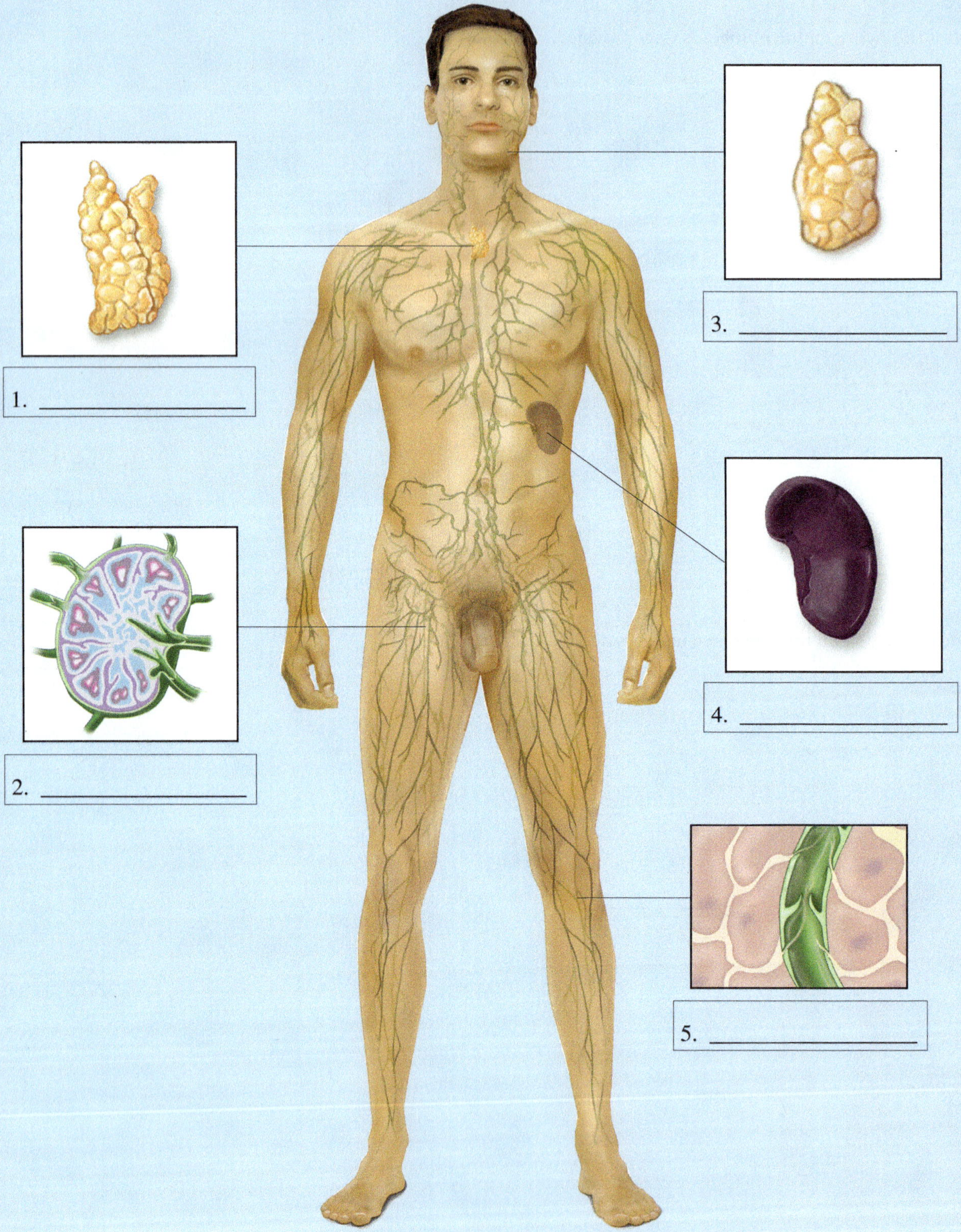

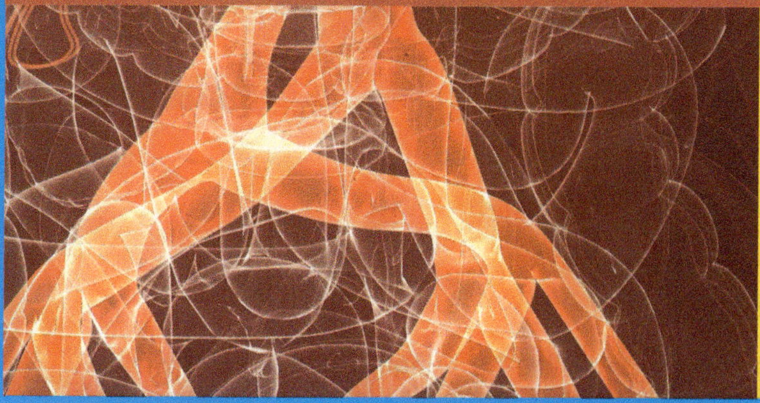

7

RESPIRATORY SYSTEM

Learning Objectives

Upon completion of this chapter, you will be able to

- Identify and define the combining forms and suffixes introduced in this chapter.
- Correctly spell and pronounce medical terms and major anatomical structures relating to the respiratory system.
- Locate and describe the major organs of the respiratory system and their functions.
- List and describe the lung volumes and capacities.
- Describe the process of respiration.
- Identify and define respiratory system anatomical terms.
- Identify and define selected respiratory system pathology terms.
- Identify and define selected respiratory system diagnostic procedures.
- Identify and define selected respiratory system therapeutic procedures.
- Identify and define selected medications relating to the respiratory system.
- Define selected abbreviations associated with the respiratory system.

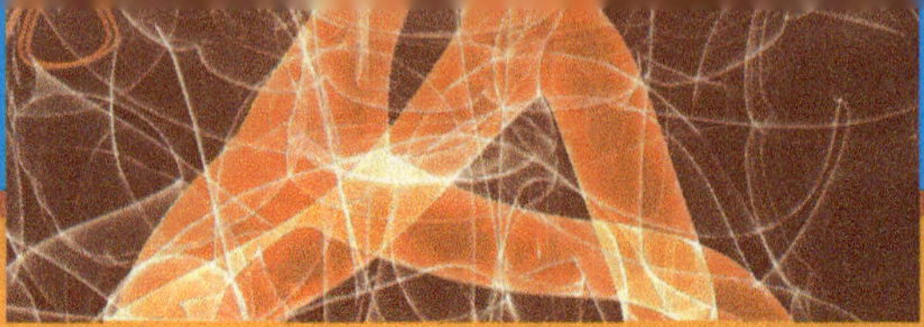

Respiratory System at a Glance

Function

The organs of the respiratory system are responsible for bringing fresh air into the lungs, exchanging oxygen for carbon dioxide between the air sacs of the lungs and the blood stream, and exhaling the stale air.

Structures

Here are the primary structures that comprise the respiratory system.

nasal cavity
pharynx
larynx
trachea
bronchial tubes
lungs

Word Parts

Here are the most common word parts (with their meanings) used to build respiratory system terms. For a more comprehensive list, refer to the Terminology section of this chapter.

Combining Forms

aer/o	air	**orth/o**	straight, upright
alveol/o	alveolus; air sac	**ox/o, ox/i**	oxygen
anthrac/o	coal	**pharyng/o**	pharynx
atel/o	incomplete	**pleur/o**	pleura
bronch/o	bronchus	**pneum/o**	lung, air
bronchi/o	bronchus	**pneumon/o**	lung, air
bronchiol/o	bronchiole	**pulmon/o**	lung
coni/o	dust	**rhin/o**	nose
diaphragmat/o	diaphragm	**sept/o**	wall
epiglott/o	epiglottis	**sinus/o**	sinus
laryng/o	larynx	**spir/o**	breathing
lob/o	lobe	**trache/o**	trachea, windpipe
nas/o	nose	**tuss/o**	cough
muc/o	mucus		

Suffixes

-capnia	carbon dioxide	**-pnea**	breathing
-osmia	smell	**-ptysis**	spitting
-phonia	voice	**-spasm**	involuntary muscle contraction
-plegia	paralysis	**-thorax**	chest

Respiratory System Illustrated

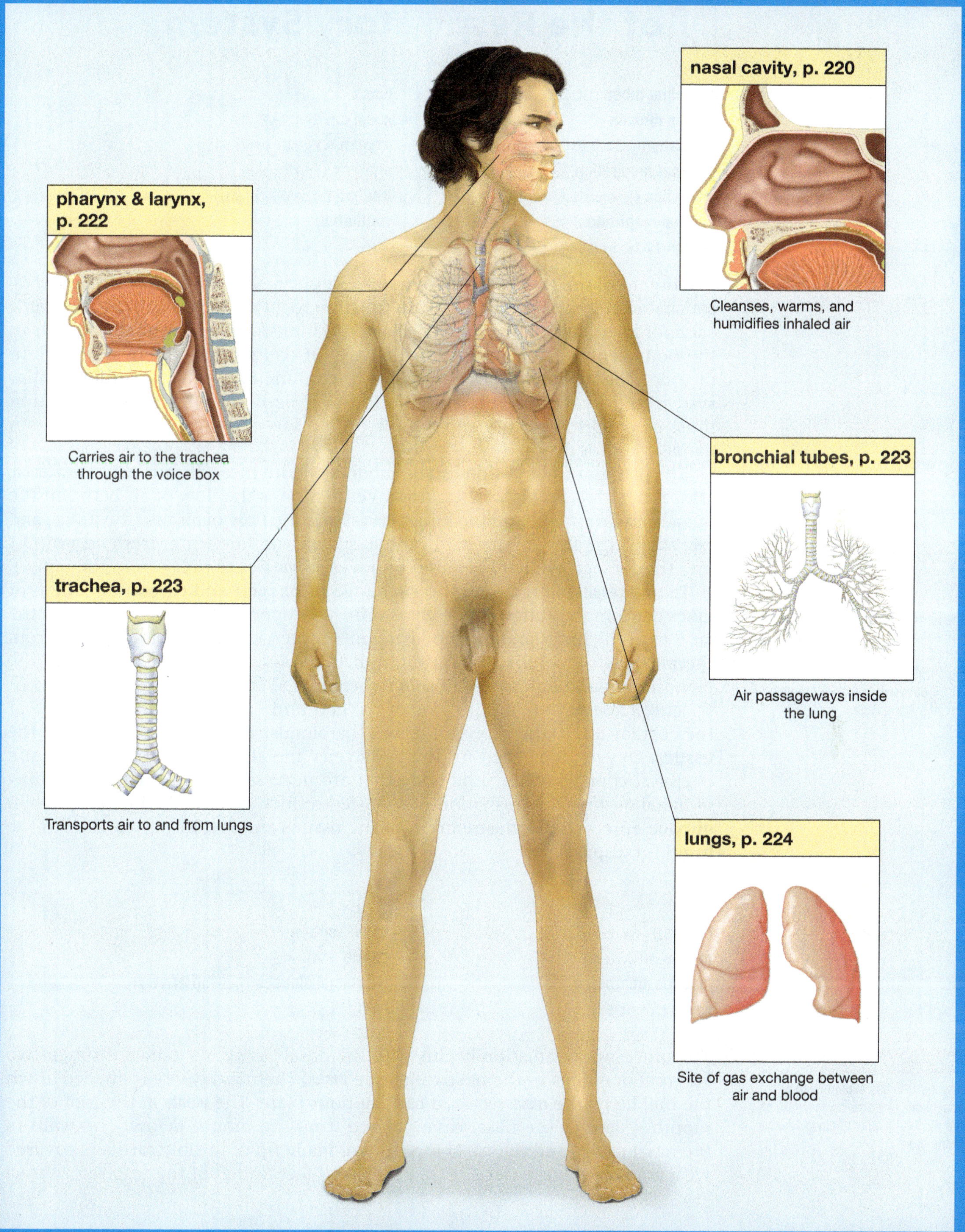

Anatomy and Physiology of the Respiratory System

bronchial tubes (BRONG-key-all)
carbon dioxide
exhalation (eks-hah-LAY-shun)
external respiration
inhalation (in-hah-LAY-shun)
internal respiration
larynx (LAIR-inks)
lungs
nasal cavity (NAY-zl)
oxygen (OK-sih-jen)
pharynx (FAIR-inks)
trachea (TRAY-kee-ah)
ventilation

The organs of the respiratory system include the **nasal cavity, pharynx, larynx, trachea, bronchial tubes,** and **lungs.** These organs function together to perform the mechanical and, for the most part, unconscious mechanism of respiration. The cells of the body require the continuous delivery of oxygen and removal of carbon dioxide. The respiratory system works in conjunction with the cardiovascular system to deliver oxygen to all the cells of the body. The process of respiration must be continuous; interruption for even a few minutes can result in brain damage and/or death.

The process of respiration can be subdivided into three distinct parts: **ventilation, external respiration,** and **internal respiration.** Ventilation is the flow of air between the outside environment and the lungs. **Inhalation** is the flow of air into the lungs, and **exhalation** is the flow of air out of the lungs. Inhalation brings fresh **oxygen** (O_2) into the air sacs, while exhalation removes **carbon dioxide** (CO_2) from the body.

MED TERM TIP

The terms *inhalation* and *inspiration* (in- = inward + spir/o = breathing) can be used interchangeably. Similarly, the terms *exhalation* and *expiration* (ex- = outward + spir/o = breathing) are interchangeable.

External respiration refers to the exchange of oxygen and carbon dioxide that takes place in the lungs. These gases diffuse in opposite directions between the air sacs of the lungs and the bloodstream. Oxygen enters the bloodstream from the air sacs to be delivered throughout the body. Carbon dioxide leaves the bloodstream and enters the air sacs to be exhaled from the body.

Internal respiration is the process of oxygen and carbon dioxide exchange at the cellular level when oxygen leaves the bloodstream and is delivered to the tissues. Oxygen is needed for the body cells' metabolism, all the physical and chemical changes within the body that are necessary for life. The by-product of metabolism is the formation of a waste product, carbon dioxide. The carbon dioxide enters the bloodstream from the tissues and is transported back to the lungs for disposal.

Nasal Cavity

cilia (SIL-ee-ah)
mucus (MYOO-kus)
mucous membrane
nares (NAIR-eez)
nasal septum
palate (PAL-at)
paranasal sinuses (pair-ah-NAY-zl)

MED TERM TIP

Anyone who has experienced a nosebleed, or *epistaxis,* is aware of the plentiful supply of blood vessels in the nose.

The process of ventilation begins with the nasal cavity. Air enters through two external openings in the nose called the **nares.** The nasal cavity is divided down the middle by the **nasal septum,** a cartilaginous plate. The **palate** in the roof of the mouth separates the nasal cavity above from the mouth below. The walls of the nasal cavity and the nasal septum are made up of flexible cartilage covered with **mucous membrane** (see Figure 7.1 ■). In fact, much of the respiratory tract

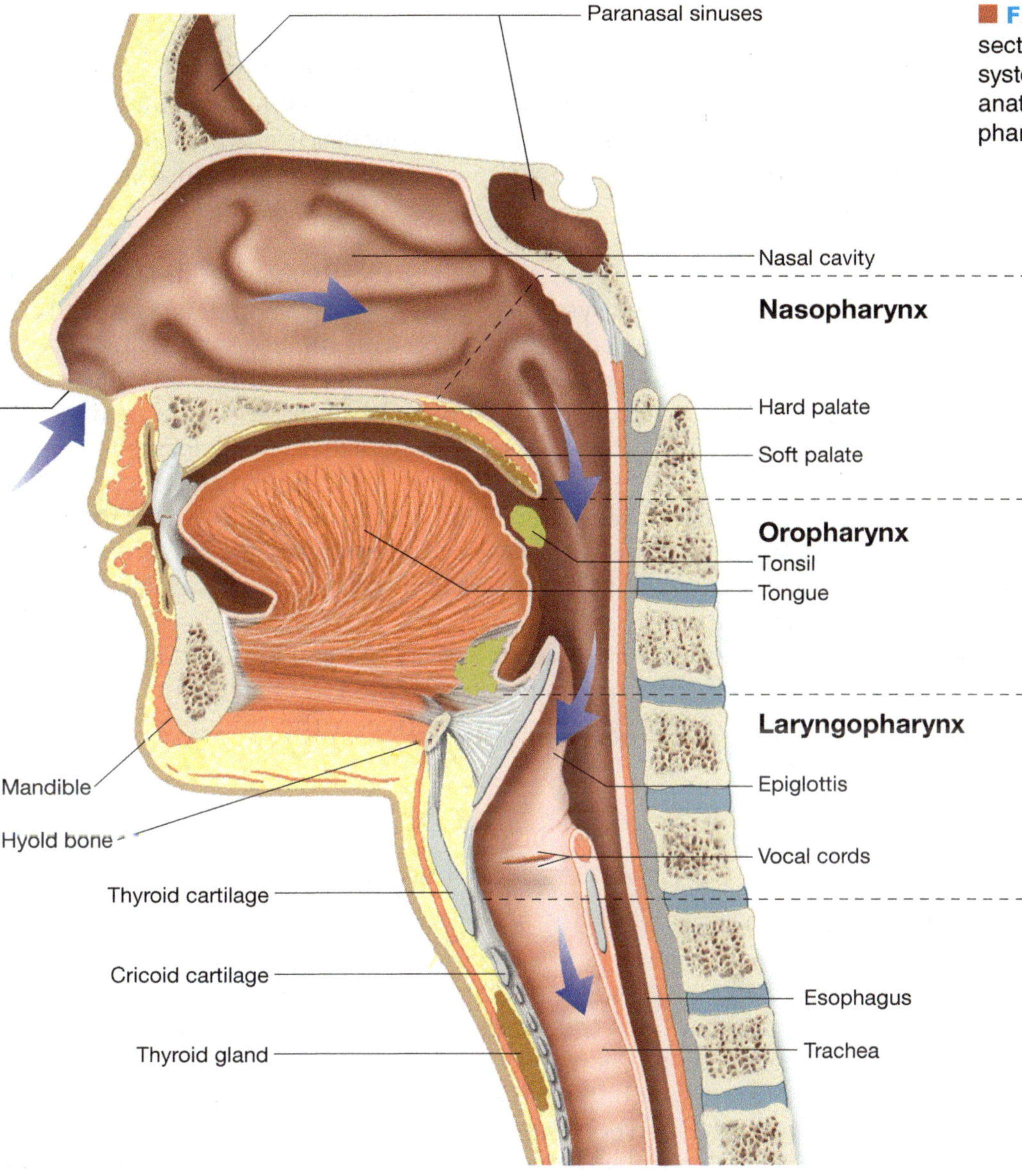

Figure 7.1 Sagittal section of upper respiratory system illustrating the internal anatomy of the nasal cavity, pharynx, larynx, and trachea.

is covered with mucous membrane, which secretes a sticky fluid, **mucus,** to help cleanse the air by trapping dust and bacteria. Since this membrane is also wet, it moisturizes inhaled air as it passes by the surface of the cavity. Very small hairs or **cilia** line the opening to the nose (as well as much of the airways), and filter out large dirt particles before they can enter the lungs. Capillaries in the mucous membranes warm inhaled air as it passes through the airways. Additionally, several **paranasal sinuses,** or air-filled cavities, are located within the facial bones. The sinuses act as an echo chamber during sound production and give resonance to the voice.

MED TERM TIP

Word Watch: The term *cilia* means hair, and there are other body systems that have cilia or cilia-like processes. For example, when discussing the eye, *cilia* means eyelashes.

Pharynx

adenoids (ADD-eh-noydz)
auditory tube
eustachian tube (yoo-STAY-she-en)
laryngopharynx (lair-ring-goh-FAIR-inks)
lingual tonsils (LING-gwal)
nasopharynx (nay-zoh-FAIR-inks)
oropharynx (or-oh-FAIR-inks)
palatine tonsils (PAL-ah-tine)
pharyngeal tonsils (fair-IN-jee-al)

Air next enters the pharynx, also called the *throat,* which is used by both the respiratory and digestive systems. At the end of the pharynx, air enters the trachea while food and liquids are shunted into the esophagus.

The pharynx is roughly a 5-inch-long tube consisting of three parts: the upper **nasopharynx,** middle **oropharynx,** and lower **laryngopharynx** (see again Figure 7.1). Three pairs of tonsils (collections of lymphatic tissue) are located in the pharynx. Tonsils are strategically placed to help keep pathogens from entering the body through either the air breathed or food and liquid swallowed. The nasopharynx, behind the nose, contains the **adenoids** or **pharyngeal tonsils.** The oropharynx, behind the mouth, contains the **palatine tonsils** and the **lingual tonsils.** Tonsils are considered a part of the lymphatic system.

MED TERM TIP

In the early 1970s it was common practice to remove the tonsils and adenoids in children suffering from repeated infections. However, it is now understood how important these organs are to remove pathogens from the air we breathe and the food we eat. Antibiotic treatment has also reduced the severity of infections.

The opening of the **eustachian** or **auditory tube** is also found in the nasopharynx. The other end of this tube is in the middle ear. Each time you swallow, this tube opens to equalize air pressure between the middle ear and the outside atmosphere.

Larynx

epiglottis (ep-ih-GLOT-iss)
glottis (GLOT-iss)
thyroid cartilage (THIGH-royd / CAR-tih-lij)
vocal cords

The larynx, or *voice box,* is a muscular structure located between the pharynx and the trachea and contains the **vocal cords** (see again Figure 7.1 and Figure 7.2 ■). The vocal cords are not actually cordlike in structure, but rather they are folds of membranous tissue that produce sound by vibrating as air passes through the **glottis,** the opening between the two vocal cords.

MED TERM TIP

Stuttering may actually result from faulty neuromuscular control of the larynx. Some stutterers can sing or whisper without difficulty. Both singing and whispering involve movements of the larynx that differ from those required for regular speech.

A flap of cartilaginous tissue, the **epiglottis,** sits above the glottis and provides protection against food and liquid being inhaled into the lungs. The epiglottis covers the larynx and trachea during swallowing and shunts food and liquid from the pharynx into the esophagus. The walls of the larynx are composed of several cartilage plates held together with ligaments and muscles. One of these cartilages, the **thyroid cartilage,** forms what is known as the *Adam's apple.* The thyroid cartilage is generally larger in males than in females and helps to produce the deeper male voice.

MED TERM TIP

The term *Adam's apple* is thought to come from a fable that when Adam realized he had sinned in the Garden of Eden, he was unable to swallow the apple in his throat.

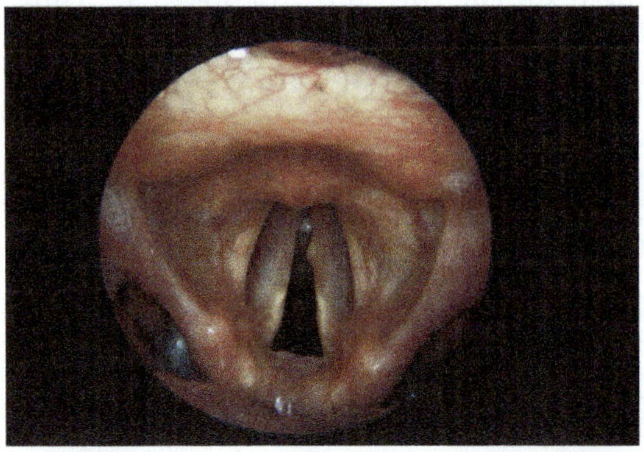

■ **Figure 7.2** The vocal cords within the larynx, superior view from the pharynx. *(CNRI/Photo Researchers, Inc.)*

Trachea

The trachea, also called the *windpipe,* is the passageway for air that extends from the pharynx and larynx down to the main bronchi (see Figure 7.3 ■). Measuring approximately 4 inches in length, it is composed of smooth muscle and cartilage rings and is lined by mucous membrane and cilia. Therefore, it also assists in cleansing, warming, and moisturizing air as it travels to the lungs.

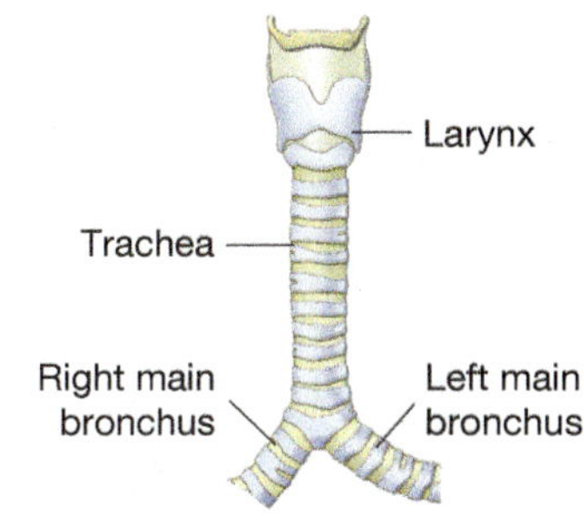

■ **Figure 7.3** Structure of the trachea, which extends from the larynx above to the main bronchi below.

Bronchial Tubes

alveoli (al-VEE-oh-lye)
bronchioles (BRONG-key-ohlz)
bronchus (BRONG-kus)
pulmonary capillaries
respiratory membrane

The distal end of the trachea divides to form the left and right main (primary) bronchi. Each **bronchus** enters one of the lungs and branches repeatedly to form secondary and tertiary bronchi. Each branch becomes narrower until the narrowest branches, the **bronchioles,** are formed (see Figure 7.4 ■). Each bronchiole terminates in a small group of air sacs, called **alveoli.** Each lung has approximately 150 million alveoli. The walls of alveoli are elastic, giving them the ability to expand to hold air and then recoil to their original size. A network of **pulmonary capillaries** from the pulmonary blood vessels tightly encases each alveolus (see Figure 7.5 ■). In fact, the walls of the alveoli and capillaries are so tightly associated with each other they are referred to as a single unit, the **respiratory membrane.** The exchange of oxygen and carbon dioxide between the air within the alveolus and the blood inside the capillaries takes place across the respiratory membrane.

MED TERM TIP

The respiratory system can be thought of as an upside-down tree and its branches. The trunk of the tree consists of the pharynx, larynx, and trachea. The trachea then divides into two branches, the bronchi. Each bronchus divides into smaller and smaller branches. In fact, this branching system of tubes is referred to as the *bronchial tree.*

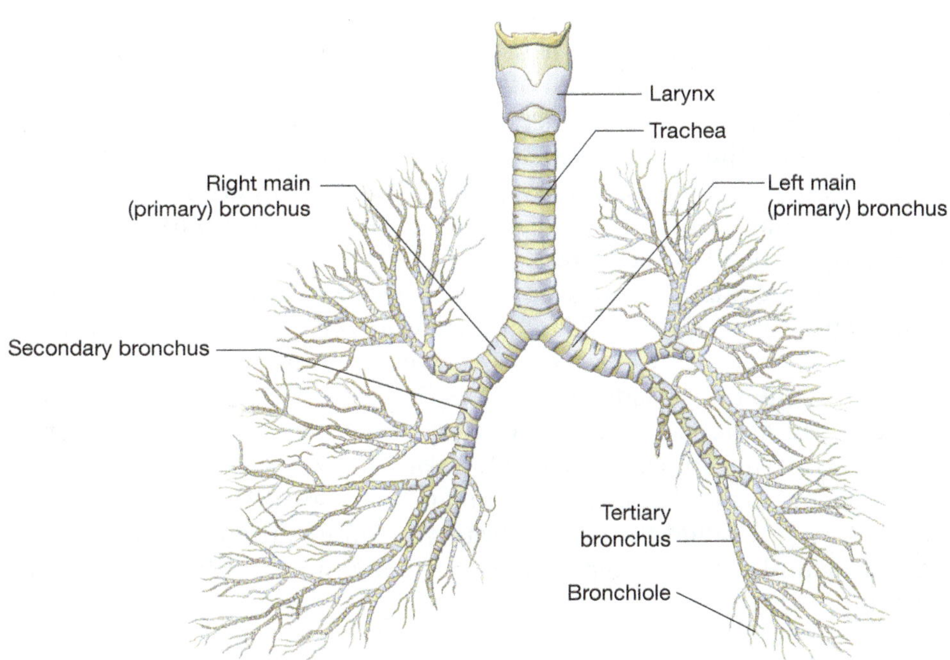

■ **Figure 7.4** The bronchial tree. Note how each main bronchus enters a lung and then branches into smaller and smaller primary bronchi, secondary bronchi, and bronchioles.

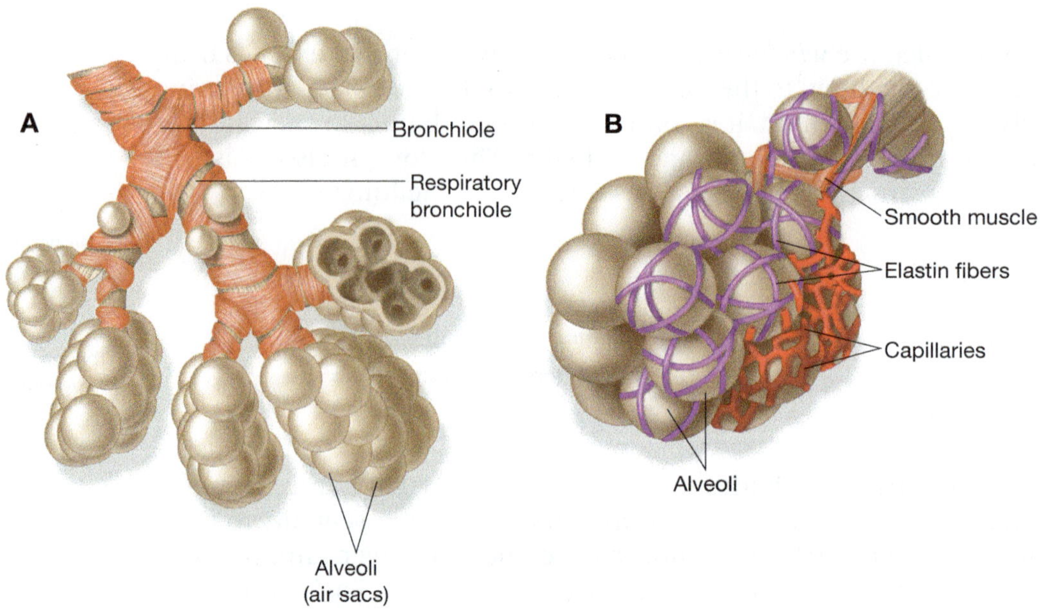

■ **Figure 7.5** (A) Each bronchiole terminates in an alveolar sac, a group of alveoli; (B) alveoli encased by network capillaries, forming the respiratory membrane.

Lungs

apex
base
hilum (HYE-lum)
lobes
mediastinum (mee-dee-ass-TYE-num)
parietal pleura (pah-RYE-eh-tal)
pleura (PLOO-rah)
pleural cavity
serous fluid (SEER-us)
visceral pleura (VISS-er-al)

Each lung is the total collection of the bronchi, bronchioles, and alveoli. They are spongy to the touch because they contain air. The lungs are protected by a double membrane called the **pleura.** The pleura's outer membrane is the **parietal pleura,** which also lines the wall of the chest cavity. The inner membrane, or **visceral pleura,** adheres to the surface of the lungs. The pleural membrane is folded in such a way that it forms a sac around each lung, referred to as the **pleural cavity.** There is normally slippery, watery **serous fluid** between the two layers of the pleura that reduces friction when the two layers rub together as the lungs repeatedly expand and contract.

MED TERM TIP

Some of the abnormal lung sounds heard with a stethoscope, such as crackling and rubbing, are made when the parietal and/or visceral pleura become inflamed and rub against one another.

The lungs contain divisions or **lobes.** There are three lobes in the larger right lung (right upper, right middle, and right lower lobes) and two in the left lung (left upper and left lower lobes). The pointed superior portion of each lung is the **apex,** while the broader lower area is the **base.** Entry of structures like the bronchi, pulmonary blood vessels, and nerves into each lung occurs along its medial border in an area called the **hilum.** The lungs within the thoracic cavity are protected from puncture and damage by the ribs. The area between the right and left lung is called the **mediastinum** and contains the heart, aorta, esophagus, thymus gland, and trachea. See Figure 7.6 ■ for an illustration of the lungs within the chest cavity.

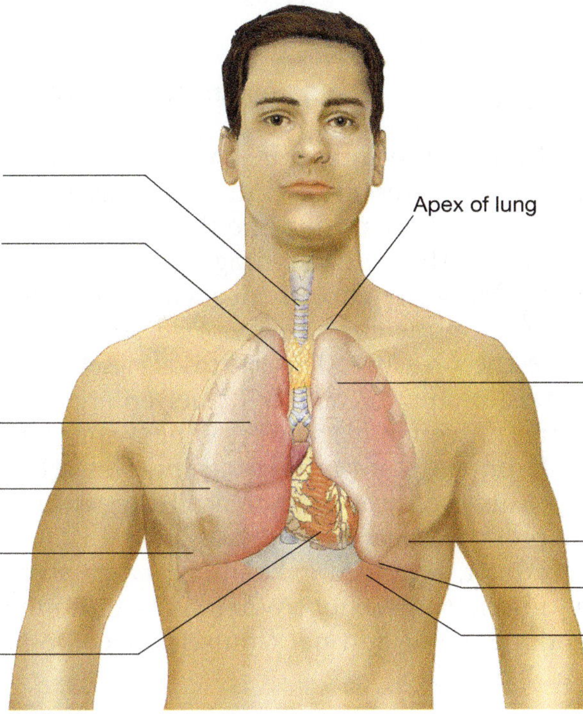

■ **Figure 7.6** Position of the lungs within the thoracic cavity; anterior view illustrating regions of the lungs and their relationship to other thoracic organs.

Lung Volumes and Capacities

pulmonary function test **respiratory therapist**

For some types of medical conditions, like emphysema, it is important to measure the volume of air flowing in and out of the lungs to determine lung capacity. Lung volumes are measured by **respiratory therapists** to aid in determining the functioning level of the respiratory system. Collectively, these measurements are called **pulmonary function tests.** Table 7.1 ■ lists and defines the four lung volumes and four lung capacities.

Table 7.1 Lung Volumes and Capacities

TERM	DEFINITION
Tidal volume (TV)	The amount of air that enters the lungs in a single inhalation or leaves the lungs in a single exhalation of quiet breathing. In an adult this is normally 500 mL.*
Inspiratory reserve volume (IRV)	The amount of air that can be forcibly inhaled after a normal inspiration. Also called *complemental air;* generally measures around 3,000 mL.*
Expiratory reserve volume (ERV)	The amount of air that can be forcibly exhaled after a normal quiet exhalation. This is also called *supplemental air;* approximately 1,000 mL.*
Residual volume (RV)	The air remaining in the lungs after a forced exhalation; about 1,500 mL* in the adult.
Inspiratory capacity (IC)	The volume of air inhaled after a normal exhale.
Functional residual capacity (FRC)	The air that remains in the lungs after a normal exhalation has taken place.
Vital capacity (VC)	The total volume of air that can be exhaled after a maximum inhalation. This amount will be equal to the sum of TV, IRV, and ERV.
Total lung capacity (TLC)	The volume of air in the lungs after a maximal inhalation.

*There is a normal range for measurements of the volume of air exchanged. The numbers given are for the average measurement.

Respiratory Muscles

diaphragm **intercostal muscles** (in-ter-COS-tal)

Air moves in and out of the lungs due to the difference between the atmospheric pressure and the pressure within the chest cavity. The **diaphragm,** the muscle separating the abdomen from the thoracic cavity, produces this difference in pressure. To do this, the diaphragm contracts and moves downward. This increase in thoracic cavity volume causes a decrease in pressure, or negative thoracic pressure, within the chest cavity. Air then flows into the lungs (inhalation) to equalize the pressure. The **intercostal muscles** between the ribs assist in inhalation by raising the rib cage to further enlarge the thoracic cavity. See Figure 7.7 ■ for an illustration of the role of the diaphragm in inhalation. Similarly, when the diaphragm and intercostal muscles relax, the thoracic cavity becomes smaller. This produces an increase in pressure within the cavity, or positive thoracic pressure, and air flows out of the lungs, resulting in exhalation. Therefore, a quiet, unforced exhalation is a passive process since it does not require any muscle contraction. When a forceful inhalation or exhalation is required, additional chest and neck muscles become active to create larger changes in thoracic pressure.

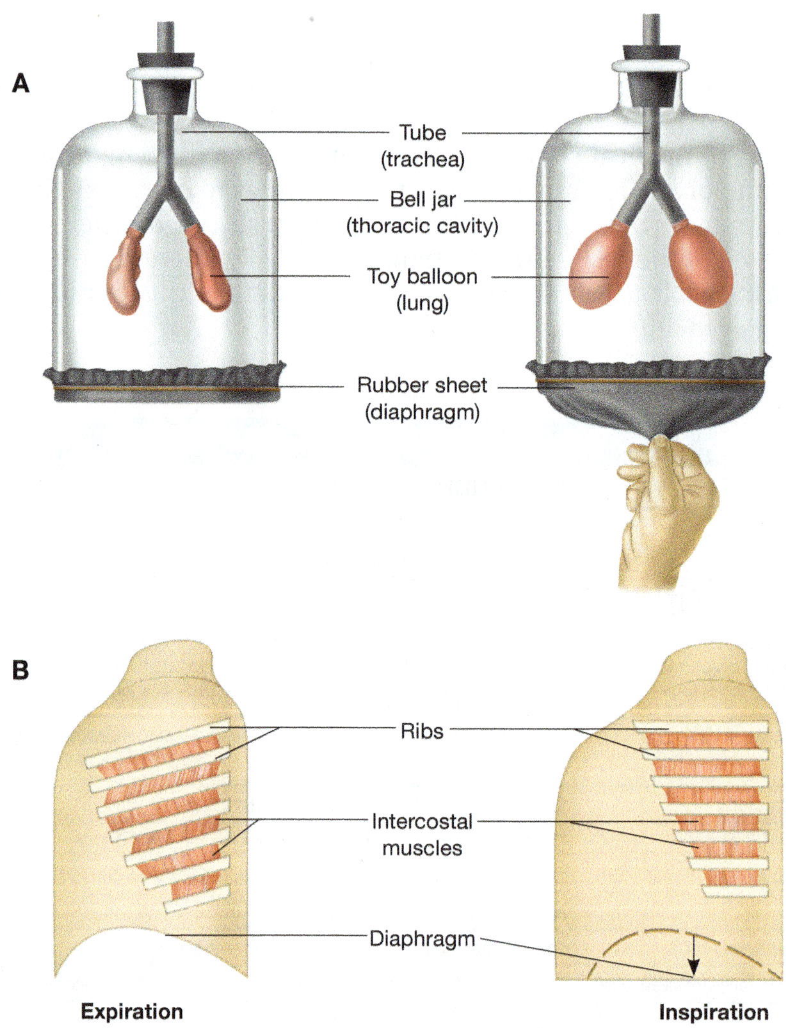

■ **Figure 7.7** (A) Bell jar apparatus demonstrating how downward movement of the diaphragm results in air flowing into the lungs; (B) action of the intercostal muscles lifts the ribs to assist the diaphragm in enlarging the volume of the thoracic cavity.

Respiratory Rate

vital signs

Respiratory rate (measured in breaths per minute) is one of our **vital signs** (VS), along with heart rate, temperature, and blood pressure. The respiratory rate is normally regulated by the level of CO_2 in the blood. When the CO_2 level is high, we breathe more rapidly to expel the excess. Likewise, when CO_2 levels drop, our respiratory rate will also drop.

When the respiratory rate falls outside the range of normal, it may indicate an illness or medical condition. For example, when a patient is running an elevated temperature and has shortness of breath (SOB) due to pneumonia, the respiratory rate may increase dramatically. Or a brain injury or some medications, such as those for pain, can cause a decrease in the respiratory rate. See Table 7.2 ■ for normal respiratory rate ranges for different age groups.

MED TERM TIP

Diaphragmatic breathing is taught to singers and public speakers. You can practice this type of breathing by allowing your abdomen to expand during inhalation and contract during exhalation while your shoulders remain motionless.

MED TERM TIP

When divers wish to hold their breath longer, they first hyperventilate (breath faster and deeper) in order to get rid of as much CO_2 as possible. This will hold off the urge to breathe longer, allowing a diver to stay submerged longer.

Table 7.2 Respiratory Rates for Different Age Groups

AGE	RESPIRATIONS PER MINUTE
Newborn	30–60
1-year-old	18 30
16-year-old	16–20
Adult	12–20

Terminology

Word Parts Used to Build Respiratory System Terms

The following lists contain the combining forms, suffixes, and prefixes used to build terms in the remaining sections of this chapter.

Combining Forms

aer/o	air
alveol/o	alveolus
angi/o	vessel
anthrac/o	coal
arteri/o	artery
atel/o	incomplete
bi/o	life
bronch/o	bronchus
bronchi/o	bronchus
bronchiol/o	bronchiole
carcin/o	cancer
cardi/o	heart
coni/o	dust
cortic/o	outer region, cortex
cyan/o	blue
cyst/o	cyst, bladder
cyt/o	cell
diaphragmat/o	diaphragm
embol/o	plug
epiglott/o	epiglottis
fibr/o	fibers
hem/o	blood
hist/o	tissue
laryng/o	larynx
lob/o	lobe
muc/o	mucus
nas/o	nose
orth/o	straight
ot/o	ear
ox/i	oxygen
ox/o	oxygen
pharyng/o	pharynx
pleur/o	pleura
pneum/o	air
pneumon/o	lung
pulmon/o	lung
py/o	pus
rhin/o	nose
sept/o	wall
sinus/o	sinus
somn/o	sleep
spir/o	breathing
thorac/o	chest
trache/o	trachea
tuss/o	cough

Suffixes

-al	pertaining to
-algia	pain
-ar	pertaining to
-ary	pertaining to
-capnia	carbon dioxide
-centesis	puncture to withdraw fluid
-dynia	pain
-eal	pertaining to
-ectasis	dilation
-ectomy	surgical removal
-emia	blood condition
-genic	produced by
-gram	record
-graphy	process of recording
-ia	condition

-ial	pertaining to
-ic	pertaining to
-ism	state of
-itis	inflammation
-logy	study of
-lytic	destruction
-meter	instrument to measure
-metry	process of measuring
-oma	tumor
-osis	abnormal condition
-osmia	smell
-ostomy	surgically create an opening
-otomy	cutting into
-phonia	voice

-plasm	formation
-plasty	surgical repair
-plegia	paralysis
-pnea	breathing
-ptysis	spitting
-rrhagia	abnormal flow condition
-rrhea	discharge
-scope	instrument for viewing
-scopy	process of visually examining
-spasm	involuntary muscle spasm
-stenosis	narrowing
-thorax	chest
-tic	pertaining to

Prefixes

a-	without
an-	without
anti-	against
brady-	slow
de-	without

dys-	abnormal, difficult
endo-	within
eu-	normal
hyper-	excessive

hypo-	insufficient
pan-	all
poly-	many
tachy-	fast

Anatomical Terms

TERM	WORD PARTS	DEFINITION
alveolar (al-VEE-oh-lar)	alveol/o = alveolus -ar = pertaining to	Pertaining to the alveoli.
bronchial (BRONG-ee-all)	bronch/o = bronchus -ial = pertaining to	Pertaining to a bronchus.
bronchiolar (brong-KEY-oh-lar)	bronchiol/o = bronchiole -ar = pertaining to	Pertaining to a bronchiole.
diaphragmatic (dye-ah-frag-MAT-ik)	diaphragmat/o = diaphragm -ic = pertaining to	Pertaining to the diaphragm.
epiglottic (ep-ih-GLOT-ik)	epiglott/o = epiglottis -ic = pertaining to	Pertaining to the epiglottis.
laryngeal (lair-in-GEE-all)	laryng/o = larynx -eal = pertaining to	Pertaining to the larynx.

Anatomical Terms *(continued)*

TERM	WORD PARTS	DEFINITION
nasal (NAY-zal)	nas/o = nose -al = pertaining to	Pertaining to the nose or nasal cavity.
pharyngeal (fair-in-GEE-all)	pharyng/o = pharynx -eal = pertaining to	Pertaining to the pharynx.
pleural (PLOO-ral)	pleur/o = pleura -al = pertaining to	Pertaining to the pleura.
pulmonary (PULL-mon-air-ee)	pulmon/o = lung -ary = pertaining to	Pertaining to the lung.
septal (SEP-tal)	sept/o = wall -al = pertaining to	Pertaining to the nasal septum.
thoracic (tho-RASS-ik)	thorac/o = chest -ic = pertaining to	Pertaining to the chest.
tracheal (TRAY-key-al)	trache/o = trachea -al = pertaining to	Pertaining to the trachea.

Pathology

TERM	WORD PARTS	DEFINITION
Medical Specialties		
internal medicine		Branch of medicine involving the diagnosis and treatment of diseases and conditions of internal organs such as the respiratory system. The physician is an *internist.*
otorhinolaryngology (ENT) (oh-toh-rye-noh-lair-in-GOL-oh-jee)	ot/o = ear rhin/o = nose laryng/o = larynx -logy = study of	Branch of medicine involving the diagnosis and treatment of conditions and diseases of the ear, nose, and throat region. The physician is an *otorhinolaryngologist.* This medical specialty may also be referred to as *otolaryngology.*
pulmonology (pull-mon-ALL-oh-jee)	pulmon/o = lung -logy = study of	Branch of medicine involved in the diagnosis and treatment of diseases and disorders of the respiratory system. Physician is a *pulmonologist.*
respiratory therapy	spir/o = breathing	Allied health specialty that assists patients with respiratory and cardiopulmonary disorders. Duties of a *respiratory therapist* include conducting pulmonary function tests, monitoring oxygen and carbon dioxide levels in the blood, administering breathing treatments, and ventilator management.
thoracic surgery (tho-RASS-ik)	thorac/o = chest -ic = pertaining to	Branch of medicine involving the diagnosis and treatment of conditions and diseases of the respiratory system by surgical means. Physician is a *thoracic surgeon.*

Pathology *(continued)*

TERM	WORD PARTS	DEFINITION
Signs and Symptoms		
anosmia (ah-NOZ-mee-ah)	an- = without -osmia = smell	Lack of the sense of smell.
anoxia (ah-NOK-see-ah)	an- = without ox/o = oxygen -ia = condition	Condition of receiving almost no oxygen from inhaled air.
aphonia (a-FOH-nee-ah)	a- = without -phonia = voice	Condition of being unable to produce sounds.
apnea (AP-nee-ah)	a- = without -pnea = breathing	Not breathing.
asphyxia (as-FIK-see-ah)	a- = without -ia = condition	Lack of oxygen that can lead to unconsciousness and death if not corrected immediately; also called *asphyxiation* or *suffocation*. Common causes include drowning, foreign body in the respiratory tract, poisoning, and electric shock.
aspiration (as-peer-RAY-shun)	spir/o = breathing	Refers to withdrawing fluid from a body cavity using suction. For example, using a long needle and syringe to withdraw fluid from the pleural cavity, or using a vacuum pump to remove phlegm from a patient's airways. Additionally, it refers to inhaling food, liquid, or a foreign object into the airways, which may lead to the development of pneumonia.
bradypnea (bray-DIP-nee-ah)	brady- = slow -pnea = breathing	Breathing too slowly; a low respiratory rate.
bronchiectasis (brong-key-EK-tah-sis)	bronchi/o = bronchus -ectasis = dilation	Dilated bronchus.
bronchospasm (BRONG-koh-spazm)	bronch/o = bronchus -spasm = involuntary muscle spasm	Involuntary muscle spasm of the smooth muscle in the wall of the bronchus.
Cheyne–Stokes respiration (CHAIN / STOHKS / res-pir-AY-shun)	spir/o = breathing	Abnormal breathing pattern in which there are long periods (10–60 seconds) of apnea followed by deeper, more rapid breathing. Named for John Cheyne, a Scottish physician, and Sir William Stokes, an Irish surgeon.
clubbing		Abnormal widening and thickening of the ends of the fingers and toes associated with chronic oxygen deficiency. Seen in patients with chronic respiratory conditions or circulatory problems.
crackles		Abnormal sound made during inspiration. Usually indicates the presence of fluid or mucus in the small airways. Also called *rales*.

Pathology *(continued)*

TERM	WORD PARTS	DEFINITION
cyanosis (sigh-ah-NO-sis)	cyan/o = blue -osis = abnormal condition	Refers to the bluish tint of skin that is receiving an insufficient amount of oxygen or circulation.
dysphonia (dis-FOH-nee-ah)	dys- = difficult, abnormal -phonia = voice	Condition of having difficulty producing sounds or producing abnormal sounds.
dyspnea (DISP-nee-ah)	dys- = abnormal, difficult -pnea = breathing	Term describing difficult or labored breathing.
epistaxis (ep-ih-STAKS-is)		Nosebleed.
eupnea (yoop-NEE-ah)	eu- = normal -pnea = breathing	Normal breathing and respiratory rate.
hemoptysis (hee-MOP-tih-sis)	hem/o = blood -ptysis = spitting	To cough up blood or blood-stained sputum.
hemothorax (hee-moh-THOH-raks)	hem/o = blood -thorax = chest	Presence of blood in the chest cavity.
hypercapnia (high-per-CAP-nee-ah)	hyper- = excessive -capnia = carbon dioxide	Condition of having excessive carbon dioxide in the body.
hyperpnea (high-per-NEE-ah)	hyper- = excessive -pnea = breathing	Taking deep breaths.
hyperventilation (HYE-per-vent-ill-a-shun)	hyper- = excessive	Breathing both too fast (tachypnea) and too deep (hyperpnea).
hypocapnia (high-poh-CAP-nee-ah)	hypo- = insufficient -capnia = carbon dioxide	An insufficient level of carbon dioxide in the body; a very serious problem because it is the presence of carbon dioxide that stimulates respiration, not the absence of oxygen. Therefore, a person with low carbon dioxide levels would respond with an increased respiratory rate.
hypopnea (high-POP-nee-ah)	hypo- = insufficient -pnea = breathing	Taking shallow breaths.
hypoventilation (HYE-poh-vent-ill-a-shun)	hypo- = insufficient	Breathing both too slow (bradypnea) and too shallow (hypopnea).
hypoxemia (high-pox-EE-mee-ah)	hypo- = insufficient ox/o = oxygen -emia = blood condition	Condition of having an insufficient amount of oxygen in the bloodstream.
hypoxia (high-POX-ee-ah)	hypo- = insufficient ox/o = oxygen -ia = condition	Condition of receiving an insufficient amount of oxygen from inhaled air.
laryngoplegia (lair-RING-goh-plee-gee-ah)	laryng/o = larynx -plegia = paralysis	Paralysis of the muscles controlling the larynx.

Pathology *(continued)*

TERM	WORD PARTS	DEFINITION
orthopnea (or-THOP-nee-ah)	orth/o = straight -pnea = breathing	Term describing dyspnea that is worsened by lying flat. The patient feels able to breath easier while sitting straight up; a common occurrence in those with pulmonary disease.
pansinusitis (pan-sigh-nus-EYE-tis)	pan- = all sinus/o = sinus -itis = inflammation	Inflammation of all the paranasal sinuses.
patent (PAY-tent)		Open or unblocked, such as a patent airway.
phlegm (FLEM)		Thick mucus secreted by the membranes lining the respiratory tract. When phlegm is coughed through the mouth, it is called *sputum.* Phlegm is examined for color, odor, and consistency and tested for the presence of bacteria, viruses, and fungi.
pleural rub (PLOO-ral)	pleur/o = pleura -al = pertaining to	Grating sound made when the two layers of the pleura rub together during respiration. It is caused when one of the surfaces becomes thicker as a result of inflammation or other disease conditions. This rub can be felt through the fingertips when placed on the chest wall or heard through a stethoscope.
pleurodynia (ploor-oh-DIN-ee-ah)	pleur/o = pleura -dynia = pain	Pleural pain.
pyothorax (pye-oh-THOH-raks)	py/o = pus -thorax = chest	Presence of pus in the chest cavity; indicates a bacterial infection.
rhinitis (rye-NYE-tis)	rhin/o = nose -itis = inflammation	Inflammation of the nasal cavity.
rhinorrhagia (rye-noh-RAH-jee-ah)	rhin/o = nose -rrhagia = abnormal flow condition	Rapid flow of blood from the nose.
rhinorrhea (rye-noh-REE-ah)	rhin/o = nose -rrhea = discharge	Discharge from the nose; commonly called a *runny nose.*
rhonchi (RONG-kigh)		Somewhat musical sound during expiration, often found in asthma or infection. Caused by spasms of the bronchial tubes. Also called *wheezing.*
shortness of breath (SOB)		Term used to indicate that a patient is having some difficulty breathing; also called *dyspnea.* The causes can range from mild SOB after exercise to SOB associated with heart disease.
sputum (SPEW-tum)		Mucus or phlegm coughed up from the lining of the respiratory tract.

MED TERM TIP

The term *sputum,* from the Latin word meaning "to spit," now refers to the material coughed up and spit out from the respiratory system.

Pathology *(continued)*

TERM	WORD PARTS	DEFINITION
stridor (STRIGH-dor)		Harsh, high-pitched, noisy breathing sound made when there is an obstruction of the bronchus or larynx. Found in conditions such as croup in children.
tachypnea (tak-ip-NEE-ah)	tachy- = fast -pnea = breathing	Breathing fast; a high respiratory rate.
thoracalgia (thor-ah-KAL-jee-ah)	thorac/o = chest -algia = pain	Chest pain. Does not refer to angina pectoris.
tracheostenosis (tray-kee-oh-steh-w-sis)	trache/o = trachea -stenosis = narrowing	Narrowing of the trachea.
Upper Respiratory System		
croup (KROOP)		Acute respiratory condition found in infants and children characterized by a barking type of cough or stridor.
diphtheria (dif-THEAR-ee-ah)	-ia = condition	Bacterial upper respiratory infection characterized by the formation of a thick membranous film across the throat and a high mortality rate. Rare now due to the DPT (diphtheria, pertussis, tetanus) vaccine.
laryngitis (lair-in-JYE-tis)	laryng/o = larynx -itis = inflammation	Inflammation of the larynx.
nasopharyngitis (nay-zoh-fair-in-JYE-tis)	nas/o = nose pharyng/o = pharynx -itis = inflammation	Inflammation of the nasal cavity and pharynx; commonly called the *common cold.*
pertussis (per-TUH-is)	tuss/o = cough	Commonly called *whooping cough,* due to the whoop sound made when coughing. An infectious bacterial disease of the upper respiratory system that children receive immunization against as part of their DPT shots.
pharyngitis (fair-in-JYE-tis)	pharyng/o = pharynx -itis = inflammation	Inflammation of the pharynx; commonly called a *sore throat.*
rhinomycosis (rye-noh-my-KOH-sis)	rhin/o = nose myc/o = fungus -osis = abnormal condition	Fungal infection of the nasal cavity.
Bronchial Tubes		
asthma (AZ-mah)		Disease caused by various conditions, like allergens, and resulting in constriction of the bronchial airways, dyspnea, coughing, and wheezing. Can cause violent spasms of the bronchi (bronchospasms) but is generally not a life-threatening condition. Medication can be very effective.

MED TERM TIP

The term *asthma,* from the Greek word meaning "panting," describes the breathing pattern of a person having an asthma attack.

Pathology (continued)

TERM	WORD PARTS	DEFINITION
bronchiectasis (brong-key-EK-tah-sis)	bronchi/o = bronchus -ectasis = dilation	Abnormal enlargement of bronchi; may be the result of a lung infection. This condition can be irreversible and result in destruction of the bronchial walls. Major symptoms include coughing up a large amount of purulent sputum, crackles, and hemoptysis.
bronchitis (brong-KIGH-tis)	bronch/o = bronchus -itis = inflammation	Inflammation of a bronchus.
bronchogenic carcinoma (brong-koh-JEN-ik / car-sin-OH-mah)	bronch/o = bronchus -genic = produced by carcin/o = cancer -oma = tumor	Malignant tumor originating in the bronchi. Usually associated with a history of cigarette smoking.

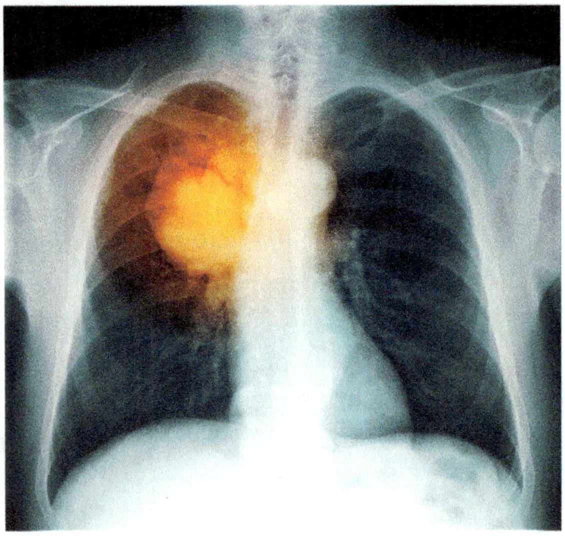

■ **Figure 7.8** Color-enhanced X-ray of large malignant tumor in the right lung. *(Du Cane Medical Imaging Ltd./Photo Researchers, Inc.)*

TERM	WORD PARTS	DEFINITION
Lungs		
adult respiratory distress syndrome (ARDS)	spir/o = breathing -al = pertaining to	Acute respiratory failure in adults characterized by tachypnea, dyspnea, cyanosis, tachycardia, and hypoxemia. May follow trauma, pneumonia, or septic infections. Also called *acute respiratory distress syndrome.*
anthracosis (an-thra-KOH-sis)	anthrac/o = coal -osis = abnormal condition	Type of pneumoconiosis that develops from the collection of coal dust in the lung. Also called *black lung* or *miner's lung.*
asbestosis (az-bes-TOH-sis)	-osis = abnormal condition	Type of pneumoconiosis that develops from collection of asbestos fibers in the lungs. May lead to the development of lung cancer.

Pathology *(continued)*

TERM	WORD PARTS	DEFINITION
atelectasis (at-eh-LEK-tah-sis)	atel/o = incomplete -ectasis = dilation	Condition in which the alveoli in a portion of the lung collapse, preventing the respiratory exchange of oxygen and carbon dioxide. Can be caused by a variety of conditions, including pressure on the lung from a tumor or other object. Term also used to describe the failure of a newborn's lungs to expand.
chronic obstructive pulmonary disease (COPD) (PULL-mon-air-ee)	pulmon/o = lung -ary = pertaining to	Progressive, chronic, and usually irreversible group of conditions, like emphysema, in which the lungs have a diminished capacity for inspiration (inhalation) and expiration (exhalation). The person may have dyspnea upon exertion and a cough.
cystic fibrosis (CF) (SIS-tik / fye-BROH-sis)	cyst/o = cyst, bladder -ic = pertaining to fibr/o = fibers -osis = abnormal condition	Hereditary condition causing the exocrine glands to malfunction. The patient produces very thick mucus that causes severe congestion within the lungs and digestive system. Through more advanced treatment, many children are now living into adulthood with this disease. The term *cystic* in cystic fibrosis refers to cysts that form in the pancreas.
emphysema (em-fih-SEE-mah)		Pulmonary condition characterized by the destruction of the walls of the alveoli, resulting in fewer overexpanded air sacs. Can occur as a result of long-term heavy smoking. Air pollution also worsens this disease. The patient may not be able to breathe except in a sitting or standing position.
histoplasmosis (his-toh-plaz-MOH-sis)	hist/o = tissue -plasm = formation -osis = abnormal condition	Pulmonary infection caused by the fungus *Histoplasma capsulatum,* found in dust and in the droppings of pigeons and chickens. The translation of the name of this condition reflects the microscopic appearance of the fungus.
infant respiratory distress syndrome (IRDS)	spir/o = breathing	Lung condition most commonly found in premature infants that is characterized by tachypnea and respiratory grunting. The condition is caused by a lack of surfactant necessary to keep the lungs inflated. Also called *hyaline membrane disease* (HMD) and *respiratory distress syndrome of the newborn.*
influenza (in-floo-EN-za)		Viral infection of the respiratory system characterized by chills, fever, body aches, and fatigue. Commonly called the *flu.*
Legionnaires' disease (lee-jen-AYRZ)		Severe, often fatal bacterial infection characterized by pneumonia and liver and kidney damage. Named after people who came down with it at an American Legion convention in 1976.

Pathology *(continued)*

TERM	WORD PARTS	DEFINITION
***Mycoplasma* pneumonia** (MY-koh-plaz-ma)	myc/o = fungus -plasm = formation	Less severe but longer lasting form of pneumonia caused by the *Mycoplasma pneumoniae* bacteria. Also called *walking pneumonia.* The translation of the name of this condition reflects the microscopic appearance of the bacteria.
pneumoconiosis (noo-moh-koh-nee-OH-sis)	pneum/o = lung coni/o = dust -osis = abnormal condition	Condition that is the result of inhaling environmental particles that become toxic. Can be the result of inhaling coal dust (anthracosis) or asbestos (asbestosis).
pneumocystis pneumonia (PCP) (noo-moh-SIS-tis / new-MOH-nee-ah)	pneum/o = lung cyst/o = cyst, bladder pneumon/o = lung -ia = condition	Pneumonia with a nonproductive cough, very little fever, and dyspnea caused by the fungus *Pneumocystis jiroveci.* An opportunistic infection often seen in those with weakened immune systems, such as AIDS patients.
pneumonia (new-MOH-nee-ah)	pneumon/o = lung -ia = condition	Inflammatory condition of the lung that can be caused by bacteria, viruses, fungi, and aspirated substances. Results in the filling of the alveoli and air spaces with fluid.
pulmonary edema (PULL-mon-air-ee / eh-DEE-mah)	pulmon/o = lung -ary = pertaining to	Condition in which lung tissue retains an excessive amount of fluid, especially in the alveoli. Results in dyspnea.
pulmonary embolism (PULL-mon-air-ee / EM-boh-lizm)	pulmon/o = lung -ary = pertaining to embol/o = plug -ism = state of	Obstruction of the pulmonary artery or one of its branches by an embolus (often a blood clot broken away from another area of the body). May cause an infarct in the lung tissue.
pulmonary fibrosis (fi-BROH-sis)	pulmon/o = lung -ary = pertaining to fibr/o = fibers -osis = abnormal condition	Formation of fibrous scar tissue in the lungs that leads to decreased ability to expand the lungs. May be caused by infections, pneumoconiosis, autoimmune diseases, and toxin exposure.
severe acute respiratory syndrome (SARS)	spir/o = breathing	Acute viral respiratory infection that begins like the flu but quickly progresses to severe dyspnea; high fatality rate. First appeared in China in 2003.
silicosis (sil-ih-KOH-sis)	-osis = abnormal condition	Type of pneumoconiosis that develops from the inhalation of silica (quartz) dust found in quarrying, glass works, sandblasting, and ceramics.
sleep apnea (AP-nee-ah)	a- = without -pnea = breathing	Condition in which breathing stops repeatedly during sleep long enough to cause a drop in oxygen levels in the blood.
sudden infant death syndrome (SIDS)		Unexpected and unexplained death of an apparently well infant under 1 year of age. The child suddenly stops breathing for unknown reasons.

Pathology *(continued)*

TERM	WORD PARTS	DEFINITION
tuberculosis (TB) (too-ber-kyoo-LOH-sis)	-osis = abnormal condition	Infectious disease caused by the bacteria *Mycobacterium tuberculosis.* Most commonly affects the respiratory system and causes inflammation and calcification in the lungs. Tuberculosis incidence is on the increase and is seen in many patients with weakened immune systems. Multidrug-resistant tuberculosis is a particularly dangerous form of the disease because some bacteria have developed a resistance to the standard drug therapy.
Pleural Cavity		
empyema (em-pye-EE-mah)	py/o = pus	Pus with in the pleural space usually associated with a bacterial infection. Also called *pyothorax.*
pleural effusion (PLOO-ral / eh-FYOO-zhun)	pleur/o = pleura -al = pertaining to	Abnormal accumulation of fluid in the pleural cavity preventing the lungs from fully expanding. Physicians can detect the presence of fluid by tapping the chest (percussion) or listening with a stethoscope (auscultation).
pleurisy (PLOOR-ih-see)	pleur/o = pleura	Inflammation of the pleura characterized by sharp chest pain with each breath. Also called *pleuritis.*
pneumothorax (new-moh-THOH-raks)	pneum/o = air -thorax = chest	Collection of air or gas in the pleural cavity, which may result in collapse of the lung.

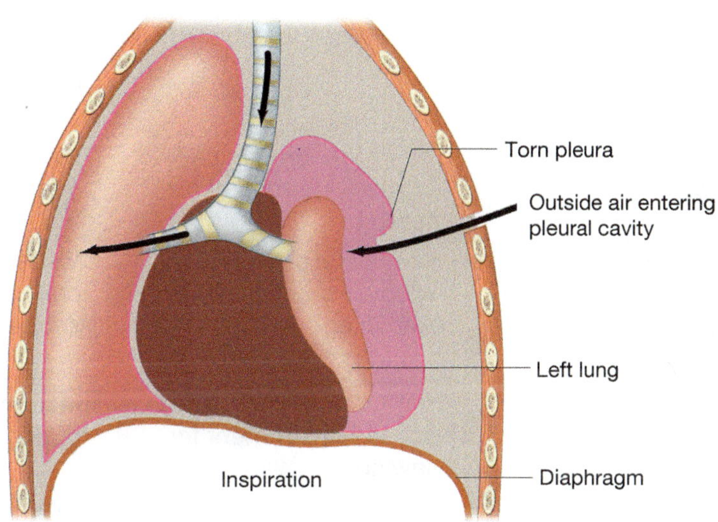

Figure 7.9 Pneumothorax. Figure illustrates how puncture of thoracic wall and tearing of pleural membrane allows air into lung and results in collapsed lung.

Diagnostic Procedures

TERM	WORD PARTS	DEFINITION
Clinical Laboratory Tests		
arterial blood gases (ABGs) (ar-TEE-ree-al)	arteri/o = artery -al = pertaining to	Testing for the gases present in the blood. Generally used to assist in determining the levels of oxygen (O_2) and carbon dioxide (CO_2) in the blood.
sputum culture and sensitivity (C&S) (SPEW-tum)		Testing sputum by placing it on a culture medium and observing any bacterial growth. The specimen is then tested to determine antibiotic effectiveness.
sputum cytology (SPEW-tum / sigh-TALL-oh-jee)	cyt/o = cell -logy = study of	Examining sputum for malignant cells.
Diagnostic Imaging		
bronchogram (BRONG-koh-gram)	bronch/o = bronchus -gram = record	X-ray record of the bronchus produced by bronchography.
bronchography (brong-KOG-rah-fee)	bronch/o = bronchus -graphy = process of recording	X-ray of the lung after a radiopaque substance has been inserted into the trachea or bronchial tube. Resulting X-ray is called a *bronchogram.*
chest X-ray (CXR)		Taking a radiographic picture of the lungs and heart from the back and sides.
pulmonary angiography (PULL-mon-air-ee / an-jee-OG-rah-fee)	pulmon/o = lung -ary = pertaining to angi/o = vessel -graphy = process of recording	Injecting dye into a blood vessel for the purpose of taking an X-ray of the arteries and veins of the lungs.
ventilation-perfusion scan (per-FUSE-shun)		Nuclear medicine diagnostic test that is especially useful in identifying pulmonary emboli. Radioactive air is inhaled for the ventilation portion to determine if air is filling the entire lung. Radioactive intravenous injection shows if blood is flowing to all parts of the lung.
Endoscopic Procedures		
bronchoscope (BRONG-koh-scope)	bronch/o = bronchus -scope = instrument for viewing	Instrument used to view inside a bronchus during a *bronchoscopy.*
bronchoscopy (Bronch) (brong-KOSS-koh-pee)	bronch/o = bronchus -scopy = process of visually examining	Visual examination of the inside of the bronchi; uses an instrument called a *bronchoscope* (see Figure 7.10 ■).
laryngoscope (lair-RING-go-scope)	laryng/o = larynx -scope = instrument for viewing	Instrument used to view inside the larynx during a *laryngoscopy.*
laryngoscopy (lair-in-GOSS-koh-pee)	laryng/o = larynx -scopy = process of visually examining	Examination of the interior of the larynx with a lighted instrument called a *laryngoscope.*

Diagnostic Procedures *(continued)*

TERM	WORD PARTS	DEFINITION

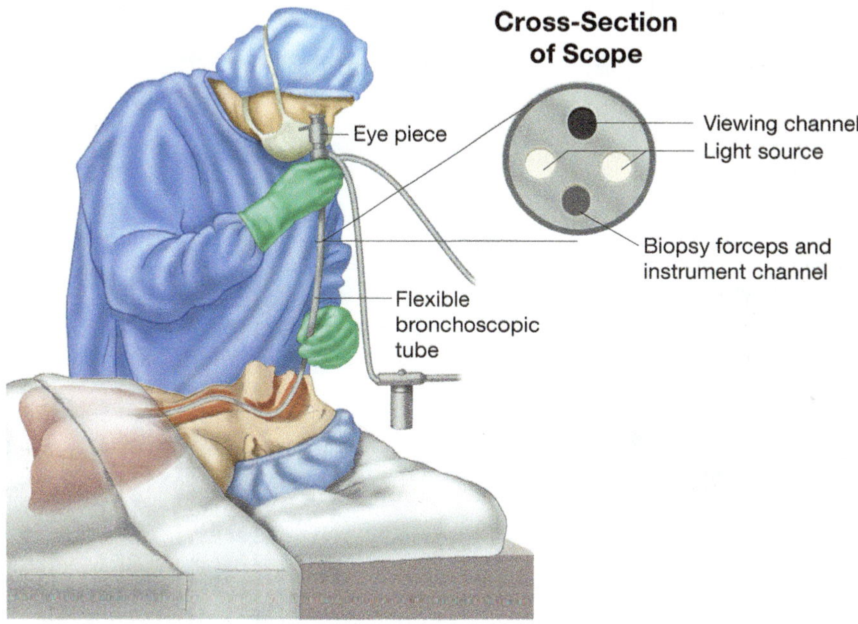

Figure 7.10 Bronchoscopy. Figure illustrates physician using a bronchoscope to inspect the patient's bronchial tubes. Advances in technology include using a videoscope, which projects the internal view of the bronchus onto a video screen.

TERM	WORD PARTS	DEFINITION
Pulmonary Function Tests		
oximeter (ox-IM-eh-ter)	ox/i = oxygen -meter = instrument to measure	Instrument that measures the amount of oxygen in the bloodstream.
oximetry (ox-IM-eh-tree)	ox/i = oxygen -metry = process of measuring	Measures the oxygen level in the blood using a device, an *oximeter,* placed on the patient's fingertip or earlobe.
pulmonary function test (PFT) (PULL-mon-air-ee)	pulmon/o = lung -ary = pertaining to	Group of diagnostic tests that give information regarding air flow in and out of the lungs, lung volumes, and gas exchange between the lungs and bloodstream.
spirometer (spy-ROM-eh-ter)	spir/o = breathing -meter = instrument to measure	Instrument to measure lung capacity used for *spirometry.*
spirometry (spy-ROM-eh-tree)	spir/o = breathing -metry = process of measuring	Procedure to measure lung capacity using a *spirometer.*
Additional Diagnostic Procedures		
polysomnography (polly-som-NOG-rah-fee)	poly- = many somn/o = sleep -graphy = process of recording	Monitoring a patient while sleeping to identify sleep apnea. Also called *sleep apnea study.*
sweat test		Test for cystic fibrosis. Patients with this disease have an abnormally large amount of salt in their sweat.
tuberculin skin tests (TB test) (too-BER-kyoo-lin)		Applying the tuberculin purified protein derivative (PPD) under the surface of the skin to determine if the patient has been exposed to tuberculosis. Also called a *Mantoux test.*

Therapeutic Procedures

TERM	WORD PARTS	DEFINITION
Respiratory Therapy		
aerosol therapy (AIR-oh-sol)	aer/o = air	Medication suspended in a mist intended for inhalation. Delivered by a *nebulizer,* which provides the mist for a period of time while the patient breathes, or a *metered-dose inhaler* (MDI), which delivers a single puff of mist.
endotracheal intubation (en-doh-TRAY-kee-al / in-too-BAY-shun)	endo- = within trache/o = trachea -al = pertaining to	Placing of a tube through the mouth, through the glottis, and into the trachea to create a patent airway.

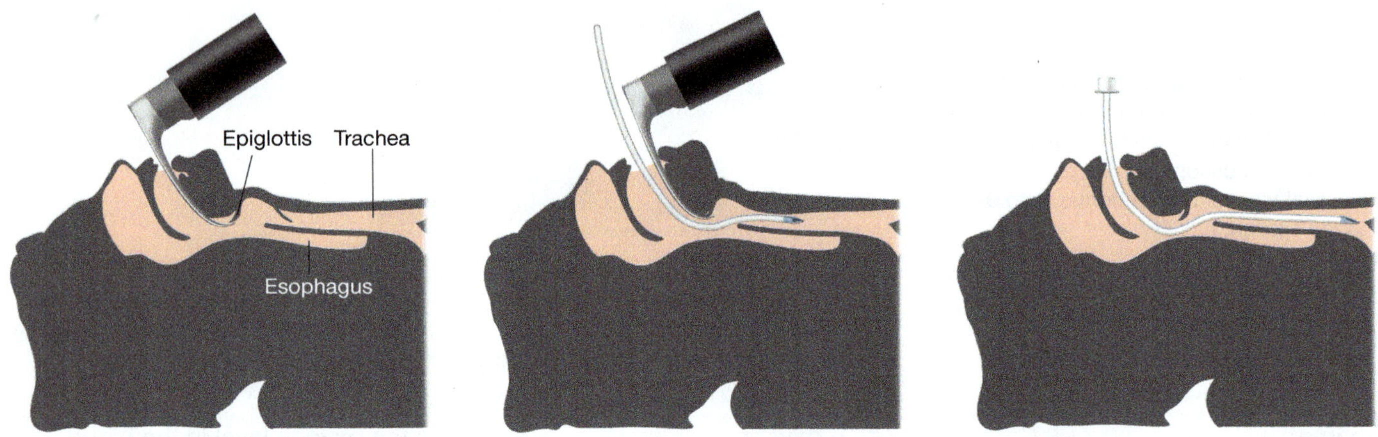

■ **Figure 7.11** Endotracheal intubation. First, a lighted scope is used to identify the trachea from the esophagus. Next, the tube is placed through the pharynx and into the trachea. Finally, the scope is removed, leaving the tube in place.

TERM	WORD PARTS	DEFINITION
intermittent positive pressure breathing (IPPB)		Method for assisting patients in breathing using a mask connected to a machine that produces an increased positive thoracic pressure.
nasal cannula (CAN-you-lah)	nas/o = nose -al = pertaining to	Two-pronged plastic device for delivering oxygen into the nose; one prong is inserted into each naris.
postural drainage	-al = pertaining to	Drainage of secretions from the bronchi by placing the patient in a position that uses gravity to promote drainage. Used for the treatment of cystic fibrosis and bronchiectasis.
supplemental oxygen therapy	-al = pertaining to	Providing a patient with additional concentration of oxygen to improve oxygen levels in the bloodstream. Oxygen may be provided by a mask or nasal cannula.
ventilator (VENT-ih-later)		Machine that provides artificial ventilation for a patient unable to breathe on his or her own. Also called a *respirator.*

Therapeutic Procedures *(continued)*

TERM	WORD PARTS	DEFINITION
Surgical Procedures		
bronchoplasty (BRONG-koh-plas-tee)	bronch/o = bronchus -plasty = surgical repair	Surgical repair of a bronchus.
laryngectomy (lair-in-JEK-toh-mee)	laryng/o = larynx -ectomy = surgical removal	Surgical removal of the larynx.
laryngoplasty (lair-RING-goh-plas-tee)	laryng/o = larynx -plasty = surgical repair	Surgical repair of the larynx.
lobectomy (loh-BEK-toh-mee)	lob/o = lobe -ectomy = surgical removal	Surgical removal of a lobe of a lung.
pleurectomy (ploor-EK-toh-mee)	pleur/o = pleura -ectomy = surgical removal	Surgical removal of the pleura.
pleurocentesis (ploor-oh-sen-TEE-sis)	pleur/o = pleura -centesis = puncture to withdraw fluid	Procedure involving insertion of a needle into the pleural space to withdraw fluid; may be a treatment for excess fluid accumulating or to obtain fluid for diagnostic examination.
rhinoplasty (RYE-noh-plas-tee)	rhin/o = nose -plasty = surgical repair	Surgical repair of the nose.
thoracentesis (thor-ah-sen-TEE-sis)	thorac/o = chest -centesis = puncture to withdraw fluid	Surgical puncture of the chest wall for the removal of fluids. Also called *thoracocentesis*.

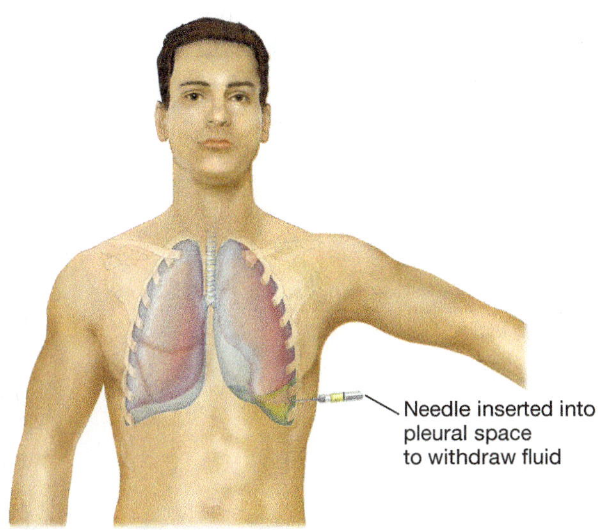

■ **Figure 7.12** Thoracentesis. A needle is inserted between the ribs to withdraw fluid from the pleural sac at the base of the left lung.

TERM	WORD PARTS	DEFINITION
thoracostomy (thor-ah-KOS-toh-mee)	thorac/o = chest -ostomy = surgically create an opening	Insertion of a tube into the chest cavity for the purpose of draining off fluid or air. Also called *chest tube*.
thoracotomy (thor-ah-KOT-oh-mee)	thorac/o = chest -otomy = cutting into	To cut into the chest cavity.

Therapeutic Procedures *(continued)*

TERM	WORD PARTS	DEFINITION
tracheotomy (tray-kee-OTT-oh-mee)	trache/o = trachea -otomy = cutting into	Surgical procedure often performed in an emergency that creates an opening directly into the trachea to allow the patient to breathe easier; also called *tracheostomy*.

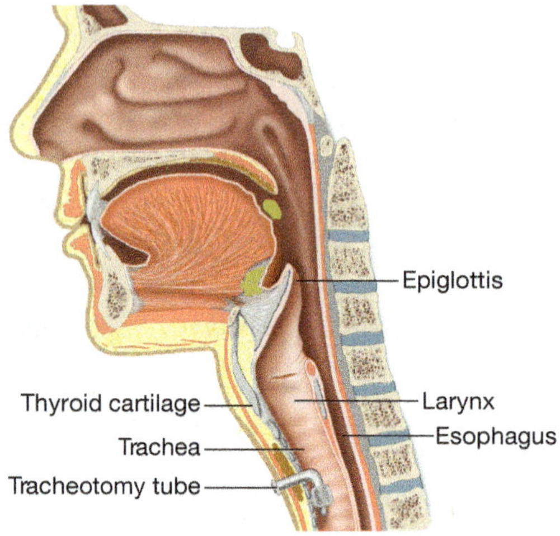

■ **Figure 7.13** A tracheotomy tube in place, inserted through an opening in the front of the neck and anchored within the trachea.

TERM	WORD PARTS	DEFINITION
Additional Procedures		
cardiopulmonary resuscitation (CPR) (car-dee-oh-PULL-mon-air-ee / ree-suss-ih-TAY-shun)	cardi/o = heart pulmon/o = lung -ary = pertaining to	Emergency treatment provided by persons trained in CPR and given to patients when their respirations and heart stop. CPR provides oxygen to the brain, heart, and other vital organs until medical treatment can restore a normal heart and pulmonary function.
Heimlich maneuver (HYME-lik)		Technique for removing a foreign body from the trachea or pharynx by exerting diaphragmatic pressure. Named for Harry Heimlich, a U.S. thoracic surgeon.
percussion (per-KUH-shun)		Use of the fingertips to tap on a surface to determine the condition beneath the surface. Determined in part by the feel of the surface as it is tapped and the sound generated.

Pharmacology

CLASSIFICATION	WORD PARTS	ACTION	EXAMPLES
antibiotic (an-tih-bye-AW-tic)	anti- = against bi/o = life -tic = pertaining to	Kills bacteria causing respiratory infections.	ampicillin; amoxicillin, Amoxil; ciprofloxacin, Cipro
antihistamine (an-tih-HIST-ah-meen)	anti- = against	Blocks the effects of histamine that has been released by the body during an allergy attack.	fexofenadine, Allegra; loratadine, Claritin; diphenhydramine, Benadryl

Pharmacology *(continued)*

CLASSIFICATION	WORD PARTS	ACTION	EXAMPLES
antitussive (an-tih-TUSS-ive)	anti- = without tuss/o = cough	Relieves the urge to cough.	hydrocodon, Hycodan; dextromethorphan, Vicks Formula 44
bronchodilator (BRONG-koh-dye-late-or)	bronch/o = bronchus	Relaxes muscle spasms in bronchial tubes. Used to treat asthma.	albuterol, Proventil, Ventolin; theophyllin, Theo-Dur
corticosteroids (core-tih-koh-STAIR-ryods)	cortic/o = outer region, cortex	Reduces inflammation and swelling in the respiratory tract.	fluticasone, Flonase; mometasone, Nasonex; triamcinolone, Azmacort
decongestant (dee-kon-JES-tant)	de- = without	Reduces stuffiness and congestion throughout the respiratory system.	oxymetazoline, Afrin, Dristan, Sinex; pseudoephedrine, Drixoral, Sudafed
expectorant (ek-SPEK-toh-rant)		Improves the ability to cough up mucus from the respiratory tract.	guaifenesin, Robitussin, Mucinex
mucolytic (myoo-koh-LIT-ik)	muc/o = mucus -lytic = destruction	Liquefies mucus so it is easier to cough and clear it from the respiratory tract.	N-acetyl-cysteine, Mucomyst

Abbreviations

ABGs	arterial blood gases
ARDS	adult (or acute) respiratory distress syndrome
Bronch	bronchoscopy
CO_2	carbon dioxide
COPD	chronic obstructive pulmonary disease
CPR	cardiopulmonary resuscitation
C&S	culture and sensitivity
CTA	clear to auscultation
CXR	chest X-ray
DOE	dyspnea on exertion
DPT	diphtheria, pertussis, tetanus injection
ENT	ear, nose, and throat
ERV	expiratory reserve volume
FRC	functional residual capacity
HMD	hyaline membrane disease
IC	inspiratory capacity
IPPB	intermittent positive pressure breathing
IRDS	infant respiratory distress syndrome
IRV	inspiratory reserve volume
LLL	left lower lobe
LUL	left upper lobe
MDI	metered-dose inhaler
O_2	oxygen
PCP	pneumocystis pneumonia
PFT	pulmonary function test
PPD	purified protein derivative
R	respiration
RA	room air
RDS	respiratory distress syndrome
RLL	right lower lobe
RML	right middle lobe
RRT	registered respiratory therapist
RV	reserve volume
RUL	right upper lobe
SARS	severe acute respiratory syndrome
SIDS	sudden infant death syndrome
SOB	shortness of breath
TB	tuberculosis
TLC	total lung capacity
TPR	temperature, pulse, and respiration
TV	tidal volume
URI	upper respiratory infection
VC	vital capacity

Chapter Review

Real-World Applications

Medical Record Analysis

This Pulmonology Consultation Report contains 12 medical terms. Underline each term and write it in the list below the report. Then define each term.

Pulmonology Consultation Report

Reason for Consultation:	Evaluation of increasingly severe asthma.
History of Present Illness:	Patient is a 10-year-old male who first presented to the Emergency Room with dyspnea, coughing, and wheezing at 7 years of age. Attacks are increasing in frequency, and there do not appear to be any precipitating factors such as exercise. No other family members are asthmatics.
Results of Physical Examination:	Patient is currently in the ER with marked dyspnea, cyanosis around the lips, prolonged expiration, and a hacking cough producing thick phlegm. Auscultation revealed rhonchi throughout lungs. ABGs indicate hypoxemia. Spirometry reveals moderately severe airway obstruction during expiration. This patient responded to Proventil and he is beginning to cough less and breathe with less effort.
Assessment:	Acute asthma attack with severe airway obstruction. There is no evidence of infection. In view of increasing severity and frequency of attacks, all his medications should be reevaluated for effectiveness and all attempts to identify precipitating factors should be made.
Recommendations:	Patient is to continue to use Proventil for relief of bronchospasms. Instructions for taking medications and controlling severity of asthma attacks were carefully reviewed with the patient and his family.

	Term	Definition
1		
2		
3		
4		
5		
6		
7		
8		
9		
10		
11		
12		

Chart Note Transcription

The chart note below contains 11 phrases that can be reworded with a medical term that you learned in this chapter. Each phrase is identified with an underline. Determine the medical term and write your answers in the space provided.

Current Complaint: A 43-year-old female was brought to the Emergency Room by her family. She complained of painful and labored breathing, (1) rapid breathing, (2) and fever. Symptoms began 3 days ago, but have become much worse during the past 12 hours.

Past History: Patient is a mother of three and a business executive. She has had no surgeries or previous serious illnesses.

Signs and Symptoms: Temperature is 103°F, respiratory rate is 20 breaths/minute, blood pressure is 165/98, and heart rate is 90 bpm. A blood test to measure the levels of oxygen in the blood (3) indicates a marked low level of oxygen in the blood. (4) The process of listening to body sounds (5) of the lungs revealed abnormal crackling sounds (6) over the left lower chest. She is producing large amounts of pus-filled (7) mucus coughed up from the respiratory tract (8) and a chest X-ray (9) shows a large cloudy patch in the lower lobe of the left lung.

Diagnosis: Left lower lobe inflammatory condition of the lungs caused by bacterial infection. (10)

Treatment: Patient was started on intravenous antibiotics. She also required a tube placed through the mouth to create an airway (11) for 3 days.

(1) ____________________

(2) ____________________

(3) ____________________

(4) ____________________

(5) ____________________

(6) ____________________

(7) ____________________

(8) ____________________

(9) ____________________

(10) ____________________

(11) ____________________

Case Study

Below is a case study presentation of a patient with a condition discussed in this chapter. Read the case study and answer the questions below. Some questions will ask for information not included within this chapter. Use your text, a medical dictionary, or any other reference material you choose to answer these questions.

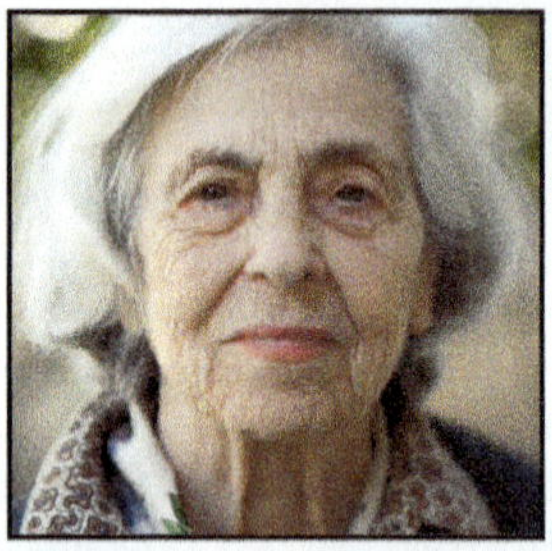

(© Francesco De Napoli/istockphoto.com)

An 88-year-old female was seen in the physician's office complaining of dyspnea, dizziness, orthopnea, elevated temperature, and a cough. Lung auscultation revealed crackles over the right bronchus. CXR revealed fluid in the RUL. The patient was sent to the hospital with an admitting diagnosis of pneumonia. Vital signs upon admission were temperature 102°F, pulse 100 BPM and rapid, respirations 24 breaths/min and labored, blood pressure 180/110. She was treated with IV antibiotics and IPPB. She responded well to treatment and was released home to her family with oral antibiotics on the third day.

1. What was this patient's admitting diagnosis? Look this condition up in a reference source and include a short description of it.

2. List and define each of the patient's presenting symptoms in your own words.

3. Define auscultation and CXR. Describe what each revealed in your own words.

4. What does the term "vital signs" mean? Describe this patient's vital signs.

5. Describe the treatments this patient received while in the hospital in your own words.

6. Explain the change in the patient's medication when she was discharged home.

Practice Exercises

A. Complete the Statement

1. The primary function of the respiratory system is ______________________.
2. The movement of air in and out of the lungs is called ______________________.
3. Define external respiration: ______________________.
4. Define internal respiration: ______________________.
5. The organs of the respiratory system are ______________________, ______________________, ______________________, ______________________, ______________________, and ______________________.
6. The passageway for food, liquids, and air is the ______________________.
7. The ______________________ helps to keep food out of the respiratory tract.
8. The function of the cilia in the nose is to ______________________.
9. The muscle that divides the thoracic cavity from the abdominal cavity is the ______________________.
10. The respiratory rate for an adult is ______________________ to ______________________ respirations per minute.
11. The respiratory rate for a newborn is ______________________ to ______________________ respirations per minute.
12. The right lung has ______________________ lobes; the left lung has ______________________ lobes.
13. The air sacs at the ends of the bronchial tree are called ______________________.
14. The term for the double membrane around the lungs is ______________________.
15. The nasal cavity is separated from the mouth by the ______________________.
16. The small branches of the bronchi are the ______________________.

B. Define the Suffix

	Definition	Example from Chapter
1. -ectasis	______________________	______________________
2. -capnia	______________________	______________________
3. -phonia	______________________	______________________
4. -thorax	______________________	______________________
5. -pnea	______________________	______________________
6. -ptysis	______________________	______________________
7. -osmia	______________________	______________________

C. Combining Form Practice

The combining form **rhin/o** refers to the nose. Use it to write a term that means:

1. inflammation of the nose ______
2. abnormal flow from the nose ______
3. discharge from the nose ______
4. surgical repair of the nose ______

The combining form **laryng/o** refers to the larynx or voice box. Use it to write a term that means:

5. inflammation of the larynx ______
6. spasm of the larynx ______
7. visual examination of the larynx ______
8. pertaining to the larynx ______
9. cutting into the larynx ______
10. removal of the larynx ______
11. surgical repair of the larynx ______
12. paralysis of the larynx ______

The combining form **bronch/o** refers to the bronchus. Use it to write a term that means:

13. pertaining to bronchus ______
14. inflammation of the bronchus ______
15. visually examine the interior of the bronchus ______
16. produced by bronchus ______
17. spasm of the bronchus ______

The combining form **thorac/o** refers to the chest. Use it to write a term that means:

18. surgical repair of the chest ______
19. cutting into the chest ______
20. chest pain ______
21. pertaining to chest ______

The combining form **trache/o** refers to the trachea. Use it to write a term that means:

22. cutting into the trachea ______

23. surgical repair of the trachea ____________________

24. narrowing of the trachea ____________________

25. pertaining to inside the trachea ____________________

26. inflammation of the trachea ____________________

D. Define the Combining Form

	Definition	Example from Chapter
1. **trache/o**	____________________	____________________
2. **laryng/o**	____________________	____________________
3. **bronch/o**	____________________	____________________
4. **spir/o**	____________________	____________________
5. **pneum/o**	____________________	____________________
6. **rhin/o**	____________________	____________________
7. **coni/o**	____________________	____________________
8. **pleur/o**	____________________	____________________
9. **epiglott/o**	____________________	____________________
10. **alveol/o**	____________________	____________________
11. **pulmon/o**	____________________	____________________
12. **ox/o**	____________________	____________________
13. **sinus/o**	____________________	____________________
14. **lob/o**	____________________	____________________
15. **nas/o**	____________________	____________________

E. Suffix Practice

The suffix **-pnea** means breathing. Use this suffix to write a medical term that means:

1. normal breathing ____________________
2. difficult or labored breathing ____________________
3. rapid breathing ____________________
4. can breathe only in an upright position ____________________
5. lack of breathing ____________________

F. Name That Term

1. the process of breathing in ____________________
2. spitting up of blood ____________________
3. blood clot in the pulmonary artery ____________________
4. inflammation of a sinus ____________________
5. sore throat ____________________
6. air in the pleural cavity ____________________
7. whooping cough ____________________
8. cutting into the pleura ____________________
9. pain in the pleural region ____________________
10. common cold ____________________

G. What's the Abbreviation?

1. upper respiratory infection ____________________
2. pulmonary function test ____________________
3. left lower lobe ____________________
4. oxygen ____________________
5. carbon dioxide ____________________
6. intermittent positive pressure breathing ____________________
7. chronic obstructive pulmonary disease ____________________
8. bronchoscopy ____________________
9. total lung capacity ____________________
10. tuberculosis ____________________
11. infant respiratory distress syndrome ____________________

H. What Does it Stand For?

1. CXR ____________________
2. TV ____________________
3. TPR ____________________
4. ABGs ____________________

5. DOE ____________________

6. RUL ____________________

7. SIDS ____________________

8. TLC ____________________

9. ARDS ____________________

10. MDI ____________________

11. CTA ____________________

12. SARS ____________________

I. Terminology Matching

Match each term to its definition.

1.	_______ inhaling environmental particles	a.	polysomnography
2.	_______ whooping cough	b.	Mantoux test
3.	_______ may result in collapsed lung	c.	oximetry
4.	_______ test to identify sleep apnea	d.	epistaxis
5.	_______ respiratory tract mucus	e.	pneumoconiosis
6.	_______ sweat test	f.	emphysema
7.	_______ measures oxygen levels in blood	g.	walking pneumonia
8.	_______ *Mycoplasma* pneumonia	h.	pneumothorax
9.	_______ disease with overexpanded air sacs	i.	empyema
10.	_______ tuberculin test	j.	phlegm
11.	_______ nosebleed	k.	pertussis
12.	_______ pus in the pleural space	l.	test for cystic fibrosis

J. Define the Term

1. total lung capacity ____________________

2. tidal volume ____________________

3. residual volume ____________________

K. Fill in the Blank

anthracosis	sputum cytology	cardiopulmonary resuscitation	patent
thoracentesis	respirator	ventilation-perfusion scan	rhonchi
supplemental oxygen	hyperventilation		

1. When the patient's breathing and heart stopped, the paramedics began ______________________.
2. The physician performed a ______________________ to remove fluid from the chest.
3. A ______________________ is also called a ventilator.
4. The patient received ______________________ through a nasal cannula.
5. An endotracheal intubation was performed to establish a ______________________ airway.
6. A ______________________ is a particularly useful test to identify a pulmonary embolus.
7. The result of the ______________________ was negative for cancer.
8. ______________________ involves tachypnea and hyperpnea.
9. ______________________ are wheezing lung sounds.
10. Miners are at risk of developing ______________________.

L. Pharmacology Challenge

Fill in the classification for each drug description, then match the brand name.

	Drug Description	Classification		Brand Name
1.	_______ Reduces stuffiness and congestion	______________________	a.	Hycodan
2.	_______ Relieves the urge to cough	______________________	b.	Flonase
3.	_______ Kills bacteria	______________________	c.	Cipro
4.	_______ Improves ability to cough up mucus	______________________	d.	Ventolin
5.	_______ Liquefies mucus	______________________	e.	Allegra
6.	_______ Relaxes bronchial muscle spasms	______________________	f.	Afrin
7.	_______ Blocks allergy attack	______________________	g.	Robitussin
8.	_______ Reduces inflammation and swelling	______________________	h.	Mucomyst

M. Ethics

Write an essay about how you would report an illegal or unethical incident at your school. Who would you tell? What would you say?

Would it matter if you knew the person who did the unethical or illegal activity? In your essay, explain why it is important to report these incidents, and how reporting them helps keeps everyone in your school environment safe.

N. Career Plan

A career plan is a tool that shows you how to achieve your career goals. Working with your teacher, a counselor, or a family member, develop a career plan that starts now. The plan may be part of an academic plan that you have already completed, or it may be a separate document. If your school has a form for the career plan, use it. Otherwise, develop the plan on a sheet of paper. Be sure to state a realistic and attainable long-term career goal that matches your skills, interests, and abilities. Also include short-term education and career goals that map out the steps you will take to achieve your ultimate career goal. Add the plan to your vocational portfolio.

Labeling Exercise

Image A

Write the labels for this figure on the numbered lines provided.

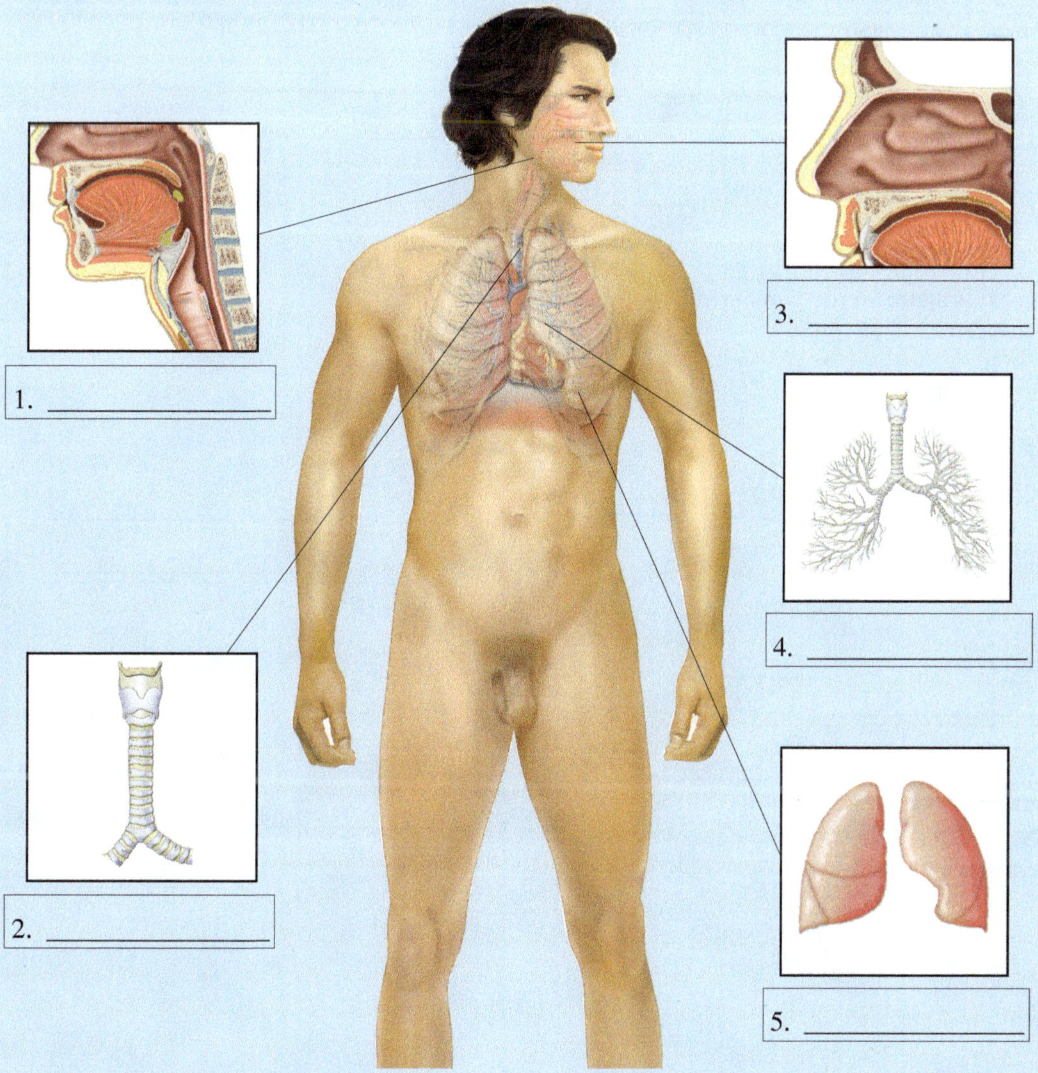

Image B

Write the labels for this figure on the numbered lines provided.

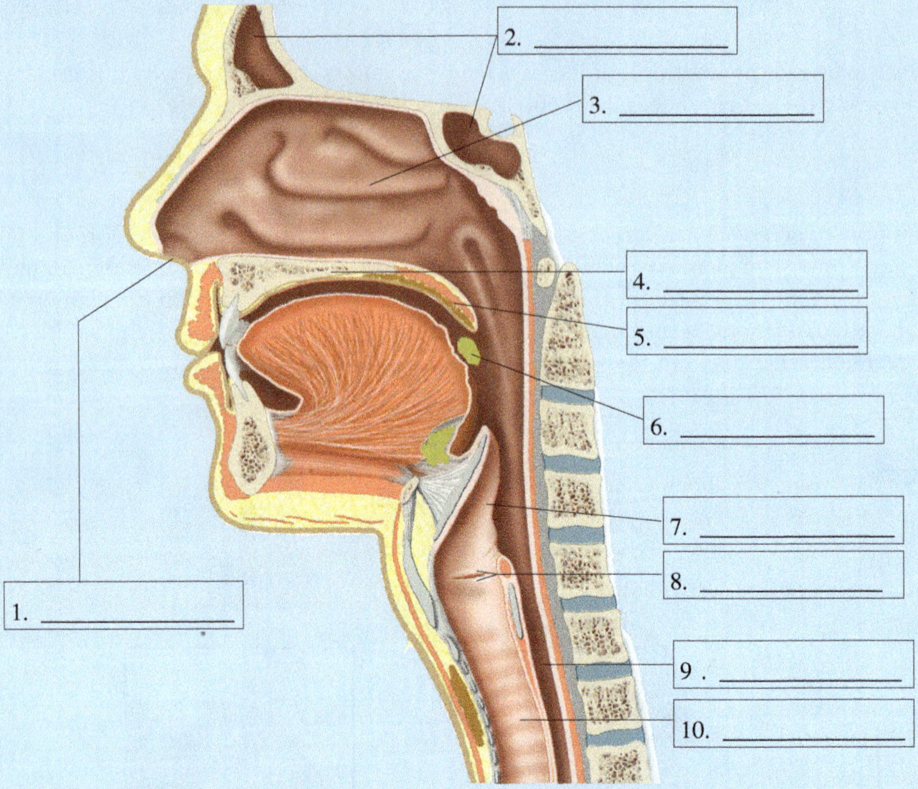

Image C

Write the labels for this figure on the numbered lines provided.

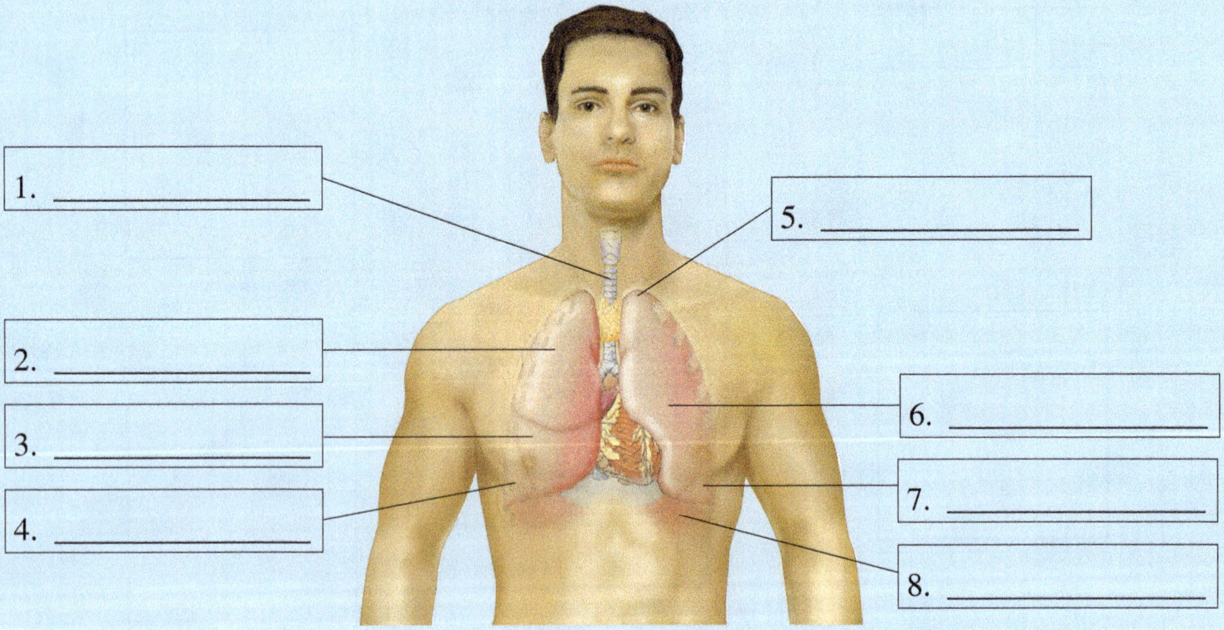

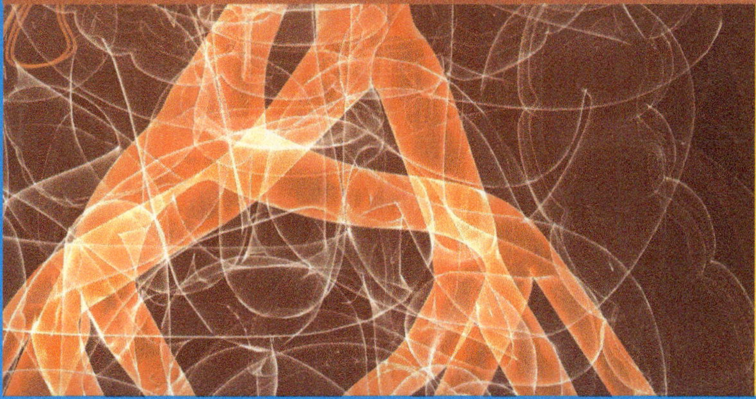

8

DIGESTIVE SYSTEM

Learning Objectives

Upon completion of this chapter, you will be able to

- Identify and define the combining forms and suffixes introduced in this chapter.
- Correctly spell and pronounce medical terms and major anatomical structures relating to the digestive system.
- Locate and describe the major organs of the digestive system and their functions.
- Describe the function of the accessory organs of the digestive system.
- Identify the shape and function of each type of tooth.
- Identify and define digestive system anatomical terms.
- Identify and define selected digestive system pathology terms.
- Identify and define selected digestive system diagnostic procedures.
- Identify and define selected digestive system therapeutic procedures.
- Identify and define selected medications relating to the digestive system.
- Define selected abbreviations associated with the digestive system.

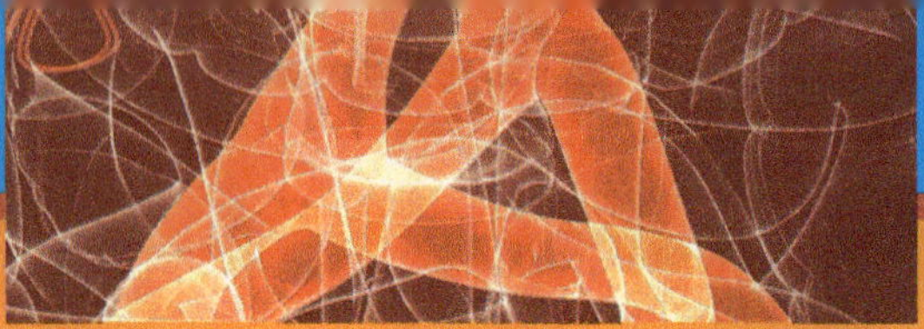

Digestive System at a Glance

Function

The digestive system begins breaking down food through mechanical and chemical digestion. After being digested, nutrient molecules are absorbed into the body and enter the bloodstream; any food not digested or absorbed is eliminated as solid waste.

Structures

Here are the primary structures that comprise the digestive system.

colon	**pancreas**
esophagus	**pharynx**
gallbladder (GB)	**salivary glands**
liver	**small intestine**
oral cavity	**stomach**

Word Parts

Here are the most common word parts (with their meanings) used to build digestive system terms. For a more comprehensive list, refer to the Terminology section of this chapter.

Combining Forms

an/o	anus	gloss/o	tongue
append/o	appendix	hepat/o	liver
appendic/o	appendix	ile/o	ileum
bar/o	weight	jejun/o	jejunum
bucc/o	cheek	labi/o	lip
cec/o	cecum	lapar/o	abdomen
cholangi/o	bile duct	lingu/o	tongue
chol/e	bile, gall	lith/o	stone
cholecyst/o	gallbladder	odont/o	tooth
choledoch/o	common bile duct	or/o	mouth
cirrh/o	yellow	palat/o	palate
col/o	colon	pancreat/o	pancreas
colon/o	colon	pharyng/o	pharynx (throat)
dent/o	tooth	polyp/o	polyp
diverticul/o	pouch	proct/o	anus and rectum
duoden/o	duodenum	pylor/o	pylorus
enter/o	small intestine	pyr/o	fire
esophag/o	esophagus	rect/o	rectum
gastr/o	stomach	sialaden/o	salivary gland
gingiv/o	gums	sigmoid/o	sigmoid colon

Suffixes

-emesis	vomit	-pepsia	digestion
-istry	specialty of	-phagia	eat, swallow
-lithiasis	condition of stones	-prandial	pertaining to a meal
-orexia	appetite	-tripsy	surgical crushing

Digestive System Illustrated

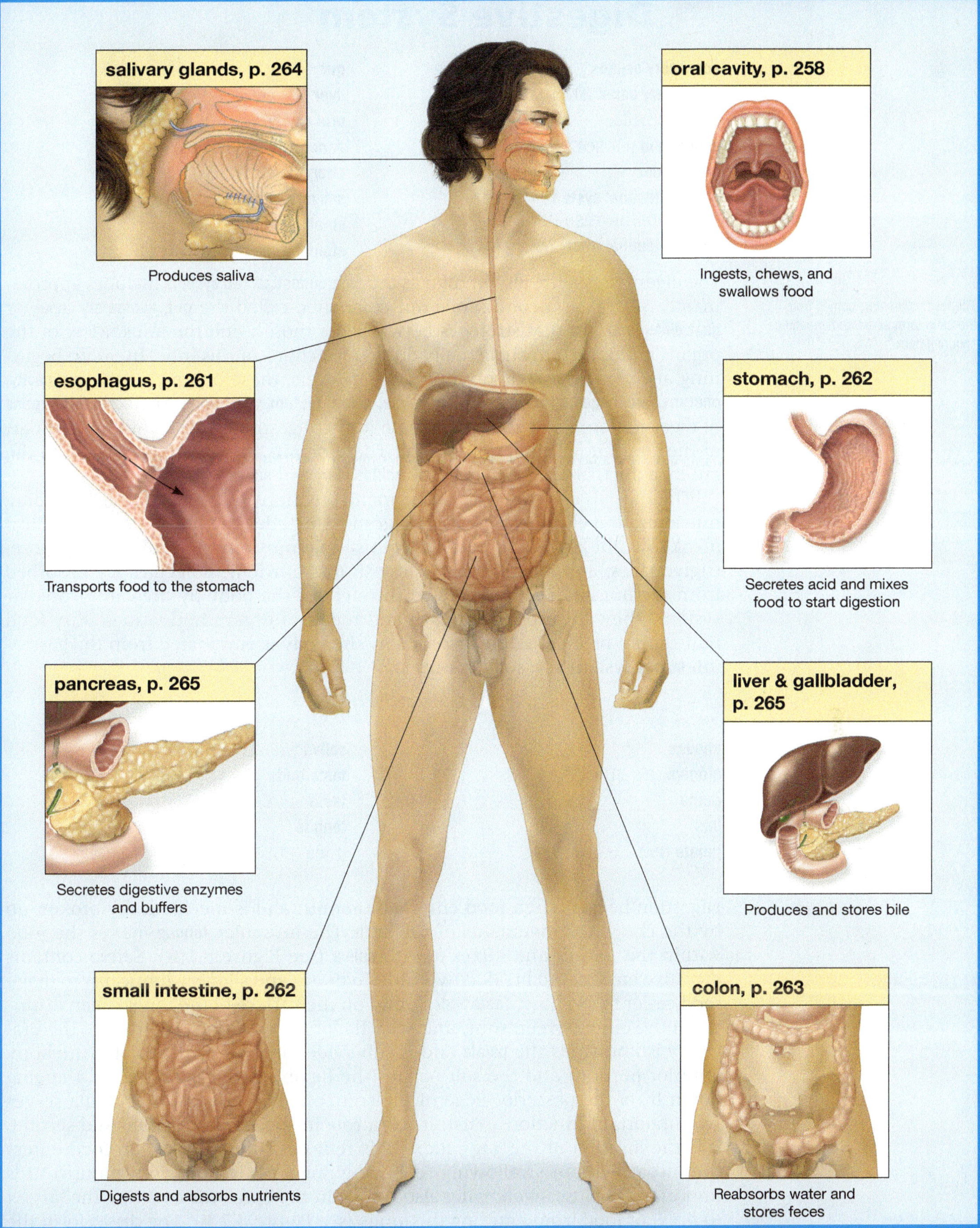

Anatomy and Physiology of the Digestive System

accessory organs
alimentary canal (al-ih-MEN-tar-ree)
colon (COH-lon)
esophagus (eh-SOFF-ah-gus)
gallbladder
gastrointestinal system (gas-troh-in-TESS-tih-nal)
gastrointestinal tract
gut
liver
oral cavity
pancreas (PAN-kree-ass)
pharynx (FAIR-inks)
salivary glands (SAL-ih-vair-ee)
small intestine
stomach (STUM-ak)

MED TERM TIP

The term *alimentary* comes from the Latin term *alimentum* meaning "nourishment."

The digestive system, also known as the **gastrointestinal (GI) system,** includes approximately 30 feet of a continuous muscular tube called the **gut, alimentary canal,** or **gastrointestinal tract** that stretches between the mouth and the anus. Most of the organs in this system are actually different sections of this tube. In order, beginning at the mouth and continuing to the anus, these organs are the **oral cavity, pharynx, esophagus, stomach, small intestine, colon, rectum,** and **anus.** The **accessory organs** of digestion are those that participate in the digestion process, but are not part of the continuous alimentary canal. These organs, which are connected to the gut by a duct, are the **liver, pancreas, gallbladder,** and **salivary glands.**

The digestive system has three main functions: digesting food, absorbing nutrients, and eliminating waste. Digestion includes the physical and chemical breakdown of large food particles into simple nutrient molecules like glucose, triglycerides, and amino acids. These simple nutrient molecules are absorbed from the intestines and circulated throughout the body by the cardiovascular system. They are used for growth and repair of organs and tissues. Any food that cannot be digested or absorbed by the body is eliminated from the gastrointestinal system as a solid waste.

Oral Cavity

cheeks
gingiva (JIN-jih-veh)
gums
lips
palate (PAL-at)
saliva (suh-LYE-vah)
taste buds
teeth
tongue
uvula (YU-vyu-lah)

Digestion begins when food enters the mouth and is mechanically broken up by the chewing movements of the **teeth.** The muscular **tongue** moves the food within the mouth and mixes it with **saliva** (see Figure 8.1 ■). Saliva contains digestive enzymes to break down carbohydrates and slippery lubricants to make food easier to swallow. **Taste buds,** found on the surface of the tongue, can distinguish the bitter, sweet, sour, and salty flavors in our food. The roof of the oral cavity is known as the **palate** and is subdivided into the hard palate (the bony anterior portion) and the soft palate (the flexible posterior portion). Hanging down from the posterior edge of the soft palate is the **uvula.** The uvula serves two important functions. First, it has a role in speech production, and second, it is the location of the gag reflex. This reflex is stimulated when food enters the throat without swallowing (e.g., laughing with food in your mouth). It is important because swallowing also results in the epiglottis covering the larynx to prevent food from entering the lungs (see Figure 8.2 ■). The **cheeks** form the

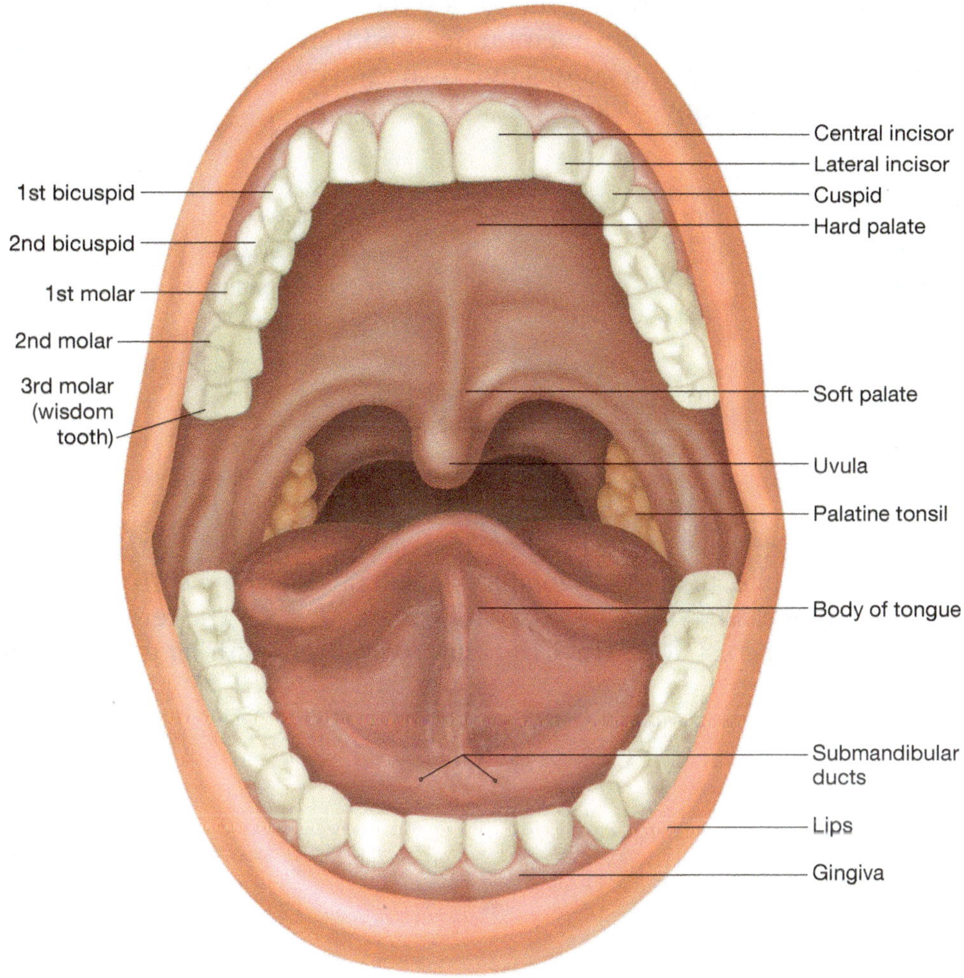

■ **Figure 8.1** Anatomy of structures of the oral cavity.

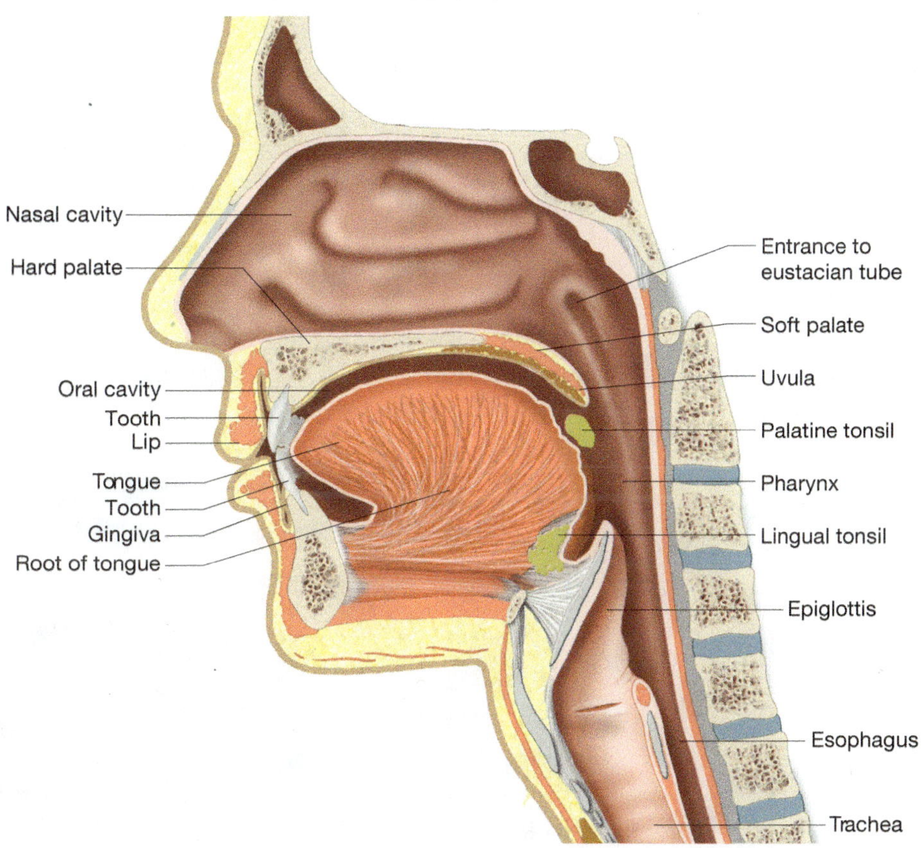

■ **Figure 8.2** Structures of the oral cavity, pharynx, and esophagus.

lateral walls of this cavity and the **lips** are the anterior opening. The entire oral cavity is lined with mucous membrane, a portion of which forms the **gums,** or **gingiva,** that combine with connective tissue to cover the jaw bone and seal off the teeth in their bony sockets.

Teeth

bicuspids (bye-CUSS-pids)
canines (KAY-nines)
cementum (see-MEN-tum)
crown
cuspids (CUSS-pids)
deciduous teeth (dee-SID-yoo-us)
dentin (DEN-tin)
enamel
incisors (in-SIGH-zors)
molars (MOH-lars)
periodontal ligaments (pair-ee-on-DON-tal)
permanent teeth
premolars (pree-MOH-lars)
pulp cavity
root
root canal

MED TERM TIP

There are three different molars, simply referred to as the first, second, or third molars. However, the third molar has a more common name, the wisdom tooth. Not every person ever forms all four wisdom teeth. Unfortunately, most people do not have enough room in their jaws for the third molars to properly erupt through the gum, a condition requiring surgical removal of the third molar, referred to as an *impacted wisdom tooth.*

Teeth are an important part of the first stage of digestion. The teeth in the front of the mouth bite, tear, or cut food into small pieces. These cutting teeth include the **cuspids** (or **canines**) and the **incisors** (see Figure 8.3 ■). The remaining posterior teeth grind and crush food into even finer pieces. These grinding teeth include the

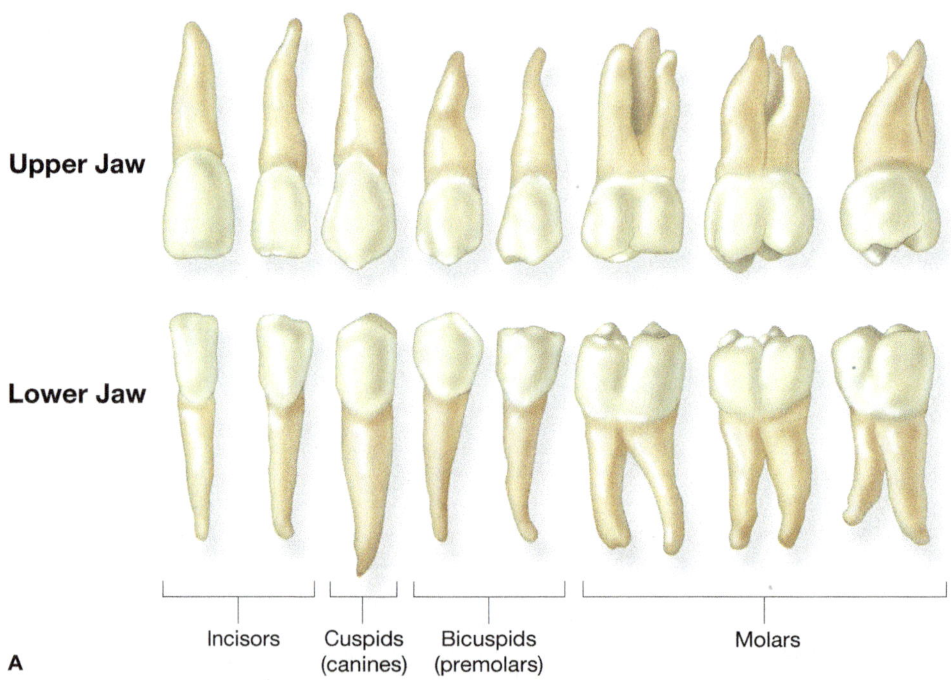

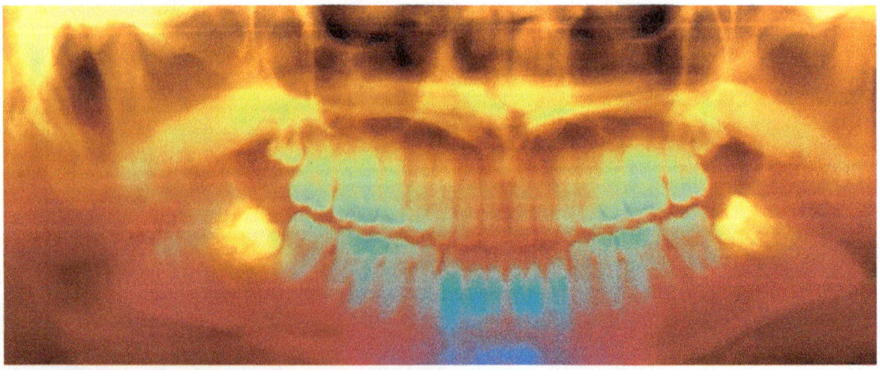

■ **Figure 8.3** (A) The name and shape of the adult teeth. These teeth represent those found in the right side of the mouth. Those of the left side would be a mirror image. The incisors and cuspids are cutting teeth. The bicuspids and molars are grinding teeth. (B) Color-enhanced X-ray of all teeth. Note the four wisdom teeth (third molars) that have not erupted. *(Photo Researchers, Inc.)*

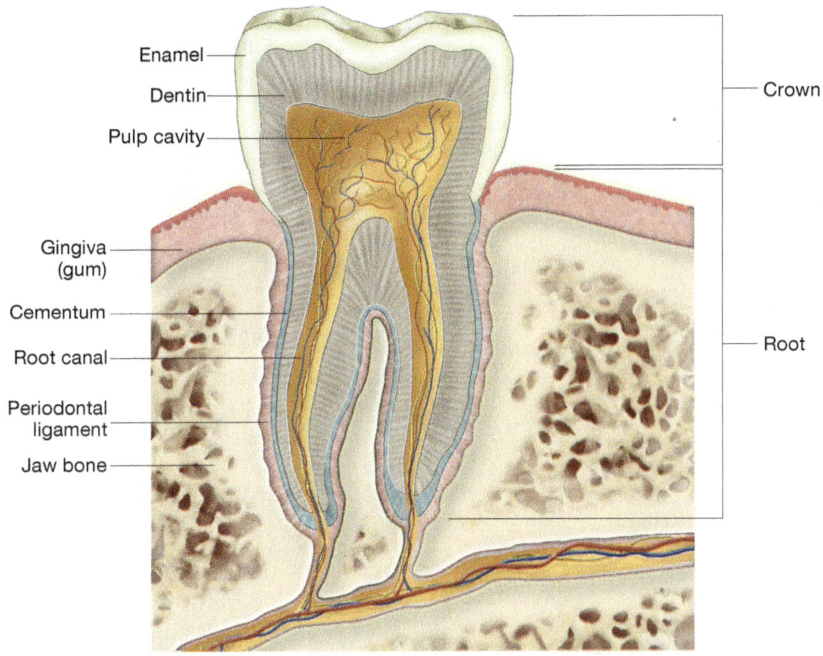

■ **Figure 8.4** An adult tooth, longitudinal view showing internal structures of the crown and root.

bicuspids (or **premolars**) and the **molars.** A tooth can be subdivided into the **crown** and the **root.** The crown is that part of the tooth visible above the gum line; the root is below the gum line. The root is anchored in the bony socket of the jaw by **cementum** and tiny **periodontal ligaments.** The crown of the tooth is covered by a layer of **enamel,** the hardest substance in the body. Under the enamel layer is **dentin,** the substance that makes up the main bulk of the tooth. The hollow interior of a tooth is called the **pulp cavity** in the crown and the **root canal** in the root. These cavities contain soft tissue made up of blood vessels, nerves, and lymph vessels (see Figure 8.4 ■).

Humans have two sets of teeth. The first set, often referred to as baby teeth, are **deciduous teeth.** There are 20 teeth in this set that erupt through the gums between the ages of 6 and 28 months. At approximately 6 years of age, these teeth begin to fall out and are replaced by the 32 **permanent teeth.** This replacement process continues until about 18–20 years of age.

MED TERM TIP

The combining form *dent/o* means teeth. Hence we have terms such as dentist and dentistry. The combining form *odont/o* also means teeth and when combined with *orth/o,* which means straight, we have the specialty of *orthodontics,* or straightening teeth.

Pharynx

epiglottis (ep-ih-GLOT-iss)
oropharynx
laryngopharynx

When food is swallowed, it enters the **oropharynx** and then the **laryngopharynx** (see again Figure 8.2). Remember from your study of the respiratory system that air is also traveling through these portions of the pharynx. The **epiglottis** is a cartilaginous flap that folds down to cover the larynx and trachea so that food is prevented from entering the respiratory tract and instead continues into the esophagus.

Esophagus

peristalsis (pair-ih-STALL-sis)

The esophagus is a muscular tube of about 10 inches long in adults. Food entering the esophagus is carried through the thoracic cavity and diaphragm and into the abdominal cavity where it enters the stomach (see Figure 8.5 ■). Food is propelled along the esophagus by wavelike muscular contractions called **peristalsis.** In fact, peristalsis works to push food through the entire gastrointestinal tract.

MED TERM TIP

It takes about 10 seconds for swallowed food to reach the stomach.

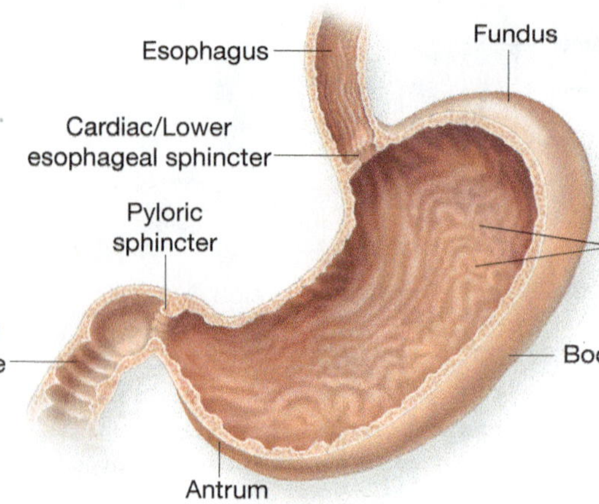

■ **Figure 8.5** The stomach. Longitudinal view showing regions and internal structures.

Stomach

antrum (AN-trum)
body
cardiac sphincter (CAR-dee-ak / SFINGK-ter)
chyme (KIGHM)
fundus (FUN-dus)
hydrochloric acid
lower esophageal sphincter (eh-soff-ah-JEE-al / SFINGK-ter)
pyloric sphincter (pigh-LOR-ik / SFINGK-ter)
rugae (ROO-gay)
sphincters (SFINGK-ters)

The stomach, a J-shaped muscular organ that acts as a bag or sac to collect and churn food with digestive juices, is composed of three parts: the **fundus** or upper region, the **body** or main portion, and the **antrum** or lower region (see again Figure 8.5). The folds in the lining of the stomach are called **rugae.** When the stomach fills with food, the rugae stretch out and disappear. **Hydrochloric acid** (HCl) is secreted by glands in the mucous membrane lining of the stomach. Food mixes with hydrochloric acid and other gastric juices to form a liquid mixture called **chyme,** which then passes through the remaining portion of the digestive system.

Entry into and exit from the stomach is controlled by muscular valves called **sphincters.** These valves open and close to ensure that food can only move forward down the gut tube. The **cardiac sphincter,** named for its proximity to the heart, is located between the esophagus and the fundus; also called the **lower esophageal sphincter** (LES), it keeps food from flowing backward into the esophagus.

The antrum tapers off into the **pyloric sphincter,** which regulates the passage of food into the small intestine. Only a small amount of the chyme is allowed to enter the small intestine with each opening of the sphincter for two important reasons. First, the small intestine is much narrower than the stomach and cannot hold as much as the stomach can. Second, the chyme is highly acidic and must be thoroughly neutralized as it leaves the stomach.

MED TERM TIP

It is easier to remember the function of the pyloric sphincter when you note that *pylor/o* means "gatekeeper." This gatekeeper controls the forward movement of food. Sphincters are rings of muscle that can be opened and closed to control entry and exit from hollow organs like the stomach, colon, and bladder.

Small Intestine

duodenum (doo-oh-DEE-num / doo-OD-eh-num)
ileocecal valve (ill-ee-oh-SEE-kal)
ileum (ILL-ee-um)
jejunum (jee-JOO-num)

The small intestine, or small bowel, is the major site of digestion and absorption of nutrients from food. It is located between the pyloric sphincter and the colon (see Figure 8.6 ■). Because the small intestine is concerned with absorption of food products, an abnormality in this organ can cause malnutrition. The small intestine, with an average length of 20 feet, is the longest portion of the alimentary canal and has three sections: the **duodenum,** the **jejunum,** and the **ileum.**

MED TERM TIP

Word Watch: Be careful not to confuse the word root *ile/o* meaning "ileum," a portion of the small intestines, and *ili/o* meaning "ilium," a pelvic bone.

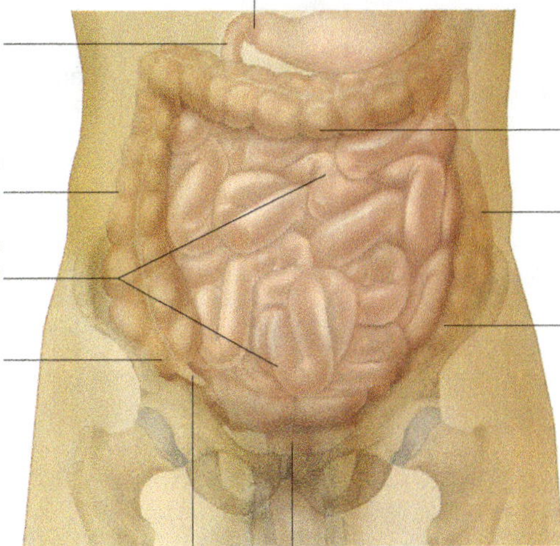

Figure 8.6 The small intestine. Anterior view of the abdominopelvic cavity illustrating how the three sections of small intestine—duodenum, jejunum, and ileum—begin at the pyloric sphincter and end at the colon, but are not arranged in an orderly fashion.

- The duodenum extends from the pyloric sphincter to the jejunum, and is about 10–12 inches long. Digestion is completed in the duodenum after the liquid chyme from the stomach is mixed with digestive juices from the pancreas and gallbladder.
- The jejunum, or middle portion, extends from the duodenum to the ileum and is about 8 feet long.
- The ileum is the last portion of the small intestine and extends from the jejunum to the colon. At 12 feet in length, it is the longest portion of the small intestine. The ileum connects to the colon with a sphincter called the **ileocecal valve.**

MED TERM TIP

We can survive without a portion of the small intestine. For example, in cases of cancer, much of the small intestine and/or colon may have to be removed. The surgeon then creates an opening between the remaining intestine and the abdominal wall. The combining form for the section of intestine connected to the abdominal wall and the suffix *-ostomy* are used to describe this procedure. For example, if a person has a *jejunostomy*, the jejunum is connected to the abdominal wall and the ileum (and remainder of the gut tube) has been removed.

Colon

anal sphincter (AY-nal / SFINGK-ter)
anus (AY-nus)
ascending colon
cecum (SEE-kum)
defecation
descending colon
feces (FEE-seez)
rectum (REK-tum)
sigmoid colon (SIG-moyd)
transverse colon
vermiform appendix (VER-mih-form / ah-PEN-diks)

Fluid that remains after the complete digestion and absorption of nutrients in the small intestine enters the colon or large intestine (see Figure 8.7 ■). Most of this fluid is water that is reabsorbed into the body. The material that remains after absorption is solid waste called **feces** (or stool). This is the product evacuated in bowel movements (BM).

The colon is approximately 5 feet long and extends from the **cecum** to the **anus.** The cecum is a pouch or saclike area in the first 2–3 inches at the beginning of the colon. The **vermiform appendix** is a small worm-shaped outgrowth at the end of the cecum. The remaining colon consists of the **ascending colon, transverse colon, descending colon,** and **sigmoid colon.** The ascending colon on the right side extends from the cecum to the lower border of the liver. The transverse colon begins where the ascending colon leaves off and moves horizontally across the upper abdomen toward the spleen. The descending colon then travels down the left side of the body to where the sigmoid colon begins. The sigmoid colon curves in an S-shape back to the midline of the body and ends at the **rectum.** The rectum, where feces is stored, leads into the anus, which contains the **anal sphincter.** This sphincter consists of rings of voluntary and involuntary muscles to control the evacuation of feces or **defecation.**

MED TERM TIP

The term *colon* refers to the large intestine. However, you should be aware that many people use it incorrectly as a general term referring to the entire intestinal system, both small and large intestines.

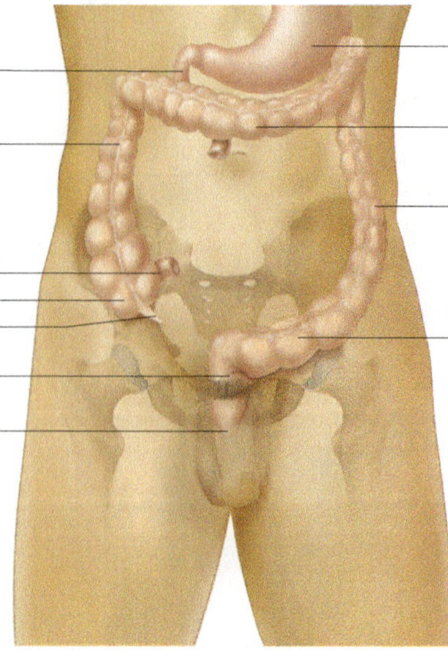

■ **Figure 8.7** The regions of the colon beginning with the cecum and ending at the anus.

Accessory Organs of the Digestive System

MED TERM TIP

In anatomy the term *accessory* generally means that the structure is auxiliary to a more important structure. This is not true for these organs. Digestion would not be possible without the digestive juices produced by these organs.

As described earlier, the accessory organs of the digestive system are the salivary glands, the liver, the pancreas, and the gallbladder. In general, these organs function by producing much of the digestive fluids and enzymes necessary for the chemical breakdown of food. Each is attached to the gut tube by a duct.

Salivary Glands

amylase (AM-ill-ace)
bolus
parotid glands (pah-ROT-id)
sublingual glands (sub-LING-gwal)
submandibular glands (sub-man-DIB-yoo-lar)

Salivary glands in the oral cavity produce saliva. This very watery and slick fluid allows food to be swallowed with less danger of choking. Saliva mixed with food in the mouth forms a **bolus,** chewed food that is ready to swallow. Saliva also contains the digestive enzyme **amylase** that begins the digestion of carbohydrates. There are three pairs of salivary glands. The **parotid glands** are in front of the ears, and the **submandibular glands** and **sublingual glands** are in the floor of the mouth (see Figure 8.8 ■).

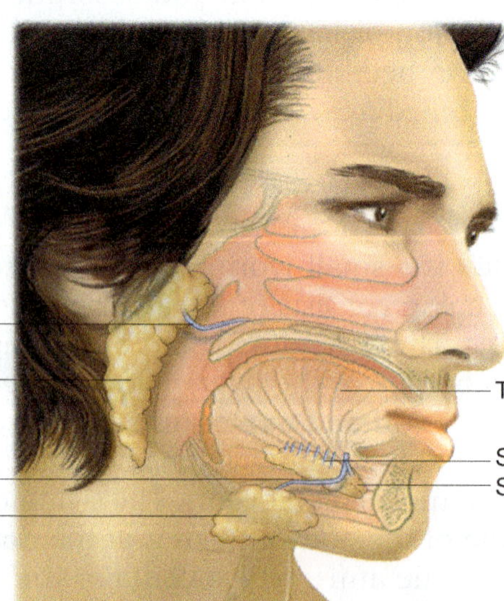

■ **Figure 8.8** The salivary glands, parotid, sublingual, and submandibular. This image shows the position of each gland and its duct emptying into the oral cavity.

Liver

bile (BYE-al) **emulsification** (ee-mull-sih-fih-KAY-shun)

The liver, a large organ located in the right upper quadrant of the abdomen, has several functions including processing the nutrients absorbed by the intestines, detoxifying harmful substances in the body, and producing **bile** (see Figure 8.9 ■). Bile is important for the digestion of fats and lipids because it breaks up large fat globules into much smaller droplets, making them easier to digest in the watery environment inside the intestines. The process is called **emulsification.**

MED TERM TIP

The liver weighs about 4 pounds and has so many important functions that people cannot live without it. It has become a major transplant organ. The liver is also able to regenerate itself. You can lose more than half of your liver, and it will regrow.

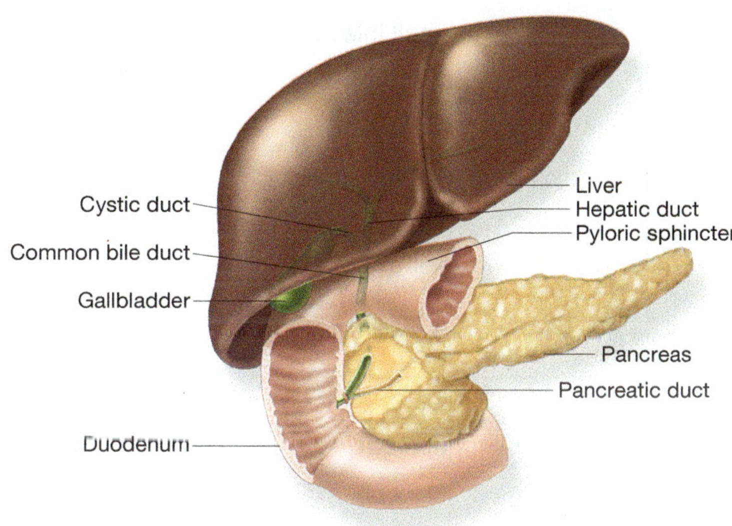

■ **Figure 8.9** The accessory organs of the digestive system: the liver, gallbladder, and pancreas. Image shows the relationship of these three organs and their ducts to the duodenum.

Gallbladder

common bile duct **cystic duct** (SIS-tik)
hepatic duct (hep-PAT-tik)

Bile produced by the liver is stored in the gallbladder (GB). As the liver produces bile, it travels down the **hepatic duct** and up the **cystic duct** into the gallbladder (see again Figure 8.9). In response to the presence of fat in the chyme, the muscular wall of the gallbladder contracts and sends bile back down the cystic duct and into the **common bile duct** (CBD), which carries bile to the duodenum where it is able to emulsify the fat in chyme.

Pancreas

buffers **pancreatic duct** (pan-kree-AT-ik)
pancreatic enzymes (pan-kree-AT-ik / EN-zimes)

The pancreas, connected to the duodenum by the **pancreatic duct,** produces two important secretions for digestion: **buffers** and **pancreatic enzymes** (see again Figure 8.9). Buffers neutralize acidic chyme that has just left the stomach, and pancreatic enzymes chemically digest carbohydrates, fats, and proteins. The pancreas is also an endocrine gland that produces the hormones insulin and glucagon, which play a role in regulating the level of glucose in the blood.

Terminology

Word Parts Used to Build Digestive System Terms

The following lists contain the combining forms, suffixes, and prefixes used to build terms in the remaining sections of this chapter.

Combining Forms

an/o	anus
append/o	appendix
appendic/o	appendix
bar/o	weight
bucc/o	cheek
carcin/o	cancer
cec/o	cecum
chol/e	bile
cholangi/o	bile duct
cholecyst/o	gallbladder
choledoch/o	common bile duct
cirrh/o	yellow
col/o	colon
colon/o	colon
cutane/o	skin
dent/o	tooth
diverticul/o	pouch
duoden/o	duodenum
enter/o	small intestine
esophag/o	esophagus
gastr/o	stomach
gingiv/o	gums
gloss/o	tongue
hem/o	blood
hemat/o	blood
hepat/o	liver
ile/o	ileum
jejun/o	jejunum
labi/o	lip
lapar/o	abdomen
lingu/o	tongue
lith/o	stone
nas/o	nose
odont/o	tooth
or/o	mouth
orth/o	straight
palat/o	palate
pancreat/o	pancreas
pharyng/o	pharynx
polyp/o	polyp
proct/o	anus and rectum
pylor/o	pylorus
pyr/o	fire
rect/o	rectum
sialaden/o	salivary gland
sigmoid/o	sigmoid colon
ven/o	vein

Suffixes

-al	pertaining to
-algia	pain
-centesis	process of removing fluid
-eal	pertaining to
-ectomy	surgical removal
-emesis	vomiting
-gram	record
-graphy	process of recording
-ic	pertaining to
-istry	specialty of
-itis	inflammation
-lithiasis	condition of stones
-logy	study of
-oma	tumor
-orexia	appetite
-osis	abnormal condition
-ostomy	create a new opening
-otomy	cutting into
-ous	pertaining to
-pepsia	digestion
-pexy	surgical fixation
-phagia	eating
-plasty	surgical repair
-plegia	paralysis
-prandial	a meal
-ptosis	drooping
-scope	instrument to view
-scopy	process of viewing
-tic	pertaining to
-tripsy	surgical crushing

Prefixes

a-	without
an-	without
anti-	against
brady-	slow
dys-	abnormal
endo-	within
hyper-	excessive
hypo-	under
intra-	within
per-	through
peri-	around
poly-	many
post-	after
retro-	backwards
sub-	under
trans-	across

Anatomical Terms

TERM	WORD PARTS	DEFINITION
anal	an/o = anus -al = pertaining to	Pertaining to the anus. **MED TERM TIP** Word Watch: Be careful when using the combining form *an/o* meaning "anus" and the prefix *an* meaning "none."
buccal (BYOO-kal)	bucc/o = cheek -al = pertaining to	Pertaining to the cheeks.
buccolabial (BYOO-koh-labe-ee-all)	bucc/o = cheek labi/o = lip -al = pertaining to	Pertaining to the cheeks and lips.
cecal (SEE-kal)	cec/o = cecum -al = pertaining to	Pertaining to the cecum.
cholecystic (koh-lee-SIS-tik)	cholecyst/o = gallbladder -ic = pertaining to	Pertaining to the gallbladder.
colonic (koh-LON-ik)	colon/o = colon -ic = pertaining to	Pertaining to the colon.
colorectal (kohl-oh-REK-tall)	col/o = colon rect/o = rectum -al = pertaining to	Pertaining to the colon and rectum.
dental (DENT-all)	dent/o = tooth -al = pertaining to	Pertaining to the teeth.
duodenal (duo-DEN-all / do-ODD-in-all)	duoden/o = duodenum -al = pertaining to	Pertaining to the duodenum.
enteric (en-TARE-ik)	enter/o = small intestine -ic = pertaining to	Pertaining to the small intestine.
esophageal (eh-soff-ah-JEE-al)	esophag/o = esophagus -eal = pertaining to	Pertaining to the esophagus.
gastric (GAS-trik)	gastr/o = stomach -ic = pertaining to	Pertaining to the stomach.
gingival (JIN-jih-vul)	gingiv/o = gums -al = pertaining to	Pertaining to the gums.
glossal (GLOSS-all)	gloss/o = tongue -al = pertaining to	Pertaining to the tongue.

Anatomical Terms *(continued)*

TERM	WORD PARTS	DEFINITION
hepatic (hep-AT-ik)	hepat/o = liver -ic = pertaining to	Pertaining to the liver.
hypoglossal (high-poe-GLOSS-all)	hypo- = under gloss/o = tongue -al = pertaining to	Pertaining to under the tongue.
ileal (ILL-ee-all)	ile/o = ileum -al = pertaining to	Pertaining to the ileum.
jejunal (jih-JUNE-all)	jejun/o = jejunum -al = pertaining to	Pertaining to the jejunum.
nasogastric (nay-zoh-GAS-trik)	nas/o = nose gastr/o = stomach -ic = pertaining to	Pertaining to the nose and stomach.
oral (OR-ral)	or/o = mouth -al = pertaining to	Pertaining to the mouth.
pancreatic (pan-kree-AT-ik)	pancreat/o = pancreas -ic = pertaining to	Pertaining to the pancreas.
pharyngeal (fair-in-JEE-all)	pharyng/o = pharynx -eal = pertaining to	Pertaining to the pharynx.
pyloric (pie-LORE-ik)	pylor/o = pylorus -ic = pertaining to	Pertaining to the pylorus.
rectal (RECK-tall)	rect/o = rectum -al = pertaining to	Pertaining to the rectum.
sigmoidal (sig-MOYD-all)	sigmoid/o = sigmoid colon -al = pertaining to	Pertaining to the sigmoid colon.
sublingual (sub-LING-gwal)	sub- = under lingu/o = tongue -al = pertaining to	Pertaining to under the tongue.

Pathology

TERM	WORD PARTS	DEFINITION
Medical Specialties		
dentistry	dent/o = tooth -istry = specialty of	Branch of healthcare involved with the prevention, diagnosis, and treatment of conditions involving the teeth, jaw, and mouth. Practitioner is a *dentist.*
gastroenterology (gas-troh-en-ter-ALL-oh-jee)	gastr/o = stomach enter/o = small intestine -logy = study of	Branch of medicine involved in diagnosis and treatment of diseases and disorders of the digestive system. Physician is a *gastroenterologist.*
oral surgery	or/o = mouth -al = pertaining to	Branch of dentistry that uses surgical means to treat dental conditions. Specialist is an *oral surgeon.*

Pathology *(continued)*

TERM	WORD PARTS	DEFINITION
orthodontics (or-thoh-DON-tiks)	orth/o = straight odont/o = tooth -ic = pertaining to	Branch of dentistry concerned with correction of problems with tooth alignment. Specialist is an *orthodontist.*
periodontics (pair-ee-oh-DON-tiks)	peri- = around odont/o = tooth -ic = pertaining to	Branch of dentistry concerned with treating conditions involving the gums and tissues surrounding the teeth. Specialist is a *periodontist.*
proctology (prok-TOL-oh-jee)	proct/o = anus and rectum -logy = study of	Branch of medicine involved in diagnosis and treatment of diseases and disorders of the anus and rectum. Physician is a *proctologist.*
Signs and Symptoms		
anorexia (an-oh-REK-see-ah)	an- = without -orexia = appetite	General term meaning loss of appetite that may accompany other conditions. Also used to refer to *anorexia nervosa,* which is an eating disorder involving the refusal to eat.
aphagia (ah-FAY-jee-ah)	a- = without -phagia = eating	Being unable to swallow or eat.
ascites (ah-SIGH-teez)		Collection or accumulation of fluid in the peritoneal cavity.
bradypepsia (brad-ee-PEP-see-ah)	brady- = slow -pepsia = digestion	Having a slow digestive system.
cachexia (ka-KEK-see-ah)		Loss of weight and generalized wasting that occurs during a chronic disease.
cholecystalgia (koh-lee-sis-TAL-jee-ah)	cholecyst/o = gallbladder -algia = pain	Having gallbladder pain.
constipation (kon-stih-PAY-shun)		Experiencing difficulty in defecation or infrequent defecation.
dentalgia (dent-AL-gee-ah)	dent/o = tooth -algia = pain	Tooth pain.
diarrhea (dye-ah-REE-ah)		Passing of frequent, watery, or bloody bowel movements. Usually accompanies gastrointestinal (GI) disorders.
dysorexia (dis-oh-REKS-ee-ah)	dys- = abnormal -orexia = appetite	Abnormal appetite; usually a diminished appetite.
dyspepsia (dis-PEP-see-ah)	dys- = difficult -pepsia = digestion	"Upset stomach"; indigestion.
dysphagia (dis-FAY-jee-ah)	dys- = abnormal -phagia = eating	Having difficulty swallowing or eating.
emesis (EM-eh-sis)		Vomiting.
gastralgia (gas-TRAL-jee-ah)	gastr/o = stomach -algia = pain	Stomach pain.
hematemesis (hee-mah-TEM-eh-sis)	hemat/o = blood -emesis = vomiting	Vomiting blood.
hematochezia (he-mat-oh-KEY-zee-ah)	hemat/o = blood	Passing bright red blood in the stools.

Pathology *(continued)*

TERM	WORD PARTS	DEFINITION
hyperemesis (high-per-EM-eh-sis)	hyper- = excessive -emesis = vomiting	Excessive vomiting.
jaundice (JAWN-diss)		Yellow cast to the skin, mucous membranes, and the whites of the eyes caused by the deposit of bile pigment from too much bilirubin in the blood. Bilirubin is a waste product produced when worn-out red blood cells are broken down. May be a symptom of a disorder such as gallstones blocking the common bile duct or carcinoma of the liver. Also called *icterus.*
melena (me-LEE-nah)		Passage of dark tarry stools. Color is the result of digestive enzymes working on blood in the gastrointestinal tract.
nausea (NAW-see-ah)	**MED TERM TIP** The term *nausea* comes from the Greek word for "seasickness."	Urge to vomit.
obesity		Body weight that is above a healthy level. A person whose weight interferes with normal activity and body function has *morbid obesity.*
polyphagia (pall-ee-FAY-jee-ah)	poly- = many -phagia = eating	Excessive eating; eating too much.
postprandial (post-PRAN-dee-all)	post- = after -prandial = a meal	After a meal.
pyrosis (pie-ROW-sis)	pyr/o = fire -osis = abnormal condition	Pain and burning sensation usually caused by stomach acid splashing up into the esophagus. Commonly called *heartburn.*
regurgitation (ree-gur-jih-TAY-shun)		Return of fluids and solids from the stomach into the mouth.
Oral Cavity		
aphthous ulcers (AF-thus)		Painful ulcers in the mouth of unknown cause. Commonly called *canker sores.*
cleft lip (CLEFT)		Congenital anomaly in which the upper lip and jaw bone fail to fuse in the midline, leaving an open gap. Often seen along with a cleft palate. Corrected with surgery.
cleft palate (CLEFT / PAL-at)		Congenital anomaly in which the roof of the mouth has a split or fissure. Corrected with surgery.
dental caries (KAIR-eez)	dent/o = tooth -al = pertaining to	Gradual decay and disintegration of teeth caused by bacteria; may lead to abscessed teeth. Commonly called a *tooth cavity.*
gingivitis (jin-jih-VIGH-tis)	gingiv/o = gums -itis = inflammation	Inflammation of the gums.

Pathology *(continued)*

TERM	WORD PARTS	DEFINITION
herpes labialis (HER-peez / lay-bee-AL-iz)	labi/o = lip	Infection of the lip by the herpes simplex virus type 1 (HSV-1). Also called *fever blisters* or *cold sores.*
periodontal disease (pair-ee-oh-DON-tal)	peri- = around odont/o = tooth -al = pertaining to	Disease of the supporting structures of the teeth, including the gums and bones; the most common cause of tooth loss.
sialadenitis (sigh-al-add-eh-NIGH-tis)	sialaden/o = salivary gland -itis = inflammation	Inflammation of a salivary gland.
Pharynx and Esophagus		
esophageal varices (eh-soff-ah-JEE-al / VAIR-ih-seez)	esophag/o = esophagus -eal = pertaining to	Enlarged and swollen varicose veins in the lower end of the esophagus. If these rupture, serious hemorrhage results; often related to liver disease.
gastroesophageal reflux disease (GERD) (gas-troh-ee-sof-ah-GEE-all / REE-fluks)	gastr/o = stomach esophag/o = esophagus -eal = pertaining to	Acid from the stomach flows backward up into the esophagus causing inflammation and pain.
pharyngoplegia (fair-in-goh-PLEE-jee-ah)	pharyng/o = pharynx plegia = paralysis	Paralysis of the throat muscles.
Stomach		
gastric carcinoma (GAS-trik / car-si-NOH-mah)	gastr/o = stomach -ic = pertaining to	Cancerous tumor in the stomach.
gastritis (gas-TRY-tis)	gastr/o = stomach -itis = inflammation	Stomach inflammation.
gastroenteritis (gas-troh-en-ter-EYE-tis)	gastr/o = stomach enter/o = small intestines -itis = inflammation	Inflammation of stomach and small intestine.
hiatal hernia (high-AY-tal / HER-nee-ah)	-al = pertaining to	Protrusion of the stomach through the diaphragm (also called a *diaphragmatocele*) and extending into the thoracic cavity; gastroesophageal reflux disease is a common symptom.

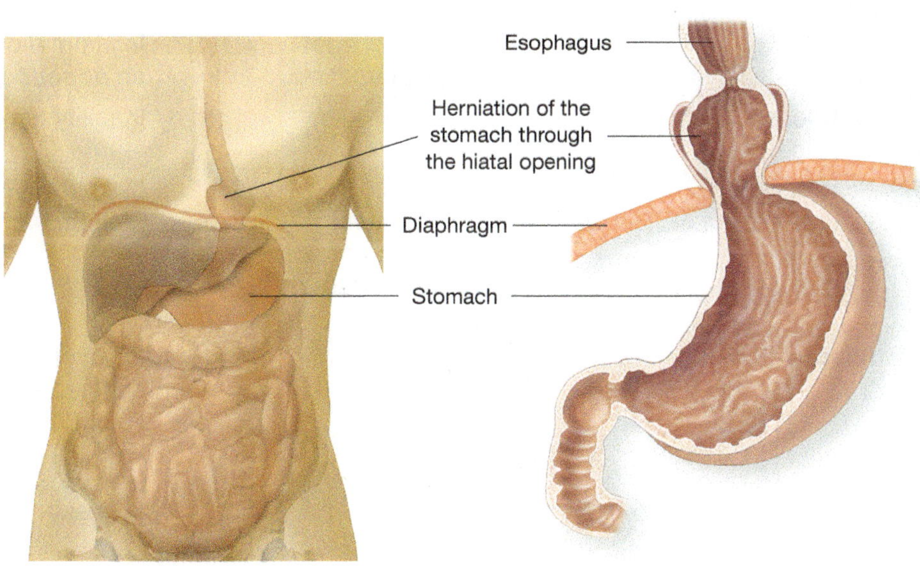

■ **Figure 8.10** A hiatal hernia or diaphragmatocele. A portion of the stomach protrudes through the diaphragm into the thoracic cavity.

Pathology *(continued)*

TERM	WORD PARTS	DEFINITION
peptic ulcer disease (PUD) (PEP-tik / ULL-sir)	-ic = pertaining to	Ulcer occurring in the lower portion of the esophagus, stomach, and/or duodenum; thought to be caused by the acid of gastric juices. Initial damage to the protective lining of the stomach may be caused by a *Helicobacter pylori* (*H. pylori*) bacterial infection. If the ulcer extends all the way through the wall of the stomach, it is called a *perforated ulcer,* which requires immediate surgery to repair.

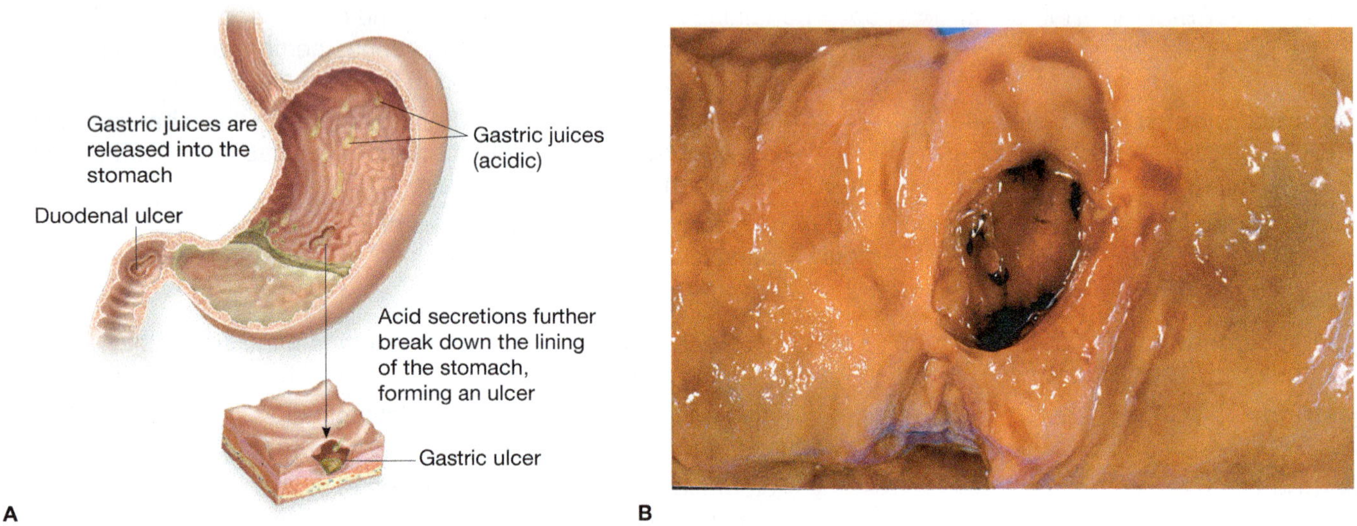

Figure 8.11 (A) Figure illustrating the location and appearance of a peptic ulcer in both the stomach and the duodenum; (B) photomicrograph illustrating a gastric ulcer. *(Dr. E. Walker/Science Photo Library/Photo Researchers, Inc.)*

TERM	WORD PARTS	DEFINITION
Small Intestine and Colon		
anal fistula (FIH-styoo-lah)	-al = pertaining to	Abnormal tube-like passage from the surface around the anal opening directly into the rectum.
appendicitis (ah-pen-dih-SIGH-tis)	appendic/o = appendix -itis = inflammation	Inflammation of the appendix; may require an *appendectomy.*
bowel incontinence (in-CON-tih-nence)		Inability to control defecation.
colorectal carcinoma (kohl-oh-REK-tall / car-ci-NOH-mah)	col/o = colon rect/o = rectum -al = pertaining to carcin/o = cancer -oma = tumor	Cancerous tumor originating in the colon or rectum.
Crohn's disease (KROHNZ)		Form of chronic inflammatory bowel disease affecting primarily the ileum and/or colon. Also called *regional ileitis.* This autoimmune condition affects all the layers of the bowel wall and results in scarring and thickening of the gut wall.

Pathology *(continued)*

TERM	WORD PARTS	DEFINITION
diverticulitis (dye-ver-tik-yoo-LYE-tis)	diverticul/o = pouch -itis = inflammation	Inflammation of a *diverticulum* (an out-pouching off the gut), especially in the colon. Inflammation often results when food becomes within the pouch.
diverticulosis (dye-ver-tik-yoo-LOW-sis)	diverticul/o = pouch -osis = abnormal condition	Condition of having diverticula (outpouches off the gut). May lead to *diverticulitis* if one becomes inflamed.
dysentery (dis-in-TARE-ee)		Disease characterized by diarrhea, often with mucus and blood, severe abdominal pain, fever, and dehydration. Caused by ingesting food or water contaminated by chemicals, bacteria, protozoans, or parasites.
enteritis (en-ter-EYE-tis)	enter/o = small intestine -itis = inflammation	Inflammation of the small intestines.
hemorrhoids (HEM-oh-roydz)	hem/o = blood	Varicose veins in the rectum and anus.
ileus (ILL-ee-us)		Severe abdominal pain, inability to pass stools, vomiting, and abdominal distension as a result of an intestinal blockage. The blockage can be a physical block such as a tumor or the failure of bowel contents to move forward due to loss of peristalsis (a nonmechanical blockage). May require surgery to reverse the blockage.
inguinal hernia (ING-gwih-nal / HER-nee-ah)	-al = pertaining to	Hernia or protrusion of a loop of small intestines into the inguinal (groin) region through a weak spot in the abdominal muscle wall that develops into a hole. May become *incarcerated* or *strangulated* if the muscle tightens down around the loop of intestines and cuts off its blood flow. See Figure 8.13 ■.

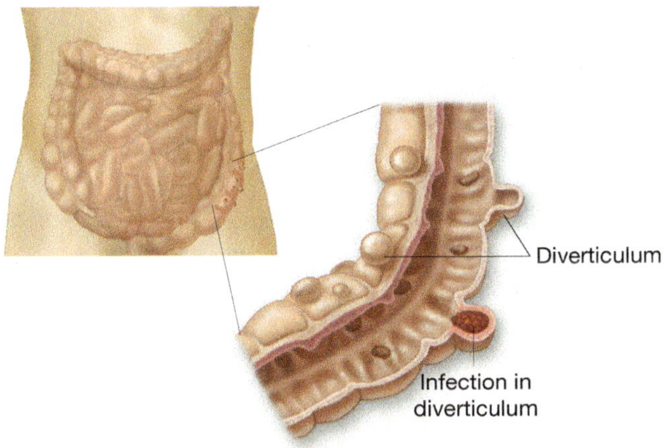

■ **Figure 8.12** Diverticulosis. Figure illustrates external and internal appearance of diverticula.

Pathology *(continued)*

TERM	WORD PARTS	DEFINITION

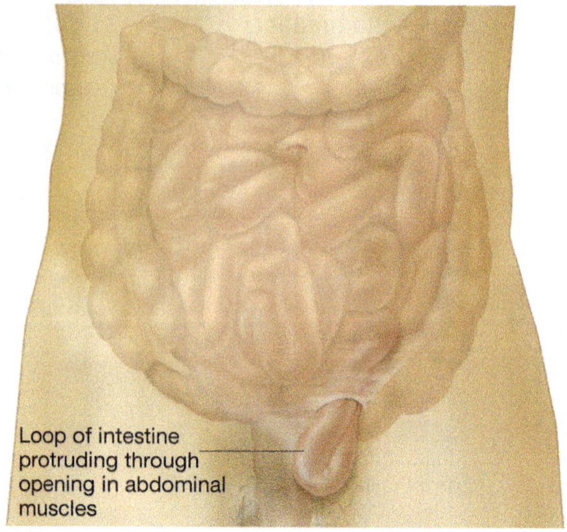

■ **Figure 8.13** An inguinal hernia. A portion of the small intestine is protruding through the abdominal muscles into the groin region.

TERM	WORD PARTS	DEFINITION
intussusception (in-tuh-suh-SEP-shun)		Result of the intestine slipping or telescoping into another section of intestine just below it. More common in children.

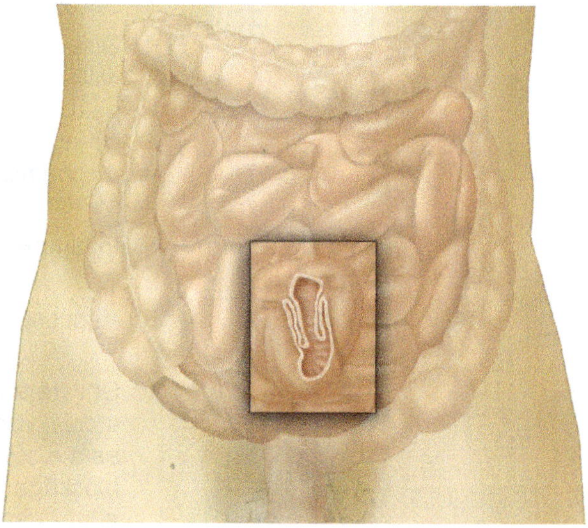

■ **Figure 8.14** Intussusception. A short length of small intestine has telescoped into itself.

TERM	WORD PARTS	DEFINITION
irritable bowel syndrome (IBS)		Disturbance in the functions of the intestine from unknown causes. Symptoms generally include abdominal discomfort and an alteration in bowel activity. Also called *spastic colon* or *functional bowel syndrome.*
polyposis (pall-ee-POH-sis)	polyp/o = polyp -osis = abnormal condition	Presence of small tumors, called **polyps,** containing a pedicle or stemlike attachment in the mucous membranes of the large intestine (colon); may be precancerous. See Figure 8.15 ■.

Pathology *(continued)*

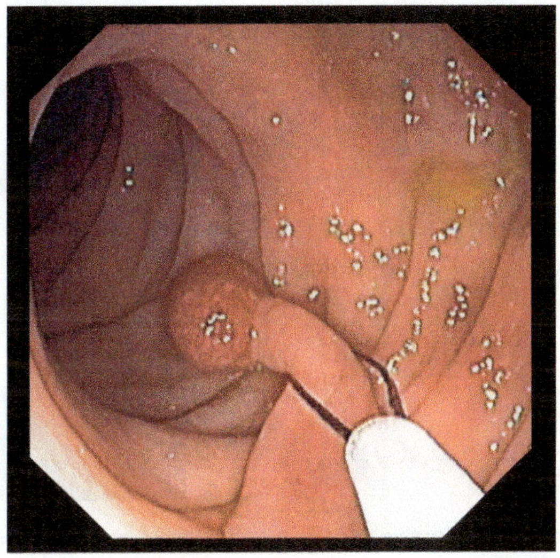

Figure 8.15 Endoscopic view of a polyp in the colon. Note the mushroom-like shape, an enlarged top growing at the end of a stem. It is being removed by means of a wire loop slipped over the polyp and then tightened to cut it off. *(David M. Martin, M.D./ Photo Researchers, Inc.)*

TERM	WORD PARTS	DEFINITION
proctoptosis (prok-top-TOH-sis)	proct/o = rectum and anus -ptosis = drooping	Prolapsed or drooping rectum.
ulcerative colitis (ULL-sir-ah-tiv / koh-LYE-tis)	col/o = colon -itis = inflammation	Chronic inflammatory condition resulting in numerous ulcers formed on the mucous membrane lining of the colon; the cause is unknown. Also known as *inflammatory bowel disease* (IBD).
volvulus (VOL-vyoo-lus)		Condition in which the bowel twists upon itself causing an obstruction; painful and requires immediate surgery.

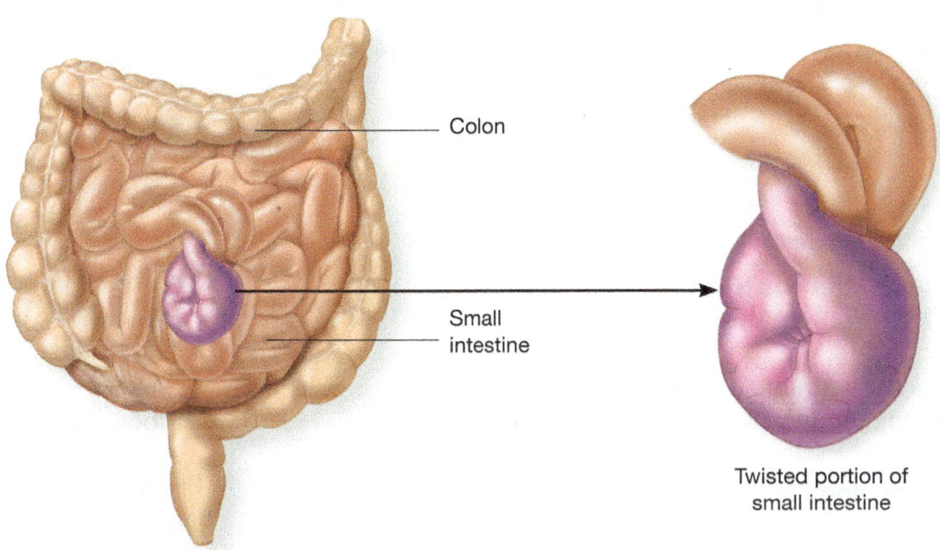

Figure 8.16 Volvulus. A length of small intestine has twisted around itself, cutting off blood circulation to the twisted loop.

Accessory Organs

TERM	WORD PARTS	DEFINITION
cholecystitis (koh-lee-sis-TYE-tis)	cholecyst/o = gallbladder -itis = inflammation	Inflammation of the gallbladder; most commonly caused by gallstones in the gallbladder or common bile duct that block the flow of bile.

Pathology *(continued)*

TERM	WORD PARTS	DEFINITION
cholelithiasis (koh-lee-lih-THIGH-ah-sis)	chol/e = bile -lithiasis = condition of stones	Presence of gallstones; may or may not cause symptoms such as *cholecystalgia*.

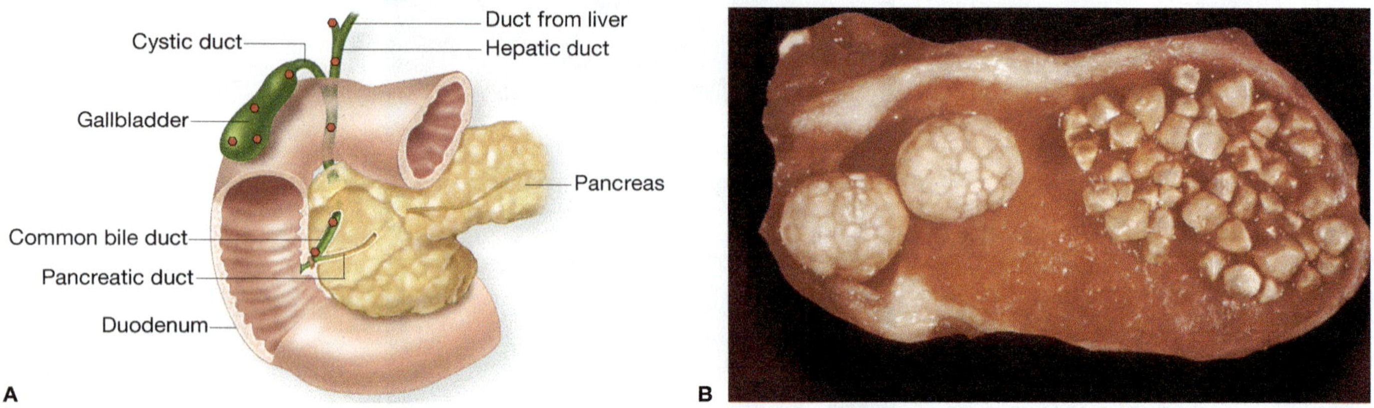

Figure 8.17 (A) Common sites for cholelithiasis; (B) a gallbladder specimen with multiple gallstones *(Biophoto Associates/Photo Researchers, Inc.).*

TERM	WORD PARTS	DEFINITION
cirrhosis (sih-ROH-sis)	cirrh/o = yellow -osis = abnormal condition	Chronic disease of the liver associated with failure of the liver to function properly.
hepatitis (hep-ah-TYE-tis)	hepat/o = liver -itis = inflammation	Inflammation of the liver, usually due to a viral infection. Different viruses are transmitted by different routes, such as sexual contact or from exposure to blood or fecally contaminated water or food.
hepatoma (hep-ah-TOH-mah)	hepat/o = liver -oma = tumor	Liver tumor.
pancreatitis (pan-kree-ah-TYE-tis)	pancreat/o = pancreas -itis = inflammation	Inflammation of the pancreas.

Diagnostic Procedures

TERM	WORD PARTS	DEFINITION
Clinical Laboratory Tests		
alanine transaminase (ALT) (AL-ah-neen / trans-AM-in-nase)		Enzyme normally present in the blood. Blood levels are increased in persons with liver disease.
aspartate transaminase (AST) (ass-PAR-tate / trans-AM-in-nase)		Enzyme normally present in the blood. Blood levels are increased in persons with liver disease.
fecal occult blood test (FOBT) (uh-CULT)	-al = pertaining to	Laboratory test on the feces to determine if microscopic amounts of blood are present. Also called *hemoccult* or *stool guaiac.*
ova and parasites (O&P) (OH-vah / PAR-ah-sights)		Laboratory examination of feces with a microscope for the presence of parasites or their eggs.
serum bilirubin (SEE-rum / BILLY-rubin)		Blood test to determine the amount of the waste product bilirubin in the bloodstream. Elevated levels indicate liver disease.

Diagnostic Procedures *(continued)*

TERM	WORD PARTS	DEFINITION
stool culture		Laboratory test of feces to determine if any pathogenic bacteria are present.
Diagnostic Imaging		
bite-wing X-ray		X-ray taken with a part of the film holder held between the teeth and parallel to the teeth.
cholecystogram (koh-lee-SIS-toh-gram)	cholecyst/o = gallbladder -gram = record	X-ray image of the gallbladder.
intravenous cholecystography (in-trah-VEE-nus / koh-lee-sis-TOG-rah-fee)	intra- = within ven/o = vein -ous = pertaining to cholecyst/o = gallbladder -graphy = process of recording	Dye is administered intravenously to the patient allowing for X-ray visualization of the gallbladder and bile ducts.
lower gastrointestinal series (lower GI series)	gastr/o = stomach -al = pertaining to	X-ray image of the colon and rectum is taken after the administration of barium (a radiopaque dye) by enema. Also called a *barium enema (BE)*.
percutaneous transhepatic cholangiography (PTC) (per-kyoo-TAY-nee-us / trans-heh-PAT-ik / koh-lan-jee-OG-rah-fee)	per- = through cutane/o = skin -ous = pertaining to trans- = across hepat/o = liver -ic = pertaining to cholangi/o = bile duct -graphy = process of recording	Procedure in which contrast medium is injected directly into the liver to visualize the bile ducts. Used to detect obstructions such as gallstones in the common bile duct.

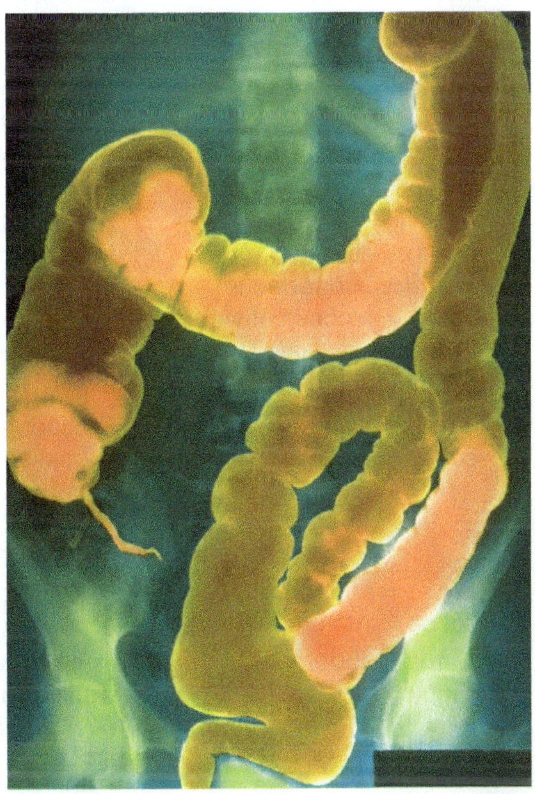

Figure 8.18 Color-enhanced X-ray of the colon taken during a barium enema. *(CNRI/Science Photo Library/Photo Researchers, Inc.)*

Diagnostic Procedures *(continued)*

TERM	WORD PARTS	DEFINITION
upper gastrointestinal (UGI) **series**	gastr/o = stomach -al = pertaining to	Patient is administered a barium contrast material orally and then X-rays are taken to visualize the esophagus, stomach, and duodenum. Also called a *barium swallow.*
Endoscopic Procedures		
colonoscope (koh-LON-oh-scope)	colon/o = colon -scope = instrument to view	Instrument used to view the colon.
colonoscopy (koh-lon-OSS-koh-pee)	colon/o = colon -scopy = process of viewing	Flexible fiberscope called a *colonoscope* is passed through the anus, rectum, and colon; used to examine the upper portion of the colon. Polyps and small growths can be removed during this procedure (see again Figure 8.15).
endoscopic retrograde cholangiopancreatography (ERCP) (en-doh-SKOP-ik / RET-roh-grayd / koh-lan-jee-oh-pan-kree-ah-TOG-rah-fee)	endo- = within -scopy = process of viewing -ic = pertaining to retro- = backwards cholangi/o = bile duct pancreat/o = pancreas -graphy = process of recording	Procedure using an endoscope to visually examine the hepatic duct, common bile duct, and pancreatic duct. First an endoscope is passed through the patient's mouth, esophagus, and stomach until it reaches the duodenum where the pancreatic and common bile ducts empty. Then a thin catheter is passed through the endoscope and into the ducts (in the retrograde direction). Contrast dye is then used to visualize these ducts on an X-ray.
esophagogastroduodenoscopy (EGD) (eh-soff-ah-go-gas-troh-duo-den-OS-koh-pee)	esophag/o = esophagus gastr/o = stomach duoden/o = duodenum -scopy = process of viewing	Use of a flexible fiberoptic endoscope to visually examine the esophagus, stomach, and beginning of the duodenum.
gastroscope (GAS-troh-scope)	gastr/o = stomach -scope = instrument to view	Instrument used to view inside the stomach.
gastroscopy (gas-TROS-koh-pee)	gastr/o = stomach -scopy = process of viewing	Procedure in which a flexible *gastroscope* is passed through the mouth and down the esophagus in order to visualize inside the stomach. Used to diagnose peptic ulcers and gastric carcinoma.
laparoscope (LAP-ah-roh-scope)	lapar/o = abdomen -scope = instrument to view	Instrument used to view inside the abdomen.
laparoscopy (lap-ar-OSS-koh-pee)	lapar/o = abdomen -scopy = process of viewing	*Laparoscope* is passed into the abdominal wall through a small incision. The abdominal cavity is then visually examined for tumors and other conditions with this lighted instrument. Also called *peritoneoscopy.*
sigmoidoscope (sig-MOYD-oh-scope)	sigmoid/o = sigmoid colon -scope = instrument to view	Instrument used to view inside the sigmoid colon.
sigmoidoscopy (sig-moid-OS-koh-pee)	sigmoid/o = sigmoid colon -scopy = process of viewing	Procedure using a flexible *sigmoidoscope* to visually examine the sigmoid colon. Commonly done to diagnose cancer and polyps.
Additional Diagnostic Procedures		
paracentesis (pair-ah-sin-TEE-sis)	-centesis = process of removing fluid	Insertion of a needle into the abdominal cavity to withdraw fluid. Tests to diagnose diseases may be conducted on the fluid.

Therapeutic Procedures

TERM	WORD PARTS	DEFINITION
Dental Procedures		
bridge		Dental appliance to replace missing teeth. It is attached to adjacent teeth for support.
crown		Artificial covering for a tooth that is created to replace the original enamel covering of the tooth.
denture (DEN-chur)	dent/o = tooth	Partial or complete set of artificial teeth that are set in plastic materials. Acts as a substitute for the natural teeth and related structures.
extraction	ex- = outward	Removing or "pulling" of teeth.
implant (IM-plant)		Prosthetic device placed in the jaw to which a tooth or denture may be anchored.
root canal	-al = pertaining to	Dental treatment involving the pulp cavity of the root of a tooth. Procedure is used to save a tooth that is badly infected or abscessed.
Medical Procedures		
gavage (guh-VAHZH)		Use of a nasogastric (NG) tube to place liquid nourishment directly into the stomach.
lavage (lah-VAHZH)		Use of a nasogastric (NG) tube to wash out the stomach. For example, after ingestion of dangerous substances.
nasogastric intubation (NG tube) (NAY-zo-gas-trik / in-two-BAY-shun)	nas/o = nose gastr/o = stomach -ic = pertaining to	Procedure in which a flexible catheter is inserted into the nose and down the esophagus to the stomach. May be used for feeding or to suction out stomach fluids.
total parenteral nutrition (TPN) (pair-in-TARE-all)	-al = pertaining to	Providing 100% of a patient's nutrition intravenously. Used when a patient is unable to eat.
Surgical Procedures		
anastomosis (ah-nas-toh-MOH-sis)		To surgically create a connection between two organs or vessels. For example, joining together two cut ends of the intestines after a section is removed.
appendectomy (ap-en-DEK-toh-mee)	append/o = appendix -ectomy = surgical removal	Surgical removal of the appendix.
bariatric surgery (bear-ee-AT-rik)	bar/o = weight	Group of surgical procedures such as stomach stapling and restrictive banding to reduce the size of the stomach. A treatment for morbid (extreme) obesity.
cholecystectomy (koh-lee-sis-TEK-toh-mee)	cholecyst/o = gallbladder -ectomy = surgical removal	Surgical removal of the gallbladder.
choledocholithotripsy (koh-led-oh-koh-LITH-oh-trip-see)	choledoch/o = common bile duct lith/o = stone -tripsy = surgical crushing	Crushing of a gallstone in the common bile duct.
colectomy (koh-LEK-toh-mee)	col/o = colon -ectomy = surgical removal	Surgical removal of the colon.

Therapeutic Procedures *(continued)*

TERM	WORD PARTS	DEFINITION
colostomy (koh-LOSS-toh-mee)	col/o = colon -ostomy = create a new opening	Surgical creation of an opening of some portion of the colon through the abdominal wall to the outside surface. Fecal material (stool) drains into a bag worn on the abdomen.

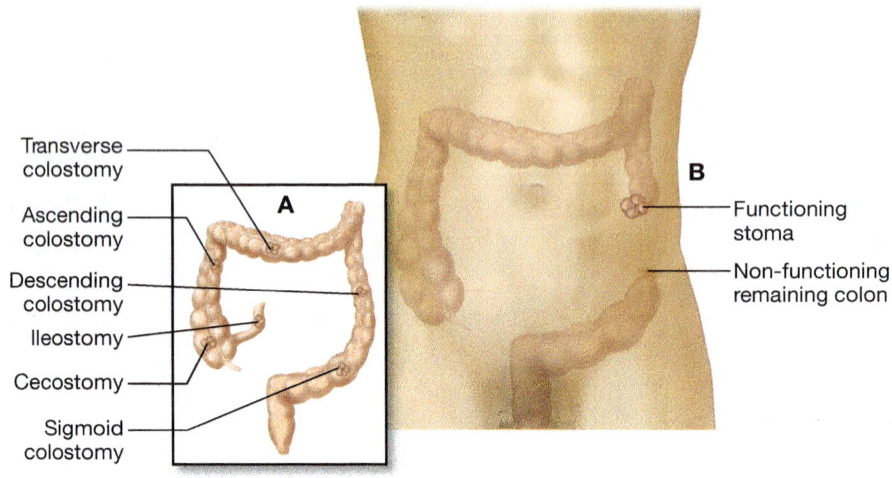

■ **Figure 8.19** (A) The colon illustrating various ostomy sites; (B) colostomy in the descending colon, illustrating functioning stoma and nonfunctioning distal sigmoid colon and rectum.

TERM	WORD PARTS	DEFINITION
diverticulectomy (dye-ver-tik-yoo-LEK-toh-mee)	diverticul/o = pouch -ectomy = surgical removal	Surgical removal of a diverticulum.
exploratory laparotomy (ek-SPLOR-ah-tor-ee / lap-ah-ROT-oh-mee)	lapar/o = abdomen -otomy = cutting into	Abdominal operation for the purpose of examining the abdominal organs and tissues for signs of disease or other abnormalities.
fistulectomy (fis-tyoo-LEK-toh-mee)	-ectomy = surgical removal	Removal of a fistula.
gastrectomy (gas-TREK-toh-mee)	gastr/o = stomach -ectomy = surgical removal	Surgical removal of the stomach.
gastric stapling	gastr/o = stomach -ic = pertaining to	Procedure that closes off a large section of the stomach with rows of staples. Results in a much smaller stomach to assist very obese patients to lose weight.
gastrostomy (gas-TROSS-toh-mee)	gastr/o = stomach -ostomy = create a new opening	Surgical procedure to create an opening in the stomach.
hemorrhoidectomy (hem-oh-royd-EK-toh-mee)	-ectomy = surgical removal	Surgical removal of hemorrhoids from the anorectal area.
hernioplasty (her-nee-oh-PLAS-tee)	-plasty = surgical repair	Surgical repair of a hernia. Also called *herniorrhaphy*.
ileostomy (ill-ee-OSS-toh-mee)	ile/o = ileum -ostomy = create a new opening	Surgical creation of an opening in the ileum.
laparoscopic cholecystectomy (lap-ar-oh-SKOP-ik / koh-lee-sis-TEK-toh-mee)	lapar/o = abdomen -scopy = process of viewing -ic = pertaining to cholecyst/o = gallbladder -ectomy = surgical removal	Surgical removal of the gallbladder through a very small abdominal incision with the assistance of a laparoscope.

Therapeutic Procedures *(continued)*

TERM	WORD PARTS	DEFINITION
laparotomy (lap-ah-ROT-oh-mee)	lapar/o = abdomen -otomy = cutting into	Surgical incision into the abdomen.
liver transplant		Transplant of a liver from a donor.
palatoplasty (pa-LOT-toh-plas-tee)	palat/o = palate -plasty = surgical repair	Surgical repair of the palate.
pharyngoplasty (fair-ING-oh-plas-tee)	pharyng/o = pharynx -plasty = surgical repair	Surgical repair of the throat.
proctopexy (PROK-toh-pek-see)	proct/o = rectum and anus -pexy = surgical fixation	Surgical fixation of the rectum and anus.

Pharmacology

CLASSIFICATION	WORD PARTS	ACTION	EXAMPLES
anorexiant (an-oh-REKS ee-ant)	an- = without -orexia = appetite	Treats obesity by suppressing appetite.	phendimetrazine, Adipost, Obezine; phentermine, Zantryl, Adipex
antacid	anti- = against	Used to neutralize stomach acids.	calcium carbonate, Tums; aluminum hydroxide and magnesium hydroxide, Maalox, Mylanta
antidiarrheal (an-tee-dye-ah-REE-all)	anti- = against -al = pertaining to	Used to control diarrhea.	loperamide, Imodium; diphenoxylate and atropine, Lomotil; kaolin/pectin, Kaopectate
antiemetic (an-tye-ee-MEH-tik)	anti- = against -emesis = vomit -tic = pertaining to	Treats nausea, vomiting, and motion sickness.	prochlorperazine, Compazine; promethazine, Phenergan
antivirals	anti- = against	Treats herpes simplex infection.	valacyclovir, Valtrex; famcyclovir, Famvir; acyclovir, Zovirax
H_2-receptor antagonist	anti- = against	Used to treat peptic ulcers and gastroesophageal reflux disease. When stimulated, H_2-receptors increase the production of stomach acid. Using an antagonist to block these receptors results in a low acid level in the stomach.	ranitidine, Zantac; cimetidine, Tagamet; famotidine, Pepcid
laxative MED TERM TIP The term *laxative* refers to a medication to stimulate a bowel movement; comes from the Latin term meaning "to relax."		Treats constipation by stimulating a bowel movement.	senosides, Senokot; psyllium, Metamucil
proton pump inhibitors		Used to treat peptic ulcers and gastroesophageal reflux disease. Blocks the stomach's ability to secrete acid.	esomeprazole, Nexium; omeprazole, Prilosec

Abbreviations

ac	before meals
ALT	alanine transaminase
AST	aspartate transaminase
Ba	barium
BE	barium enema
BM	bowel movement
BS	bowel sounds
CBD	common bile duct
EGD	esophagogastroduodenoscopy
ERCP	endoscopic retrograde cholangio-pancreatography
FOBT	fecal occult blood test
GB	gallbladder
GERD	gastroesophageal reflux disease
GI	gastrointestinal
HAV	hepatitis A virus
HBV	hepatitis B virus
HCl	hydrochloric acid
HCV	hepatitis C virus
HDV	hepatitis D virus
HEV	hepatitis E virus
HSV-1	herpes simplex virus type 1
IBD	inflammatory bowel disease
IBS	irritable bowel syndrome
IVC	intravenous cholangiography
n&v	nausea and vomiting
NG	nasogastric (tube)
NPO	nothing by mouth
O&P	ova and parasites
pc	after meals
PO	by mouth
pp	postprandial
PTC	percutaneous transhepatic cholangiography
PUD	peptic ulcer disease
TPN	total parenteral nutrition
UGI	upper gastrointestinal series

Chapter Review

Real-World Applications

Medical Record Analysis

This Gastroenterology Consultation Report contains 12 medical terms. Underline each term and write it in the list below the report. Then define each term.

Gastroenterology Consultation Report

Reason for Consultation:	Evaluation of recurrent epigastric pain with anemia and melena.
History of Present Illness:	Patient is a 56-year-old male. He reports a long history of mild dyspepsia characterized by burning epigastric pain, especially when his stomach is empty. This pain has been relieved by over-the-counter antacids. Approximately two weeks ago, the pain became significantly worse and he noted that his stools were dark and tarry.
Results of Physical Examination:	CBC indicates anemia, and a fecal occult blood test is positive for blood. A blood test for *Helicobacter pylori* is positive. Gastroscopy located an ulcer in the lining of the stomach. This ulcer is 1.5 cm in diameter and deep. There is evidence of active bleeding from the ulcer.
Assessment:	Peptic ulcer disease.
Recommendations:	A gastrectomy to remove the ulcerated portion of stomach is indicated because the ulcer is already bleeding.

	Term	Definition
1	______	______
2	______	______
3	______	______
4	______	______
5	______	______
6	______	______
7	______	______
8	______	______
9	______	______
10	______	______
11	______	______
12	______	______

Chart Note Transcription

The chart note below contains 12 phrases that can be reworded with a medical term that you learned in this chapter. Each phrase is identified with an underline. Determine the medical term and write your answers in the space provided.

Current Complaint: Patient is a 74-year-old female seen by a physician who specializes in the treatment of the gastrointestinal tract ❶ with complaints of severe lower abdominal pain and extreme difficulty with having a bowel movement. ❷

Past History: Patient has a history of the presence of gallstones ❸, requiring surgical removal of the gallbladder ❹ 10 years ago and chronic acid backing up from the stomach into the esophagus. ❺

Signs and Symptoms: The patient's abdomen is distended with fluid collecting in the abdominal cavity. ❻ X-ray of the colon after inserting barium dye with an enema ❼ revealed the presence of multiple small tumors growing on a stalk ❽ throughout the colon. Visual examination of the colon by a scope inserted through the rectum ❾ was performed, and biopsies taken for microscopic examination located a tumor.

Diagnosis: Carcinoma of the section of colon between the descending colon and the rectum. ❿

Treatment: Surgical removal of the colon ⓫ between the descending colon and the rectum with the surgical creation of an opening of the colon through the abdominal wall. ⓬

❶ ______________________

❷ ______________________

❸ ______________________

❹ ______________________

❺ ______________________

❻ ______________________

❼ ______________________

❽ ______________________

❾ ______________________

❿ ______________________

⓫ ______________________

⓬ ______________________

Case Study

Below is a case study presentation of a patient with a condition discussed in this chapter. Read the case study and answer the questions below. Some questions will ask for information not included within this chapter. Use your text, a medical dictionary, or any other reference material you choose to answer these questions.

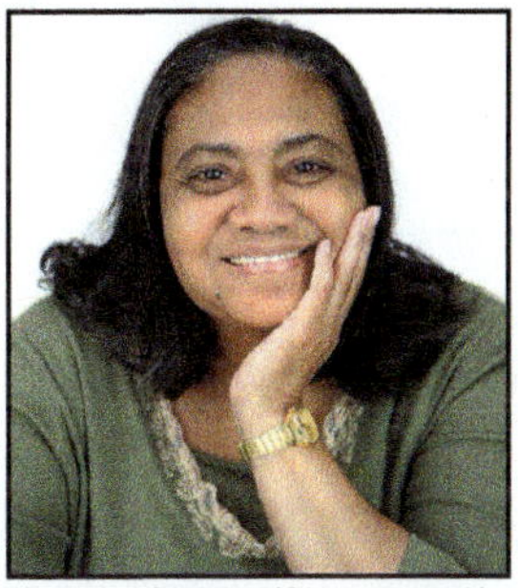

(© Rob Marmion/Shutterstock)

A 60-year-old obese female has come into the ER due to severe RUQ pain for the past 2 hours. Patient also reports increasing nausea but denies emesis. Patient states she has been told she has cholelithiasis by her family physician following a milder episode of this pain 2 years ago. In addition to severe pain, patient displays a moderate degree of scleral jaundice. Abdominal ultrasound identified acute cholecystitis and a large number of gallstones. Because of the jaundice a PTC was performed and confirmed choledocholithiasis. Patient was sent to surgery for laparoscopic cholecystectomy to remove the gallbladder and all gallstones. She recovered without incident.

1. Define each of the patient's symptoms.

____

____

2. The patient has severe RUQ pain. What organs are located in the RUQ?

____

____

3. After reading the definition of jaundice, what is most likely causing this patient to have it?

____

____

4. Describe the diagnostic imaging procedures this patient received.

____

____

5. What is the difference between cholelithiasis and cholecystitis?

____

____

6. The patient's gallbladder was removed laparoscopically. What does that mean?

____

____

Practice Exercises

A. Complete the Statement

1. The digestive system is also known as the ____________________ system.
2. The continuous muscular tube of the digestive system is called the ____________________ or ____________________ and stretches between the ____________________ and ____________________.
3. The accessory organs of the digestive system are the ____________________, ____________________, ____________________, and ____________________.
4. The three main functions of the digestive system are ____________________, ____________________, and ____________________.
5. The incisors are examples of ____________________ teeth and the molars are examples of ____________________ teeth.
6. Food is propelled through the gut by wavelike muscular contractions called ____________________.
7. Food in the stomach is mixed with ____________________ and other gastric juices to form a watery mixture called ____________________.
8. The three sections of small intestine in order are the ____________________, ____________________, and ____________________.
9. The S-shaped section of colon that curves back toward the rectum is called the ____________________ colon.
10. ____________________ produced by the liver is responsible for the ____________________ of fats. It is stored in the ____________________.

B. Combining Form Practice

The combining form **gastr/o** refers to the stomach. Use it to write a term that means:

1. inflammation of the stomach ____________________
2. study of the stomach and small intestines ____________________
3. removal of the stomach ____________________
4. visual exam of the stomach ____________________
5. stomach pain ____________________
6. enlargement of the stomach ____________________
7. cutting into the stomach ____________________

The combining form **esophag/o** refers to the esophagus. Use it to write a term that means:

8. inflammation of the esophagus ____________________
9. visual examination of the esophagus ____________________

10. surgical repair of the esophagus ______

11. pertaining to the esophagus ______

12. stretched-out esophagus ______

The combining form **proct/o** refers to the rectum and anus. Use it to write a term that means:

13. surgical fixation of the rectum and anus ______

14. drooping of the rectum and anus ______

15. inflammation of the rectum and anus ______

16. specialist in the study of the rectum and anus ______

The combining form **cholecyst/o** refers to the gallbladder. Use it to write a term that means:

17. removal of the gallbladder ______

18. condition of having gallbladder stones ______

19. gallbladder stone surgical crushing ______

20. gallbladder inflammation ______

The combining form **lapar/o** refers to the abdomen. Use it to write a term that means:

21. instrument to view inside the abdomen ______

22. cutting into the abdomen ______

23. visual examination of the abdomen ______

The combining form **hepat/o** refers to the liver. Use it to write a term that means:

24. liver tumor ______

25. enlargement of the liver ______

26. pertaining to the liver ______

27. inflammation of the liver ______

The combining form **pancreat/o** refers to the pancreas. Use it to write a term that means:

28. inflammation of the pancreas ______

29. pertaining to the pancreas ______

The combining form **col/o** refers to the colon. Use it to write a term that means:

30. create an opening in the colon ______

31. inflammation of the colon ______

C. Define the Combining Form

	Definition	Example from Chapter
1. esophag/o	______	______
2. hepat/o	______	______
3. ile/o	______	______
4. proct/o	______	______
5. gloss/o	______	______
6. labi/o	______	______
7. jejun/o	______	______
8. sigmoid/o	______	______
9. rect/o	______	______
10. gingiv/o	______	______
11. cholecyst/o	______	______
12. duoden/o	______	______
13. an/o	______	______
14. enter/o	______	______
15. dent/o	______	______

D. Suffix Practice

Use the following suffixes to create a medical term for the following definitions.

-orexia	-phagia	-pepsia	-prandial
-emesis	-lithiasis		

1. after meals ______
2. condition of having gallstones ______
3. no appetite ______
4. difficulty swallowing ______
5. vomiting blood ______
6. slow digestion ______

E. What Does it Stand For?

1. BM ______________________________

2. UGI ______________________________

3. BE ______________________________

4. BS ______________________________

5. n & v ______________________________

6. O & P ______________________________

7. PO ______________________________

8. CBD ______________________________

9. NPO ______________________________

10. pp ______________________________

F. Terminology Matching

Match each term to its definition.

1.	________ dentures	a.	excess body weight
2.	________ anorexia	b.	chronic liver disease
3.	________ hematemesis	c.	heartburn
4.	________ pyrosis	d.	small colon tumors
5.	________ obesity	e.	fluid accumulation in abdominal cavity
6.	________ constipation	f.	vomit blood
7.	________ melena	g.	bowel twists on self
8.	________ ascites	h.	set of artificial teeth
9.	________ cirrhosis	i.	loss of appetite
10.	________ spastic colon	j.	difficulty having BM
11.	________ polyposis	k.	irritable bowel syndrome
12.	________ volvulus	l.	black tarry stool
13.	________ hiatal hernia	m.	yellow skin color
14.	________ ulcerative colitis	n.	bloody diarrhea
15.	________ dysentery	o.	diaphragmatocele
16.	________ jaundice	p.	inflammatory bowel disease

G. What's the Abbreviation?

1. nasogastric ______________________
2. gastrointestinal ______________________
3. hepatitis B virus ______________________
4. fecal occult blood test ______________________
5. inflammatory bowel disease ______________________
6. herpes simplex virus type 1 ______________________
7. aspartate transaminase ______________________
8. after meals ______________________
9. peptic ulcer disease ______________________
10. gastroesophageal reflux disease ______________________

H. Define the Term

1. colonoscopy ______________________
2. bite wing X-ray ______________________
3. hematochezia ______________________
4. serum bilirubin ______________________
5. cachexia ______________________
6. lavage ______________________
7. hernioplasty ______________________
8. extraction ______________________
9. choledocholithotripsy ______________________
10. anastomosis ______________________

I. Fill in the Blank

colonoscopy	barium swallow	lower GI series
gastric stapling	colostomy	colectomy
total parenteral nutrition	choledocholithotripsy	liver biopsy
ileostomy	fecal occult blood test	intravenous cholecystography

1. Excising a small piece of hepatic tissue for microscopic examination is called a(n) ______________________.
2. When a surgeon performs a total or partial colectomy for cancer, she may have to create an opening on the surface of the skin for fecal matter to leave the body. This procedure is called a(n) ______________________.
3. Another name for an upper GI series is a(n) ______________________.
4. Mr. White has had a radiopaque material placed into his large bowel by means of an enema for the purpose of viewing his colon. This procedure is called a(n) ______________________.

5. A(n) ______________________ is the surgical removal of the colon.
6. Jessica has been on a red meat-free diet in preparation for a test of her feces for the presence of hidden blood. This test is called a(n) ______________________.
7. Dr. Mendez uses equipment to crush gallstones in the common bile duct. This procedure is called a(n) ______________.
8. Mrs. Alcazar required ______________________ because she could not eat following her intestinal surgery.
9. Mr. Bright had a(n) ______________________ to treat his morbid obesity.
10. Visualizing the gallbladder and bile ducts by injecting a dye into the patient's arm is called a(n) ______________________.
11. Passing an instrument into the anus and rectum in order to see the colon is called a(n) ______________________.
12. Ms. Fayne suffers from Crohn's disease, which has necessitated the removal of much of her small intestine. She has had a surgical passage created for the external disposal of waste material from the ileum. This is called a(n) ________________.

J. Terminology Matching

Match each term to its definition.

1. _______ dentures	a. tooth decay
2. _______ cementum	b. prosthetic device used to anchor a tooth
3. _______ root canal	c. inflammation of the gums
4. _______ crown	d. full set of artificial teeth
5. _______ bridge	e. portion of the tooth covered by enamel
6. _______ implant	f. replacement for missing teeth
7. _______ gingivitis	g. anchors root in bony socket of jaw
8. _______ dental caries	h. surgery on the tooth pulp

K. Pharmacology Challenge

Fill in the classification for each drug description, then match the brand name.

Drug Description	Classification	Brand Name
1. _______ Controls diarrhea	______________________	a. Pepcid
2. _______ Blocks stomach's ability to secrete acid	______________________	b. Obezine
3. _______ Treats motion sickness	______________________	c. Metamucil
4. _______ Blocks acid-producing receptors	______________________	d. Compazine
5. _______ Suppresses appetite	______________________	e. Maalox
6. _______ Stimulates a bowel movement	______________________	f. Imodium
7. _______ Neutralizes stomach acid	______________________	g. Nexium

L. Technology

The impact of technology on all areas of health care is tremendous. Select one of the five career pathways in the Health Science career cluster (diagnostic, therapeutic, health informatics, support services, or biotechnology research and development systems), and research and identify how a worker in that field would use technology on the job. What type of technological equipment would the worker use? Write a brief paper describing your findings.

M. Team Building

In order for a team to function well, it is important to build relationships with all of your teammates. One way to develop a relationship is to find common bonds. For example, you and another team member might both enjoy playing soccer. Or, you might both have brothers or sisters. Or, you might both play the guitar. Discovering common bonds helps you understand the other person so you can work together successfully as a team.

In teams of four, identify at least five common bonds among you. How would the things you all have in common help you function better as a team?

N. Career Connection

Research professions related to the Digestive Systems and report on the following:

1. Profession description to include job responsibilities
2. Educational requirements
3. Job opportunities
4. Opportunities outside of the hospital setting
5. Salary range
6. Licensure and continuing education requirements

Present your findings to the class.

O. Research Project: Professional Organizations and Trends in Health Care

Joining a professional organization provides you with opportunities to learn more about your industry, strengthen your job skills, achieve accreditation or certification in your field, and expand your network of personal contacts. To an employer, it shows that you are motivated to look beyond the workplace to find new and innovative ideas that can help you and your organization be more productive.

One way that a professional organization helps its members is by distributing information about the industry through Web sites, newsletters, or magazines. Working in teams of three or four, select a health care career and create a two-page publication, report, or research article for a professional organization that would serve it.

Using medical journals, professional publications, and the Internet, research current trends, policies, or events affecting the health care industry. Be sure to gather information on the organization's accreditation and certification procedures, if applicable, and how they prepare members to achieve the credentials necessary for certification and/or licensure in their field.

Give the publication a suitable name, and write three or four articles that the members would find useful. Include medical terminology as appropriate when developing the publication. Cite all sources accessed using conventional citation methods used in medical literature. Share your project with a peer for feedback. Revise the publication as necessary. When your project is complete, print it to share with the class, or publish it on your class Web site.

Labeling Exercise

Image A

Write the labels for this figure on the numbered lines provided.

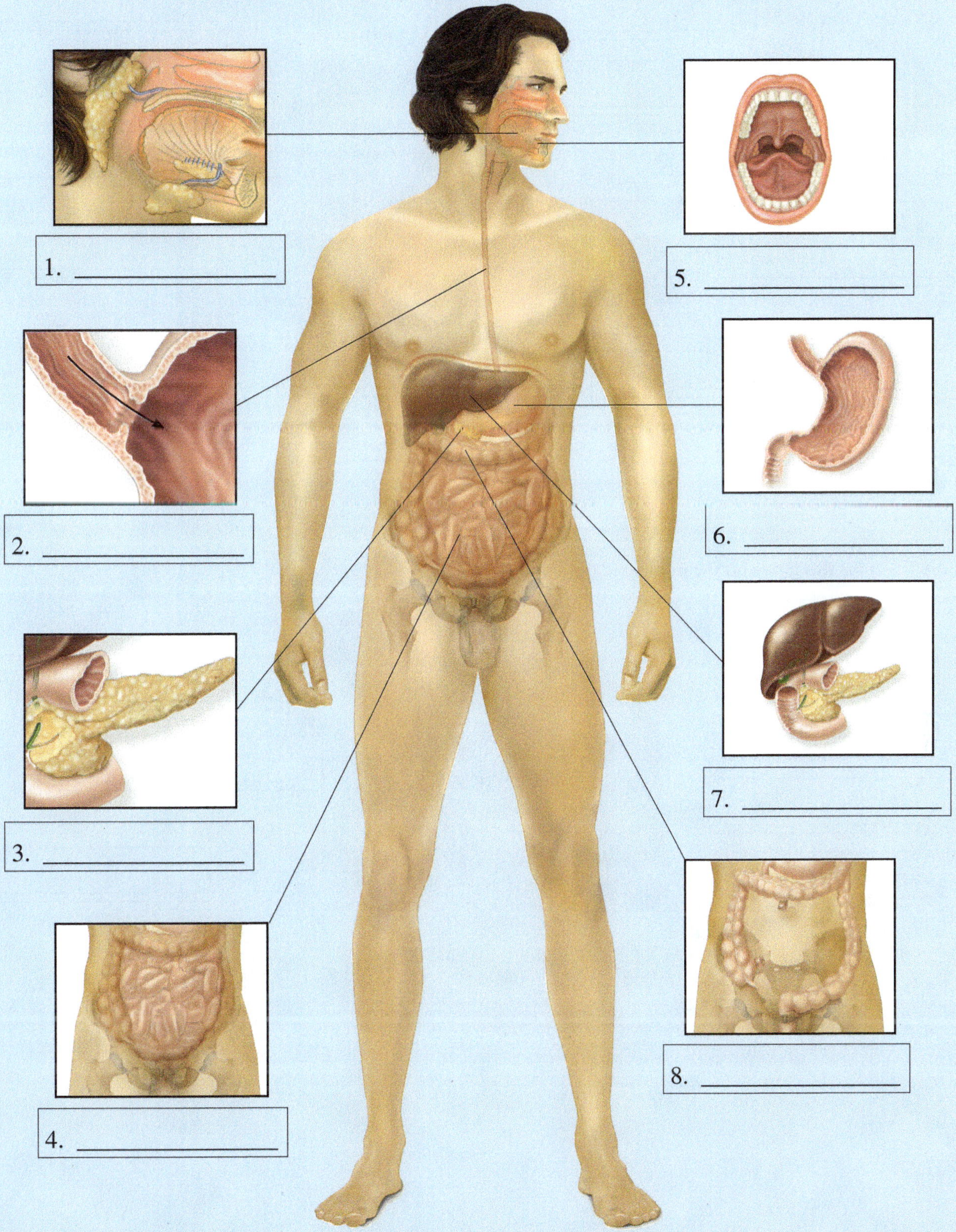

Image B

Write the labels for this figure on the numbered lines provided.

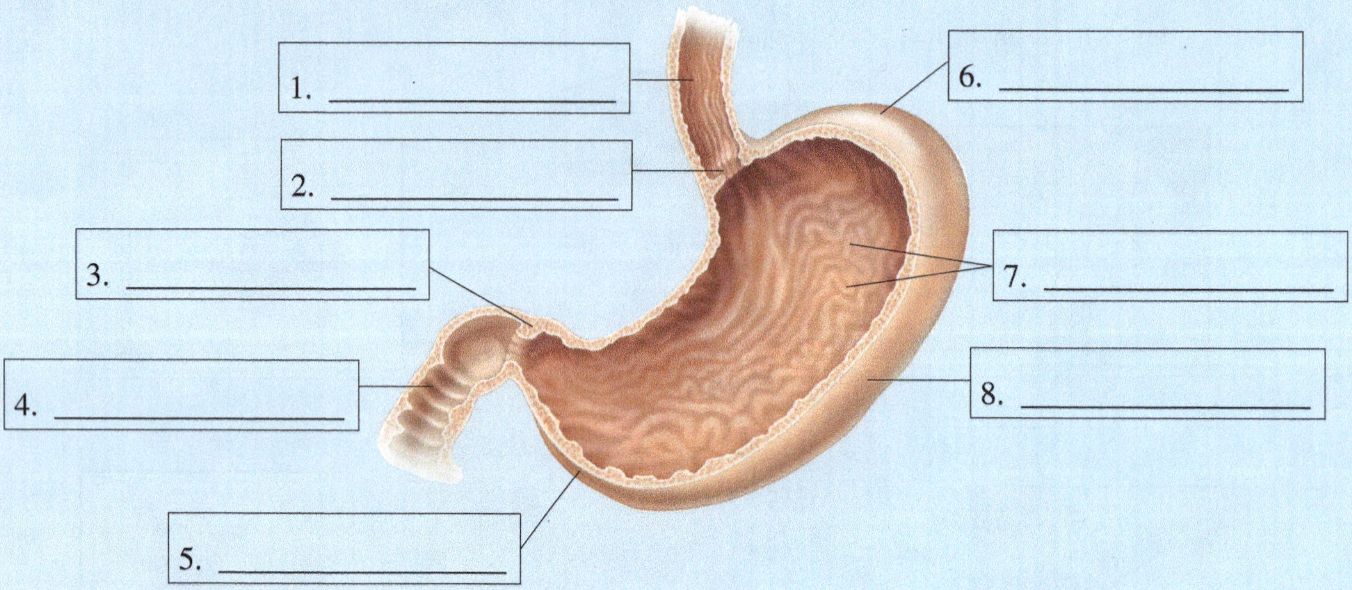

Image C

Write the labels for this figure on the numbered lines provided.

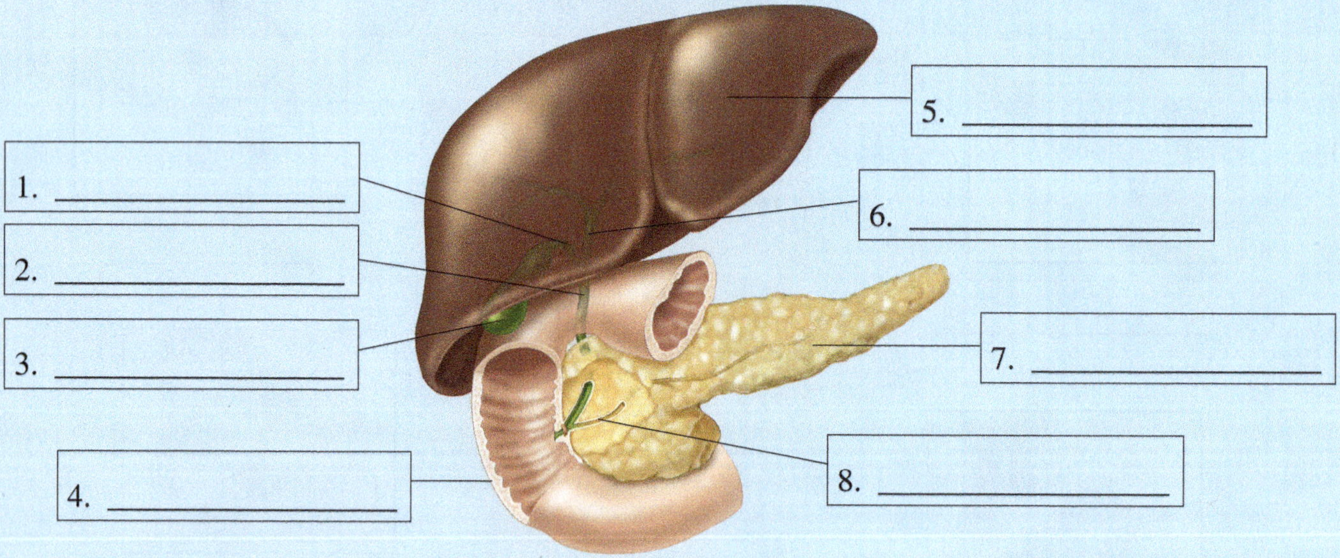

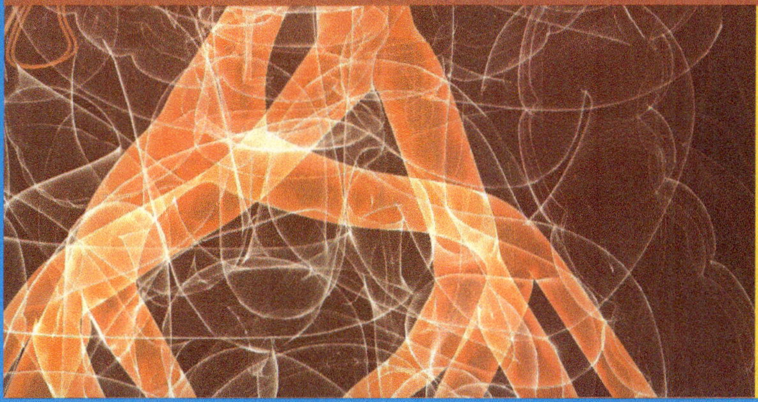

9

URINARY SYSTEM

Learning Objectives

Upon completion of this chapter, you will be able to

- Identify and define the combining forms and suffixes introduced in this chapter.
- Correctly spell and pronounce medical terms and major anatomical structures relating to the urinary system.
- Locate and describe the major organs of the urinary system and their functions.
- Describe the nephron and the mechanisms of urine production.
- Identify the characteristics of urine and a urinalysis.
- Identify and define urinary system anatomical terms.
- Identify and define selected urinary system pathology terms.
- Identify and define selected urinary system diagnostic procedures.
- Identify and define selected urinary system therapeutic procedures.
- Identify and define selected medications relating to the urinary system.
- Define selected abbreviations associated with the urinary system.

Urinary System at a Glance

Function

The urinary system is responsible for maintaining a stable internal environment for the body. In order to achieve this state, the urinary system removes waste products, adjusts water and electrolyte levels, and maintains the correct pH.

Structures

Here are the primary structures that comprise the urinary system.

kidneys
ureters
urethra
urinary bladder

Word Parts

Here are the most common word parts (with their meanings) used to build urinary system terms. For a more comprehensive list, refer to the Terminology section of this chapter.

Combining Forms

azot/o	nitrogenous waste
bacteri/o	bacteria
cyst/o	bladder, pouch
glomerul/o	glomerulus
glycos/o	sugar, glucose
keton/o	ketones
lith/o	stone
meat/o	meatus
nephr/o	kidney
noct/i	night
olig/o	scanty
protein/o	protein
pyel/o	renal pelvis
ren/o	kidney
ureter/o	ureter
urethr/o	urethra
urin/o	urine
ur/o	urine

Suffixes

-lith	stone
-lithiasis	condition of stones
-ptosis	drooping
-tripsy	surgical crushing
-uria	condition of the urine

Urinary System Illustrated

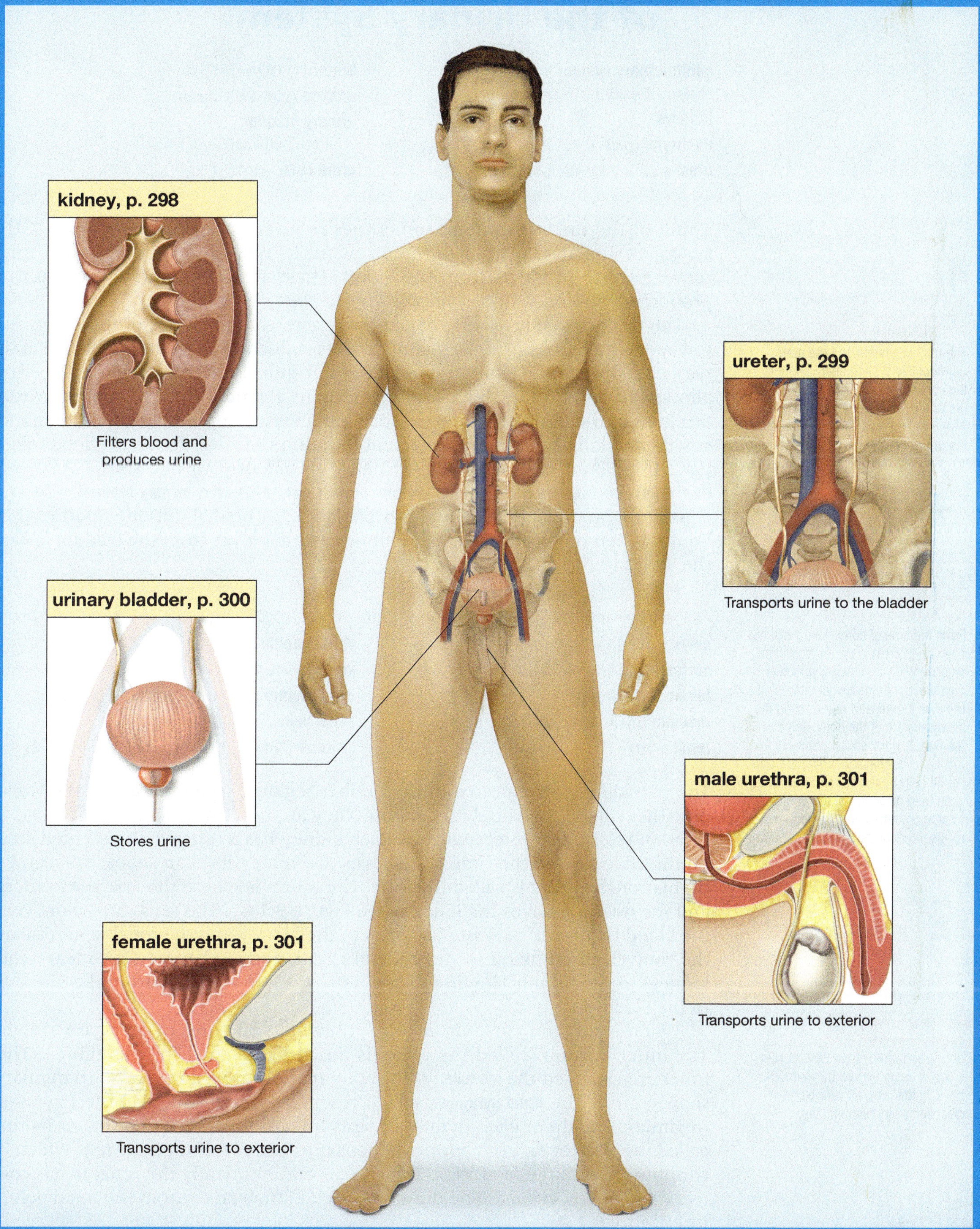

Anatomy and Physiology of the Urinary System

genitourinary system (jen-ih-toh-YOO-rih-nair-ee)
kidneys
nephrons (NEF-ronz)
uremia (yoo-REE-mee-ah)
ureters (YOO-reh-ters)
urethra (yoo-REE-thrah)
urinary bladder (YOO-rih-nair-ee)
urine (YOO-rin)

Think of the urinary system, sometimes referred to as the **genitourinary** (GU) **system,** as similar to a water filtration plant. Its main function is to filter and remove waste products from the blood. These waste materials result in the production and excretion of **urine** from the body.

The urinary system is one of the hardest working systems of the body. All the body's metabolic processes result in the production of waste products. These waste products are a natural part of life but quickly become toxic if they are allowed to build up in the blood, resulting in a condition called **uremia.** Waste products in the body are removed through a very complicated system of blood vessels and kidney tubules. The actual filtration of wastes from the blood takes place in millions of **nephrons,** which make up each of your two **kidneys.** As urine drains from each kidney, the **ureters** transport it to the **urinary bladder.** We are constantly producing urine, and our bladders can hold about one quart of this liquid. When the urinary bladder empties, urine moves from the bladder down the **urethra** to the outside of the body.

MED TERM TIP

The urinary system and the male reproductive system share some of the same organs, particularly the urethra. Hence the term *genitourinary* (GU) is sometimes used to describe the urinary system.

Kidneys

calyx (KAY-liks)
cortex (KOR-teks)
hilum (HIGH-lum)
medulla (meh-DULL-ah)
renal artery
renal papilla (pah-PILL-ah)
renal pelvis
renal pyramids
renal vein
retroperitoneal (ret-roh-pair-ih-toh-NEE-al)

MED TERM TIP

From the time of early man, there has been an interest in urine. Drawings on cave walls and hieroglyphics in Egyptian pyramids reveal interest in urine as a means of determining the physical state of the body. Some of the first doctors, called *pisse prophets,* believed that examining the urine would help treat a patient. Now urologists treat disorders of the urinary tract in both men and women, as well as disorders of the male reproductive tract.

The two kidneys are located in the lumbar region of the back above the waist on either side of the vertebral column. They are not inside the peritoneal sac, a location referred to as **retroperitoneal.** Each kidney has a concave or indented area on the edge toward the center that gives the kidney its bean shape. The center of this concave area is called the **hilum.** The hilum is where the **renal artery** enters and the **renal vein** leaves the kidney (see Figure 9.1 ■). The renal artery delivers the blood that is full of waste products to the kidney and the renal vein returns the now cleansed blood to the general circulation. The ureters also leave the kidneys at the hilum. The ureters are narrow tubes that lead from the kidneys to the bladder.

When a surgeon cuts into a kidney, several structures or areas are visible. The outer portion, called the **cortex,** is much like a shell for the kidney. The inner area is called the **medulla.** Within the medulla are a dozen or so triangular-shaped areas, the **renal pyramids,** which resemble their namesake, the Egyptian pyramids. The tip of each pyramid points inward toward the hilum. At its tip, called the **renal papilla,** each pyramid opens into a **calyx** (plural is *calyces*), which is continuous with the **renal pelvis.** The calyces and ultimately the renal pelvis collect urine as it is formed. The ureter for each kidney arises from the renal pelvis (see Figure 9.2 ■).

MED TERM TIP

At any one time, about 20% of your blood is being filtered by your kidneys. In this way, all your blood is cleansed every few minutes.

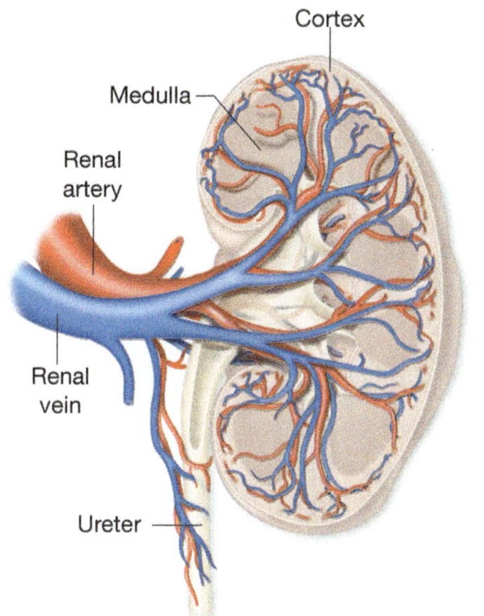

Figure 9.1 Kidney structure. Longitudinal section showing the renal artery entering and the renal vein and ureter exiting at the hilium of the kidney.

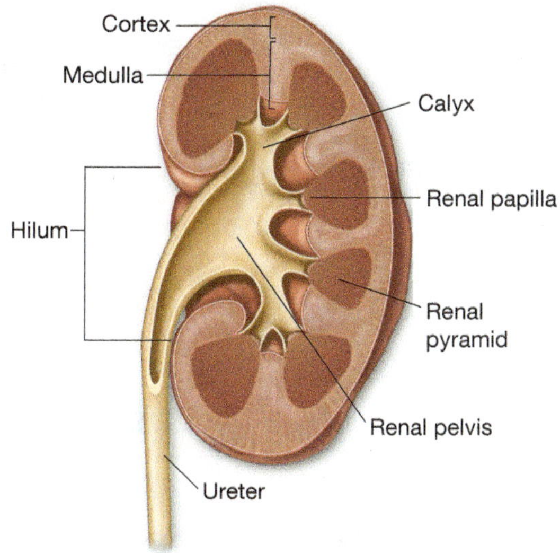

Figure 9.2 Longitudinal section of a kidney illustrating the internal structures.

Nephrons

afferent arteriole (AFF-er-ent)
Bowman's capsule
collecting tubule
distal convoluted tubule (DISS-tall / con-voh-LOOT-ed)
efferent arteriole (EF-er-ent)
glomerular capsule (glom-AIR-yoo-lar)
glomerulus (glom-AIR-yoo-lus)
loop of Henle
nephron (NEF-ron)
nephron loop
proximal convoluted tubule (PROK-sim-al / con-voh-LOOT-ed)
renal corpuscle (KOR-pus-ehl)
renal tubule

The functional or working unit of the kidney is the **nephron**. There are more than one million of these microscopic structures in each human kidney. Each nephron consists of the **renal corpuscle** and the **renal tubule** (see Figure 9.3 ■). The renal corpuscle is the blood-filtering portion of the nephron. It has a double-walled cuplike structure called the **glomerular capsule** (also known as **Bowman's capsule**) that encases a ball of capillaries called the **glomerulus.** An **afferent arteriole** carries blood to the glomerulus, and an **efferent arteriole** carries blood away from the glomerulus.

Water and substances that were removed from the bloodstream in the renal corpuscle flow into the renal tubules to finish the urine production process. This continuous tubule is divided into four sections: the **proximal convoluted tubule,** followed by the narrow **nephron loop** (also known as the **loop of Henle**), then the **distal convoluted tubule,** and finally the **collecting tubule.**

MED TERM TIP

The kidney bean is so named because it resembles a kidney in shape. Each organ weighs 4–6 ounces, is 2–3 inches wide and approximately 1 inch thick, and is about the size of your fist. In most people the left kidney is slightly higher and larger than the right kidney. Functioning kidneys are necessary for life, but it is possible to live with only one functioning kidney.

MED TERM TIP

Afferent, meaning moving toward, and *efferent*, meaning moving away from, are terms used when discussing moving either toward or away from the central point in many systems. For example, there are afferent and efferent nerves in the nervous system.

Ureters

As urine drains out of the renal pelvis it enters the ureter, which carries it down to the urinary bladder (see Figure 9.4 ■). Ureters are very narrow tubes measuring less than ¼-inch wide and 10–12 inches long that extend from the renal pelvis to the urinary bladder. Mucous membrane lines the ureters just as it lines most passages that open to the external environment.

■ **Figure 9.3** The structure of a nephron, illustrating the nephron structure in relation to the circulatory system.

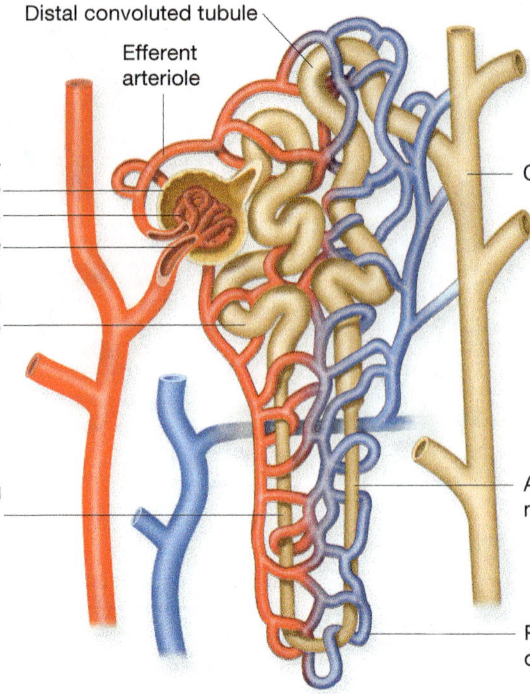

MED TERM TIP

The terms *ureter* and *urethra* are frequently confused. Remember that there are two ureters carrying urine from the kidneys into the bladder. There is only one urethra, and it carries urine from the bladder to the outside of the body.

MED TERM TIP

Terms such as *micturition, voiding,* and *urination* all mean basically the same thing—the process of releasing urine from the body.

Urinary Bladder

external sphincter (SFINGK-ter)
internal sphincter
rugae (ROO-gay)
urination

The urinary bladder is an elastic muscular sac that lies in the base of the pelvis just behind the pubic symphysis (see Figure 9.5 ■). It is composed of three layers of smooth muscle tissue lined with mucous membrane containing **rugae** or folds that allow it to stretch. The bladder receives the urine directly from the ureters, stores it, and excretes it by **urination** through the urethra.

Generally, an adult bladder will hold 250 mL of urine. This amount then creates an urge to void or empty the bladder. Involuntary muscle action causes the bladder to contract and the **internal sphincter** to relax. The internal sphincter protects us from having our bladder empty at the wrong time. Voluntary action

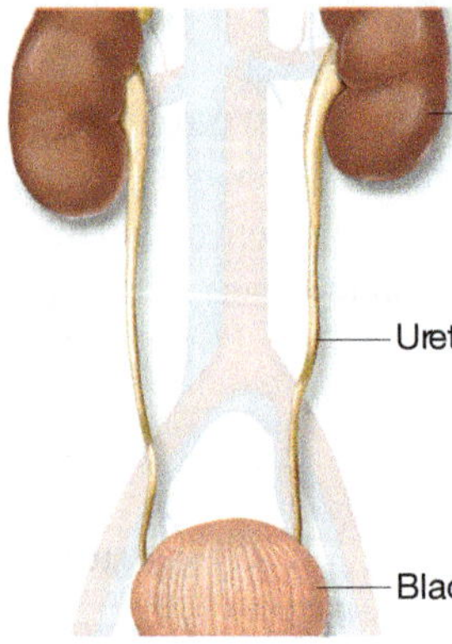

■ **Figure 9.4** The ureters extend from the kidneys to the urinary bladder.

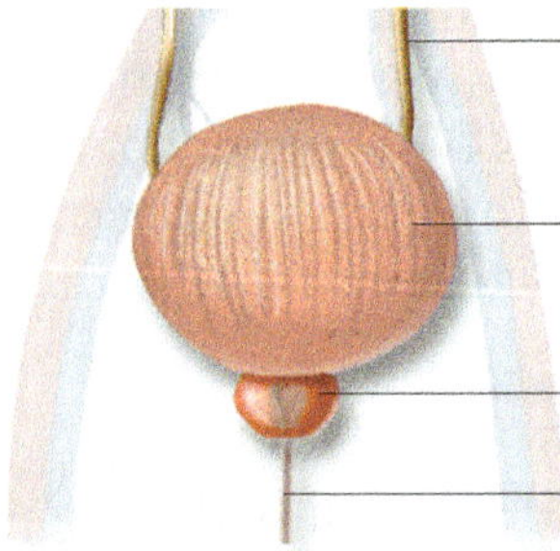

■ **Figure 9.5** The structure of the urinary bladder. (Note the prostate gland.)

controls the **external sphincter,** which opens on demand to allow the intentional emptying of the bladder. The act of controlling the emptying of urine is developed sometime after a child is 2 years of age.

Urethra

urinary meatus (mee-AY-tus)

The urethra is a tubular canal that carries the flow of urine from the bladder to the outside of the body (see Figure 9.6 ■ for the male urethra). The external opening through which urine passes out of the body is called the **urinary meatus.** Mucous membrane also lines the urethra as it does other structures of the urinary system. This is one of the reasons that infection spreads up the urinary tract. The urethra is 1–2 inches long in the female and 8 inches long in the male. In a woman it functions only as the outlet for urine and is in front of the vagina. In the male, however, it has two functions: an outlet for urine and the passageway for semen to leave the body.

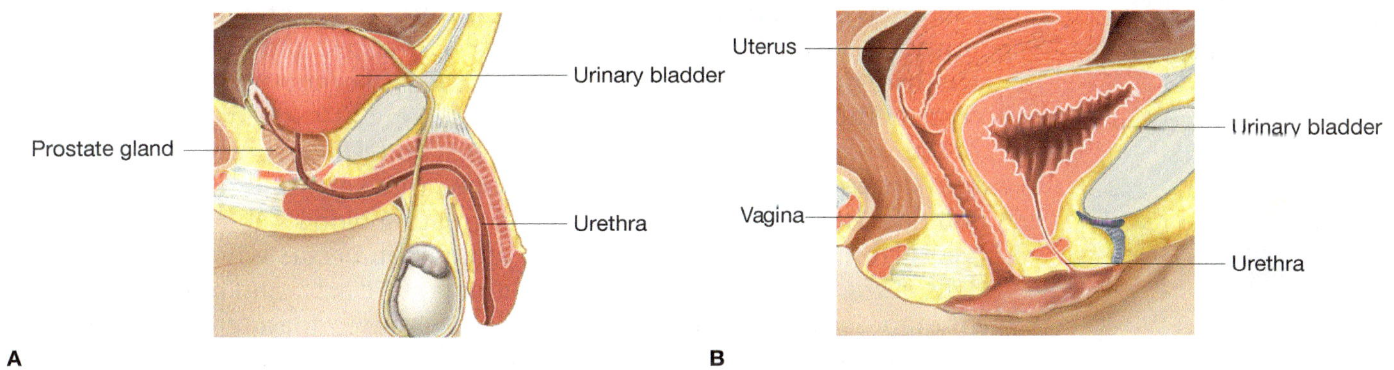

■ **Figure 9.6** (A) The male urethra extends from the urinary bladder in the floor of the pelvis through the penis to the urinary meatus; (B) the much shorter female urethra extends from the urinary bladder to the floor of the pelvis and exits just in front of the vaginal opening.

Role of Kidneys in Homeostasis

electrolytes (ee-LEK-troh-lites) **homeostasis** (hoh-mee-oh-STAY-sis)

The kidneys are responsible for **homeostasis** or balance in the body. They continually adjust the chemical conditions in the body, allowing us to survive. Because of its interaction with the bloodstream and its ability to excrete substances from the body, the urinary system maintains the body's proper balance of water and chemicals. If the body is low on water, the kidneys conserve it, or in the opposite case, if there is excess water in the body, the kidneys excrete the excess. In adition to water, the kidneys regulate the level of **electrolytes**—small biologically important molecules such as sodium (Na^+), potassium (K^+), chloride (Cl^-), and bicarbonate (HCO_3^-). Finally, the kidneys play an important role in maintaining the correct pH range within the body, making sure we do not become too acidic or too alkaline. The kidneys accomplish these important tasks through the production of urine.

MED TERM TIP

Mucous membranes will carry infections up the urinary tract from the urinary meatus and urethra into the bladder and eventually up the ureters and the kidneys if not stopped. It is never wise to ignore a simple bladder infection or what is called *cystitis.*

Stages of Urine Production

filtration
glomerular filtrate
peritubular capillaries
reabsorption
secretion

As wastes and unnecessary substances are removed from the bloodstream by the nephrons, many desirable molecules are also removed initially. Waste products are eliminated from the body, but other substances such as water, electrolytes, and nutrients must be returned to the bloodstream. Urine, in its final form ready for elimination from the body, is the ultimate product of this entire process.

Urine production occurs in three stages: **filtration, reabsorption,** and **secretion.** Each of these steps is performed by a different section of the nephrons (see Figure 9.7 ■).

MED TERM TIP

The amount of water and other fluids processed by the kidneys each day is astonishing. Approximately 190 quarts of fluid are filtered out of the glomerular blood every day. Most of this fluid returns to the body through the reabsorption process. About 99% of the water that leaves the blood each day through the filtration process returns to the blood by proximal tubule reabsorption.

1. **Filtration.** The first stage is the filtering of particles, which occurs in the renal corpuscle. The pressure of blood flowing through the glomerulus forces material out of the bloodstream, through the wall of the glomerular capsule, and into the renal tubules. This fluid in the tubules is called the **glomerular filtrate** and consists of water, electrolytes, nutrients such as glucose and amino acids, wastes, and toxins.
2. **Reabsorption.** After filtration, the filtrate passes through the four sections of the tubule. As the filtrate moves along its twisted journey, most of the water and much of the electrolytes and nutrients are reabsorbed into the **peritubular capillaries,** a capillary bed that surrounds the renal tubules. They can then reenter the circulating blood.
3. **Secretion.** The final stage of urine production occurs when the special cells of the renal tubules secrete ammonia, uric acid, and other waste substances directly into the renal tubule. Urine formation is now finished; it passes into the collecting tubules, renal papilla, calyx, renal pelvis, and ultimately into the ureter.

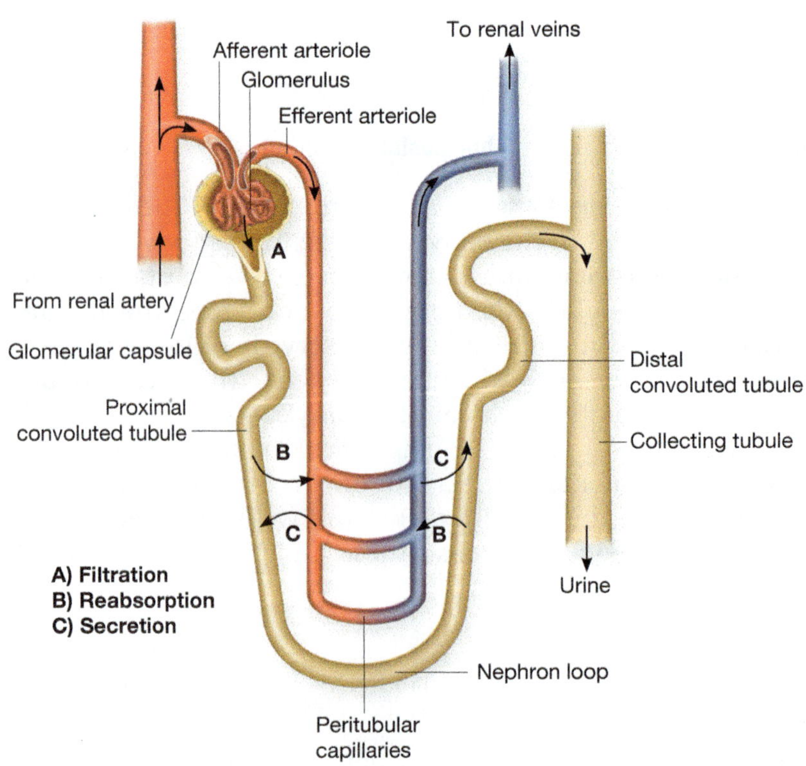

■ **Figure 9.7** The three stages of urine production: filtration, reabsorption, and secretion.

Urine

albumin (al-BEW-min)
nitrogenous wastes (nigh-TROJ-eh-nus)
specific gravity
urinalysis (yoo-rih-NAL-ih-sis)

Urine is normally straw-colored to clear, and sterile. Although it is 95% water, it also contains many dissolved substances, such as electrolytes, toxins, and **nitrogenous wastes,** the by-products of muscle metabolism. At times the urine also contains substances that should not be there, such as glucose, blood, or **albumin,** a protein that should remain in the blood. This is the reason for performing a **urinalysis,** a physical and chemical analysis of urine, which gives medical personnel important information regarding disease processes occurring in a patient. Normally, during a 24-hour period the output of urine will be 1,000–2,000 mL, depending on the amount of fluid consumed and the general health of the person. Normal urine is acidic because this is one way our bodies dispose of excess acids. **Specific gravity** indicates the amount of dissolved substances in urine. The specific gravity of pure water is 1.000. The specific gravity of urine varies from 1.001 to 1.030. Highly concentrated urine has a higher specific gravity, while the specific gravity of very dilute urine is close to that of water. See Table 9.1 ■ for the normal values for urine testing and Table 9.2 ■ for abnormal findings.

MED TERM TIP

The color, odor, volume, and sugar content of urine have been examined for centuries. Color charts for urine were developed by 1140, and "taste testing" was common in the late seventeenth century. By the nineteenth century, urinalysis was a routine part of a physical examination.

Table 9.1 Values for Urinalysis Testing

ELEMENT	NORMAL FINDINGS
Color	Straw-colored, pale yellow to deep gold
Odor	Aromatic
Appearance	Clear
Specific gravity	1.001–1.030
pH	5.0–8.0
Protein	Negative to trace
Glucose	None
Ketones	None
Blood	Negative

Table 9.2 Abnormal Urinalysis Findings

ELEMENT	IMPLICATIONS
Color	Color varies depending on the patient's fluid intake and output or medication. Brown or black urine color indicates a serious disease process.
Odor	A fetid or foul odor may indicate infection. While a fruity odor may be found in diabetes mellitus, dehydration, or starvation. Other odors may be due to medication or foods.
Appearance	Cloudiness may mean that an infection is present.
Specific gravity	Concentrated urine has a higher specific gravity. Dilute urine, such as can be found with diabetes insipidus, acute tubular necrosis, or salt-restricted diets, has a lower specific gravity.
pH	A pH value below 7.0 (acidic) is common in urinary tract infections, metabolic or respiratory acidosis, diets high in fruits or vegetables, or administration of some drugs. A pH higher than 7.0 (basic or alkaline) is common in metabolic or respiratory alkalosis, fever, high-protein diets, and taking ascorbic acid.
Protein	Protein may indicate glomerulonephritis or preeclampsia in a pregnant woman.
Glucose	Small amounts of glucose may be present as the result of eating a high-carbohydrate meal, stress, pregnancy, and taking some medications, such as aspirin or corticosteroids. Higher levels may indicate poorly controlled diabetes, Cushing's syndrome, or infection.
Ketones	The presence of ketones may indicate poorly controlled diabetes, dehydration, starvation, or ingestion of large amounts of aspirin.
Blood	Blood may indicate glomerulonephritis, cancer of the urinary tract, some types of anemia, taking of some medications (such as blood thinners), arsenic poisoning, reactions to transfusion, trauma, burns, and convulsions.

Terminology

Word Parts Used to Build Urinary System Terms

The following lists contain the combining forms, suffixes, and prefixes used to build terms in the remaining sections of this chapter.

Combining Forms

azot/o	nitrogenous waste
bacteri/o	bacteria
bi/o	life
carcin/o	cancer
corpor/o	body
cyst/o	bladder, pouch
glomerul/o	glomerulus
glycos/o	sugar
hem/o	blood
hemat/o	blood

keton/o	ketones
lith/o	stone
meat/o	meatus
necr/o	death
nephr/o	kidney
neur/o	nerve
noct/i	night
olig/o	scanty
peritone/o	peritoneum
protein/o	protein

py/o	pus
pyel/o	renal pelvis
ren/o	kidney
ur/o	urine
ureter/o	ureter
urethr/o	urethra
urin/o	urine
ven/o	vein

Suffixes

-al	pertaining to
-algia	pain
-ar	pertaining to
-ary	pertaining to
-cele	protrusion
-eal	pertaining to
-ectasis	dilated
-ectomy	surgical removal
-emia	blood condition
-genic	produced by
-gram	record
-graphy	process of recording
-ic	pertaining to
-itis	inflammation
-lith	stone

-lithiasis	condition of stones
-logist	one who studies
-logy	study of
-lysis	to destroy (to break down)
-malacia	softening
-megaly	enlarged
-meter	instrument to measure
-oma	tumor
-ory	pertaining to
-osis	abnormal condition
-ostomy	create a new opening
-otomy	cutting into
-ous	pertaining to

-pathy	disease
-pexy	surgical fixation
-plasty	surgical repair
-ptosis	drooping
-rrhagia	abnormal flow condition
-sclerosis	hardening
-scope	instrument to visually examine
-scopy	process of visually examining
-stenosis	narrowing
-tic	pertaining to
-tripsy	surgical crushing
-uria	urine condition

Prefixes

an-	without
anti-	against
dys-	abnormal, difficult

extra-	outside of
hydro-	water
intra-	within

poly-	many
retro-	backward

Anatomical Terms

TERM	WORD PARTS	DEFINITION
cystic (SIS-tik)	cyst/o = bladder -ic = pertaining to	Pertaining to the bladder.
renal (REE-nal)	ren/o = kidney -al = pertaining to	Pertaining to the kidney.
ureteral (yoo-REE-ter-all)	ureter/o = ureter -al = pertaining to	Pertaining to the ureter.
urethral (yoo-REE-thral)	urethr/o = urethra -al = pertaining to	Pertaining to the urethra.
urinary (yoo-rih-NAIR-ee)	urin/o = urine -ary = pertaining to	Pertaining to urine.

MED TERM TIP

Word Watch: Be particularly careful when using the three very similar combining forms: *uter/o* meaning "uterus," *ureter/o* meaning "ureter," and *urethr/o* meaning "urethra."

Pathology

TERM	WORD PARTS	DEFINITION
Medical Specialties		
nephrology (neh-FROL-oh-jee)	nephr/o = kidney -logy = study of	Branch of medicine involved in diagnosis and treatment of diseases and disorders of the kidney. Physician is a *nephrologist.*
urology (yoo-RAL-oh-jee)	ur/o = urine -logy = study of	Branch of medicine involved in diagnosis and treatment of diseases and disorders of the urinary system (and male reproductive system). Physician is a *urologist.*
Signs and Symptoms		
anuria (an-YOO-ree-ah)	an- = without -uria = urine condition	Complete suppression of urine formed by the kidneys and a complete lack of urine excretion.
azotemia (a-zo-TEE-mee-ah)	azot/o = nitrogenous waste -emia = blood condition	Accumulation of nitrogenous waste in the bloodstream. Occurs when the kidney fails to filter these wastes from the blood.
bacteriuria (back-teer-ree-YOO-ree-ah)	bacteri/o = bacteria -uria = urine condition	Presence of bacteria in the urine.

Pathology *(continued)*

TERM	WORD PARTS	DEFINITION
calculus (KAL-kew-lus)		Stone formed within an organ by an accumulation of mineral salts. Found in the kidney, renal pelvis, ureters, bladder, or urethra. Plural is *calculi*.

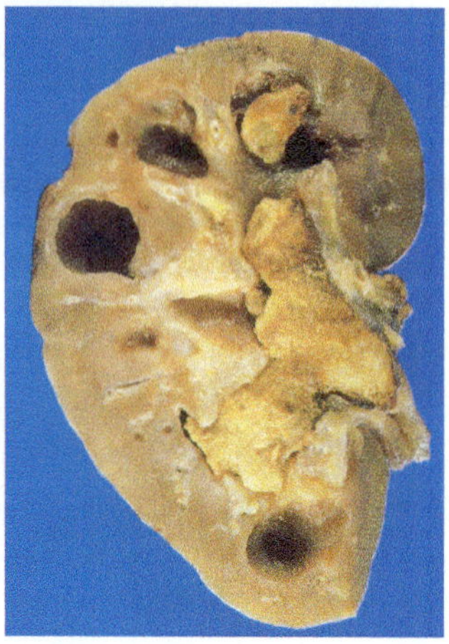

Figure 9.8 Photograph of sectioned kidney specimen illustrating extensive renal calculi. *(Photo Researchers, Inc.)*

TERM	WORD PARTS	DEFINITION
cystalgia (sis-TAL-jee-ah)	cyst/o = bladder -algia = pain	Urinary bladder pain.

MED TERM TIP

Word Watch: Be careful using the combining forms *cyst/o* meaning "bladder" and *cyt/o* meaning "cell."

TERM	WORD PARTS	DEFINITION
cystolith (SIS-toh-lith)	cyst/o = bladder -lith = stone	Bladder stone.
cystorrhagia (sis-toh-RAH-jee-ah)	cyst/o = bladder -rrhagia = abnormal flow condition	Profuse bleeding from the urinary bladder.
diuresis (dye-yoo-REE-sis)		Increased formation and excretion of urine.
dysuria (dis-YOO-ree-ah)	dys- = abnormal, difficult -uria = urine condition	Difficult or painful urination.
enuresis (en-yoo-REE-sis)		Involuntary discharge of urine after the age by which bladder control should have been established. This usually occurs by the age of 5. *Nocturnal enuresis* refers to bed-wetting at night.
frequency		Greater-than-normal occurrence in the urge to urinate, without an increase in the total daily volume of urine. Frequency is an indication of inflammation of the bladder or urethra.
glycosuria (glye-kohs-YOO-ree-ah)	glycos/o = sugar -uria = urine condition	Presence of sugar in the urine.
hematuria (hee-mah-TOO-ree-ah)	hemat/o = blood -uria = urine condition	Presence of blood in the urine.

Pathology *(continued)*

TERM	WORD PARTS	DEFINITION
hesitancy		Decrease in the force of the urine stream, often with difficulty initiating the flow. It is often a symptom of a blockage along the urethra, such as an enlarged prostate gland.
ketonuria (key-tone-YOO-ree-ah)	keton/o = ketones -uria = urine condition	Presence of ketones in the urine. This occurs when the body burns fat instead of glucose for energy, such as in uncontrolled diabetes mellitus.
nephrolith (NEF-roh-lith)	nephr/o = kidney -lith = stone	Kidney stone.
nephromalacia (nef-roh-mah-LAY-she-ah)	nephr/o = kidney -malacia = softening	Kidney is abnormally soft.
nephromegaly (nef-roh-MEG-ah-lee)	nephr/o = kidney -megaly = enlarged	Kidney is enlarged.
nephrosclerosis (nef-roh-skleh-ROH-sis)	nephr/o = kidney -sclerosis = hardening	Kidney tissue has become hardened.
nocturia (nok-TOO-ree-ah)	noct/i = night -uria = urine condition	Having to urinate frequently during the night.
oliguria (ol-ig-YOO-ree-ah)	olig/o = scanty -uria = urine condition	Producing too little urine.
polyuria (pol-ee-YOO-ree-ah)	poly- = many -uria = urine condition	Producing an unusually large volume of urine.
proteinuria (pro-ten-YOO-ree-ah)	protein/o = protein -uria = urine condition	Presence of protein in the urine.
pyuria (pye-YOO-ree-ah)	py/o = pus -uria = urine condition	Presence of pus in the urine.
renal colic (KOL-ik)	ren/o = kidney -al = pertaining to -ic = pertaining to	Pain caused by a kidney stone. Can be an excruciating pain and generally requires medical treatment.
stricture (STRIK-chur)		Narrowing of a passageway in the urinary system.
uremia (yoo-REE-me-ah)	ur/o = urine -emia = blood condition	Accumulation of waste products (especially nitrogenous wastes) in the bloodstream. Associated with renal failure.
ureterectasis (yoo-ree-ter-EK-tah-sis)	ureter/o = ureter -ectasis = dilated	Ureter is stretched out or dilated.
ureterolith (yoo-REE-teh-roh-lith)	ureter/o = ureter -lith = stone	Stone in the ureter.
ureterostenosis (yoo-ree-ter-oh-sten-OH-sis)	ureter/o = ureter -stenosis = narrowing	Ureter has become narrow.
urethralgia (yoo-ree-THRAL-jee-ah)	urethr/o = urethra -algia = pain	Urethral pain.

Pathology (continued)

TERM	WORD PARTS	DEFINITION
urethrorrhagia (yoo-ree-throh-RAH-jee-ah)	urethr/o = urethra -rrhagia = abnormal flow condition	Profuse bleeding from the urethra.
urethrostenosis (yoo-ree-throh-steh-NOH-sis)	urethr/o = urethra -stenosis = narrowing	Urethra has become narrow.
urgency (ER-jen-see)		Feeling the need to urinate immediately.
urinary incontinence (in-CON-tin-ens)	urin/o = urine -ary = pertaining to	Involuntary release of urine. In some patients an indwelling catheter is inserted into the bladder for continuous urine drainage.

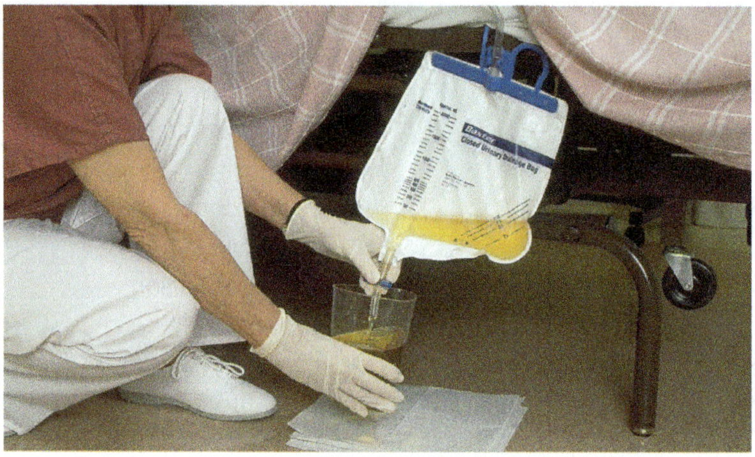

■ **Figure 9.9** Healthcare worker draining urine from a bladder catheter bag.

TERM	WORD PARTS	DEFINITION
urinary retention	urin/o = urine -ary = pertaining to	Inability to fully empty the bladder, often indicates a blockage in the urethra.
Kidney		
acute tubular necrosis (ATN) (ne-KROH-sis)	-ar = pertaining to necr/o = death -osis = abnormal condition	Damage to the renal tubules due to presence of toxins in the urine or to ischemia. Results in oliguria.
diabetic nephropathy (ne-FROH-path-ee)	-ic = pertaining to nephr/o = kidney -pathy = disease	Accumulation of damage to the glomerulus capillaries due to the chronic high blood sugars of diabetes mellitus.
glomerulonephritis (gloh-mair-yoo-loh-neh-FRYE-tis)	glomerul/o = glomerulus nephr/o = kidney -itis = inflammation	Inflammation of the kidney (primarily of the glomerulus). Since the glomerular membrane is inflamed, it becomes more permeable and will allow protein and blood cells to enter the filtrate. Results in protein in the urine (proteinuria) and hematuria.
hydronephrosis (high-droh-neh-FROH-sis)	hydro- = water nephr/o = kidney -osis = abnormal condition	Distention of the renal pelvis due to urine collecting in the kidney; often a result of the obstruction of a ureter.
nephritis (neh-FRYE-tis)	nephr/o = kidney -itis = inflammation	Kidney inflammation.

Pathology *(continued)*

TERM	WORD PARTS	DEFINITION
nephrolithiasis (nef-roh-lith-EE-a-sis)	nephr/o = kidney -lithiasis = condition of stones	Presence of calculi in the kidney. Usually begins with the solidification of salts present in the urine.
nephroma (neh-FROH-ma)	nephr/o = kidney -oma = tumor	Kidney tumor.
nephropathy (neh-FROP-ah-thee)	nephr/o = kidney -pathy = disease	General term describing the presence of kidney disease.
nephroptosis (nef-rop-TOH-sis)	nephr/o = kidney -ptosis = drooping	Downward displacement of the kidney out of its normal location; commonly called a *floating kidney.*
nephrotic syndrome (NS)	nephr/o = kidney -tic = pertaining to	Damage to the glomerulus resulting in protein appearing in the urine, proteinuria, and the corresponding decrease in protein in the bloodstream. Also called *nephrosis.*
polycystic kidneys (POL-ee-sis-tik)	poly- = many cyst/o = pouch -tic = pertaining to	Formation of multiple cysts within the kidney tissue. Results in the destruction of normal kidney tissue and uremia.

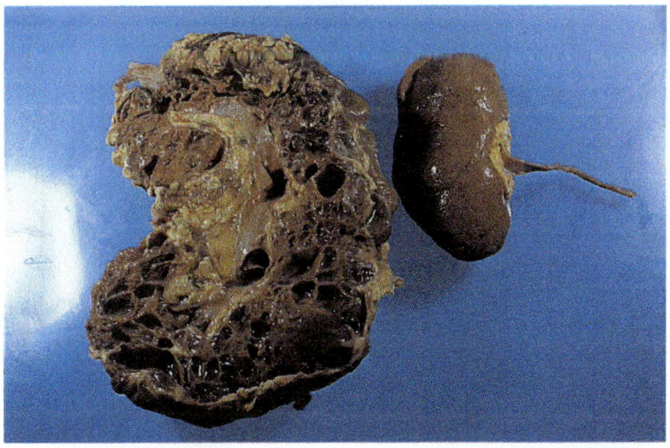

Figure 9.10 Photograph of a polycystic kidney on the left compared to a normal kidney on the right. *(Simon Fraser/Royal Victoria Infirmary, Newcastle/Science Photo Library/Photo Researchers, Inc.)*

TERM	WORD PARTS	DEFINITION
pyelitis (pye-eh-LYE-tis)	pyel/o = renal pelvis -itis = inflammation	Renal pelvis inflammation.
pyelonephritis (pye-eh-loh-neh-FRYE-tis)	pyel/o = renal pelvis nephr/o = kidney -itis = inflammation	Inflammation of the renal pelvis and the kidney. One of the most common types of kidney disease. It may be the result of a lower urinary tract infection that moved up to the kidney by way of the ureters. There may be large quantities of white blood cells and bacteria in the urine. Blood (hematuria) may even be present in the urine in this condition. Can occur with any untreated or persistent case of cystitis.
renal cell carcinoma	ren/o = kidney -al = pertaining to carcin/o = cancer -oma = tumor	Cancerous tumor that arises from kidney tubule cells.

Pathology *(continued)*

TERM	WORD PARTS	DEFINITION
renal failure	ren/o = kidney -al = pertaining to	Inability of the kidneys to filter wastes from the blood resulting in uremia. May be acute or chronic. Major reason for a patient being placed on dialysis.
Wilm's tumor (VILMZ)		Malignant kidney tumor found most often in children.
Urinary Bladder		
bladder cancer		Cancerous tumor that arises from the cells lining the bladder; major sign is hematuria.
bladder neck obstruction (BNO)		Blockage of the bladder outlet. Often caused by an enlarged prostate gland in males.
cystitis (sis-TYE-tis)	cyst/o = bladder -itis = inflammation	Urinary bladder inflammation.
cystocele (SIS-toh-seel)	cyst/o = bladder -cele = protrusion	Hernia or protrusion of the urinary bladder into the wall of the vagina.
interstitial cystitis (in-ter-STISH-al / sis-TYE-tis)	-al = pertaining to cyst/o = bladder -itis = inflammation	Disease of unknown cause in which there is inflammation and irritation of the bladder. Most commonly seen in middle-aged women.
neurogenic bladder (noo-roh-JEN-ik)	neur/o = nerve -genic = produced by	Loss of nervous control that leads to retention; may be caused by spinal cord injury or multiple sclerosis.
urinary tract infection (UTI)	urin/o = urine -ary = pertaining to	Infection, usually from bacteria, of any organ of the urinary system. Most often begins with cystitis and may ascend into the ureters and kidneys. Most common in women because of their shorter urethra.

Diagnostic Procedures

TERM	WORD PARTS	DEFINITION
Clinical Laboratory Tests		
blood urea nitrogen (BUN) (yoo-REE-ah / NIGH-troh-jen)		Blood test to measure kidney function by the level of nitrogenous waste (urea) that is in the blood.
clean catch specimen (CC)		Urine sample obtained after cleaning off the urinary opening and catching or collecting a urine sample in midstream (halfway through the urination process) to minimize contamination from the genitalia.

Diagnostic Procedures *(continued)*

TERM	WORD PARTS	DEFINITION
creatinine clearance (kree-AT-tih-neen)		Test of kidney function. Creatinine is a waste product cleared from the bloodstream by the kidneys. For this test, urine is collected for 24 hours, and the amount of creatinine in the urine is compared to the amount of creatinine that remains in the bloodstream.
urinalysis (U/A, UA) (yoo-rih-NAL-ih-sis)	urin/o = urine -lysis = to destroy (to break down)	Laboratory test consisting of the physical, chemical, and microscopic examination of urine.
urine culture and sensitivity (C&S)		Laboratory test of urine for bacterial infection. Attempt to grow bacteria on a culture medium in order to identify it and determine which antibiotics it is sensitive to.
urinometer (yoo-rin-OH-meter)	urin/o = urine -meter = instrument to measure	Instrument to measure the specific gravity of urine; part of a urinalysis.
Diagnostic Imaging		
cystogram (SIS-toh-gram)	cyst/o = bladder -gram = record	X-ray record of the urinary bladder.
cystography (sis-TOG-rah-fee)	cyst/o = bladder -graphy = process of recording	Process of instilling a contrast material or dye into the bladder by catheter to visualize the urinary bladder on X-ray.
excretory urography (EU) (EKS-kreh-tor-ee / yoo-ROG-rah-fee)	-ory = pertaining to ur/o = urine -graphy = process of recording	Injecting dye into the bloodstream and then taking an X-ray to trace the action of the kidney as it excretes the dye.
intravenous pyelography (IVP) (in-trah-VEE-nus / pye-eh-LOG-rah-fee)	intra- = within ven/o = vein -ous = pertaining to pyel/o = renal pelvis -graphy = process of recording	Diagnostic X-ray procedure in which a dye is injected into a vein and then X-rays are taken to visualize the renal pelvis as the dye is removed by the kidneys.
kidneys, ureters, bladder (KUB)		X-ray taken of the abdomen demonstrating the kidneys, ureters, and bladder without using any contrast dye. Also called a *flat-plate abdomen*.
nephrogram (NEH-fro-gram)	nephr/o = kidney -gram = record	X-ray record of the kidney.
pyelogram (PYE-eh-loh-gram)	pyel/o = renal pelvis -gram = record	X-ray record of the renal pelvis.

Diagnostic Procedures *(continued)*

TERM	WORD PARTS	DEFINITION
retrograde pyelography (RP) (RET-roh-grayd/ pye-eh-LOG-rah-fee)	retro- = backward pyel/o = renal pelvis -graphy = process of recording	Diagnostic X-ray procedure in which dye is inserted through the urethra to outline the bladder, ureters, and renal pelvis.
voiding cystourethrography (VCUG) (sis-toh-yoo-ree-THROG-rah-fee)	cyst/o = bladder urethr/o = urethra -graphy = process of recording	X-ray taken to visualize the urethra while the patient is voiding after a contrast dye has been placed in the bladder.
Endoscopic Procedure		
cystoscope (SIS-toh-scope)	cyst/o = bladder -scope = instrument to visually examine	Instrument used to visually examine the inside of the urinary bladder.
cystoscopy (cysto) (sis-TOSS-koh-pee)	cyst/o = bladder -scopy = process of visually examining	Visual examination of the urinary bladder using an instrument called a *cystoscope.*
urethroscope (yoo-REE-throh-scope)	urethr/o = urethra -scope = instrument to visually examine	Instrument to visually examine the inside of the urethra.

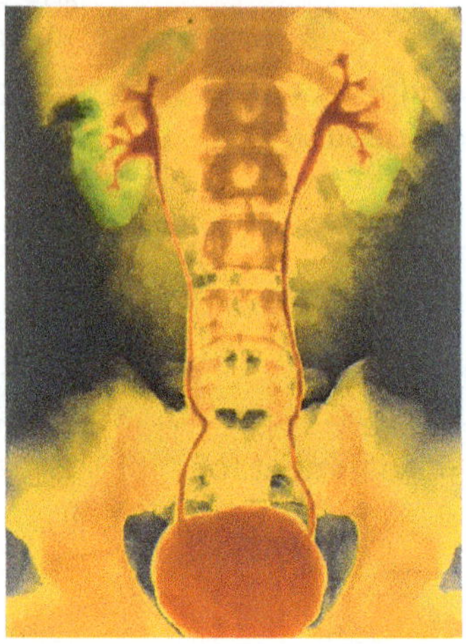

■ **Figure 9.11** Color-enhanced retrograde pyelogram X-ray. Radiopaque dye outlines urinary bladder, ureters, and renal pelvis. *(Clinique Ste. Catherine/CNRI/Science Photo Library/Photo Researchers, Inc.)*

Therapeutic Procedures

TERM	WORD PARTS	DEFINITION
Medical Treatments		
catheter (KATH-eh-ter)		Flexible tube inserted into the body for the purpose of moving fluids into or out of the body. Most commonly used to refer to a tube threaded through the urethra into the bladder to withdraw urine (see again Figure 9.9).
catheterization (cath) (kath-eh-ter-ih-ZAY-shun)		Insertion of a tube through the urethra and into the urinary bladder for the purpose of withdrawing urine or inserting dye.

Therapeutic Procedures *(continued)*

TERM	WORD PARTS	DEFINITION
extracorporeal shockwave lithotripsy (ESWL) (eks-trah-cor-POR-ee-al / shockwave / LITH-oh-trip-see)	extra- = outside of corpor/o = body -eal = pertaining to lith/o = stone -tripsy = surgical crushing	Use of ultrasound waves to break up stones. Process does not require invasive surgery.

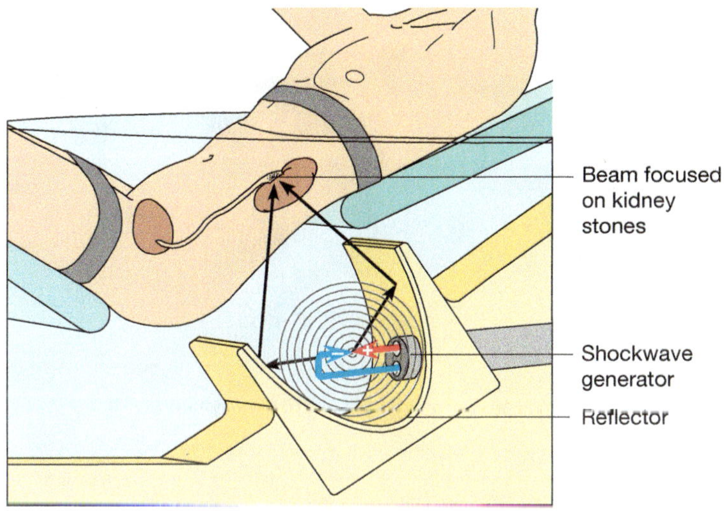

■ **Figure 9.12** Extracorporeal shockwave lithotripsy, a noninvasive procedure using high-frequency sound waves to shatter kidney stones.

TERM	WORD PARTS	DEFINITION
hemodialysis (HD) (hee-moh-dye-AL-ih-sis)	hem/o = blood	Use of an artificial kidney machine that filters the blood of a person to remove waste products. Use of this technique in patients who have defective kidneys is lifesaving.

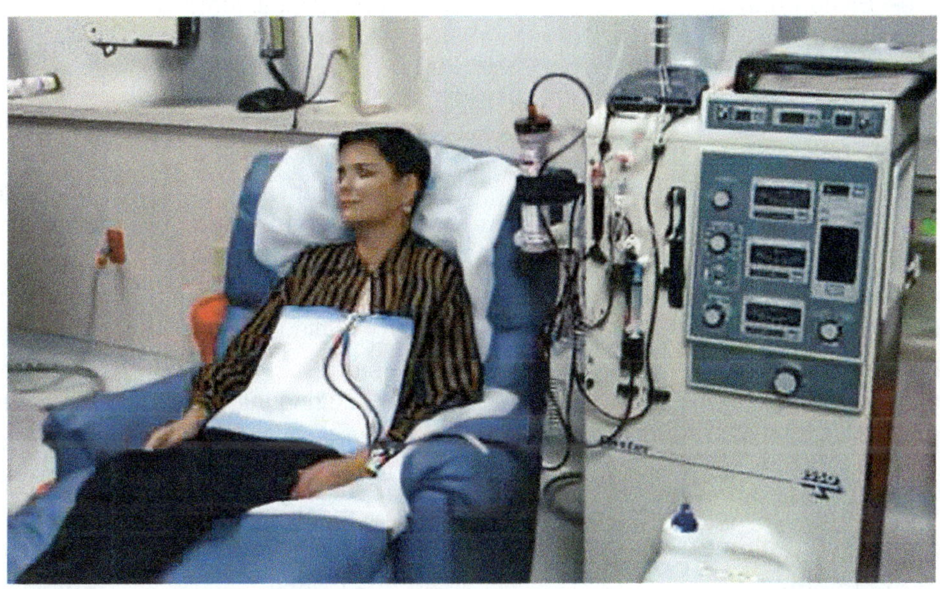

■ **Figure 9.13** Patient undergoing hemodialysis. Patient's blood passes through hemodialysis machine for cleansing and is then returned to her body.

Therapeutic Procedures *(continued)*

TERM	WORD PARTS	DEFINITION
peritoneal dialysis (pair-ih-TOH-nee-al / dye-AL-ih-sis)	peritone/o = peritoneum -eal = pertaining to	Removal of toxic waste substances from the body by placing warm chemically balanced solutions into the peritoneal cavity. Wastes are filtered out of the blood across the peritoneum. Used in treating renal failure and certain poisonings.

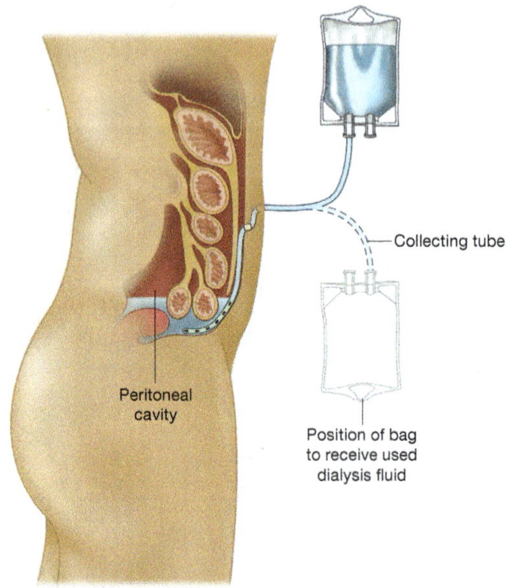

Figure 9.14 Peritoneal dialysis. Chemically balanced solution is placed into the abdominal cavity to draw impurities out of the bloodstream. It is removed after several hours.

Surgical Treatments

TERM	WORD PARTS	DEFINITION
cystectomy (sis-TEK-toh-me)	cyst/o = bladder -ectomy = surgical removal	Surgical removal of the urinary bladder.
cystopexy (SIS-toh-pek-see)	cyst/o = bladder -pexy = surgical fixation	Surgical fixation of the urinary bladder.
cystoplasty (SIS-toh-plas-tee)	cyst/o = bladder -plasty = surgical repair	To repair the urinary bladder by surgical means.
cystostomy (sis-TOSS-toh-mee)	cyst/o = bladder -ostomy = create a new opening	To create a new opening into the urinary bladder through the abdominal wall.
cystotomy (sis-TOT-oh-mee)	cyst/o = bladder -otomy = cutting into	To cut into the urinary bladder.
lithotomy (lith-OT-oh-me)	lith/o = stone -otomy = cutting into	To cut into an organ for the purpose of removing a stone.
lithotripsy (LITH-oh-trip-see)	lith/o = stone -tripsy = surgical crushing	Destroying or crushing stones in the bladder or urethra.
meatotomy (mee-ah-TOT-oh-me)	meat/o = meatus -otomy = cutting into	To cut into the meatus in order to enlarge the opening of the urethra.
nephrectomy (ne-FREK-toh-mee)	nephr/o = kidney -ectomy = surgical removal	Surgical removal of a kidney.
nephrolithotomy (nef-roh-lith-OT-oh-mee)	nephr/o = kidney lith/o = stone -otomy = cutting into	To cut into the kidney in order to remove stones.

Therapeutic Procedures *(continued)*

TERM	WORD PARTS	DEFINITION
nephropexy (NEF-roh-pek-see)	nephr/o = kidney -pexy = surgical fixation	Surgical fixation of a kidney; to anchor it in its normal anatomical position.
nephrostomy (neh-FROS-toh-mee)	nephr/o = kidney -ostomy = create a new opening	To create a new opening into the kidney through the abdominal wall.
nephrotomy (neh-FROT-oh-mee)	nephr/o = kidney -otomy = cutting into	To cut into the kidney.
pyeloplasty (PIE-ah-loh-plas-tee)	pyel/o = renal pelvis -plasty = surgical repair	To repair the renal pelvis by surgical means.
renal transplant	ren/o = kidney -al = pertaining to	Surgical placement of a donor kidney.

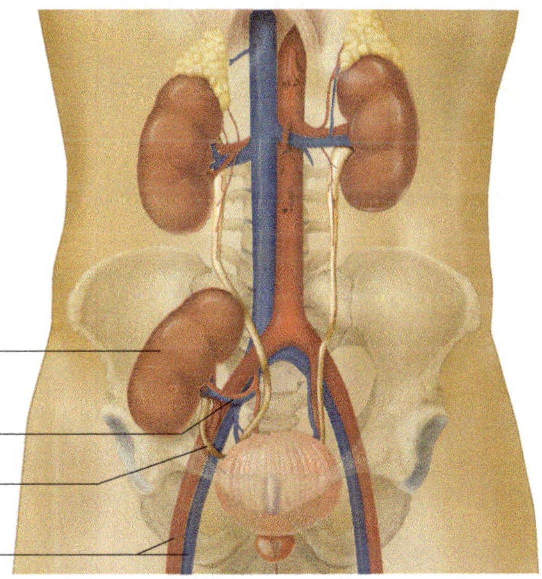

Figure 9.15 Figure illustrates location utilized for implantation of donor kidney.

Pharmacology

CLASSIFICATION	WORD PARTS	ACTION	EXAMPLES
antibiotic	anti- = against bi/o = life -tic = pertaining to	Used to treat bacterial infections of the urinary tract.	ciprofloxacin, Cipro; nitrofurantoin, Macrobid
antispasmodic (an-tye-spaz-MAH-dik)	anti- = against -ic = pertaining to	Medication to prevent or reduce bladder muscle spasms.	oxybutynin, Ditropan; neostigmine, Prostigmine
diuretic (dye-yoo-REH-tiks)	-tic = pertaining to	Medication that increases the volume of urine produced by the kidneys. Useful in the treatment of edema, kidney failure, heart failure, and hypertension.	furosemide, Lasix; spironolactone, Aldactone

Abbreviations

AGN	acute glomerulonephritis	**HD**	hemodialysis
ARF	acute renal failure	**H_2O**	water
ATN	acute tubular necrosis	**I&O**	intake and output
BNO	bladder neck obstruction	**IPD**	intermittent peritoneal dialysis
BUN	blood urea nitrogen	**IVP**	intravenous pyelogram
CAPD	continuous ambulatory peritoneal dialysis	**K^+**	potassium
cath	catheterization	**KUB**	kidneys, ureters, bladder
CC	clean catch urine specimen	**mL**	milliliter
Cl^-	chloride	**Na^+**	sodium
CRF	chronic renal failure	**NS**	nephrotic syndrome
C&S	culture and sensitivity	**pH**	acidity or alkalinity of urine
cysto	cystoscopy	**RP**	retrograde pyelogram
ESRD	end-stage renal disease	**SG, sp. gr.**	specific gravity
ESWL	extracorporeal shockwave lithotripsy	**U/A, UA**	urinalysis
EU	excretory urography	**UC**	urine culture
GU	genitourinary	**UTI**	urinary tract infection
HCO_3^-	bicarbonate	**VCUG**	voiding cystourethrography

Chapter Review

Real-World Applications

Medical Record Analysis

This Discharge Summary contains 13 medical terms. Underline each term and write it in the list below the report. Then define each term.

Discharge Summary

Admitting Diagnosis:	Severe right side pain and hematuria.
Final Diagnosis:	Pyelonephritis right kidney, complicated by chronic cystitis.
History of Present Illness:	Patient has long history of frequent bladder infections, but denies any recent lower pelvic pain or dysuria. Earlier today he had rapid onset of severe right side pain and is unable to stand fully erect. His temperature was 101°F, and his skin was sweaty and flushed. He was admitted from the ER for further testing and diagnosis.
Summary of Hospital Course:	Clean catch urinalysis revealed gross hematuria and pyuria, but no albuminuria. A culture and sensitivity was ordered to identify the pathogen and an antibiotic was started. Cystoscopy showed evidence of chronic cystitis, bladder irritation, and a bladder neck obstruction. The obstruction appears to be congenital and the probable cause of the chronic cystitis. The patient was catheterized to ensure complete emptying of the bladder, and fluids were encouraged. Patient responded well to the antibiotic therapy and fluids, and his symptoms improved.
Discharge Plans:	Patient was discharged home after 3 days in the hospital. He was switched to an oral antibiotic for the pyelonephritis and chronic cystitis. A repeat urinalysis is scheduled for next week. After all inflammation is corrected, will repeat cystoscopy to reevaluate bladder neck obstruction.

	Term	Definition
1	______________	______________________________
2	______________	______________________________
3	______________	______________________________
4	______________	______________________________
5	______________	______________________________
6	______________	______________________________
7	______________	______________________________
8	______________	______________________________
9	______________	______________________________
10	______________	______________________________
11	______________	______________________________
12	______________	______________________________
13	______________	______________________________

Chart Note Transcription

The chart note below contains 11 phrases that can be reworded with a medical term that you learned in this chapter. Each phrase is identified with an underline. Determine the medical term and write your answers in the space provided.

Current Complaint:	A 36-year-old male was seen by the specialist in the treatment of diseases of the urinary system ❶ because of right flank pain and blood in the urine. ❷
Past History:	Patient has a history of bladder infection; ❸ denies experiencing any symptoms for 2 years.
Signs and Symptoms:	A technique used to obtain an uncontaminated urine sample ❹ obtained for laboratory analysis of the urine ❺ revealed blood in the urine, but no pus in the urine. ❻ A kidney X-ray made after inserting dye into the bladder ❼ was normal on the left, but dye was seen filling the right tube between the kidney and bladder ❽ only halfway to the kidney.
Diagnosis:	Stone in the tube between the kidney and the bladder ❾ on the right.
Treatment:	Patient underwent the use of ultrasound waves to break up stones. ❿ Pieces of dissolved kidney stones ⓫ were flushed out, after which symptoms resolved.

❶ ______________________________

❷ ______________________________

❸ ______________________________

❹ ______________________________

❺ ______________________________

❻ ______________________________

❼ ______________________________

❽ ______________________________

❾ ______________________________

❿ ______________________________

⓫ ______________________________

Case Study

Below is a case study presentation of a patient with a condition discussed in this chapter. Read the case study and answer the questions below. Some questions will ask for information not included within this chapter. Use your text, a medical dictionary, or any other reference material you choose to answer these questions.

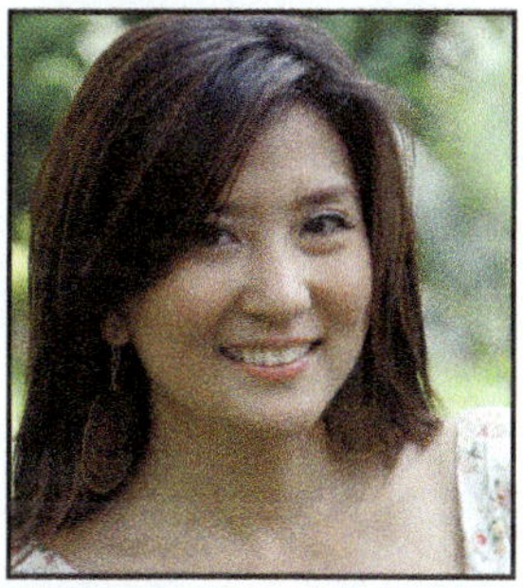
(Gina Smith/Shutterstock)

A 32-year-old female is seen in the urologist's office because of a fever, chills, and generalized fatigue. She also reported urgency, frequency, dysuria, and hematuria. In addition, she noticed that her urine was cloudy with a fishy odor. The physician ordered the following tests: a clean catch specimen for a U/A, a urine C&S, and a KUB. The U/A revealed pyuria, bacteriuria, and a slightly acidic pH. A common type of bacteria was grown in the culture. X-rays reveal acute pyelonephritis resulting from cystitis, which has spread up to the kidney from the bladder. The patient was placed on an antibiotic and encouraged to "push fluids" by drinking 2L of water a day.

Questions

1. This patient has two urinary system infections in different locations; name them. Which one caused the other and how?

____

____

2. List and define each of the patient's presenting symptoms in your own words.

____

____

3. What diagnostic tests did the urologist order? Describe them in your own words.

____

____

4. Explain the results of each diagnostic test in your own words.

____

____

5. What were the physician's treatment instructions for this patient? Explain the purpose of each treatment.

____

____

6. Describe the normal appearance of urine.

____

____

Practice Exercises

A. Complete the Statement

1. The functional or working units of the kidneys are the ______________________.
2. The three stages of urine production are ______________________, ______________________, and ______________________.
3. Na^+, K^+, and Cl^- are collectively known as ______________________.
4. The term that describes the location of the kidneys is ______________________.
5. The center of the concave side of the kidney is the ______________________.
6. The glomerular capsule surrounds the ______________________.
7. The tip of each renal pyramid opens into a(n) ______________________.
8. There are ______________________ ureters and ______________________ urethra.
9. Urination can also be referred to as ______________________ or ______________________.
10. A(n) ______________________ is the physical and chemical analysis of urine.

B. Combining Form Practice

The combining form **nephr/o** refers to the kidney. Use it to write a term that means:

1. surgical fixation of the kidney ______________________
2. X-ray record of the kidney ______________________
3. condition of kidney stones ______________________
4. removal of a kidney ______________________
5. inflammation of the kidney ______________________
6. kidney disease ______________________
7. hardening of the kidney ______________________

The combining form **cyst/o** refers to the urinary bladder. Use it to write a term that means:

8. inflammation of the bladder ______________________
9. abnormal flow condition from the bladder ______________________
10. surgical repair of the bladder ______________________
11. instrument to view inside the bladder ______________________
12. bladder pain ______________________

The combining form **pyel/o** refers to the renal pelvis. Use it to write a term that means:

13. surgical repair of the renal pelvis ______________________

14. inflammation of the renal pelvis ______________________

15. X-ray record of the renal pelvis ______________________

The combining form **ureter/o** refers to one or both of the ureters. Use it to write a term that means:

16. a ureteral stone ______________________

17. ureter dilation ______________________

18. ureter narrowing ______________________

The combining form **urethr/o** refers to the urethra. Use it to write a term that means:

19. urethra inflammation ______________________

20. instrument to view inside the urethra ______________________

C. Define the Combining Form

	Definition	Example from Chapter
1. **ur/o**	______________	______________
2. **meat/o**	______________	______________
3. **cyst/o**	______________	______________
4. **ren/o**	______________	______________
5. **pyel/o**	______________	______________
6. **glycos/o**	______________	______________
7. **noct/i**	______________	______________
8. **olig/o**	______________	______________
9. **ureter/o**	______________	______________
10. **glomerul/o**	______________	______________

D. Pharmacology Challenge

Fill in the classification for each drug description, then match the brand name.

	Drug Description	Classification	Brand Name
1.	_______ Reduces bladder muscle spasms	______________	a. Lasix
2.	_______ Treats bacterial infections	______________	b. Ditropan
3.	_______ Increases volume of urine produced	______________	c. Cipro

E. Define the Term

1. micturition ______________________
2. diuretic ______________________
3. renal colic ______________________
4. catheterization ______________________
5. pyelitis ______________________
6. glomerulonephritis ______________________
7. lithotomy ______________________
8. enuresis ______________________
9. meatotomy ______________________
10. diabetic nephropathy ______________________
11. urinalysis ______________________
12. hesitancy ______________________

F. Name That Term

1. absence of urine ______________________
2. blood in the urine ______________________
3. kidney stone ______________________
4. crushing a stone ______________________
5. inflammation of the urethra ______________________
6. pus in the urine ______________________
7. bacteria in the urine ______________________
8. painful urination ______________________
9. ketones in the urine ______________________
10. protein in the urine ______________________
11. (too) much urine ______________________

G. What's the Abbreviation?

1. potassium ______________________________
2. sodium ______________________________
3. urinalysis ______________________________
4. blood urea nitrogen ______________________________
5. specific gravity ______________________________
6. intravenous pyelogram ______________________________
7. bladder neck obstruction ______________________________
8. intake and output ______________________________
9. acute tubular necrosis ______________________________
10. end stage renal disease ______________________________

H. What Does it Stand For?

1. KUB ______________________________
2. cath ______________________________
3. cysto ______________________________
4. GU ______________________________
5. ESWL ______________________________
6. UTI ______________________________
7. UC ______________________________
8. RP ______________________________
9. ARF ______________________________
10. BUN ______________________________
11. CRF ______________________________
12. H_2O ______________________________

I. Terminology Matching

Match each term to its definition.

1. _______ Wilm's tumor
2. _______ electrolytes
3. _______ nephrons
4. _______ nephron loop
5. _______ calyx
6. _______ incontinence
7. _______ hydronephrosis
8. _______ urgency
9. _______ nephrolithiasis
10. _______ polycystic kidneys

a. kidney stones
b. feeling the need to urinate immediately
c. childhood malignant kidney tumor
d. swelling of the kidney due to urine collecting in the renal pelvis
e. involuntary release of urine
f. collects urine as it is produced
g. sodium and potassium
h. functional unit of the kidneys
i. part of the renal tubule
j. multiple cysts in the kidneys

J. Define the Suffix

	Definition	Example from Chapter
1. -ptosis	______________________	______________________
2. -uria	______________________	______________________
3. -lith	______________________	______________________
4. -tripsy	______________________	______________________
5. -lithiasis	______________________	______________________

K. Converting Between Units of Volume in the Metric System

All health care workers need a basic understanding of the metric system in order to complete daily duties. For example, a dental assistant may be asked to measure and mix materials when completing such tasks as creating study models. In order to measure volume, a dental assistant may use units such as milliliters, cubic centimeters, liters, and cubic liters.

Volume is the amount of space in a three-dimensional object. Volume can be measured with things such as beakers, measuring cups, measuring spoons, and graduated cylinders.

The following lists conversion information to change to different units of volume:

- 1,000 milliliters (mL) = 1 liter (L)
- 1 cubic centimeter (cm^3) = 1 milliliter (mL)
- 1,000 liters (1 L) = 1 cubic meter (m^3)

Example 1: Convert 3000 milliliters to liters.

1,000 mL = 1 L
1,000 × 3 = 1 L × 3
3,000 mL = 3 L

Example 2: Convert 500 cubic centimeters into liters.

Since 1 cm^3 = 1 mL then 500 cm^3 = 500 mL

You can use this information to help you figure out the answer:

1,000 mL = 1 L
1,000 / 2 = 1 / 2
500 mL = .5 L

If 500 mL equal .5 L then 500 cm^3 also equals .5 L.

a. Convert 10 cubic centimeters to milliliters.

b. Convert 2 cubic meters to liters.

c. Convert .25 liter to cubic centimeters.

What types of things might be measured in volume in a dental office? List the materials used to create study models. What are the appropriate quantities for each material?

Why is it important that the quantities are exact?

L. Fill in the Blank

renal transplant	ureterectomy	intravenous pyelogram (IVP)
cystostomy	pyelolithectomy	nephropexy
renal biopsy	cystoscopy	urinary tract infection

1. Juan suffered from chronic renal failure. His sister, Maria, donated one of her normal kidneys to him, and he had a(n) ______________________.
2. Anesha's floating kidney needed surgical fixation. Her physician performed a surgical procedure known as ______________________.
3. Kenya's physician stated that she had a general infection that he referred to as a UTI. The full name for this infection is ______________________.
4. The surgeons operated on Robert to remove calculi from his renal pelvis. The name of this surgery is ______________________.
5. Charles had to have a small piece of his kidney tissue removed so that the physician could perform a microscopic evaluation. This procedure is called a(n) ______________________.
6. Naomi had to have one of her ureters removed due to a stricture. This procedure is called ______________________.
7. The physician had to create a temporary opening between Eric's bladder and his abdominal wall. This procedure is called ______________________.
8. Sally's bladder was visually examined using a special instrument. This procedure is called a(n) ______________________.
9. The doctors believe that Jacob has a tumor of the right kidney. They are going to do a test called a(n) ______________________ that requires them to inject a radiopaque contrast medium intravenously so that they can see the kidney on X-ray.

Labeling Exercise

Image A

Write the labels for this figure on the numbered lines provided.

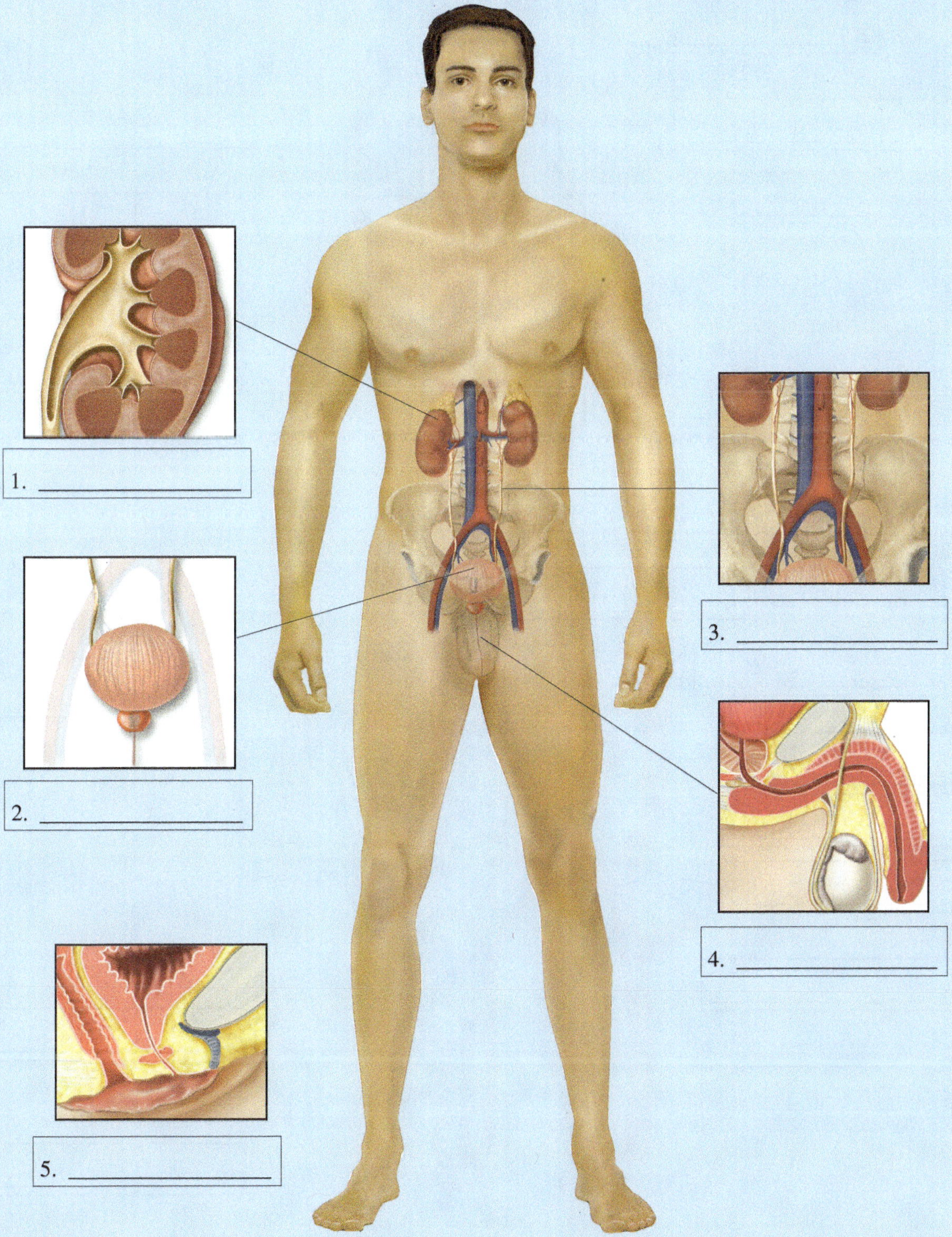

Image B

Write the labels for this figure on the numbered lines provided.

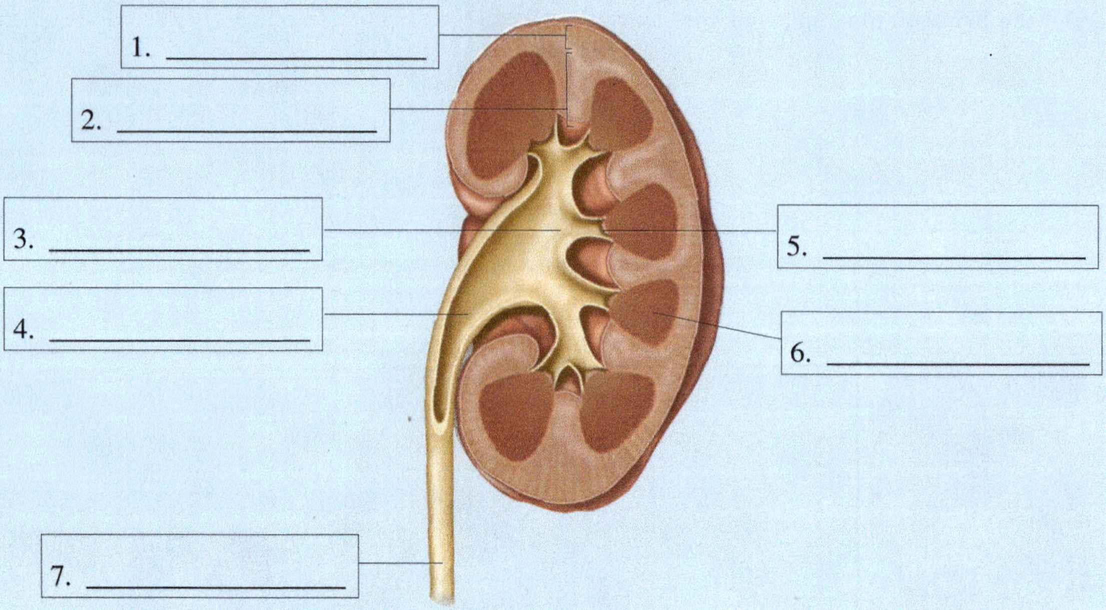

Image C

Write the labels for this figure on the numbered lines provided.

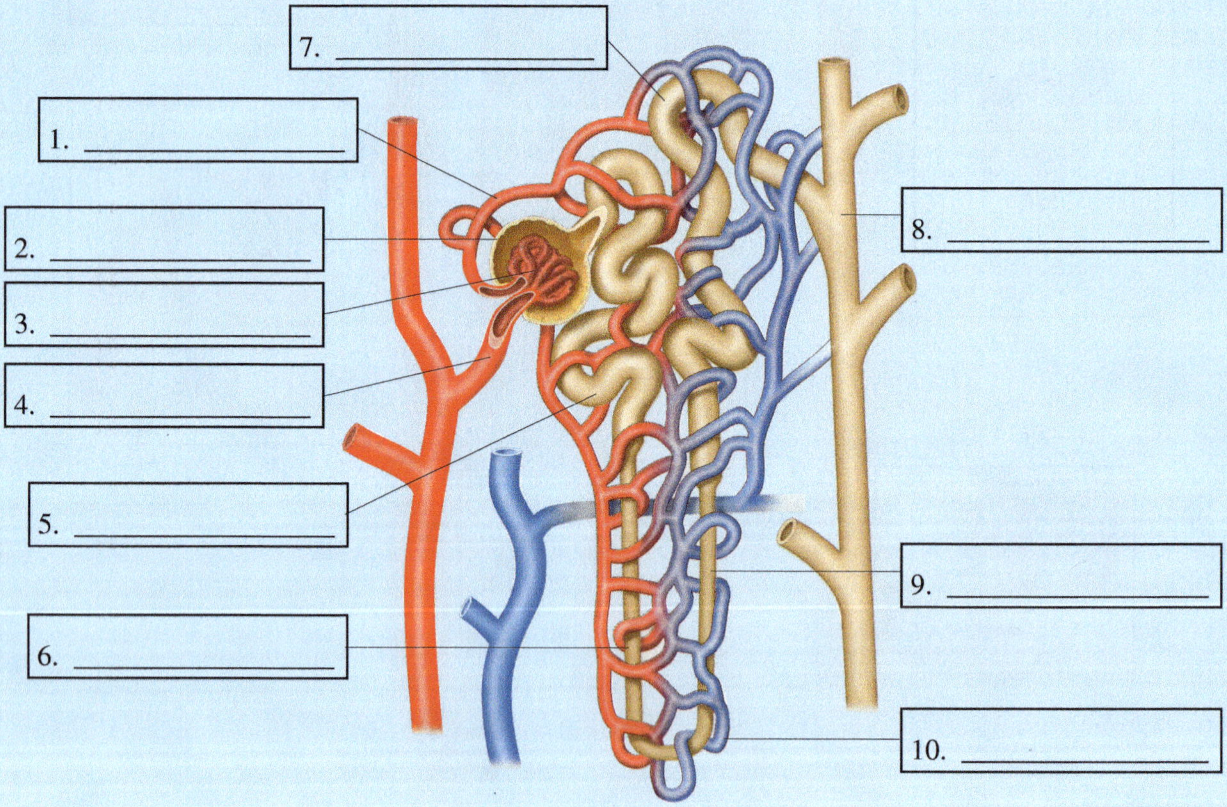

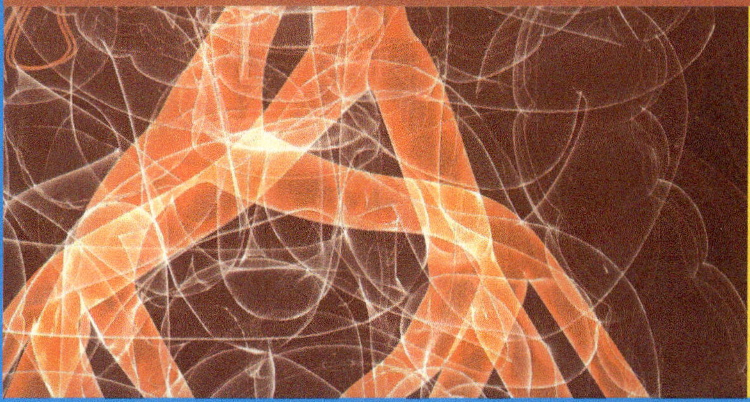

10

REPRODUCTIVE SYSTEM

Learning Objectives

Upon completion of this chapter, you will be able to

- Identify and define the combining forms and suffixes introduced in this chapter.
- Correctly spell and pronounce medical terms and major anatomical structures relating to the reproductive systems.
- Locate and describe the major organs of the reproductive systems and their functions.
- Use medical terms to describe circumstances relating to pregnancy.
- Identify the symptoms and origin of sexually transmitted diseases.
- Identify and define reproductive system anatomical terms.
- Identify and define selected reproductive system pathology terms.
- Identify and define selected reproductive system diagnostic procedures.
- Identify and define selected reproductive system therapeutic procedures.
- Identify and define selected medications relating to the reproductive systems.
- Define selected abbreviations associated with the reproductive systems.

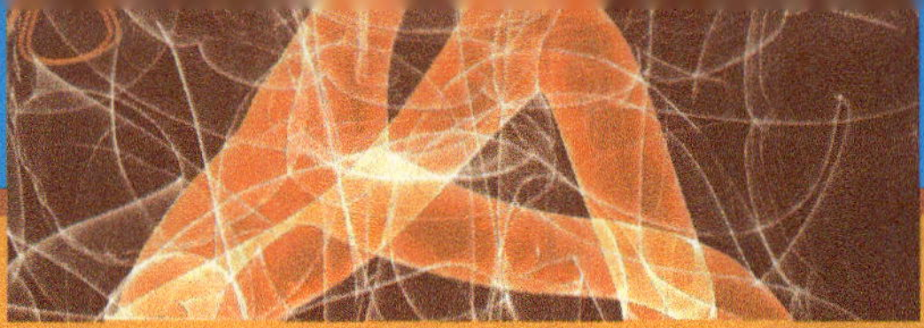

Section I: Female Reproductive System at a Glance

Function

The female reproductive system produces ova (the female reproductive cells), provides a location for fertilization and growth of a baby, and secretes female sex hormones. In addition, the breasts produce milk to nourish the newborn.

Structures

Here are the primary structures that comprise the female reproductive system.

breasts
uterine tubes
ovaries
uterus
vagina
vulva

Word Parts

Here are the most common word parts (with their meanings) used to build female reproductive system terms. For a more comprehensive list, refer to the Terminology section of this chapter.

Combining Forms

Combining Form	Meaning
amni/o	amnion
cervic/o	neck, cervix
chori/o	chorion
colp/o	vagina
culd/o	cul-de-sac
embry/o	embryo
episi/o	vulva
fet/o	fetus
gynec/o	woman, female
hymen/o	hymen
hyster/o	uterus
lact/o	milk
mamm/o	breast
mast/o	breast
men/o	menses, menstruation
metr/o	uterus
nat/o	birth
o/o	egg
oophor/o	ovary
ovari/o	ovary
perine/o	perineum
salping/o	uterine tubes, fallopian tubes
uter/o	uterus
vagin/o	vagina
vulv/o	vulva

Suffixes

Suffix	Meaning
-arche	beginning
-cyesis	state of pregnancy
-gravida	pregnancy
-para	to bear (offspring)
-partum	childbirth
-salpinx	uterine tube
-tocia	labor, childbirth

Female Reproductive System Illustrated

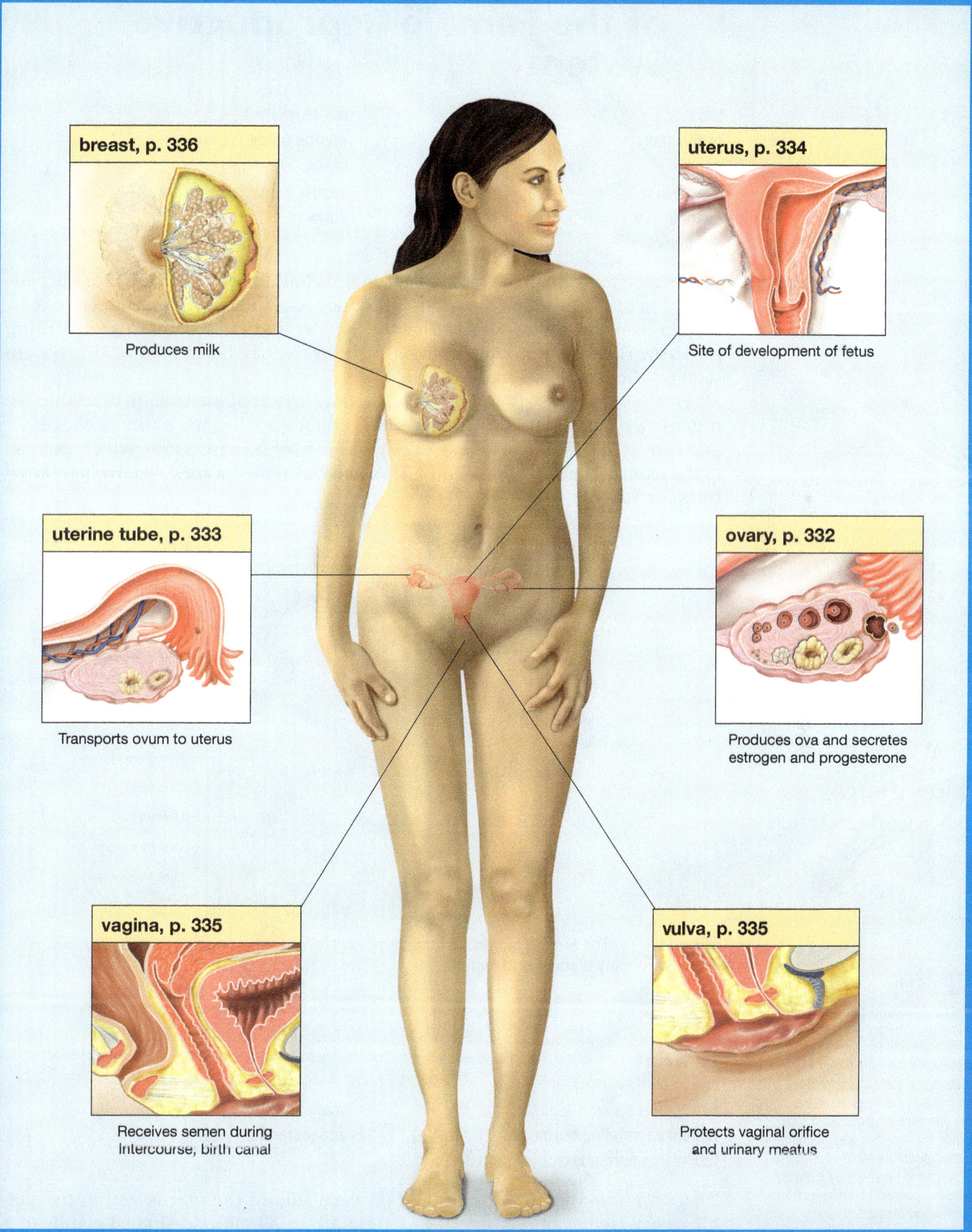

Anatomy and Physiology of the Female Reproductive System

breasts
fertilization
genitalia (jen-ih-TAY-lee-ah)
ova (OH-vah)
ovaries (OH-vah-reez)
pregnancy
sex hormones
uterine tubes (YOO-ter-in)
uterus (YOO-ter-us)
vagina (vah-JIGH-nah)
vulva (VULL-vah)

The female reproductive system plays many vital functions that ensure the continuation of the human race. First, it produces **ova,** the female reproductive cells. It then provides a place for **fertilization** to occur and for a baby to grow during **pregnancy.** The **breasts** provide nourishment for the newborn. Finally, this system secretes the female **sex hormones.**

This system consists of both internal and external **genitalia,** or reproductive organs (see Figure 10.1 ■). The internal genitalia are located in the pelvic cavity and consist of the **uterus,** two **ovaries,** two **uterine tubes,** and the **vagina,** which extends to the external surface of the body. The external genitalia are collectively referred to as the **vulva.**

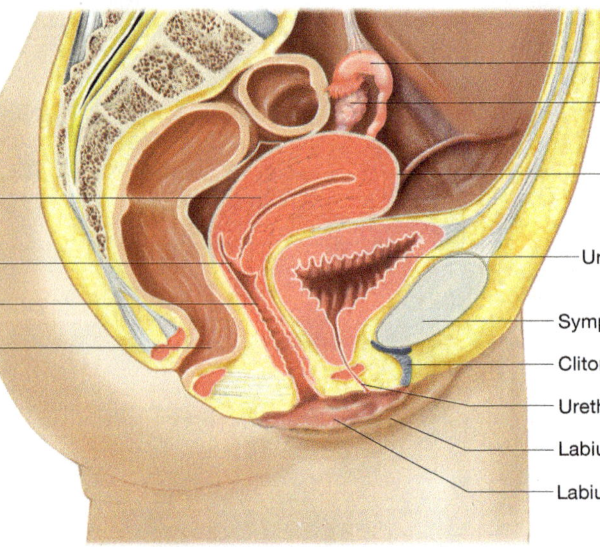

■ **Figure 10.1** The female reproductive system, sagittal view showing organs of the system in relation to the urinary bladder and rectum.

MED TERM TIP

The singular for egg is *ovum.* The plural term for many eggs is *ova.* The term *ova* is not used exclusively when discussing the human reproductive system. For instance, testing the stool for ova and parasites is used to detect the presence of parasites or their ova in the digestive tract, a common cause for severe diarrhea. Ova are produced in the ovary by a process called *oogenesis* (*o/o* = egg and *-genesis* = produced).

Internal Genitalia

Ovaries

estrogen (ESS-troh-jen)
follicle stimulating hormone (FOLL-ih-kl)
luteinizing hormone (loo-teh-NIGH-zing)
ovulation (ov-yoo-LAY-shun)
progesterone (proh-JES-ter-ohn)

There are two ovaries, one located on each side of the uterus within the pelvic cavity (see again Figure 10.1). These are small almond-shaped glands that produce ova (singular is *ovum*) and the female sex hormones (see Figure 10.2 ■). In humans approximately every 28 days hormones from the anterior pituitary, **follicle stimulating hormone** (FSH) and **luteinizing hormone** (LH), stimulate maturation of ovum and trigger **ovulation,** the process by which one ovary releases an ovum (see Figure 10.3 ■). The principal female sex hormones produced by the ovaries, **estrogen** and **progesterone,** stimulate the lining of the uterus to be prepared to receive a fertilized ovum. These hormones are also responsible for the female secondary sexual characteristics.

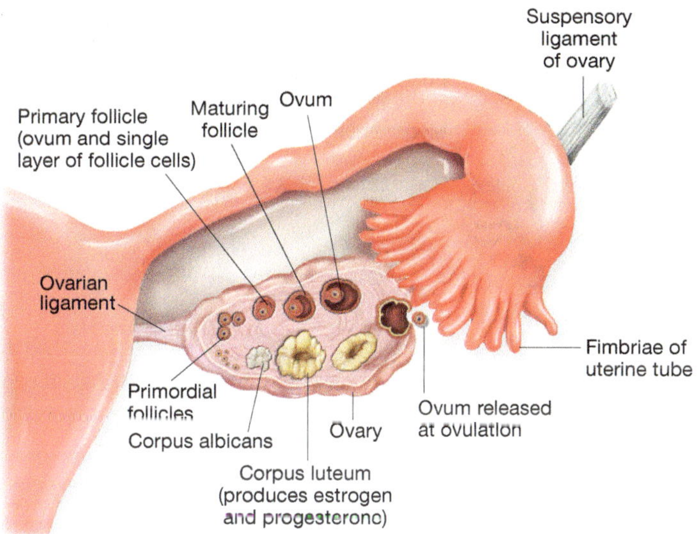

■ **Figure 10.2** Structure of the ovary and uterine (fallopian) tube. Figure illustrates stages of ovum development and the relationship of the ovary to the uterine tube.

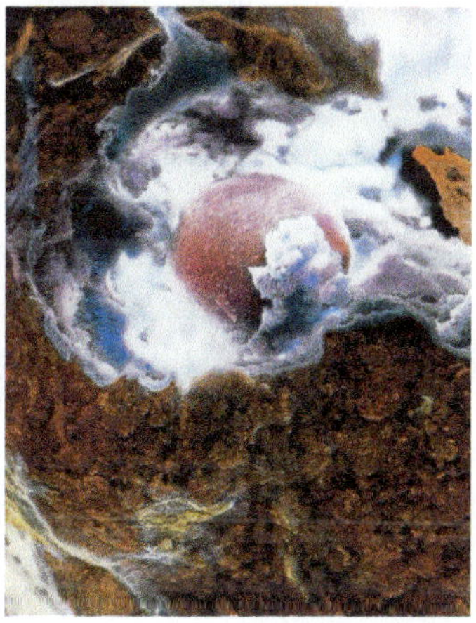

■ **Figure 10.3** Color-enhanced scanning electron micrograph showing an ovum (pink) released by the ovary at ovulation surrounded by follicle (white) tissue. The external surface of the ovary is brown in this photo. *(P.M. Motta and J. Van Blekrom/Science Photo Library/Photo Researchers, Inc.)*

Uterine Tubes

conception (con-SEP-shun)
fallopian tubes (fah-LOH-pee-an)
fimbriae (FIM-bree-ay)
oviducts (OH-vih-ducts)

The uterine tubes, also called the **fallopian tubes** or **oviducts,** are approximately 5 1/2 inches long and run from the area around each ovary to either side of the upper portion of the uterus (see Figures 10.4 ■ and 10.5 ■). As they near the ovaries,

MED TERM TIP

When the fertilized egg adheres or implants to the uterine tube instead of moving into the uterus, a condition called *tubal pregnancy* exists. There is not enough room in the uterine tube for the fetus to grow normally. Implantation of the fertilized egg in any location other than the uterus is called an *ectopic pregnancy. Ectopic* is a general term meaning "in the wrong place."

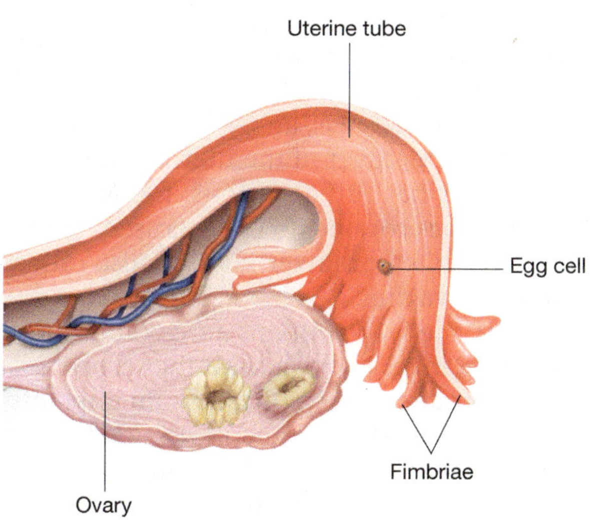

■ **Figure 10.4** Uterine (fallopian) tube, showing released ovum within the uterine tube.

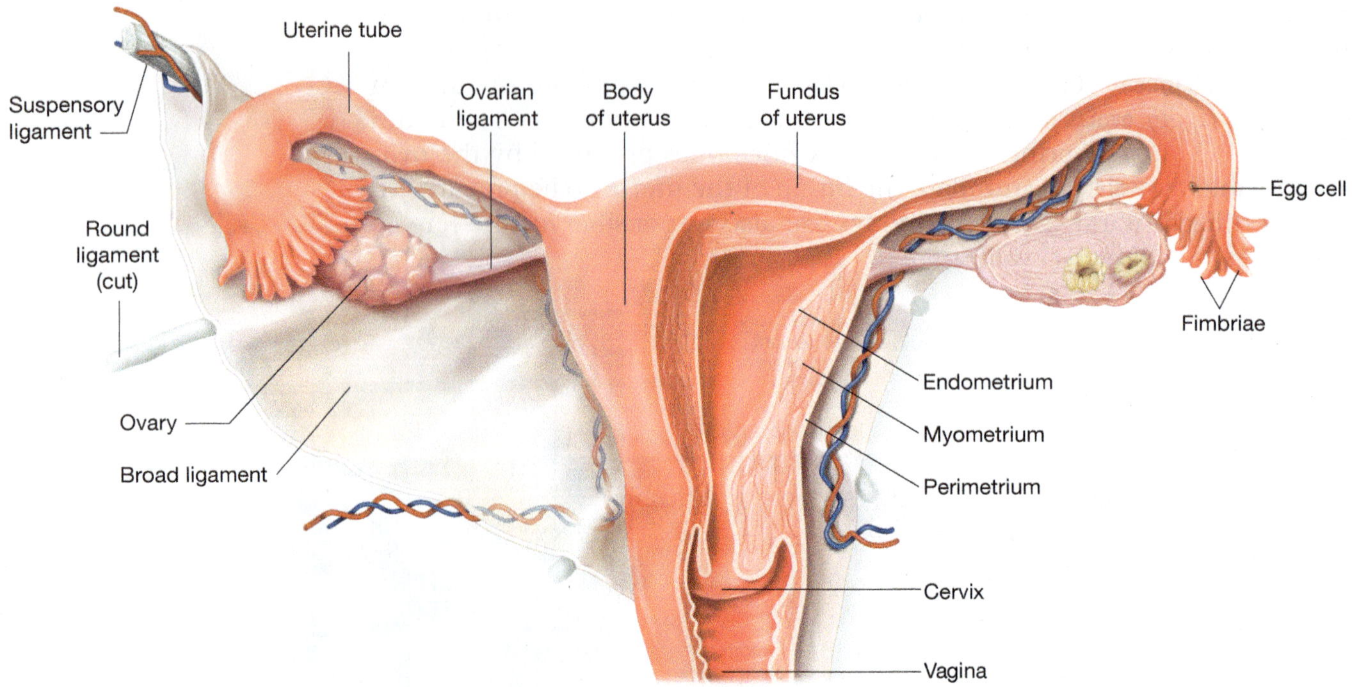

Figure 10.5 The uterus. Cutaway view shows regions of the uterus and cervix and its relationship to the uterine (fallopian) tubes and vagina.

the unattached ends of these two tubes expand into finger-like projections called **fimbriae.** The fimbriae catch an ovum after ovulation and direct it into the uterine tube. The uterine tube can then propel the ovum from the ovary to the uterus so that it can implant. The meeting of the egg and sperm, called fertilization or **conception,** normally takes place within the upper one-half of the uterine tubes.

Uterus

anteflexion (an-tee-FLEK-shun)
cervix (SER-viks)
corpus (KOR-pus)
endometrium (en-doh-MEE-tre-um)
fundus (FUN-dus)
menarche (men-AR-kee)
menopause (MEN-oh-pawz)
menstrual period (MEN-stroo-all)
menstruation (men-stroo-AY-shun)
myometrium (my-oh-MEE-tre-um)
perimetrium (pear-ee-MEE-tre-um)
puberty (PEW-ber-tee)

MED TERM TIP

During pregnancy, the height of the fundus is an important measurement for estimating the stage of pregnancy and the size of the fetus. Following birth, massaging the fundus with pressure applied in a circular pattern stimulates the uterine muscle to contract to help stop bleeding. Patients may be more familiar with a common term for uterus, *womb*. However, the correct medical term is uterus.

The uterus is a hollow, pear-shaped organ that contains a thick muscular wall, a mucous membrane lining, and a rich supply of blood (see again Figure 10.5). It lies in the center of the pelvic cavity between the bladder and the rectum. It is normally bent slightly forward, which is called **anteflexion,** and is held in position by strong fibrous ligaments anchored in the outer layer of the uterus, called the **perimetrium** (see again Figure 10.1). The uterus has three sections: the **fundus** or upper portion, between where the uterine tubes connect to the uterus; **corpus** or body, which is the central portion; and **cervix** (Cx), or lower portion, also called the neck of the uterus, which opens into the vagina.

The inner layer, or **endometrium,** of the uterine wall contains a rich blood supply. The endometrium reacts to hormonal changes every month that prepare it to receive a fertilized ovum. In a normal pregnancy the fertilized ovum implants in the endometrium, which can then provide nourishment and protection for the developing fetus. Contractions of the thick muscular walls of the uterus, called the **myometrium,** assist in propelling the fetus through the birth canal at delivery.

If a pregnancy is not established, the endometrium is sloughed off, resulting in **menstruation** or the **menstrual period.** During a pregnancy, the lining of the uterus does not leave the body but remains to nourish the fetus. A girl's first menstrual period occurs during **puberty** (the sequence of events by which a child becomes a young adult capable of reproduction) and is called **menarche** (*men/o* = menstruation, *-arche* = beginning), while the ending of menstrual activity and childbearing years is called **menopause.** This generally occurs between the ages of 40 and 55.

MED TERM TIP

Word Watch: Be careful using the combining forms *uter/o* meaning "uterus" and *ureter/o* meaning "ureter."

Vagina

Bartholin's glands (BAR-toh-linz)
hymen (HIGH-men)
vaginal orifice (VAJ-ih-nal / OR-ih-fis)

The vagina is a muscular tube lined with mucous membrane that extends from the cervix of the uterus to the outside of the body (see Figure 10.6 ■). The vagina allows for the passage of the menstrual flow. In addition, during intercourse, it receives the male's penis and semen, which is the fluid containing sperm. The vagina also serves as the birth canal through which the baby passes during a normal vaginal birth.

The **hymen** is a thin membranous tissue that partially covers the external vaginal opening or **vaginal orifice.** This membrane is broken by the use of tampons, during physical activity, or during sexual intercourse. A pair of glands (called **Bartholin's glands**) are located on either side of the vaginal orifice and secrete mucus for lubrication during intercourse.

Vulva

MED TERM TIP

Word Watch: Be careful using the combining forms *colp/o* meaning "vagina" and *culd/o* meaning "cul-de-sac (rectouterine pouch)."

clitoris (KLIT-oh-ris)
erectile tissue (ee-REK-tile)
labia majora (LAY-bee-ah / mah-JOR-ah)
labia minora (LAY-bee-ah / min-NOR-ah)
perineum (pair-ih-NEE-um)
urinary meatus (YOO-rih-nair-ee / mee-AY-tus)

The vulva is a general term that refers to the group of structures that make up the female external genitalia. The **labia majora** and **labia minora** are folds of skin that serve as protection for the genitalia, the vaginal orifice, and the **urinary meatus** (see Figure 10.7 ■). Since the urinary tract and the reproductive organs are located in proximity to one another and each contains mucous membranes that can transport infection, there is a danger of infection entering the urinary tract. The

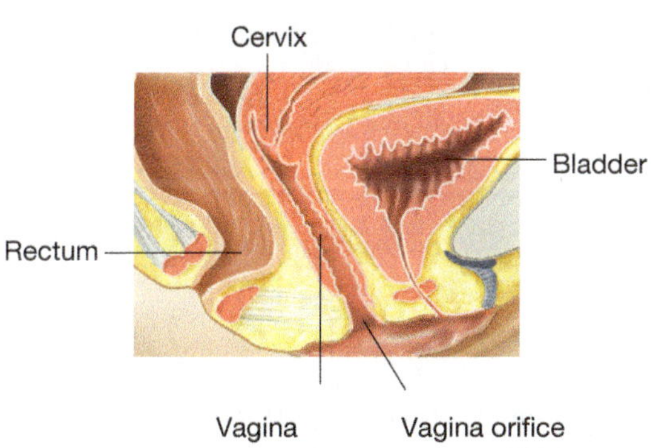

■ **Figure 10.6** The vagina, sagittal section showing the location of the vagina and its relationship to the cervix, uterus, rectum, and bladder.

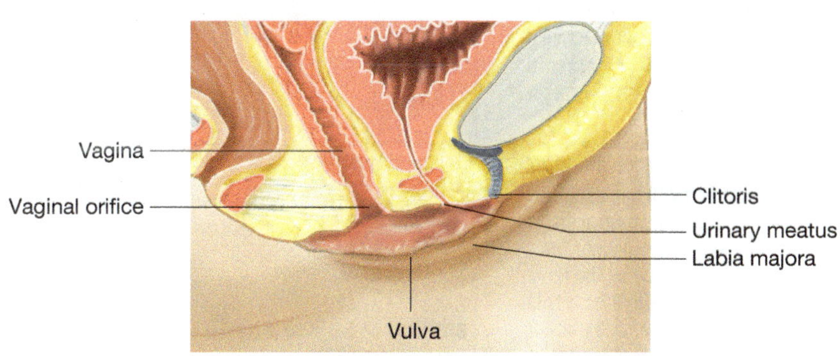

■ **Figure 10.7** The vulva, sagittal section illustrating how the labia majora and labia minora cover and protect the vaginal orifice, clitoris, and urinary meatus.

clitoris is a small organ containing sensitive **erectile tissue** that is aroused during sexual stimulation and corresponds to the penis in the male. The region between the vaginal orifice and the anus is referred to as the **perineum.**

Breast

areola (ah-REE-oh-la)
lactation (lak-TAY-shun)
lactiferous ducts (lak-TIF-er-us)
lactiferous glands (lak-TIF-er-us)
mammary glands (MAM-ah-ree)
nipple
nurse

The breasts, or **mammary glands,** play a vital role in the reproductive process because they produce milk, a process called **lactation,** to nourish the newborn. The size of the breasts, which varies greatly from woman to woman, has no bearing on the ability to **nurse** or feed a baby. Milk is produced by the **lactiferous glands** and is carried to the **nipple** by the **lactiferous ducts** (see Figure 10.8 ■). The **areola** is the pigmented area around the nipple. As long as the breast is stimulated by the nursing infant, the breast will continue to secrete milk.

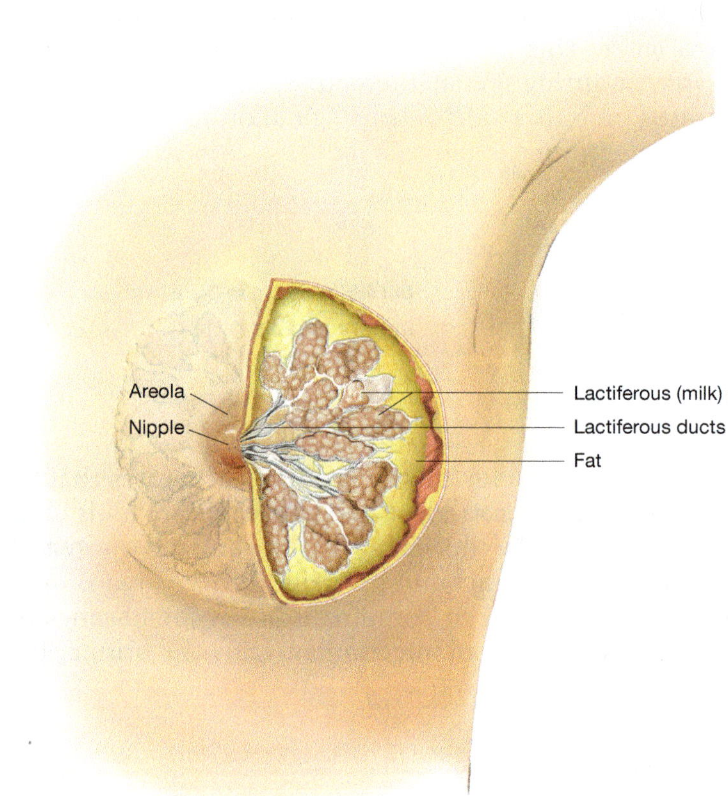

■ **Figure 10.8** The breast, cutaway view showing both internal and external features.

MED TERM TIP

The term *abortion* (AB) has different meanings for medical professionals and the general population. The general population equates the term *abortion* specifically with the planned termination of a pregnancy. However, to the medical community, abortion is a broader medical term meaning that a pregnancy has ended before a fetus is *viable*, meaning before it can live on its own.

Pregnancy

amnion (AM-nee-on)
amniotic fluid (am-nee-OT-ik)
chorion (KOR-ree-on)
embryo (EM-bree-oh)
fetus (FEE-tus)
gestation (jess-TAY-shun)
placenta (plah-SEN-tah)
premature
umbilical cord (um-BILL-ih-kal)

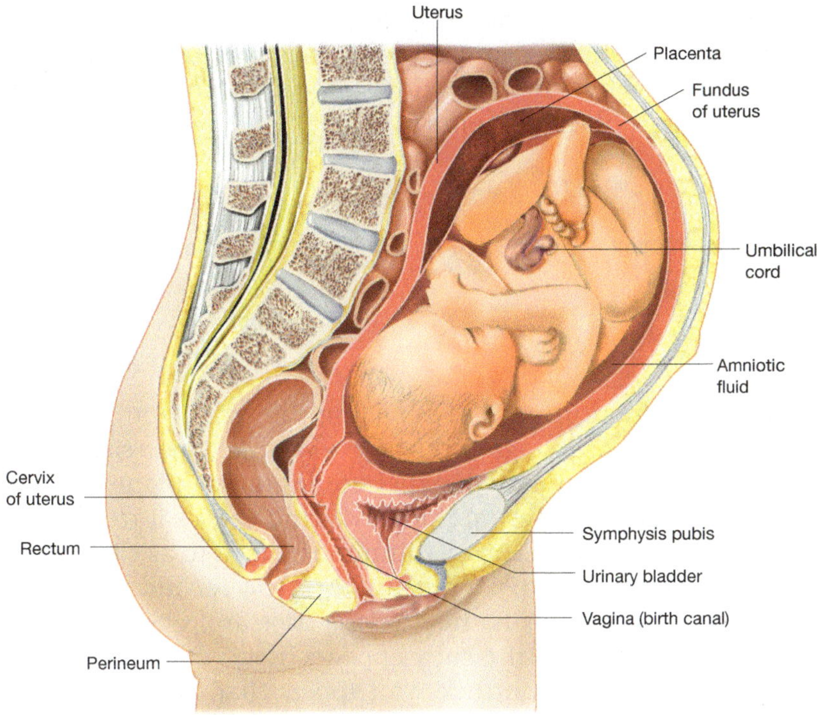

■ **Figure 10.9** A full-term pregnancy. Image illustrates position of the fetus and the structures associated with pregnancy.

Pregnancy refers to the period of time during which a fetus grows and develops in its mother's uterus (see Figure 10.9 ■). The normal length of time for a pregnancy (**gestation**) is 40 weeks. If a baby is born before completing at least 37 weeks of gestation, it is considered **premature.**

During pregnancy the female body undergoes many changes. In fact, all of the body systems become involved in the development of a healthy infant. From the time the fertilized egg implants in the uterus until approximately the end of the eighth week, the infant is referred to as an **embryo** (see Figure 10.10 ■). During this period all the major organs and body systems are formed. Following the embryo stage and lasting until birth, the infant is called a **fetus** (see Figure 10.11 ■). During this time, the longest period of gestation, the organs mature and begin to function.

MED TERM TIP

During the embryo stage of gestation, the organs and organ systems of the body are formed. Therefore, this is a very common time for *congenital anomalies*, or birth defects, to occur. This may happen before the woman is even aware of being pregnant.

The fetus receives nourishment from its mother by way of the **placenta,** which is a spongy, blood-filled organ that forms in the uterus next to the fetus. The placenta is commonly referred to as the afterbirth. The fetus is attached to the

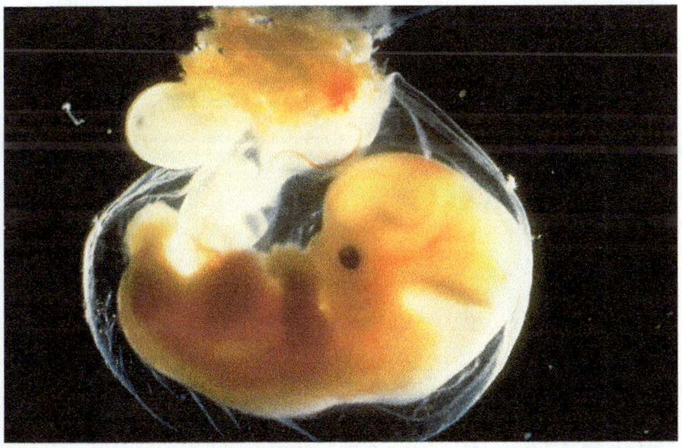

■ **Figure 10.10** Photograph illustrating the development of an embryo. *(Photo Researchers, Inc.)*

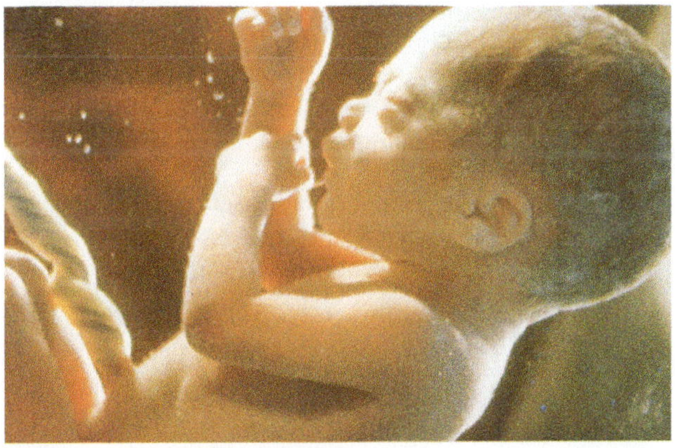

■ **Figure 10.11** Photograph illustrating the development of a fetus. *(Petit Format/Photo Researchers, Inc.)*

placenta by way of the **umbilical cord** and is surrounded by two membranous sacs, the **amnion** and the **chorion.** The amnion is the innermost sac, and it holds the **amniotic fluid** in which the fetus floats. The chorion is an outer, protective sac and also forms part of the placenta.

Labor and Delivery

breech presentation
crowning
delivery
dilation stage (dye-LAY-shun)
effacement (eh-FACE-ment)
expulsion stage (ex-PULL-shun)
labor
placental stage (plah-SEN-tal)

Labor is the actual process of expelling the fetus from the uterus and through the vagina. The first stage is referred to as the **dilation stage,** in which the uterine muscle contracts strongly to expel the fetus (see Figure 10.12A ■). During this process the fetus presses on the cervix and causes it to dilate or expand. As the cervix dilates, it also becomes thinner, referred to as **effacement.** When the cervix is completely dilated to 10 centimeters, the second stage of labor begins (see Figure 10.12B ■). This is the **expulsion stage** and ends with **delivery** of the baby. Generally, the head of the baby appears first, which is referred to as **crowning.** In some cases the baby's buttocks will appear first, and this is referred to as a **breech presentation** (see Figure 10.13 ■). The last stage of labor is the **placental stage** (see Figure 10.12C ■). Immediately after childbirth, the uterus continues to contract, causing the placenta to be expelled through the vagina.

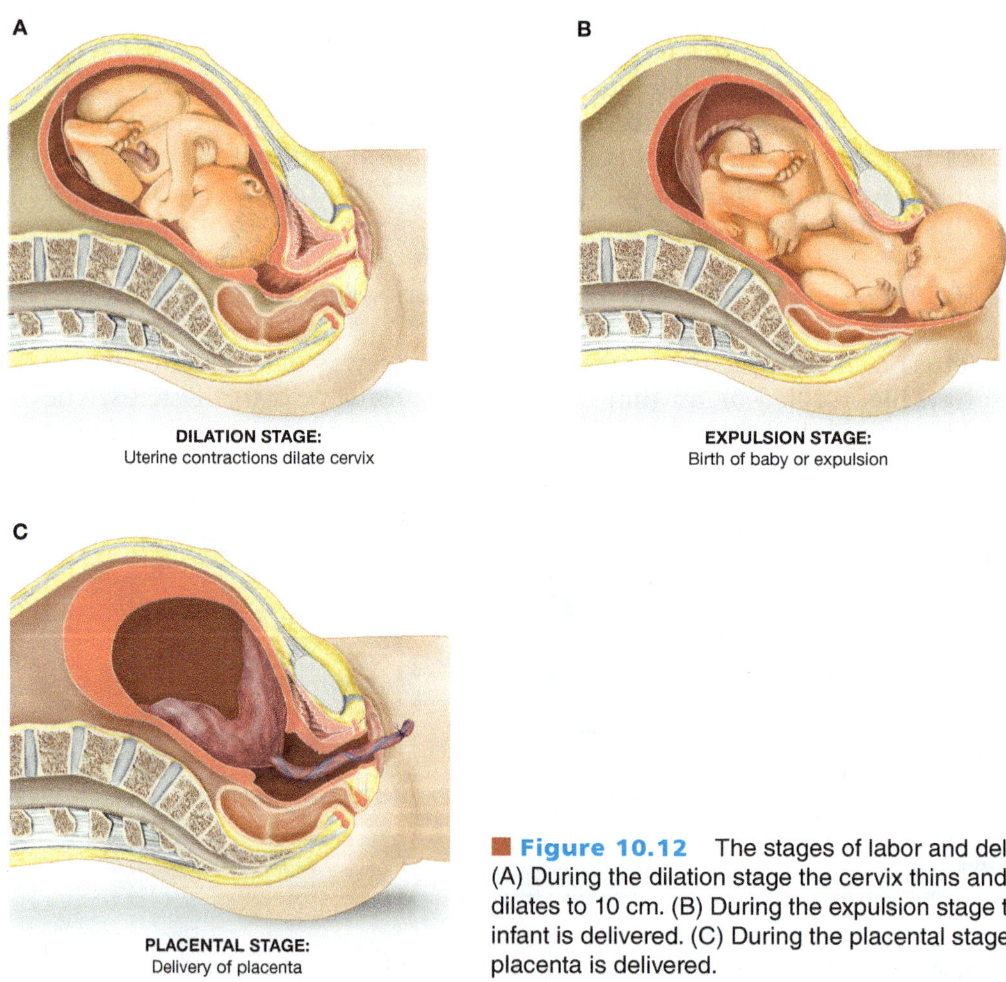

■ **Figure 10.12** The stages of labor and delivery. (A) During the dilation stage the cervix thins and dilates to 10 cm. (B) During the expulsion stage the infant is delivered. (C) During the placental stage the placenta is delivered.

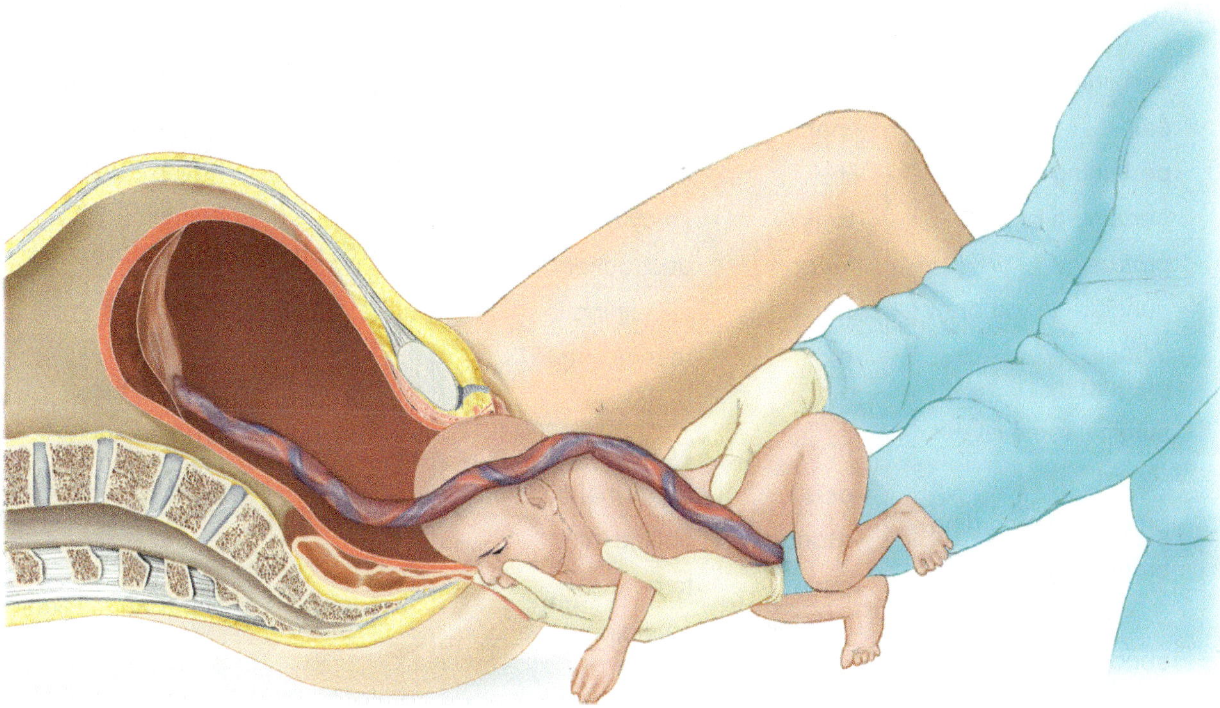

■ **Figure 10.13** A breech birth. This image illustrates a newborn that has been delivered buttocks first.

Terminology

Word Parts Used to Build Female Reproductive System Terms

The following lists contain the combining forms, suffixes, and prefixes used to build terms in the remaining sections of this chapter.

Combining Forms

abdomin/o	abdomen
amni/o	amnion
bi/o	life
carcin/o	cancer
cervic/o	cervix
chori/o	chorion
colp/o	vagina
culd/o	cul-de-sac
cyst/o	bladder, pouch
embry/o	embryo
episi/o	vulva
fet/o	fetus
fibr/o	fibers
gynec/o	woman

hem/o	blood
hemat/o	blood
hymen/o	hymen
hyster/o	uterus
lact/o	milk
lapar/o	abdomen
later/o	side
mamm/o	breast
mast/o	breast
men/o	menstruation
metr/o	uterus
nat/o	birth
olig/o	scanty
oophor/o	ovary

or/o	mouth
ovari/o	ovary
pelv/o	pelvis
perine/o	perineum
py/o	pus
rect/o	rectum
salping/o	uterine tube
son/o	sound
tox/o	poison
uter/o	uterus
vagin/o	vagina
vulv/o	vulva

Suffixes

-al	pertaining to
-algia	pain
-an	pertaining to
-ary	pertaining to
-cele	protrusion
-centesis	puncture to withdraw fluid
-cyesis	pregnancy
-ectomy	surgical removal
-gram	record
-graphy	process of recording
-gravida	pregnancy
-ia	condition
-iasis	abnormal condition
-ic	pertaining to
-ine	pertaining to
-itis	inflammation
-logy	study of
-lytic	destruction
-nic	pertaining to
-oid	resembling
-oma	tumor
-opsy	to view
-osis	abnormal condition
-otomy	cutting into
-para	to bear
-partum	childbirth
-pexy	surgical fixation
-plasty	surgical repair
-rrhagia	abnormal flow condition
-rrhaphy	suture
-rrhea	discharge
-rrhexis	rupture
-salpinx	uterine tube
-scope	instrument for viewing
-scopy	process of viewing
-tic	pertaining to
-tocia	labor and childbirth

Prefixes

a-	without
ante-	before
bi-	two
contra-	against
dys-	abnormal, difficult
endo-	within
in-	not
intra-	inside
multi-	many
neo-	new
nulli-	none
peri-	around
post-	after
pre-	before
primi-	first
pseudo-	false
ultra-	beyond

Anatomical Terms

TERM	WORD PARTS	DEFINITION
amniotic (am-nee-OT-ik)	amni/o = amnion -tic = pertaining to	Pertaining to the amnion.
cervical (SER-vih-kal)	cervic/o = cervix -al = pertaining to	Pertaining to the cervix.
chorionic (koh-ree-ON-ik)	chori/o = chorion -nic = pertaining to	Pertaining to the chorion.
embryonic (em-bree-ON-ik)	embry/o = embryo -nic = pertaining to	Pertaining to the embryo.
fetal (FEE-tall)	fet/o = fetus -al = pertaining to	Pertaining to the fetus.
lactic (LAK-tik)	lact/o = milk -ic = pertaining to	Pertaining to milk.
mammary (MAM-mah-ree)	mamm/o = breast -ary = pertaining to	Pertaining to the breast.

Anatomical Terms *(continued)*

TERM	WORD PARTS	DEFINITION
ovarian (oh-VAIR-ee-an)	ovari/o = ovary -an = pertaining to	Pertaining to the ovary.
perineal (per-ih-NEE-al)	perine/o = perineum -al = pertaining to	Pertaining to the perineum.
uterine (YOO-ter-in)	uter/o = uterus -ine = pertaining to	Pertaining to the uterus.
vaginal (VAJ-ih-nal)	vagin/o = vagina -al = pertaining to	Pertaining to the vagina.
vulvar (VUL-var)	vulv/o = vulva -ar = pertaining to	Pertaining to the vulva.

Pregnancy Terms

TERM	WORD PARTS	DEFINITION
antepartum (an-tee-PAR-tum)	ante- = before -partum = childbirth	Period of time before birth.
colostrum (kuh-LOS trum)		Thin fluid first secreted by the breast after delivery. It does not contain much protein, but is rich in antibodies.
fraternal twins	-al = pertaining to	Twins that develop from two different ova fertilized by two different sperm. Although twins, these siblings do not have identical DNA.
identical twins	-al = pertaining to	Twins that develop from the splitting of one fertilized ovum. These siblings have identical DNA.
lactorrhea (lak-toh-REE-ah)	lact/o = milk -rrhea = flow	Discharge of milk from the breast.
meconium (meh-KOH-nee-um)		First bowel movement of a newborn. It is greenish-black in color and consists of mucus and bile.
multigravida (mull-tih-GRAV-ih-dah)	multi- = many -gravida = pregnancy	A woman who has been pregnant two or more times.
multipara (mull-TIP-ah-rah)	multi- = many -para = to bear	A woman who has given birth to a live infant two or more times.
neonate (NEE-oh-nayt)	neo- = new nat/o = birth	Term for a newborn baby.
nulligravida (null-ih-GRAV-ih-dah)	nulli- = none -gravida = pregnancy	A woman who has not been pregnant.
nullipara (null-IP-ah-rah)	nulli- = none -para = to bear	A woman who has not given birth to a live infant.
postpartum (post-PAR-tum)	post- = after -partum = childbirth	Period of time shortly after birth.
primigravida (prem-ih-GRAV-ih-dah)	primi- = first -gravida = pregnancy	A woman who is pregnant for the first time.
primipara (prem-IP-ah-rah)	primi- = first -para = to bear	A woman who has given birth to a live infant once.

Pathology

TERM	WORD PARTS	DEFINITION
Medical Specialties		
gynecology (GYN) (gigh-neh-KOL-oh-jee)	gynec/o = woman -logy = study of	Branch of medicine specializing in the diagnosis and treatment of conditions of the female reproductive system. Physician is called a *gynecologist.*
neonatology (nee-oh-nay-TALL-oh-jee)	neo- = new nat/o = birth -logy = study of	Branch of medicine specializing in the diagnosis and treatment of conditions involving newborns. Physician is called a *neonatologist.*
obstetrics (OB) (ob-STET-riks)		Branch of medicine specializing in the diagnosis and treatment of women during pregnancy and childbirth, and immediately after childbirth. Physician is called an *obstetrician.*
Signs and Symptoms		
amenorrhea (ah-men-oh-REE-ah)	a- = without men/o = menstruation -rrhea = flow	Condition of having no menstrual flow.
amniorrhea (am-nee-oh-REE-ah)	amni/o = amnion -rrhea = flow	Flow of amniotic fluid when the amnion ruptures.
dysmenorrhea (dis-men-oh-REE-ah)	dys- = abnormal, painful men/o = menstruation -rrhea = flow	Condition of having abnormal or painful menstrual flow.
dystocia (dis-TOH-she-ah)	dys- = abnormal, difficult -tocia = labor and childbirth	Difficult labor and childbirth.
hematosalpinx (hee-mah-toh-SAL-pinks)	hemat/o = blood -salpinx = uterine tube	Presence of blood in a uterine tube.
mastalgia (mas-TAL-jee-ah)	mast/o = breast -algia = pain	Breast pain.
menorrhagia (men-oh-RAY-jee-ah)	men/o = menstruation -rrhagia = abnormal flow condition	Condition of having abnormally heavy menstrual flow during normal menstruation time.
metrorrhagia (meh-troh-RAY-jee-ah)	metr/o = uterus -rrhagia = abnormal flow condition	Term is used to describe uterine bleeding between menstrual periods.
metrorrhea (meh-troh-REE-ah)	metr/o = uterus -rrhea = discharge	Having a discharge (such as mucus or pus) from the uterus that is not the menstrual flow.
oligomenorrhea (ol-lih-goh-men-oh-REE-ah)	olig/o = scanty men/o = menstruation -rrhea = flow	Condition of having light menstrual flow.
Ovary		
oophoritis (oh-off-oh-RIGH-tis)	oophor/o = ovary -itis = inflammation	Inflammation of the ovary.

Pathology *(continued)*

TERM	WORD PARTS	DEFINITION
ovarian carcinoma (oh-VAY-ree-an / kar-sih-NOH-mah)	ovari/o = ovary -an = pertaining to carcin/o = cancer -oma = tumor	Cancer of the ovary.
ovarian cyst (oh-VAY-ree-an / SIST)	ovari/o = ovary -an = pertaining to	Cyst that develops within the ovary. These may be multiple cysts and may rupture, causing pain and bleeding.
Uterine Tubes		
pyosalpinx (pie-oh-SAL-pinks)	py/o = pus -salpinx = uterine tube	Presence of pus in a uterine tube.
salpingitis (sal-ping-JIGH-tis)	salping/o = uterine tube -itis = inflammation	Inflammation of the uterine tube.
Uterus		
cervical cancer (SER-vih-kal)	cervic/o = cervix -al = pertaining to	Malignant growth in the cervix. Some cases are caused by the *human papilloma virus* (HPV), a sexually transmitted virus for which there is now a vaccine. An especially difficult type of cancer to treat that causes 5% of the cancer deaths in women. Pap smear tests have helped to detect early cervical cancer.
endocervicitis (en-doh-ser-vih-SIGH-tis)	endo- = within cervic/o = cervix -itis = inflammation	Inflammation that occurs within the cervix.
endometrial cancer (en-doh-MEE-tree-al)	endo- = within metr/o = uterus -al = pertaining to	Cancer of the endometrial lining of the uterus.
endometritis (en-doh-meh-TRY-tis)	endo- = within metr/o = uterus -itis = inflammation	Inflammation of the endometrium (inner layer of the uterine wall)

MED TERM TIP

Word Watch: Be careful when using the combining form *metr/o* meaning "uterus" and the suffix *-metry* meaning "process of measuring."

TERM	WORD PARTS	DEFINITION
fibroid tumor (FIGH-broyd / TOO-mor)	fibr/o = fibers -oid = resembling	Benign tumor or growth that contains fiber-like tissue. Uterine fibroid tumors are the most common tumors in women.

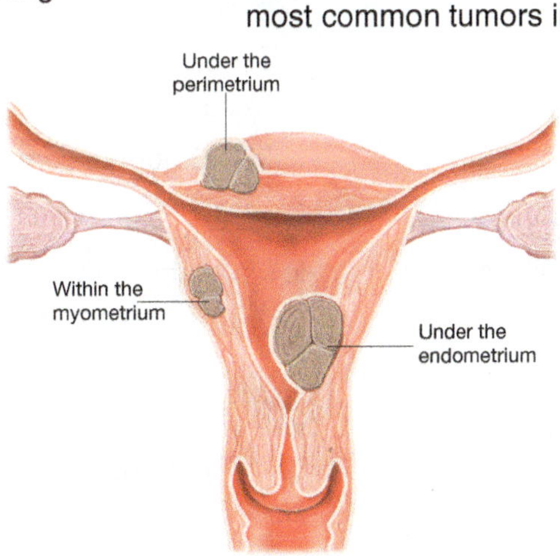

Figure 10.14 Common sites for the development of fibroid tumors.

Pathology *(continued)*

TERM	WORD PARTS	DEFINITION
hysterorrhexis (hiss-ter-oh-REK-sis)	hyster/o = uterus -rrhexis = rupture	Rupture of the uterus; may occur during labor.
menometrorrhagia (men-oh-met-thro-RAY-jee-ah)	men/o = menstruation metr/o = uterus -rrhagia = abnormal flow condition	Excessive bleeding during the menstrual period and at intervals between menstrual periods.
premenstrual syndrome (PMS) (pre-MEN-stroo-al / SIN-drohm)	pre- = before men/o = menstruation -al = pertaining to	Symptoms that develop just prior to the onset of a menstrual period, which can include irritability, headache, tender breasts, and anxiety.
prolapsed uterus (pro-LAPS'D / YOO-ter-us)		Fallen uterus that can cause the cervix to protrude through the vaginal opening. Generally caused by weakened muscles from vaginal delivery or as the result of pelvic tumors pressing down.
Vagina		
candidiasis (kan-dih-DYE-ah-sis)	-iasis = abnormal condition	Yeast infection of the skin and mucous membranes that can result in white plaques on the tongue and vagina.
MED TERM TIP The term *candida* comes from a Latin term meaning "dazzling white." Candida is the scientific name for yeast and refers to the very white discharge that is the hallmark of a yeast infection.		
cystocele (SIS-toh-seel)	cyst/o = bladder -cele = protrusion	Hernia or outpouching of the bladder that protrudes into the vagina. This may cause urinary frequency and urgency.
rectocele (REK-toh-seel)	rect/o = rectum -cele = protrusion	Protrusion or herniation of the rectum into the vagina.
toxic shock syndrome (TSS)	tox/o = poison -ic = pertaining to	Rare and sometimes fatal staphylococcus infection that generally occurs in menstruating women. Initial infection of the vagina is associated with prolonged wearing of a super-absorbent tampon.
vaginitis (vaj-ih-NIGH-tis)	vagin/o = vagina -itis = inflammation	Inflammation of the vagina.
Pelvic Cavity		
endometriosis (en-doh-mee-tree-OH-sis)	endo- = within metr/o = uterus -osis = abnormal condition	Abnormal condition of endometrium tissue appearing throughout the pelvis or on the abdominal wall. This tissue is normally found within the uterus.
pelvic inflammatory disease (PID) (PELL-vik / in-FLAM-mah-toh-ree)	pelv/o = pelvis -ic = pertaining to	Chronic or acute infection, usually bacterial, that has ascended through the female reproductive organs and out into the pelvic cavity. May result in scarring that interferes with fertility.
perimetritis (pair-ih-meh-TRY-tis)	peri- = around metr/o = uterus -itis = inflammation	Inflammation in the pelvic cavity around the outside of the uterus.

Pathology *(continued)*

TERM	WORD PARTS	DEFINITION
Breast		
breast cancer		Malignant tumor of the breast. Usually forms in the milk-producing gland tissue or the lining of the milk ducts (see Figure 10.15A ■).
fibrocystic breast disease (figh-bro-SIS-tik)	fibr/o = fibers cyst/o = pouch -ic = pertaining to	Benign cysts forming in the breast (see Figure 10.15B ■).

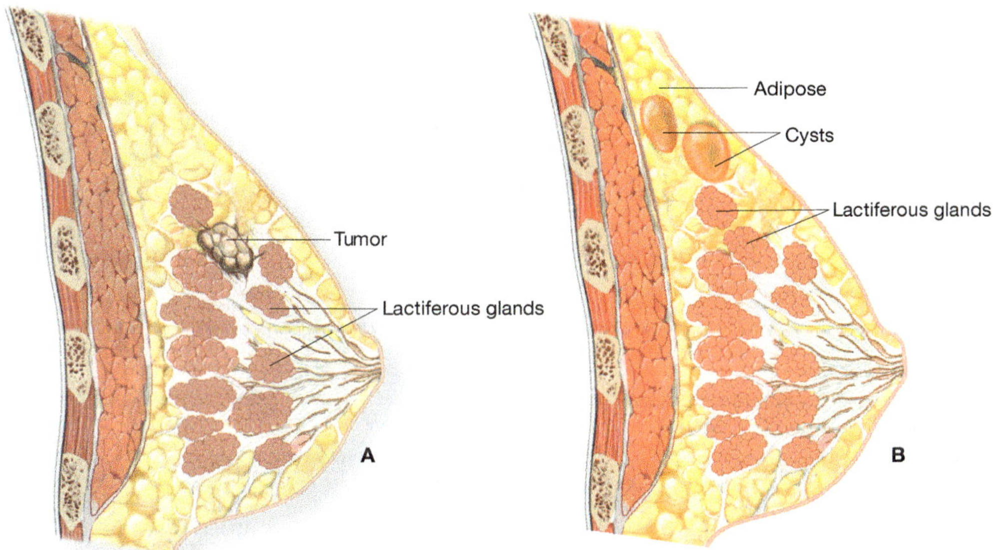

■ **Figure 10.15** Comparison of breast cancer and fibrocystic disease. (A) Breast with a malignant tumor growing in the lactiferous gland and duct; (B) the location of a fibrocystic lump in the adipose tissue covering the breast.

TERM	WORD PARTS	DEFINITION
mastitis (mas-TYE-tis)	mast/o = breast -itis = inflammation	Inflammation of the breast.
Pregnancy		
abruptio placentae (ah-BRUP-tee-oh / plah-SEN-tee)		Emergency condition in which the placenta tears away from the uterine wall prior to delivery of the infant. Requires immediate delivery of the baby.
eclampsia (eh-KLAMP-see-ah)	-ia = condition	Further worsening of preeclampsia symptoms with the addition of seizures and coma; may occur between the 20th week of pregnancy and up to 6 weeks postpartum.
hemolytic disease of the newborn (HDN) (hee-moh-LIT-ik)	hem/o = blood -lytic = destruction	Condition developing in the baby when the mother's blood type is Rh-negative and the baby's blood is Rh-positive. Antibodies in the mother's blood enter the fetus's bloodstream through the placenta and destroy the fetus's red blood cells, causing anemia, jaundice, and enlargement of the spleen. Treatment is early diagnosis and blood transfusion. Also called *erythroblastosis fetalis*.

Pathology *(continued)*

TERM	WORD PARTS	DEFINITION
infertility	in- = not	Inability to produce children. Generally defined as no pregnancy after properly timed intercourse for 1 year.
placenta previa (plah-SEN-tah / PREE-vee-ah)		A placenta that is implanted in the lower portion of the uterus and, in turn, blocks the birth canal.

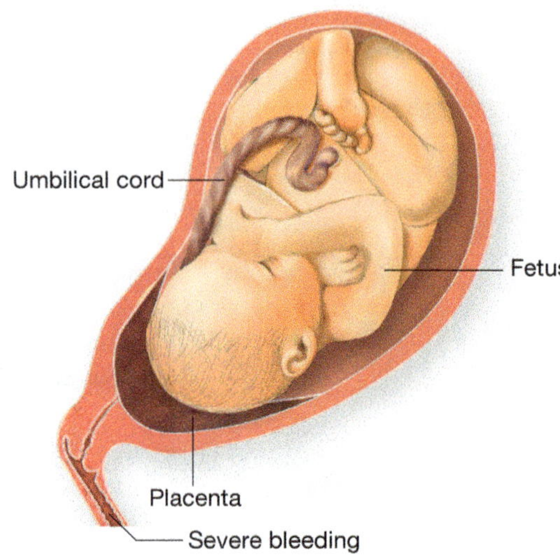

■ **Figure 10.16** Placenta previa, longitudinal section showing the placenta growing over the opening into the cervix.

TERM	WORD PARTS	DEFINITION
preeclampsia (pre-eh-KLAMP-see-ah)	pre- = before	Metabolic disease of pregnancy. If untreated, it may progress to eclampsia. Symptoms include hypertension, headaches, albumin in the urine, and edema. May occur between the 20th week of pregnancy and up to 6 weeks postpartum. Also called *toxemia* or pregnancy-induced hypertension (PIH)
prolapsed umbilical cord (pro-LAPS'D / um-BILL-ih-kal)		When the umbilical cord of the baby is expelled first during delivery and is squeezed between the baby's head and the vaginal wall. This presents an emergency situation since the baby's circulation is compromised.
pseudocyesis (soo-doh-sigh-EE-sis)	pseudo- = false -cyesis = pregnancy	Condition in which the body reacts as if there is a pregnancy (especially hormonal changes), but there is no pregnancy.
salpingocyesis (sal-ping-goh-sigh-EE-sis)	salping/o = uterine tube -cyesis = pregnancy	Pregnancy that occurs in the uterine tube instead of in the uterus.
spontaneous abortion		Unplanned loss of a pregnancy due to the death of the embryo or fetus before the time it is viable, commonly referred to as a *miscarriage.*
stillbirth		Birth in which a viable-aged fetus dies shortly before or at the time of delivery.

Diagnostic Procedures

TERM	WORD PARTS	DEFINITION
Clinical Laboratory Tests		
Pap (Papanicolaou) **smear** (pap-ah-NIK-oh-low)		Test for the early detection of cancer of the cervix named after the developer of the test, George Papanicolaou, a Greek physician. A scraping of cells is removed from the cervix for examination under a microscope.
pregnancy test (PREG-nan-see)		Chemical test that can determine a pregnancy during the first few weeks. Can be performed in a physician's office or with a home-testing kit.
Diagnostic Imaging		
hysterosalpingography (HSG) (hiss-ter-oh-sal-pin-GOG-rah-fee)	hyster/o = uterus salping/o = uterine tube -graphy = process of recording	Taking of an X-ray after injecting radiopaque material into the uterus and uterine tubes.
mammogram (MAM-moh-gram)	mamm/o = breast -gram = record	X-ray record of the breast.
mammography (mam-OG-rah-fee)	mamm/o = breast -graphy = process of recording	X-ray to diagnose breast disease, especially breast cancer.
pelvic ultrasonography (PELL-vik / ull-trah-son-OG-rah-fee)	pelv/o = pelvis -ic = pertaining to ultra- = beyond son/o = sound -graphy = process of recording	Use of high-frequency sound waves to produce an image or photograph of an organ, such as the uterus, ovaries, or fetus.
Endoscopic Procedures		
colposcope (KOL-poh-scope)	colp/o = vagina -scope = instrument for viewing	Instrument used to view inside the vagina.
colposcopy (kol-POS-koh-pee)	colp/o = vagina -scopy = process of viewing	Examination of vagina using an instrument called a *colposcope.*
culdoscopy (kul-DOS-koh-pee)	culd/o = cul-de-sac -scopy = process of viewing	Examination of the female pelvic cavity, particularly behind the uterus, by introducing an endoscope through the wall of the vagina.
laparoscope (LAP-ah-row-scope)	lapar/o = abdomen -scope = instrument for viewing	Instrument used to view inside the abdomen.
laparoscopy (lap-ar-OS-koh-pee)	lapar/o = abdomen -scopy = process of viewing	Examination of the peritoneal cavity using an instrument called a *laparoscope.* The instrument is passed through a small incision made by the surgeon into the abdominopelvic cavity.

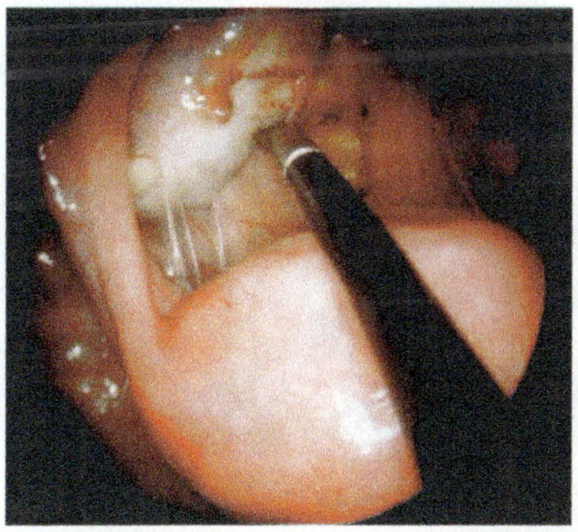

Figure 10.17 Photograph taken during a laparoscopic procedure. The fundus of the uterus is visible below the probe, the ovary is at the tip of the probe, and the uterine tube extends along the left side of the photo. *(Southern Illinois University/ Photo Researchers, Inc.)*

Diagnostic Procedures *(continued)*

TERM	WORD PARTS	DEFINITION
Obstetrical Diagnostic Procedures		
amniocentesis (am-nee-oh-sen-TEE-sis)	amni/o = amnion -centesis = puncture to withdraw fluid	Puncturing of the amniotic sac using a needle and syringe for the purpose of withdrawing amniotic fluid for testing. Can assist in determining fetal maturity, development, and genetic disorders.
Apgar score (AP-gar)		Evaluation of a neonate's adjustment to the outside world. Observes color, heart rate, muscle tone, respiratory rate, and response to stimulus at 1 minute and 5 minutes after birth.
chorionic villus sampling (CVS) (kor-ree-ON-ik / vill-us)	chori/o = chorion -nic = pertaining to	Removal of a small piece of the chorion for genetic analysis. May be done at an earlier stage of pregnancy than amniocentesis.
fetal monitoring (FEE-tal)	fet/o = fetus -al = pertaining to	Using electronic equipment placed on the mother's abdomen or the fetus' scalp to check the fetal heart rate (FHR). Also called fetal heart tone (FHT) during labor. The normal heart rate of the fetus is rapid, ranging from 120 to 160 beats per minute. A drop in the fetal heart rate indicates the fetus is in distress.
Additional Diagnostic Procedures		
cervical biopsy (SER-vih-kal / BYE-op-see)	cervic/o = cervix -al = pertaining to bi/o = life -opsy = to view	Taking a sample of tissue from the cervix to test for the presence of cancer cells.
endometrial biopsy (EMB) (en-doh-MEE-tre-al BYE-op-see)	endo- = within metr/o = uterus -al = pertaining to bi/o = life -opsy = to view	Taking a sample of tissue from the lining of the uterus to test for abnormalities.
pelvic examination (PELL-vik)	pelv/o = pelvis -ic = pertaining to	Physical examination of the vagina and adjacent organs performed by a physician placing the fingers of one hand into the vagina. An instrument called a *speculum* is used to open the vagina.

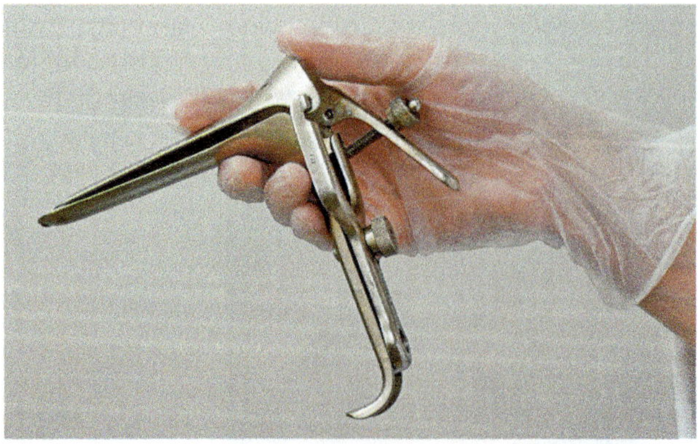

Figure 10.18 A speculum used to hold the vagina open in order to visualize the cervix.

Therapeutic Procedures

TERM	WORD PARTS	DEFINITION
Medical Procedures		
barrier contraception (kon-trah-SEP-shun)	contra- = against	Prevention of a pregnancy using a device to prevent sperm from meeting an ovum. Examples include condoms, diaphragms, and cervical caps.
hormonal contraception	-al = pertaining to contra- = against	Use of hormones to block ovulation and prevent conception. May be in the form of a pill, a patch, an implant under the skin, or an injection.
intrauterine device (IUD) (in-trah-YOO-ter-in)	intra- = inside uter/o = uterus -ine = pertaining to	Device inserted into the uterus by a physician for the purpose of contraception.

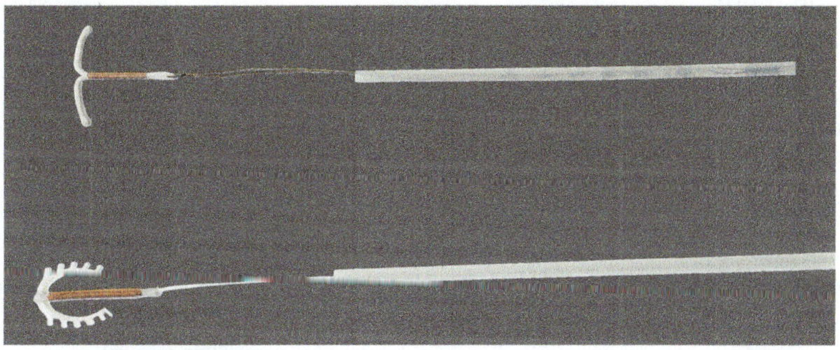

■ **Figure 10.19** Photographs illustrating the shape of two different intrauterine devices (IUDs). *(Jules Selmes and Debi Treloar/Dorling Kindersley)*

TERM	WORD PARTS	DEFINITION
Surgical Procedures		
amniotomy (am-nee-OT-oh-mee)	amni/o = amnion -otomy = cutting into	Surgically cutting open the amnion; commonly referred to as "breaking the water."
cervicectomy (ser-vih-SEK-toh-mee)	cervic/o = cervix -ectomy = surgical removal	Surgical removal of the cervix.
cesarean section (CS, C-section) (see-SAYR-ee-an)		Surgical delivery of a baby through an incision into the abdominal and uterine walls. Legend has it that the Roman emperor, Julius Caesar, was the first person born by this method.
conization (kon-ih-ZAY-shun)		Surgical removal of a core of cervical tissue. Also refers to partial removal of the cervix.
dilation and curettage (D & C) (dye-LAY-shun / koo-reh-TAHZ)		Surgical procedure in which the opening of the cervix is dilated and the uterus is scraped or suctioned of its lining or tissue. Often performed after a spontaneous abortion and to stop excessive bleeding from other causes.
elective abortion		Legal termination of a pregnancy for nonmedical reasons.
episiorrhaphy (eh-peez-ee-OR-ah-fee)	episi/o = vulva -rrhaphy = suture	To suture the perineum; procedure to repair an episiotomy postpartum. Note that the combining form *episi/o* is used even though the perineum is not part of the vulva.
episiotomy (eh-peez-ee-OT-oh-mee)	episi/o = vulva -otomy = cutting into	Surgical incision of the perineum to facilitate the delivery process. Can prevent an irregular tearing of tissue during birth. Note that the combining form *episi/o* is used even though the perineum is not part of the vulva.

Therapeutic Procedures *(continued)*

TERM	WORD PARTS	DEFINITION
hymenectomy (high-men-EK-toh-mee)	hymen/o = hymen -ectomy = surgical removal	Surgical removal of the hymen.
hysterectomy (hiss-ter-EK-toh-mee)	hyster/o = uterus -ectomy = surgical removal	Surgical removal of the uterus.
hysteropexy (HISS-ter-oh-pek-see)	hyster/o = uterus -pexy = surgical fixation	To surgically anchor the uterus to its proper location in the pelvic cavity; a treatment for a prolapsed uterus.
laparotomy (lap-ah-ROT-oh-mee)	lapar/o = abdomen -otomy = cutting into	To cut open the abdomen; performed in order to complete other surgical procedures inside the abdomen or performed during a C-section.
lumpectomy (lump-EK-toh-mee)	-ectomy = surgical removal	Removal of only a breast tumor and the tissue immediately surrounding it.
mammoplasty (MAM-moh-plas-tee)	mamm/o = breast -plasty = surgical repair	Surgical repair or reconstruction of the breast.
mastectomy (mass-TEK-toh-mee)	mast/o = breast -ectomy = surgical removal	Surgical removal of the breast.
oophorectomy (oh-off-oh-REK-toh-mee)	oophor/o = ovary -ectomy = surgical removal	Surgical removal of the ovary.
radical mastectomy (mast-EK-toh-mee)	-al = pertaining to mast/o = breast -ectomy = surgical removal	Surgical removal of the breast tissue plus chest muscles and axillary lymph nodes.
salpingectomy (sal-ping-JECK-toh-mee)	salping/o = uterine tube -ectomy = surgical removal	Surgical removal of the uterine tube.
simple mastectomy (mast-EK-toh-mee)	mast/o = breast -ectomy = surgical removal	Surgical removal of the breast tissue.
therapeutic abortion		Termination of a pregnancy for the health of the mother or another medical reason.
total abdominal hysterectomy—bilateral salpingo-oophorectomy (TAH-BSO) (hiss-ter-EK-toh-me / sal-ping-goh / oh-oh-foe-REK-toh-mee)	abdomin/o = abdomen -al = pertaining to hyster/o = uterus -ectomy = surgical removal bi- = two later/o = side -al = pertaining to salping/o = uterine tube oophor/o = ovary -ectomy = surgical removal	Removal of the entire uterus, cervix, both ovaries, and both uterine tubes.
tubal ligation (TOO-bal / lye-GAY-shun)	-al = pertaining to	Surgical tying off of the uterine tubes to prevent conception from taking place. Results in sterilization of the female.
vaginal hysterectomy (VAJ-ih-nal / hiss-ter-EK-toh-me)	vagin/o = vagina -al = pertaining to hyster/o = uterus -ectomy = surgical removal	Removal of the uterus through the vagina rather than through an abdominal incision.

Pharmacology

CLASSIFICATION	WORD PARTS	ACTION	EXAMPLES
abortifacient (ah-bore-tih-FAY-shee-ent)		Medication that terminates a pregnancy.	mifepristone, Mifeprex; dinoprostone, Prostin E2
fertility drug		Medication that triggers ovulation. Also called *ovulation stimulant.*	clomiphene, Clomid; follitropin alfa, Gonal-F
hormone replacement therapy (HRT)		Menopause or the surgical loss of the ovaries results in the lack of estrogen production. Replacing this hormone may prevent some of the consequences of menopause, especially in younger women who have surgically lost their ovaries.	conjugated estrogens, Cenestin, Premarin
oral contraceptive pills (OCPs) (kon-trah-SEP-tive)	or/o = mouth -al = pertaining to contra- = against	Birth control medication that uses low doses of female hormones to prevent conception by blocking ovulation.	desogestrel/ethinyl estradiol, Ortho-Cept; ethinyl estradiol/norgestrel, Lo/Ovral
oxytocin (ox-ee-TOH-sin)		Oxytocin is a natural hormone that begins or improves uterine contractions during labor and delivery.	oxytocin, Pitocin, Syntocinon

Abbreviations

AB	abortion
AI	artificial insemination
BSE	breast self-examination
CS, C-section	cesarean section
CVS	chorionic villus sampling
Cx	cervix
D & C	dilation and curettage
EDC	estimated date of confinement
EMB	endometrial biopsy
ERT	estrogen replacement therapy
FEKG	fetal electrocardiogram
FHR	fetal heart rate
FHT	fetal heart tone
FSH	follicle-stimulating hormone
FTND	full-term normal delivery
GI, grav I	first pregnancy
GYN, gyn	gynecology
HCG, hCG	human chorionic gonadotropin
HDN	hemolytic disease of the newborn
HPV	human papilloma virus
HRT	hormone replacement therapy
HSG	hysterosalpingography
IUD	intrauterine device
IVF	*in vitro* fertilization
LBW	low birth weight
LH	luteinizing hormone
LMP	last menstrual period
NB	newborn
OB	obstetrics
OCPs	oral contraceptive pills
Pap	Papanicolaou test
PI, para I	first delivery
PID	pelvic inflammatory disease
PIH	pregnancy-induced hypertension
PMS	premenstrual syndrome
TAH-BSO	total abdominal hysterectomy–bilateral salpingo-oophorectomy
TSS	toxic shock syndrome
UC	uterine contractions

Section II: Male Reproductive System at a Glance

Function

Similar to the female reproductive system, the male reproductive system is responsible for producing sperm, the male reproductive cell, secreting the male sex hormones, and delivering sperm to the female reproductive tract.

Structures

Here are the primary structures that comprise the male reproductive system.

bulbourethral glands
epididymis
penis
prostate gland
seminal vesicles
testes
vas deferens

Word Parts

Here are the most common word parts (with their meanings) used to build male reproductive system terms. For a more comprehensive list, refer to the Terminology section of this chapter.

Combining Forms

andr/o	male
balan/o	glans penis
crypt/o	hidden
epididym/o	epididymis
genit/o	genitals
orch/o	testes
orchi/o	testes
orchid/o	testes
pen/o	penis
prostat/o	prostate
spermat/o	sperm
testicul/o	testes
vas/o	vas deferens
vesicul/o	seminal vesicle

Suffixes

-cide	to kill
-spermia	condition of sperm

Male Reproductive System Illustrated

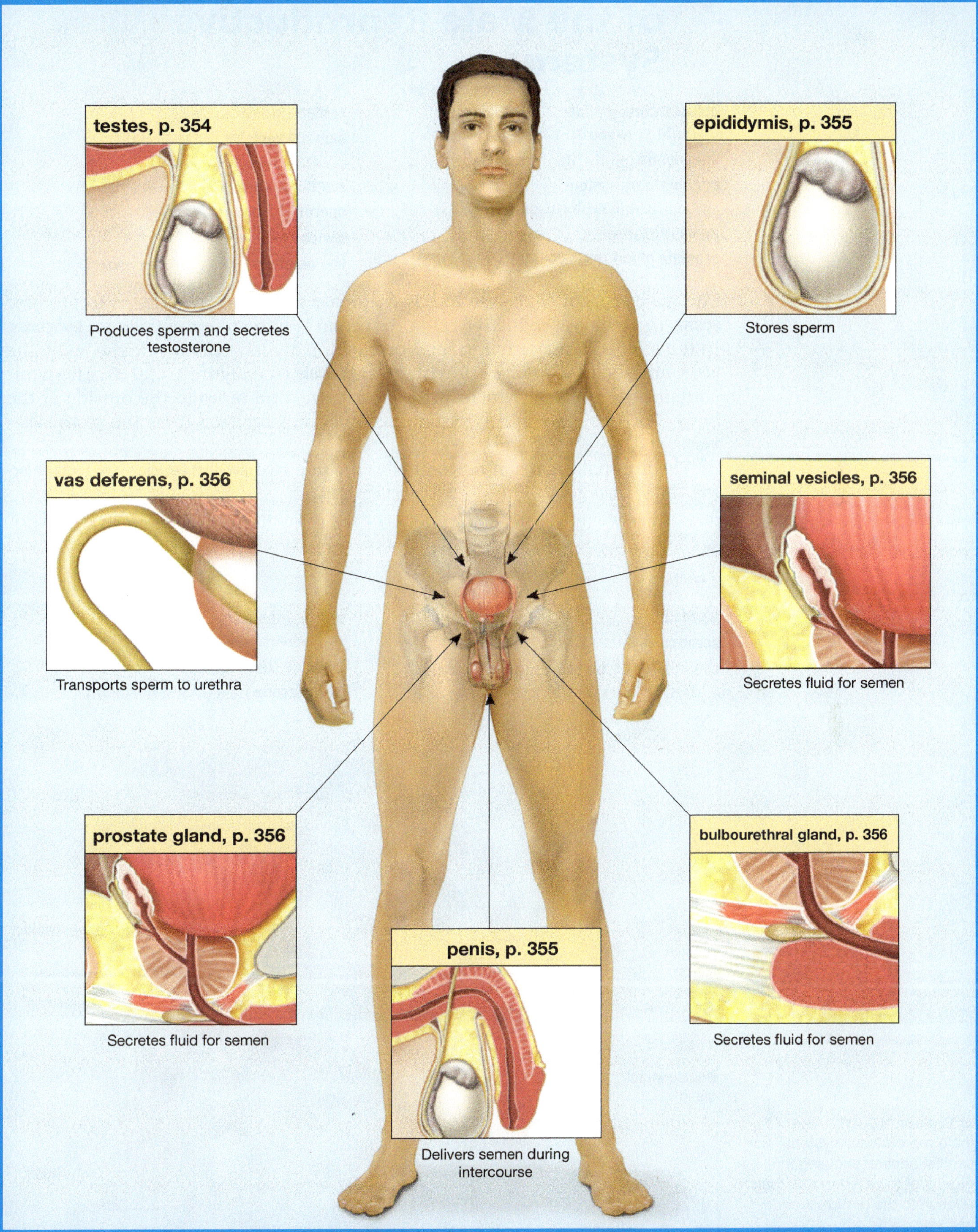

Anatomy and Physiology of the Male Reproductive System

bulbourethral glands (buhl-boh-yoo-REE-thral)
epididymis (ep-ih-DID-ih-mis)
genitourinary system (jen-ih-toh-YOO-rih-nair-ee)
penis (PEE-nis)
prostate gland (PROSS-tayt)
semen (SEE-men)
seminal vesicles (SEM-ih-nal / VESS-ih-kls)
sex hormones
sperm
testes (TESS-teez)
vas deferens (VAS / DEF-er-enz)

The male reproductive system has two main functions. The first is to produce **sperm,** the male reproductive cell; the second is to secrete the male **sex hormones.** In the male, the major organs of reproduction are located outside the body: the **penis,** and the two **testes,** each with an **epididymis** (see Figure 10.20 ■). The penis contains the urethra, which carries both urine and **semen** to the outside of the body. For this reason, this system is sometimes referred to as the **genitourinary system** (GU).

The internal organs of reproduction include two **seminal vesicles,** two **vas deferens,** the **prostate gland,** and two **bulbourethral glands.**

External Organs of Reproduction

Testes

perineum
scrotum (SKROH-tum)
seminiferous tubules (sem-ih-NIF-er-us / TOO-byools)
spermatogenesis (sper-mat-oh-JEN-eh-sis)
testicles (test-IH-kles)
testosterone (tess-TAHSS-ter-own)

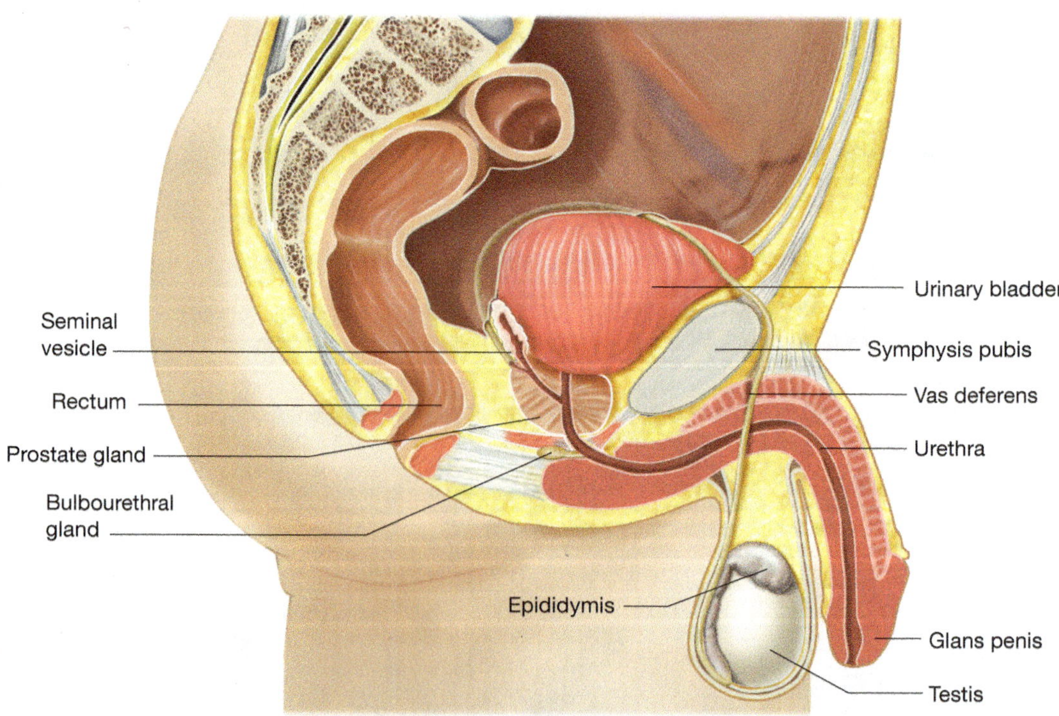

■ **Figure 10.20** The male reproductive system, sagittal section showing the organs of the system and their relation to the urinary bladder and rectum.

The testes (singular is *testis*) or **testicles** are oval in shape and are responsible for the production of sperm (see again Figure 10.20). This process, called **spermatogenesis,** takes place within the **seminiferous tubules** that make up the insides of the testes (see Figure 10.21 ■). The testes must be maintained at the proper temperature for the sperm to survive. This lower temperature level is achieved by the placement of the testes suspended in the **scrotum,** a sac outside the body. The **perineum** of the male is similar to that in the female and is the area between the scrotum and the anus. The male sex hormone **testosterone,** which is responsible for the development of the male reproductive organs, sperm, and secondary sex characteristics, is also produced by the testes.

MED TERM TIP

Spermatozoon and its plural form, *spermatozoa*, are other terms that mean "sperm." You have no doubt realized that there can be several terms with the same meaning in medical terminology. You must continue to remain flexible when working with these terms in your career. In some cases, one term will be more commonly used, depending on the type of medical specialty or even what part of the country you are in.

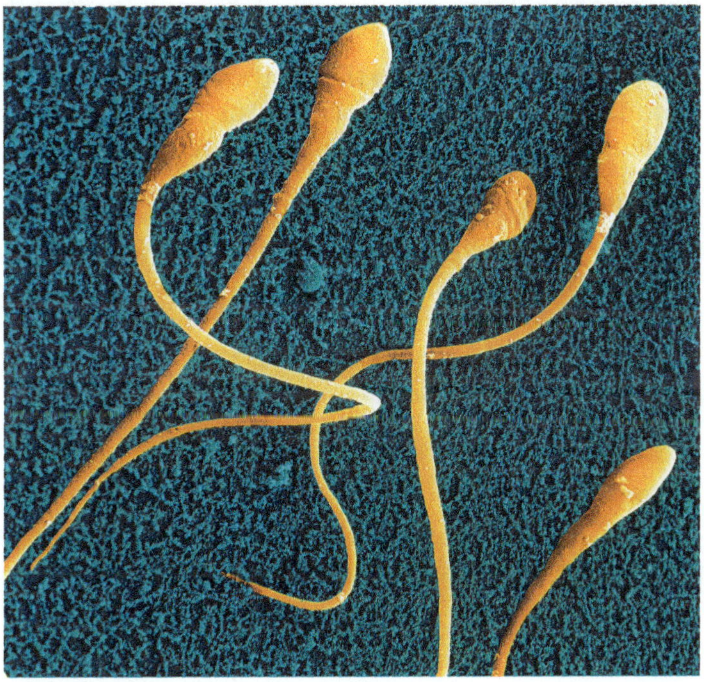

■ **Figure 10.21** Electron-micrograph of human sperm.
(Juergen Berger, Max-Planck Institute/Science Photo Library/Photo Researchers, Inc.)

Epididymis

Each epididymis is a coiled tubule that lies on top of the testes within the scrotum (see again Figure 10.20). This elongated structure serves as the location for sperm maturation and storage until they are ready to be released into the vas deferens.

Penis

circumcision (ser-kum-SIH-zhun)
ejaculation (ee-jak-yoo-LAY-shun)
erectile tissue (ee-REK-tile)
glans penis (GLANS / PEE-nis)
prepuce (PREE-pyoos)
sphincter (SFINGK-ter)
urinary meatus (YOO-rih-nair-ee / me-AY-tus)

The penis is the male sex organ containing **erectile tissue** that is encased in skin (see again Figure 10.20). This organ delivers semen into the female vagina. The soft tip of the penis is referred to as the **glans penis.** It is protected by a covering called the **prepuce** or foreskin. It is this covering of skin that is removed during the procedure known as **circumcision.** The penis becomes erect during sexual stimulation, which allows it to be placed within the female for the **ejaculation** of semen. The male urethra extends from the urinary bladder to the external opening in the penis, the **urinary meatus,** and serves a dual function: the elimination of urine and the ejaculation of semen. During the ejaculation process, a **sphincter** closes to keep urine from escaping.

MED TERM TIP

During sexual intercourse, which is also referred to as *coitus*, the male can eject up to 100 million sperm cells. The adult male produces nearly 200 million sperm daily.

Internal Organs of Reproduction

Vas Deferens

spermatic cord (sper-MAT-ik)

Each vas deferens carries sperm from the epididymis up into the pelvic cavity. They travel up in front of the urinary bladder, over the top, and then back down the posterior side of the bladder to empty into the urethra (see again Figure 10.20). They, along with nerves, arteries, veins, and lymphatic vessels running between the pelvic cavity and the testes, form the **spermatic cord.**

Seminal Vesicles

The two seminal vesicles are small glands located at the base of the urinary bladder (see again Figure 10.20). These vesicles are connected to the vas deferens just before it empties into the urethra. The seminal vesicles secrete a glucose-rich fluid that nourishes the sperm. This liquid, along with the sperm, constitutes semen, the fluid that is eventually ejaculated during sexual intercourse.

Prostate Gland

The single prostate gland is located just below the urinary bladder (see again Figure 10.20). It surrounds the urethra and when enlarged can cause difficulty in urination. The prostate is important for the reproductive process since it secretes an alkaline fluid that assists in keeping the sperm alive by neutralizing the pH of the urethra and vagina.

Bulbourethral Glands

Cowper's glands (KOW-perz)

The bulbourethral glands, also known as **Cowper's glands,** are two small glands located on either side of the urethra just below the prostate (see again Figure 10.20). They produce a mucus-like lubricating fluid that joins with semen to become a part of the ejaculate.

Terminology

Word Parts Used to Build Male Reproductive System Terms

The following lists contain the combining forms, suffixes, and prefixes used to build terms in the remaining sections of this chapter.

Combining Forms

Combining Form	Meaning
andr/o	male
balan/o	glans penis
carcin/o	cancer
crypt/o	hidden
epididym/o	epididymis
genit/o	genital
hydr/o	water
immun/o	protection
olig/o	scanty
orch/o	testes
orchi/o	testes
orchid/o	testes
pen/o	penis
prostat/o	prostate gland
rect/o	rectum
spermat/o	sperm
testicul/o	testicle
ur/o	urine
urethr/o	urethra
varic/o	dilated vein
vas/o	vas deferens
vesicul/o	seminal vesicle

Suffixes

-al	pertaining to
-ar	pertaining to
-cele	protrusion
-cide	to kill
-ectomy	surgical removal
-gen	that which produces
-iasis	abnormal condition
-ic	pertaining to
-ile	pertaining to
-ism	state of
-itis	inflammation
-logy	study of
-lysis	destruction
-oid	resembling
-oma	tumor
-osis	abnormal condition
-ostomy	create a new opening
-otomy	cutting into
-pexy	surgical fixation
-plasia	growth
-plasty	surgical repair
-rrhea	discharge
-spermia	sperm condition

Prefixes

a-	without
an-	without
anti-	against
dys-	abnormal, difficult
epi-	upon
hyper-	excessive
hypo-	below

Anatomical Terms

TERM	WORD PARTS	DEFINITION
balanic (buh-LAN-ik)	balan/o = glans penis -ic = pertaining to	Pertaining to the glans penis.
epididymal (ep-ih-DID-ih-mal)	epididym/o = epididymis -al = pertaining to	Pertaining to the epididymis.
penile (PEE-nile)	pen/o = penis -ile = pertaining to	Pertaining to the penis.
prostatic (pross-TAT-ik)	prostat/o = prostate gland -ic = pertaining to	Pertaining to the prostate gland.
spermatic (sper-MAT-ik)	spermat/o = sperm -ic = pertaining to	Pertaining to sperm.
testicular (tes-TIK-yoo-lar)	testicul/o = testes -ar = pertaining to	Pertaining to the testes.
vasal (VAY-sal)	vas/o = vas deferens -al = pertaining to	Pertaining to the vas deferens.
vesicular (veh-SIC-yoo-lar)	vesicul/o = seminal vesicle -ar = pertaining to	Pertaining to the seminal vesicle.

MED TERM TIP

Word Watch: Be careful using the combining forms *vesic/o* meaning "bladder" and *vesicul/o* meaning "seminal vesicle."

Pathology

TERM	WORD PARTS	DEFINITION
Medical Specialties		
urology (yoo-RAL-oh-jee)	ur/o = urine -logy = study of	Branch of medicine involved in diagnosis and treatment of diseases and disorders of the urinary system and male reproductive system. Physician is a *urologist.*
Signs and Symptoms		
aspermia (ah-SPER-mee-ah)	a- = without -spermia = sperm condition	Condition of having no sperm.
balanorrhea (bah-lah-noh-REE-ah)	balan/o = glans penis -rrhea = discharge	Discharge from the glans penis.
oligospermia (ol-ih-goh-SPER-mee-ah)	olig/o = scanty -spermia = sperm condition	Condition of having too few sperm, making the chances of fertilization very low.
spermatolysis (sper-mah-TOL-ih-sis)	spermat/o = sperm -lysis = destruction	Term that refers to anything that destroys sperm.
Testes		
anorchism (an-OR-kizm)	an- = without orch/o = testes -ism = condition	The absence of testes; may be congenital or as the result of an accident or surgery.
cryptorchidism (kript-OR-kid-izm)	crypt/o = hidden orchid/o = testes -ism = state of	Failure of the testes to descend into the scrotal sac before birth. Usually, the testes will descend before birth. A surgical procedure called orchidopexy may be required to bring the testes down into the scrotum permanently. Failure of the testes to descend could result in sterility in the male or an increased risk of testicular cancer.
hydrocele (HIGH-droh-seel)	hydr/o = water -cele = protrusion	Accumulation of fluid around the testes or along the spermatic cord. Common in infants.
sterility		Inability to father children due to a problem with spermatogenesis.
testicular carcinoma (kar-sih-NOH-mah)	testicul/o = testicle -ar = pertaining to carcin/o = cancer -oma = tumor	Cancer of one or both testicles; most common cancer in men under age 40.
testicular torsion	testicul/o = testicle -ar = pertaining to	Twisting of the spermatic cord.
varicocele (VAIR-ih-koh-seel)	varic/o = dilated vein -cele = protrusion	Enlargement of the veins of the spermatic cord that commonly occurs on the left side of adolescent males.
Epididymis		
epididymitis (ep-ih-did-ih-MYE-tis)	epididym/o = epididymis -itis = inflammation	Inflammation of the epididymis.

Pathology *(continued)*

TERM	WORD PARTS	DEFINITION
Prostate Gland		
benign prostatic hyperplasia (BPH) (bee-NINE / pross-TAT-ik / high-PER-troh-fee)	prostat/o = prostate gland -ic = pertaining to hyper- = excessive -plasia = growth	Noncancerous enlargement of the prostate gland commonly seen in males over age 50. Formerly called *benign prostatic hypertrophy.*
prostate cancer (PROSS-tayt)		Slow-growing cancer that affects a large number of males after age 50. The prostate-specific antigen (PSA) test is used to assist in early detection of this disease.
prostatitis (pross-tah-TYE-tis)	prostat/o = prostate gland -itis = inflammation	Inflammation of the prostate gland.
Penis		
balanitis (bal-ah-NYE-tis)	balan/o = glans penis -itis = inflammation	Inflammation of the glans penis.
epispadias (ep-ih-SPAY-dee-as)	epi- = upon	Congenital opening of the urethra on the dorsal surface of the penis.
erectile dysfunction (ED) (ee-REK-tile)	-ile = pertaining to dys- = abnormal, difficult	Inability to engage in sexual intercourse due to inability to maintain an erection. Also called *impotence.*
hypospadias (high-poh-SPAY-dee-as)	hypo- = below	Congenital opening of the male urethra on the underside of the penis.
phimosis (fih-MOH-sis)	-osis = abnormal condition	Narrowing of the foreskin over the glans penis resulting in difficulty with hygiene. This condition can lead to infection or difficulty with urination. The condition is treated with circumcision, the surgical removal of the foreskin.
priapism (pri-ah-pizm)	-ism = state of	A persistent and painful erection due to pathological causes, not sexual arousal.
Sexually Transmitted Diseases		
chancroid (SHANG-kroyd)	-oid = resembling	Highly infectious nonsyphilitic venereal ulcer.
chlamydia (klah-MID-ee-ah)		Bacterial infection causing genital inflammation in males and females. Can lead to pelvic inflammatory disease in females and eventual infertility.
genital herpes (JEN-ih-tal / HER-peez)	genit/o = genital -al = pertaining to	Spreading skin disease that can appear like a blister or vesicle on the genital region of males and females; may spread to other areas of the body. Caused by a sexually transmitted virus.

Pathology *(continued)*

TERM	WORD PARTS	DEFINITION
genital warts (JEN-ih-tal)	genit/o = genital -al = pertaining to	Growth of warts on the genitalia of both males and females that can lead to cancer of the cervix in females. Caused by the sexual transmission of the human papilloma virus (HPV).
gonorrhea (GC) (gon-oh-REE-ah)	-rrhea = discharge	Sexually transmitted bacterial infection of the mucous membranes of either sex. Can be passed on to an infant during the birth process.
human immunodeficiency virus (HIV)	immun/o = protection	Sexually transmitted virus that attacks the immune system.
sexually transmitted disease (STD)		Disease usually acquired as the result of sexual intercourse. Formerly referred to as *venereal disease* (VD).
syphilis (SIF-ih-lis)		Infectious, chronic, bacterial venereal disease that can involve any organ. May exist for years without symptoms, but is fatal if untreated. Treated with the antibiotic penicillin.
trichomoniasis (trik-oh-moh-NYE-ah-sis)	-iasis = abnormal condition	Genitourinary infection caused by a single-cell protist that is usually without symptoms (asymptomatic) in both males and females. In women the disease can produce itching and/or burning, a foul-smelling discharge, and result in vaginitis.

Diagnostic Procedures

TERM	WORD PARTS	DEFINITION
Clinical Laboratory Tests		
prostate-specific antigen (PSA) (PROSS-tayt-specific / AN-tih-jen)	anti- = against -gen = that which produces	Blood test to screen for prostate cancer. Elevated blood levels of PSA are associated with prostate cancer.
semen analysis (SEE-men / ah-NAL-ih-sis)		Procedure used when performing a fertility workup to determine if the male is able to produce sperm. Semen is collected by the patient after abstaining from sexual intercourse for a period of 3–5 days. The sperm in the semen are analyzed for number, swimming strength, and shape. Also used to determine if a vasectomy has been successful. After a period of 6 weeks, no further sperm should be present in a sample from the patient.
Additional Diagnostic Procedures		
digital rectal exam (DRE) (DIJ-ih-tal / REK-tal)	rect/o = rectum -al = pertaining to	Manual examination for an enlarged prostate gland performed by palpating (feeling) the prostate gland through the wall of the rectum.

Therapeutic Procedures

TERM	WORD PARTS	DEFINITION
Surgical Procedures		
balanoplasty (BAL-ah-noh-plas-tee)	balan/o = glans penis -plasty = surgical repair	Surgical repair of the glans penis.
castration (kass-TRAY-shun)		Removal of the testicles in the male or the ovaries in the female.
circumcision (ser-kum-SIH-zhun)		Surgical removal of the end of the prepuce or foreskin of the penis. Generally performed on the newborn male at the request of the parents. The primary reason is for ease of hygiene. Circumcision is also a ritual practice in some religions.
epididymectomy (ep-ih-did-ih-MEK-toh-mee)	epididym/o = epididymis -ectomy = surgical removal	Surgical removal of the epididymis.
orchidectomy (or-kid-EK-toh-mee)	orchid/o = testes -ectomy = surgical removal	Surgical removal of one or both testes.
orchidopexy (OR-kid-oh-peck-see)	orchid/o = testes -pexy = surgical fixation	Surgical fixation to move undescended testes into the scrotum and to attach them to prevent retraction. Used to treat cryptorchidism.
orchiectomy (or-kee-EK-toh-mee)	orchi/o = testes -ectomy = surgical removal	Surgical removal of one or both testes.
orchiotomy (or-kee-OT-oh-mee)	orchi/o = testes -otomy = cutting into	To cut into the testes.
orchioplasty (OR-kee-oh-plas-tee)	orchi/o = testes -plasty = surgical repair	Surgical repair of testes.
prostatectomy (pross-tah-TEK-toh-mee)	prostat/o = prostate gland -ectomy = surgical removal	Surgical removal of the prostate gland.
sterilization (ster-ih-lih-ZAY-shun)		Process of rendering a male or female sterile or unable to conceive children.
transurethral resection of the prostate (TUR, TURP) (trans-yoo-REE-thrall / REE-sek-shun / PROSS-tayt)	trans- = across urethr/o = urethra -al = pertaining to	Surgical removal of the part of the prostate gland that is blocking urine flow by inserting a device through the urethra and removing prostate tissue.
vasectomy (vas-EK-toh-mee)	vas/o = vas deferens -ectomy = surgical removal	Removal of a segment or all of the vas deferens to prevent sperm from leaving the male body. Used for contraception purposes. See Figure 10.22 ■.

MED TERM TIP

The vas deferens is the tubing that is severed during a procedure called a *vasectomy.* A vasectomy results in the sterilization of the male since the sperm are no longer able to travel into the urethra and out of the penis during sexual intercourse. The surgical procedure to reverse a vasectomy is a *vasovasostomy.* A new opening is created in order to reconnect one section of the vas deferens to another section of the vas deferens, thereby reestablishing an open tube for sperm to travel through.

Therapeutic Procedures *(continued)*

TERM	WORD PARTS	DEFINITION
vasovasostomy (vas-oh-vay-ZOS-toh-mee)	vas/o = vas deferens -ostomy = create a new opening	Surgical procedure to reconnect the vas deferens to reverse a vasectomy.

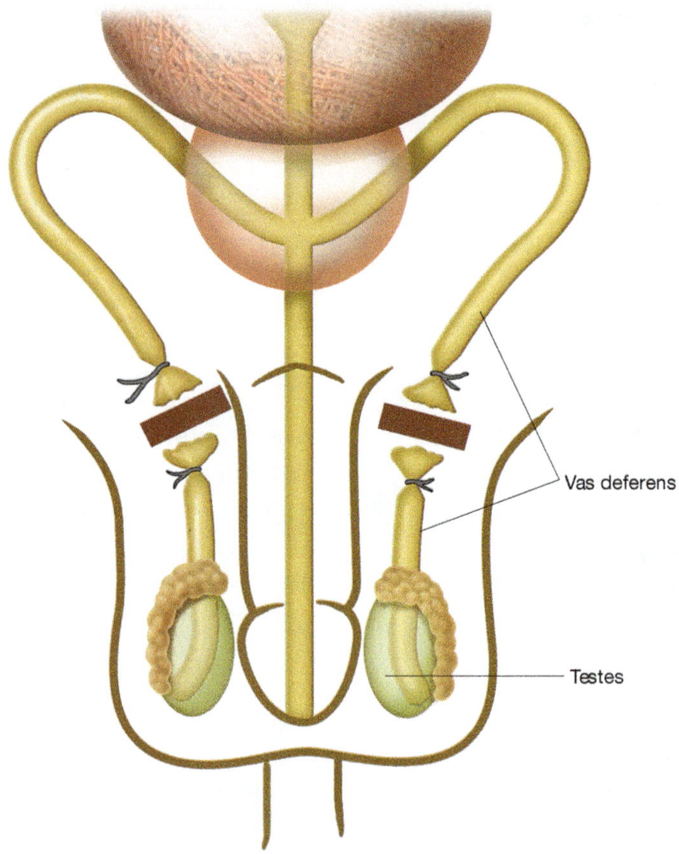

■ **Figure 10.22** A vasectomy, showing how each vas deferens is tied off in two places and then a section is removed from the middle. This prevents sperm from traveling through the vas deferens during ejaculation.

Pharmacology

CLASSIFICATION	WORD PARTS	ACTION	EXAMPLES
androgen therapy (AN-droh-jen)	andr/o = male -gen = that which produces	Replacement of male hormones to treat patients who produce insufficient hormone naturally.	testosterone cypionate, Andronate, depAndro
antiprostatic agents (an-tye-pross-TAT-ik)	anti- = against prostat/o = prostate gland -ic = pertaining to	Medication to treat early cases of benign prostatic hyperplasia. May prevent surgery for mild cases.	finasteride, Proscar; dutasteride, Avodart
erectile dysfunction agents (ee-REK-tile)	-ile = pertaining to dys- = abnormal, difficult	Medication that temporarily produces an erection in patients with erectile dysfunction.	sildenafil citrate, Viagra; tadalafil, Cialis
spermatocide (sper-mah-toh-LIT-ik)	spermat/o = sperm -cide = to kill	Destruction of sperm. One form of birth control is the use of spermatolytic creams.	octoxynol 9, Semicid, Ortho-Gynol

Abbreviations

BPH	benign prostatic hyperplasia	**RPR**	rapid plasma reagin (test for syphilis)
DRE	digital rectal exam	**SPP**	suprapubic prostatectomy
ED	erectile dysfunction	**STD**	sexually transmitted disease
GC	gonorrhea	**TUR**	transurethral resection
GU	genitourinary	**TURP**	transurethral resection of the prostate
PSA	prostate-specific antigen	**VD**	venereal disease

Chapter Review

Real-World Applications

Medical Record Analysis

This High-Risk Obstetrics Consultation Report contains 12 medical terms. Underline each term and write it in the list below the report. Then define each term.

High-Risk Obstetrics Consultation Report

Reason for Consultation:	High-risk pregnancy with late-term bleeding
History of Present Illness:	Patient is 23 years old. She is currently estimated to be at 175 days of gestation. Amniocentesis at 20 weeks shows a normally developing male fetus. She noticed a moderate degree of bleeding this morning but denies any cramping or pelvic pain. She immediately saw her obstetrician who referred her for high-risk evaluation.
Past Medical History:	This patient is multigravida but nullipara with three early miscarriages without obvious cause.
Results of Physical Examination:	Patient appears well nourished and abdominal girth appears consistent with length of gestation. Pelvic ultrasound indicates placenta previa with placenta almost completely overlying cervix. However, there is no evidence of abruptio placentae at this time. Fetal size estimate is consistent with 25 weeks of gestation. The fetal heartbeat is strong with a rate of 130 beats/minute.
Recommendations:	Fetus appears to be developing well and in no distress at this time. The placenta appears to be well attached on ultrasound, but the bleeding is cause for concern. With the extremely low position of the placenta, this patient is at very high risk for abruptio placentae. She will require C-section at onset of labor.

	Term	
1	______	______
2	______	______
3	______	______
4	______	______
5	______	______
6	______	______
7	______	______
8	______	______
9	______	______
10	______	______
11	______	______
12	______	______

Chart Note Transcription

The chart note below contains 10 phrases that can be reworded with a medical term that you learned in this chapter. Each phrase is identified with an underline. Determine the medical term and write your answers in the space provided.

Current Complaint:	Patient is a 77-year-old male seen by the urologist with complaints of nocturia and difficulty with the release of semen from the urethra. ❶
Past History:	Medical history revealed that the patient had failure of the testes to descend into the scrotum ❷ at birth, which was repaired by surgical fixation of the testes. ❸ He had also undergone elective sterilization by removal of a segment of the vas deferens ❹ at the age of 41.
Signs and Symptoms:	Patient states he first noted these symptoms about 5 years ago. They have become increasingly severe and now he is not able to sleep without waking to urinate up to 20 times a night. He has difficulty with release of semen. ❺ Palpation of the prostate gland through the rectum ❻ revealed multiple round, firm nodules in prostate gland. A needle biopsy was negative for slow-growing cancer that frequently affects males over age 50 ❼ and a blood test for prostate cancer ❽ was normal.
Diagnosis:	Noncancerous enlargement of the prostate gland. ❾
Treatment:	Patient was scheduled for a surgical removal of prostate tissue through the urethra. ❿

❶ ____________________

❷ ____________________

❸ ____________________

❹ ____________________

❺ ____________________

❻ ____________________

❼ ____________________

❽ ____________________

❾ ____________________

❿ ____________________

Case Study

Below is a case study presentation of a patient with a condition covered by this chapter. Read the case study and answer the questions below. Some questions will ask for information not included within this chapter. Use your text, a medical dictionary, or any other reference material you choose to answer these questions.

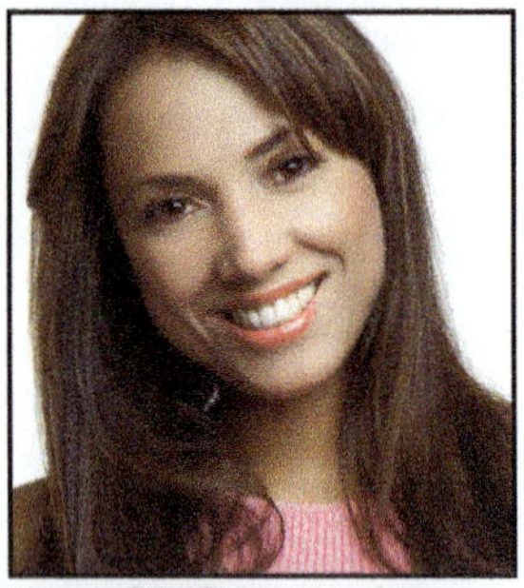

(Jason Stitt/Shutterstock)

A 22-year-old female has come into the gynecologist's office complaining of fever, malaise, dysuria, and vaginal leukorrhea. Upon examination the physician observes fluid-filled vesicles on her cervix, vulva, and perineum. Several have ruptured into ulcers with marked erythema and edema. Palpation revealed painful and enlarged inguinal lymph nodes. She also has an extragenital lesion on her mouth. Her diagnosis is genital herpes.

Questions

1. What pathological condition does this patient have? Look this condition up in a reference source and include a short description of it.

____

____

2. List and define each of the patient's presenting symptoms in your own words. Leukorrhea is a term you have not seen before. Can you give its meaning just from its word parts?

____

____

3. Describe the results of the physician's examination in your own words.

____

____

4. Explain what extragenital lesion means.

____

____

5. Explain what palpation means.

____

____

6. What is the potential effect of having this virus present in open genital lesions on the patient's future pregnancy and child birth?

____

____

Practice Exercises

A. Complete the Statement

1. The study of the female reproductive system is the medical specialty of ______________________.
2. A physician who specializes in the treatment of women is called a(n) ______________________.
3. The three stages of labor and delivery are the ______________________ stage, the ______________________ stage, and the ______________________ stage.
4. The time required for the development of a fetus is called ______________________.
5. The cessation of menstruation is called ______________________.
6. The female sex cell is a(n) ______________________.
7. The inner lining of the uterus is called the ______________________.
8. The organ in which the developing fetus resides is called the ______________________.
9. The tubes that extend from the outer edges of the uterus and assist in transporting the ova and sperm are called ______________________.
10. One of the longest terms used in medical terminology refers to the removal of the uterus, cervix, ovaries, and uterine tubes. This term is ______________________.

B. What Does it Stand For?

1. SPP ______________________
2. TUR ______________________
3. GU ______________________
4. BPH ______________________
5. DRE ______________________
6. PSA ______________________

C. Define the Term

1. spermatogenesis ______________________
2. hydrocele ______________________
3. transurethral resection of the prostate (TURP) ______________________
4. sterility ______________________
5. orchiectomy ______________________
6. vasectomy ______________________
7. castration ______________________

D. Combining Form Practice

The combining form **colp/o** refers to the vagina. Use it to write a term that means:

1. visual examination of the vagina ____________________
2. instrument used to examine the vagina ____________________

The combining form **cervic/o** refers to the cervix. Use it to write a term that means:

3. removal of the cervix ____________________
4. inflammation of the cervix ____________________
5. pertaining to the cervix ____________________

The combining form **hyster/o** also refers to the uterus. Use it to write a term that means:

6. surgical fixation of the uterus ____________________
7. removal of the uterus ____________________
8. rupture of the uterus ____________________

The combining form **oophor/o** refers to the ovaries. Use it to write a term that means:

9. inflammation of an ovary ____________________
10. removal of an ovary ____________________

The combining form **mamm/o** refers to the breasts. Use it to write a term that means:

11. pertaining to the breasts ____________________
12. record of breast ____________________
13. surgical repair of breast ____________________

The combining form **amni/o** refers to the amnion. Use it to write a term that means:

14. pertaining to the amnion ____________________
15. cutting into amnion ____________________
16. flow from amnion ____________________

E. What Does it Stand For?

1. Cx ____________________
2. LMP ____________________
3. FHR ____________________
4. PID ____________________
5. GYN ____________________

6. CS ______

7. NB ______

8. PMS ______

9. TSS ______

10. LBW ______

F. What's the Abbreviation?

1. first pregnancy ______
2. artificial insemination ______
3. uterine contractions ______
4. full-term normal delivery ______
5. intrauterine device ______
6. dilation and curettage ______
7. hormone replacement therapy ______
8. gynecology ______
9. abortion ______
10. oral contraception pills ______

G. Define the Combining Form

	Definition	Example from Chapter
1. **metr/o**	______	______
2. **hyster/o**	______	______
3. **gynec/o**	______	______
4. **episi/o**	______	______
5. **oophor/o**	______	______
6. **ovari/o**	______	______
7. **salping/o**	______	______
8. **men/o**	______	______
9. **vagin/o**	______	______
10. **mast/o**	______	______

H. Terminology Matching

Match each term to its definition.

1. ________ hemolytic disease of the newborn
2. ________ ovary
3. ________ vagina
4. ________ abruptio placentae
5. ________ placenta
6. ________ endometrium
7. ________ clitoris
8. ________ candidiasis
9. ________ Pap smear
10. ________ uterine tube
11. ________ dysmenorrhea
12. ________ breech presentation
13. ________ Apgar
14. ________ neonate
15. ________ eclampsia

a. seizures and coma during pregnancy
b. erythroblastosis fetalis
c. detached placenta
d. female erectile tissue
e. produces eggs
f. normal place for fertilization
g. buttocks first to appear in birth canal
h. birth canal
i. nourishes fetus
j. uterine lining
k. measures newborn's adjustment to outside world
l. test for cervical cancer
m. newborn
n. yeast infection
o. painful menstruation

I. Define the Suffix

	Definition	Example from Chapter
1. **-tocia**	________	________
2. **-gravida**	________	________
3. **-arche**	________	________
4. **-cyesis**	________	________
5. **-partum**	________	________
6. **-para**	________	________
7. **-salpinx**	________	________
8. **-spermia**	________	________

J. Fill in the Blank

premenstrual syndrome	stillbirth	conization	laparoscopy
D & C	puberty	endometriosis	eclampsia
fibroid tumor	cesarean section		

1. Kesha had a core of tissue from her cervix removed for testing. This is called ____________________ .
2. Joan delivered a baby that had died while still in the uterus. She had a(n) ____________________ .
3. Ashley has just started her first menstrual cycle. She is said to have entered ____________________ .
4. Kimberly is experiencing tender breasts, headaches, and some irritability just prior to her monthly menstrual cycle. This may be ____________________ .
5. Ana has been scheduled for an examination in which her physician will use an instrument to observe her abdominal cavity to rule out the diagnosis of severe endometriosis. The physician will insert the instrument through a small incision. This procedure is called a(n) ____________________ .
6. Lenora is scheduled to have a hysterectomy as a result of a long history of large benign growths in her uterus that have caused pain and bleeding. Lenora has a(n) ____________________
7. Tiffany's physician has recommended that she have a uterine scraping to stop excessive bleeding after a miscarriage. She will be scheduled for a(n) ____________________ .
8. Stacey is having frequent prenatal checkups to prevent the serious condition of pregnancy called ____________________ .
9. Marion has experienced painful menstrual periods as a result of the lining of her uterus being displaced into her pelvic cavity. This is called ____________________ .
10. Because her cervix was not dilating, Shataundra was informed that she will probably require a(n) ____________________ for her baby's delivery.

K. Complete the Statement

1. The male reproductive system is a combination of the ____________________ and ____________________ systems.
2. The male's external organs of reproduction consist of the ____________________, ____________________, and the ____________________.
3. Another term for the prepuce is the ____________________.
4. The organs responsible for developing the sperm cells are the ____________________.
5. The glands of lubrication and fluid production at each side of the male urethra are the ____________________.
6. The male sex hormone is ____________________.
7. The area between the scrotum and the anus is called the ____________________.

L. Terminology Matching

Match each term to its definition.

1. ________ gonorrhea
2. ________ genital herpes
3. ________ human immunodeficiency virus
4. ________ syphilis
5. ________ venereal disease
6. ________ genital warts
7. ________ chancroid
8. ________ chlamydia
9. ________ trichomoniasis

a. also called STD
b. caused by parasitic microorganism
c. treated with penicillin
d. caused by human papilloma virus
e. can pass to infant during birth
f. genitourinary infection
g. venereal ulcer
h. attacks the immune system
i. skin disease with vesicles

M. Combining Form Practice

The combining form **prostat/o** refers to the prostate. Use this to write a term that means:

1. removal of prostate ________
2. pertaining to the prostate ________
3. inflammation of the prostate ________

The combining form **orchi/o** refers to the testes. Use this to write a term that means:

4. removal of the testes ________
5. surgical repair of the testes ________
6. incision into the testes ________

The suffix **-spermia** refers to a sperm condition. Use this to write a term that means:

7. condition of being without sperm ________
8. condition of having too few (scanty) sperm ________

The combining form **spermat/o** refers to sperm. Use this to write a term that means:

9. sperm forming ________
10. sperm destruction ________

N. Pharmacology Challenge

Fill in the classification for each drug description, then match the brand name.

	Drug Description	Classification	Brand Name
1.	________ replacement male hormone	____________________	a. Pitocin
2.	________ improves uterine contractions	____________________	b. Avodart
3.	________ treats early BPH	____________________	c. Clomid
4.	________ blocks ovulation	____________________	d. Semicid
5.	________ kills sperm	____________________	e. Mifeprex
6.	________ produces an erection	____________________	f. Andronate
7.	________ replaces estrogen	____________________	g. Ortho-Cept
8.	________ terminates a pregnancy	____________________	h. Viagra
9.	________ triggers ovulation	____________________	i. Premarin

Labeling Exercise

Image A

Write the labels for this figure on the numbered lines provided.

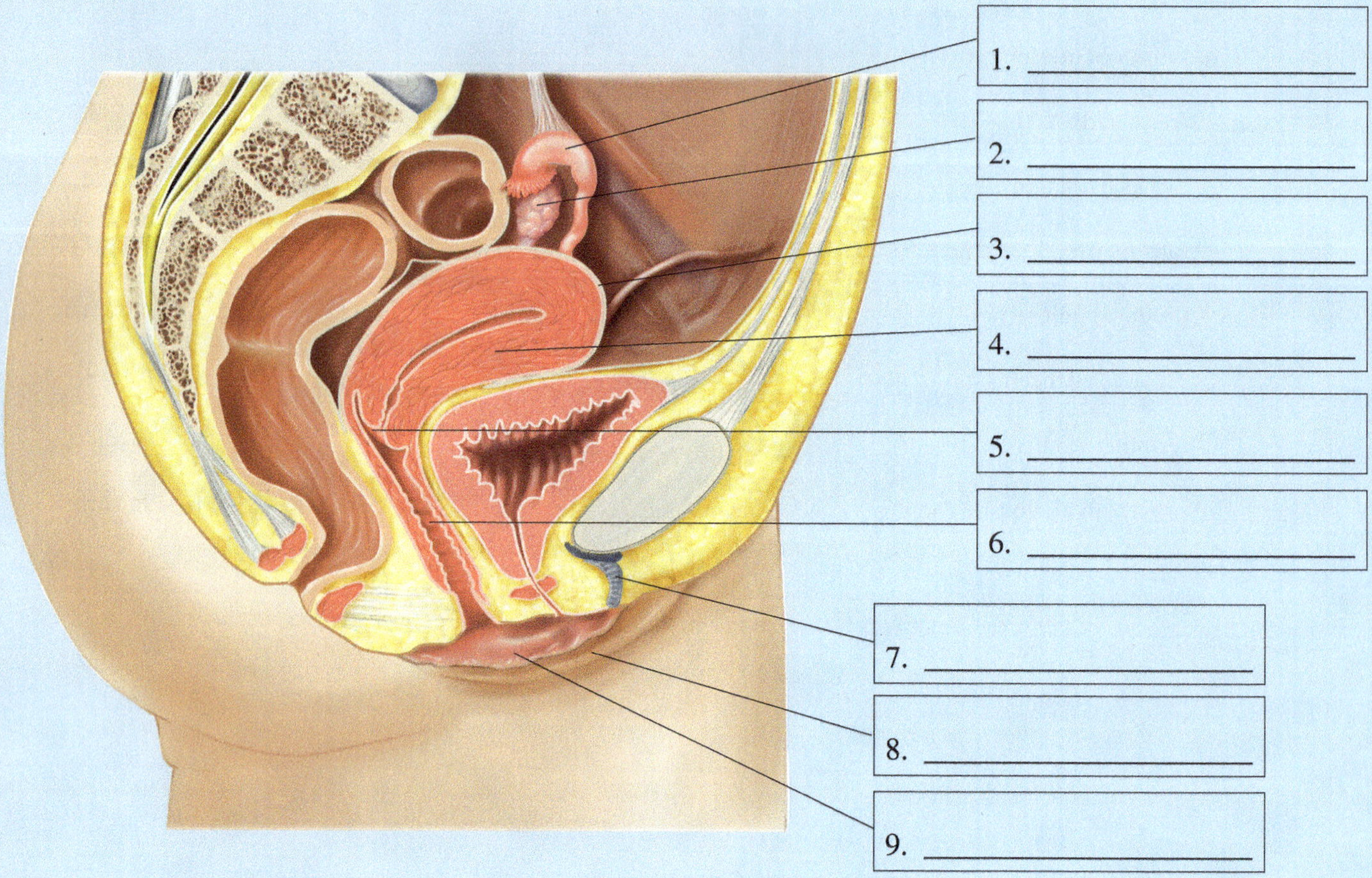

Image B

Write the labels for this figure on the numbered lines provided.

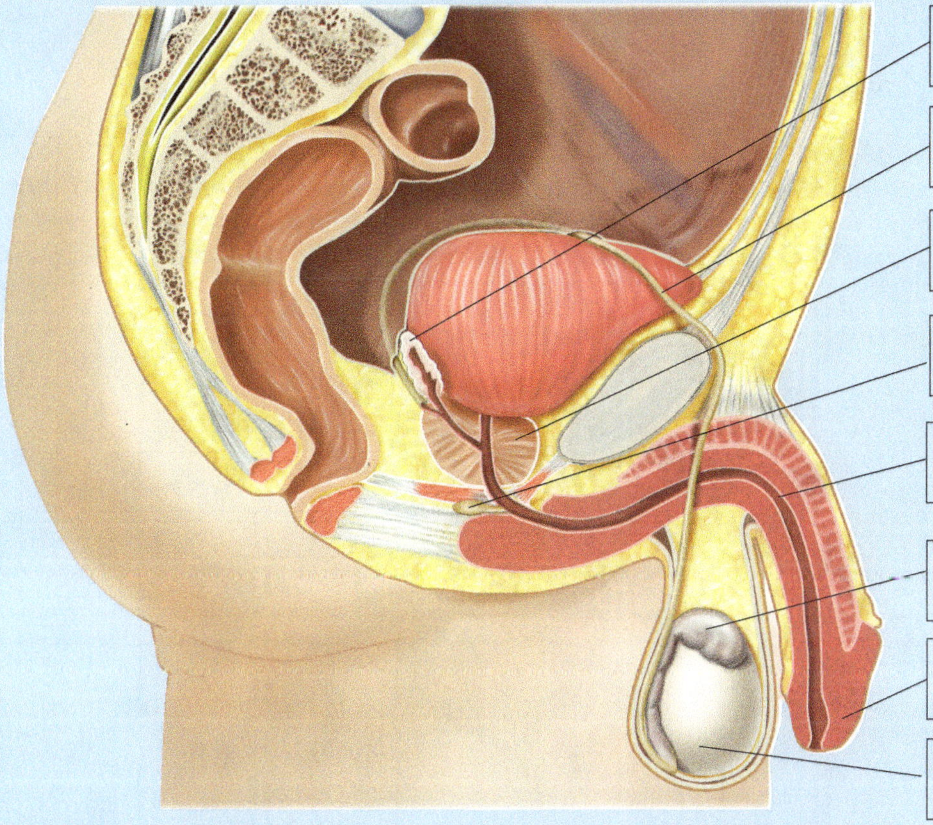

1. ______________________
2. ______________________
3. ______________________
4. ______________________
5. ______________________
6. ______________________
7. ______________________
8. ______________________

Image C

Write the labels for this figure on the numbered lines provided.

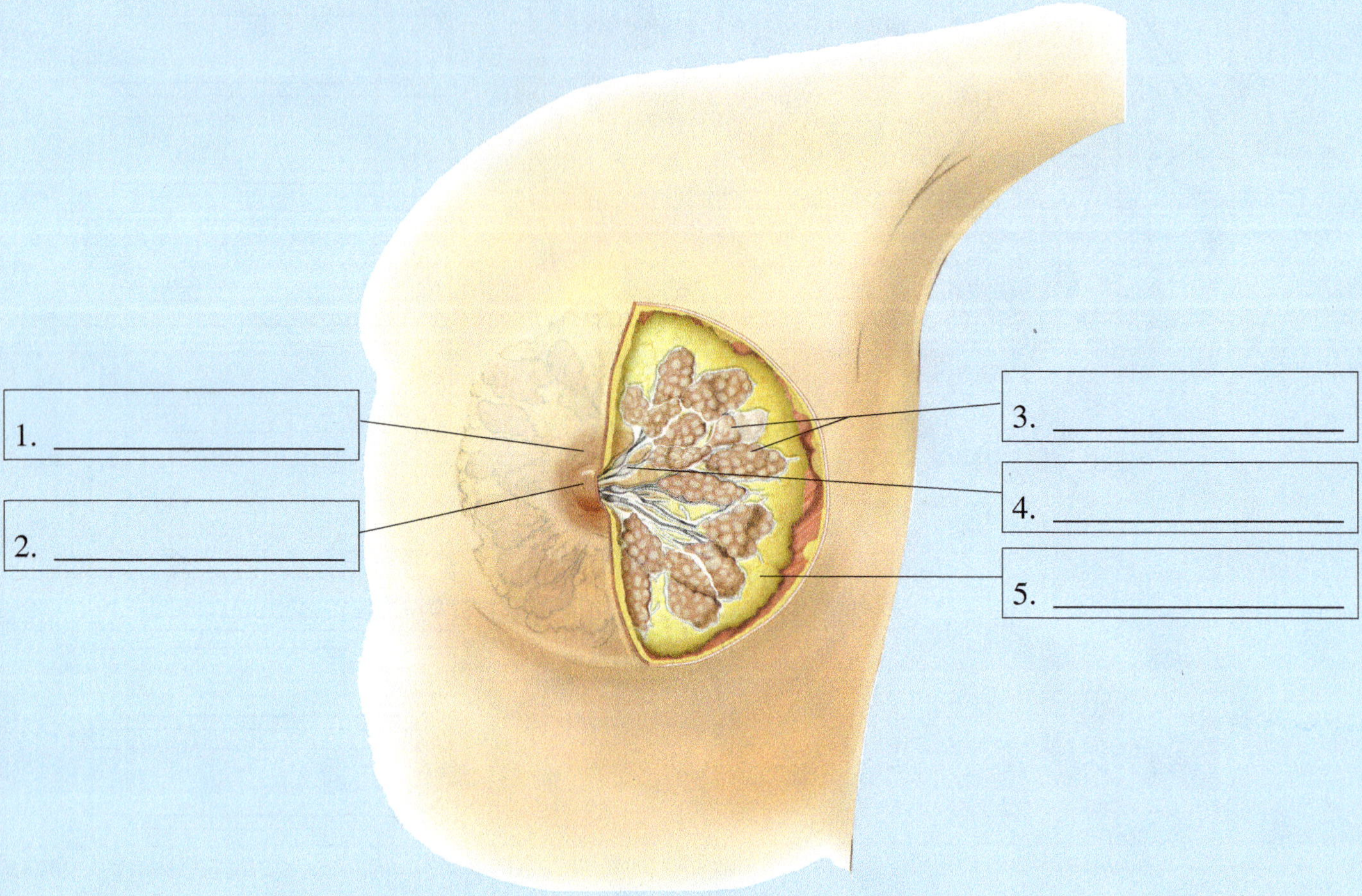

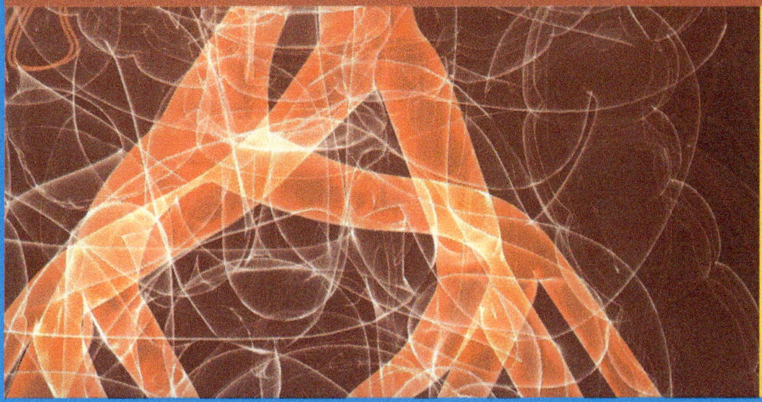

11

ENDOCRINE SYSTEM

Learning Objectives

Upon completion of this chapter, you will be able to

- Identify and define the combining forms and suffixes introduced in this chapter.
- Correctly spell and pronounce medical terms and major anatomical structures relating to the endocrine system.
- Locate and describe the major organs of the endocrine system and their functions.
- List the major hormones secreted by each endocrine gland and describe their functions.
- Identify and define endocrine system anatomical terms.
- Identify and define selected endocrine system pathology terms.
- Identify and define selected endocrine system diagnostic procedures.
- Identify and define selected endocrine system therapeutic procedures.
- Identify and define selected medications relating to the endocrine system.
- Define selected abbreviations associated with the endocrine system.

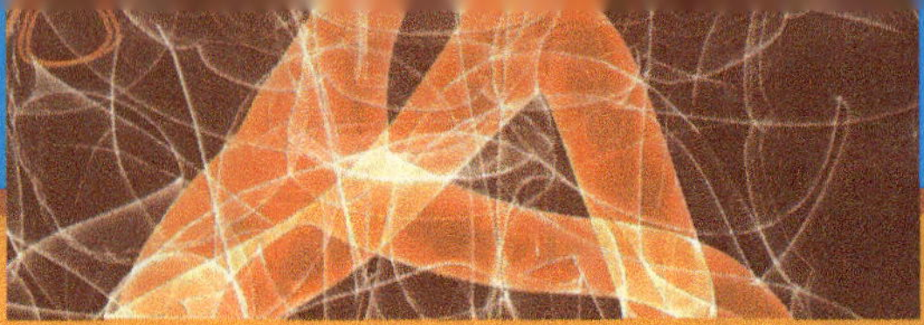

Endocrine System at a Glance

Function

Endocrine glands secrete hormones that regulate many body activities such as metabolic rate, water and mineral balance, immune system reactions, and sexual functioning.

Structures

Here are the primary structures that comprise the endocrine system.

adrenal glands
ovaries
pancreas (islets of Langerhans)
parathyroid glands
pineal gland
pituitary gland
testes
thymus gland
thyroid gland

Word Parts

Here are the most common word parts used to build endocrine system terms. For a more comprehensive list, refer to the Terminology section of this chapter.

Combining Forms

acr/o	extremities
adren/o	adrenal glands
adrenal/o	adrenal glands
andr/o	male
calc/o	calcium
crin/o	to secrete
estr/o	female
gluc/o	glucose
glyc/o	sugar
glycos/o	sugar
gonad/o	sex glands
home/o	sameness
iod/o	iodine
kal/i	potassium
ket/o	ketones
mineral/o	minerals, electrolytes
natr/o	sodium
ophthalm/o	eye
ovari/o	ovary
pancreat/o	pancreas
parathyroid/o	parathyroid gland
pineal/o	pineal gland
pituitar/o	pituitary gland
testicul/o	testes
thym/o	thymus gland
thyr/o	thyroid gland
thyroid/o	thyroid gland
toxic/o	poison

Suffixes

-dipsia	thirst
-prandial	relating to a meal
-pressin	to press down
-tropin	to stimulate

Endocrine System Illustrated

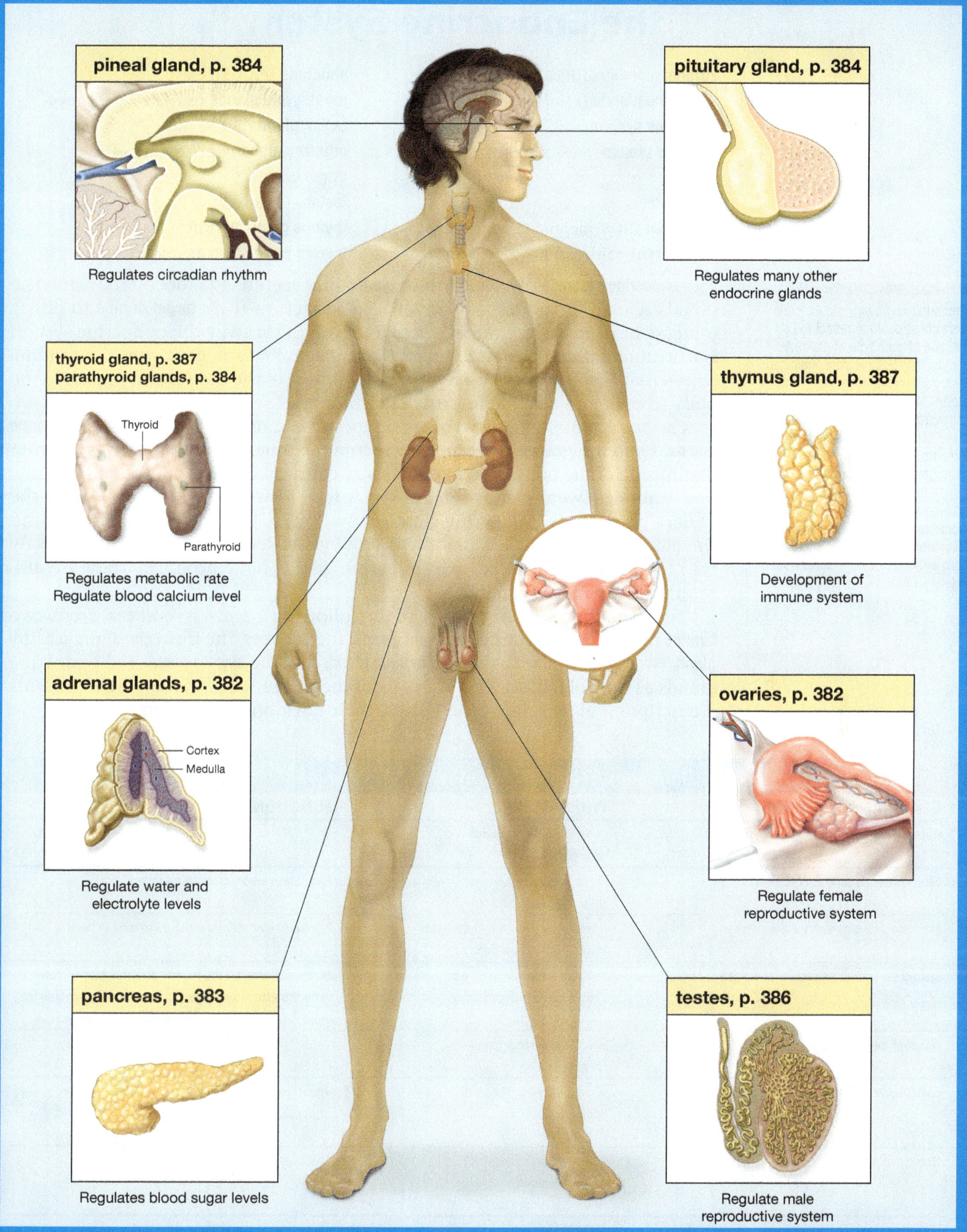

Anatomy and Physiology of the Endocrine System

adrenal glands (ad-REE-nal)
endocrine glands (EN-doh-krin)
endocrine system
exocrine glands (EKS-oh-krin)
glands
homeostasis (hoe-me-oh-STAY-sis)
hormones (HOR-mohnz)
ovaries (OH-vah-reez)
pancreas (PAN-kree-ass)
parathyroid glands (pair-ah-THIGH-royd)
pineal gland (pih-NEAL)
pituitary gland (pih-TOO-ih-tair-ee)
target organs
testes (TESS-teez)
thymus gland (THIGH-mus)
thyroid gland (THIGH-royd)

The **endocrine system** is a collection of **glands** that secrete **hormones** directly into the bloodstream. Hormones are chemicals that act on their **target organs** to either increase or decrease the target's activity level. In this way the endocrine system is instrumental in maintaining **homeostasis** (*home/o* = sameness; *-stasis* = standing still)—that is, adjusting the activity level of most of the tissues and organs of the body to maintain a stable internal environment.

The body actually has two distinct types of glands: **exocrine glands** and **endocrine glands.** Exocrine glands release their secretions into a duct that carries them to the outside of the body or to a passageway connected to the outside of the body. For example, sweat glands release sweat into a sweat duct that travels to the surface of the body. Endocrine glands, however, release hormones directly into the bloodstream. For example, the thyroid gland secretes its hormones directly into the bloodstream. Because endocrine glands have no ducts, they are also referred to as *ductless glands.*

MED TERM TIP

The terms *endocrine* and *exocrine* were constructed to reflect the function of each type of gland. As glands, they both secrete, indicated by the combining form *crin/o*. The prefix *exo-*, meaning "external" or "outward," tells us that exocrine gland secretions are carried to the outside of the body or to a passageway connected to the outside of the body. However, the prefix *endo-*, meaning "within" or "internal," indicates that endocrine gland secretions are carried to other internal body structures by the bloodstream.

The endocrine system consists of the following glands: two **adrenal glands,** two **ovaries** in the female, four **parathyroid glands,** the **pancreas,** the **pineal gland,** the **pituitary gland,** two **testes** in the male, the **thymus gland,** and the **thyroid gland.** The endocrine glands as a whole affect the functions of the entire body. Table 11.1 ■ presents a description of the endocrine glands, their hormones, and their functions.

Table 11.1 Endocrine Glands and Their Hormones

GLAND AND HORMONE	WORD PARTS	FUNCTION
Adrenal cortex	adren/o = adrenal gland -al = pertaining to	
Glucocorticoids such as cortisol	gluc/o = glucose cortic/o = outer portion	Regulates carbohydrate levels in the body.
Mineralocorticoids such as aldosterone	mineral/o = minerals, electrolytes cortic/o = outer portion	Regulates electrolytes and fluid volume in body.
Steroid sex hormones such as androgen	andr/o = male -gen = that which produces	Male sex hormones from adrenal cortex may be converted to estrogens in the bloodstream. Responsible for reproduction and secondary sexual characteristics.
Adrenal medulla	adren/o = adrenal gland -al = pertaining to	
Epinephrine (adrenaline)	epi- = above nephr/o = kidney -ine = pertaining to	Intensifies response during stress; "fight-or-flight" response.
Norepinephrine	epi- = above nephr/o = kidney -ine = pertaining to	Chiefly a vasoconstrictor.

Table 11.1 Endocrine Glands and Their Hormones (continued)

GLAND AND HORMONE	WORD PARTS	FUNCTION
Ovaries		
Estrogen	estr/o = female -gen = that which produces	Stimulates development of secondary sex characteristics in females; regulates menstrual cycle.
Progesterone	pro- = before estr/o = female	Prepares for conditions of pregnancy.
Pancreas		
Glucagon		Stimulates liver to release glucose into the blood.
Insulin		Regulates and promotes entry of glucose into cells.
Parathyroid glands		
Parathyroid hormone (PTH)		Stimulates bone breakdown; regulates calcium level in the blood.
Pituitary anterior lobe		
Adrenocorticotropic hormone (ACTH)	adren/o = adrenal gland cortic/o = outer portion -tropin = to stimulate	Regulates function of adrenal cortex.
Gonadotropins	gonad/o = gonads -tropin = to stimulate	
Follicle-stimulating hormone (FSH)		Stimulates growth of eggs in female and sperm in males.
Luteinizing hormone (LH)		Regulates function of male and female gonads and plays a role in releasing ova in females.
Growth hormone (GH)		Stimulates growth of the body.
Melanocyte-stimulating hormone (MSH)	melan/o = black -cyte = cell	Stimulates pigment in skin.
Prolactin	pro- = before lact/o = milk	Stimulates milk production.
Thyroid-stimulating hormone (TSH)		Regulates function of thyroid gland.
Pituitary posterior lobe		
Antidiuretic hormone (ADH)	anti- = against -tic = pertaining to	Stimulates reabsorption of water by the kidneys.
Oxytocin		Stimulates uterine contractions and releases milk into ducts.
Testes		
Testosterone		Promotes sperm production and development of secondary sex characteristics in males.
Thymus		
Thymosin	thym/o = thymus gland	Promotes development of cells in immune system.
Thyroid gland		
Calcitonin (CT)		Stimulates deposition of calcium into bone.
Thyroxine (T_4)	thyr/o = thyroid gland -ine = pertaining to	Stimulates metabolism in cells.
Triiodothyronine (T_3)	tri- = three iod/o = iodine thyr/o = thyroid gland -ine = pertaining to	Stimulates metabolism in cells.

Adrenal Glands

adrenal cortex (KOR-tex)
adrenal medulla (meh-DOOL-lah)
adrenaline (ah-DREN-ah-lin)
aldosterone (al-DOSS-ter-ohn)
androgens (AN-druh-jenz)
corticosteroids (kor-tih-koh-STAIR-oydz)
cortisol (KOR-tih-sal)
epinephrine (ep-ih-NEF-rin)
estrogen (ESS-troh-jen)
glucocorticoids (gloo-koh-KOR-tih-koydz)
mineralocorticoids (min-er-al-oh-KOR-tih-koydz)
norepinephrine (nor-ep-ih-NEF-rin)
progesterone (proh-JESS-ter-ohn)
steroid sex hormones (STAIR-oyd)

The two adrenal glands are located above each of the kidneys (see Figure 11.1 ■). Each gland is composed of two sections: **adrenal cortex** and **adrenal medulla.**

The outer adrenal cortex manufactures several different families of hormones: **mineralocorticoids, glucocorticoids,** and **steroid sex hormones.** However, because they are all produced by the cortex, they are collectively referred to as **corticosteroids.** The mineralocorticoid hormone, **aldosterone,** regulates sodium (Na^+) and potassium (K^+) levels in the body. The glucocorticoid hormone, **cortisol,** regulates carbohydrates in the body. The adrenal cortex of both men and women secretes steroid sex hormones, **androgens** (which may be converted to **estrogen** once released into the bloodstream). These hormones regulate secondary sexual characteristics. All hormones secreted by the adrenal cortex are steroid hormones.

The inner adrenal medulla is responsible for secreting the hormones **epinephrine,** also called **adrenaline,** and **norepinephrine.** These hormones are critical during emergency situations because they increase blood pressure, heart rate, and respiration levels. This helps the body perform better during emergencies or otherwise stressful times.

MED TERM TIP

The term *cortex* is frequently used in anatomy to indicate the outer portion of an organ such as the adrenal gland or the kidney. The term *cortex* means "bark," as in the bark of a tree. The term *medulla* means "marrow." Because marrow is found in the inner cavity of bones, the term came to stand for the middle of an organ.

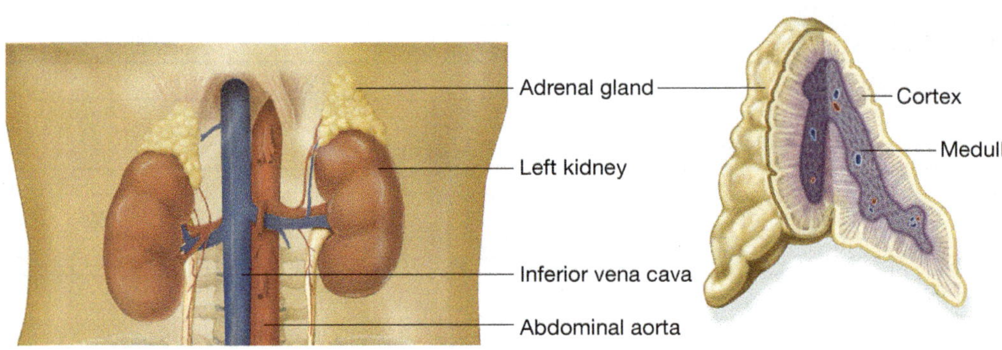

■ **Figure 11.1** The adrenal glands. These glands sit on top of each kidney. Each adrenal is subdivided into an outer cortex and an inner medulla. Each region secretes different hormones.

Ovaries

estrogen
gametes (GAM-eats)
gonads (GOH-nadz)
menstrual cycle (MEN-stroo-all)
ova
progesterone

The two ovaries are located in the lower abdominopelvic cavity of the female (see Figure 11.2 ■). They are the female **gonads.** Gonads are organs that produce **gametes** or the reproductive sex cells. In the case of females, the gametes are the **ova.** Of importance to the endocrine system, the ovaries produce the female sex hormones, **estrogen** and **progesterone.** Estrogen is responsible for the appearance of the female sexual characteristics and regulation of the **menstrual cycle.** Progesterone helps to maintain a suitable uterine environment for pregnancy.

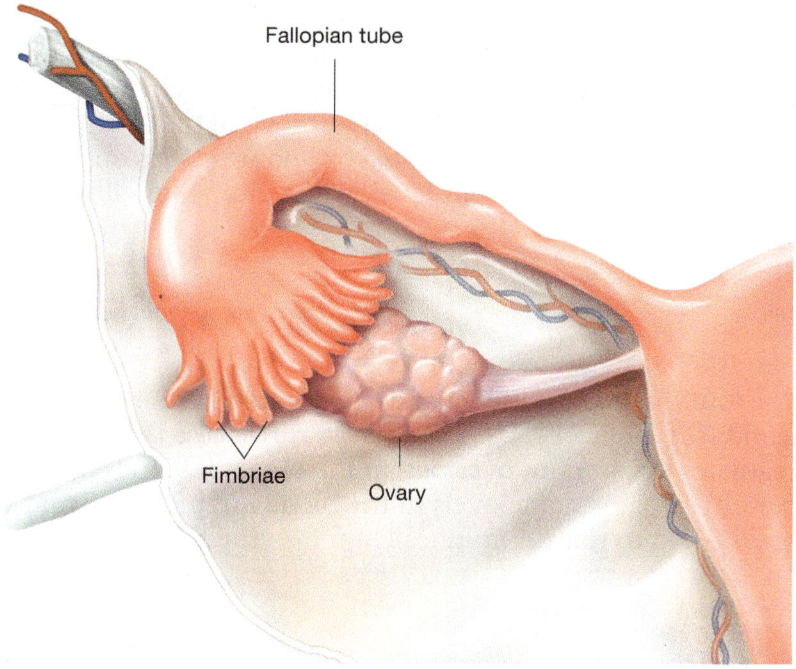

■ **Figure 11.2**
The ovaries. In addition to producing ova, the ovaries secrete the female sex hormones, estrogen and progesterone.

Pancreas

glucagon (GLOO-koh-gon)
insulin (IN-suh-lin)
islets of Langerhans (EYE-lets / of / LAHNG-er-hahnz)

The pancreas is located along the lower curvature of the stomach (see Figure 11.3A ■). It is the only organ in the body that has both endocrine and exocrine functions. The exocrine portion of the pancreas releases digestive enzymes through a duct into the duodenum of the small intestine. The endocrine sections of the pancreas, **islets of Langerhans,** are named after Dr. Paul Langerhans, a German anatomist. The islets cells produce two different hormones: **insulin** and **glucagon** (see Figure 11.3B ■). Insulin, produced by beta (β) islet cells, stimulates the cells of the body to take in glucose from the bloodstream, lowering the body's blood sugar level. This occurs after a meal has been eaten and the carbohydrates are absorbed into the bloodstream. In this way the cells obtain the glucose they need for cellular respiration.

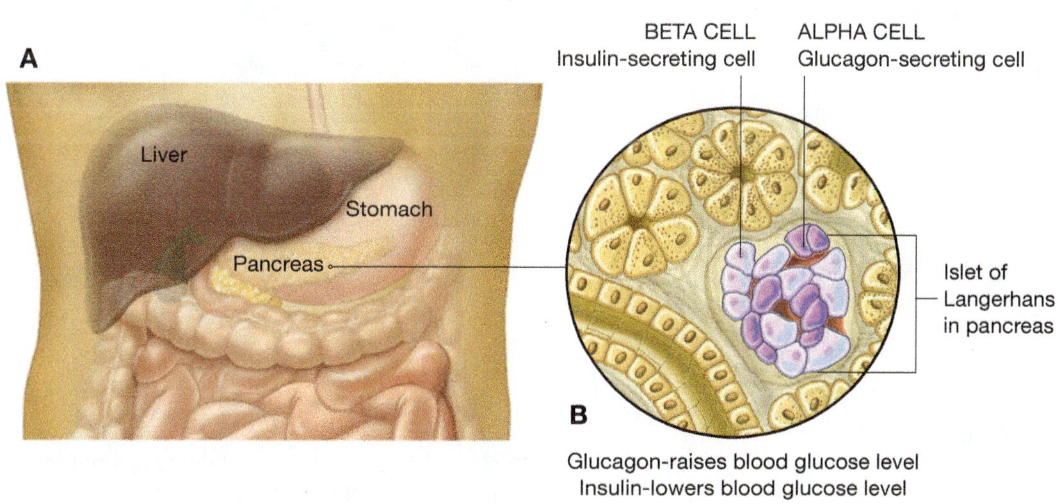

■ **Figure 11.3**
The pancreas. This organ sits just below the stomach and is both an exocrine and an endocrine gland. The endocrine regions of the pancreas are called the islets of Langerhans and they secrete insulin and glucagon.

Another set of islet cells, the alpha (α) cells, secrete a different hormone, glucagon, which stimulates the liver to release glucose, thereby raising the blood glucose level. Glucagon is released when the body needs more sugar, such as at the beginning of strenuous activity or several hours after the last meal has been digested. Insulin and glucagon have opposite effects on blood sugar level. Insulin will reduce the blood sugar level, while glucagon will increase it.

Parathyroid Glands

calcium

parathyroid hormone (pair-ah-THIGH-royd / HOR-mohn)

> **MED TERM TIP**
> A calcium deficiency in the system can result in a condition called *tetany,* or muscle excitability and tremors. If the parathyroid glands are removed during thyroid surgery, calcium replacement in the body is often necessary.

The four tiny parathyroid glands are located on the dorsal surface of the thyroid gland (see Figure 11.4 ■). The **parathyroid hormone** (PTH) secreted by these glands regulates the amount of **calcium** in the blood. If blood calcium levels fall too low, parathyroid hormone levels in the blood are increased and will stimulate bone breakdown to release more calcium into the blood.

Pineal Gland

circadian rhythm (seer-KAY-dee-an)

melatonin (mel-ah-TOH-nin)

thalamus (THALL-mus)

> **MED TERM TIP**
> The pineal gland is an example of an organ named for its shape. *Pineal* means "shaped like a pine cone."

The pineal gland is a small pine cone-shaped gland that is part of the **thalamus** region of the brain (see Figure 11.5 ■). The pineal gland secretes **melatonin,** a hormone not well understood, but that plays a role in regulating the body's **circadian rhythm.** This is the 24-hour clock that governs our periods of wakefulness and sleepiness.

Pituitary Gland

adrenocorticotropic hormone (ah-dree-noh-kor-tih-koh-TROH-pk)

anterior lobe

antidiuretic hormone (an-tye-dye-yoo-RET-ik)

follicle-stimulating hormone (FOLL-ih-kl / STIM-yoo-lay-ting)

gonadotropins (go-nad-oh-TROH-pins)

growth hormone

hypothalamus (high-poh-THAL-ah-mus)

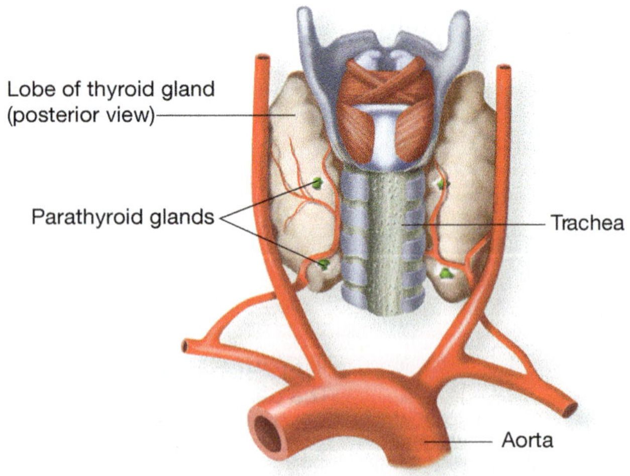

■ **Figure 11.4** The parathyroid glands. These four glands are located on the posterior side of the thyroid gland. They secrete parathyroid hormone.

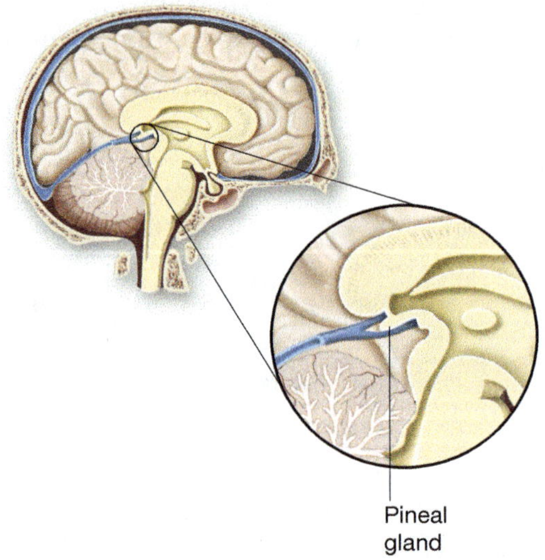

■ **Figure 11.5** The pineal gland is a part of the thalamus region of the brain. It secretes melatonin.

luteinizing hormone (LOO-tee-in-eye-zing)
melanocyte-stimulating hormone
oxytocin (ok-see-TOH-sin)
posterior lobe
prolactin (proh-LAK-tin)
somatotropin (so-mat-oh-TROH-pin)
thyroid-stimulating hormone

The pituitary gland is located underneath the brain (see Figure 11.6 ■). The small marble-shaped gland is divided into an **anterior lobe** and a **posterior lobe.** Both lobes are controlled by the **hypothalamus,** a region of the brain active in regulating automatic body responses.

The anterior pituitary secretes several different hormones (see Figure 11.7 ■). **Growth hormone** (GH), also called **somatotropin,** promotes growth of the body by stimulating cells to rapidly increase in size and divide. **Thyroid-stimulating hormone** (TSH) regulates the function of the thyroid gland. **Adrenocorticotropic hormone** (ACTH) regulates the function of the adrenal cortex. **Prolactin** (PRL) stimulates milk production in the breast following pregnancy and birth. **Follicle-stimulating hormone** (FSH) and **luteinizing hormone** (LH) both exert their influence on the male and female gonads. Therefore, these two hormones together are referred to as the **gonadotropins.** Follicle-stimulating hormone is responsible for the development of ova in ovaries and sperm in testes. It also stimulates the ovary to secrete estrogen. Luteinizing hormone stimulates secretion of sex hormones in both males and females and plays a role in releasing ova in females. **Melanocyte-stimulating hormone** (MSH) stimulates melanocytes to produce more melanin, thereby darkening the skin.

The posterior pituitary secretes two hormones, **antidiuretic hormone** (ADH) and **oxytocin.** Antidiuretic hormone promotes water reabsorption by the kidney tubules. Oxytocin stimulates uterine contractions during labor and delivery, and after birth the release of milk from the mammary glands.

MED TERM TIP

The pituitary gland is sometimes referred to as the "master gland" because several of its secretions regulate other endocrine glands.

MED TERM TIP

Many people use the term *diabetes* to refer to diabetes mellitus (DM). But there is another type of diabetes, called *diabetes insipidus* (DI), that is a result of the inadequate secretion of the antidiuretic hormone (ADH) from the pituitary gland.

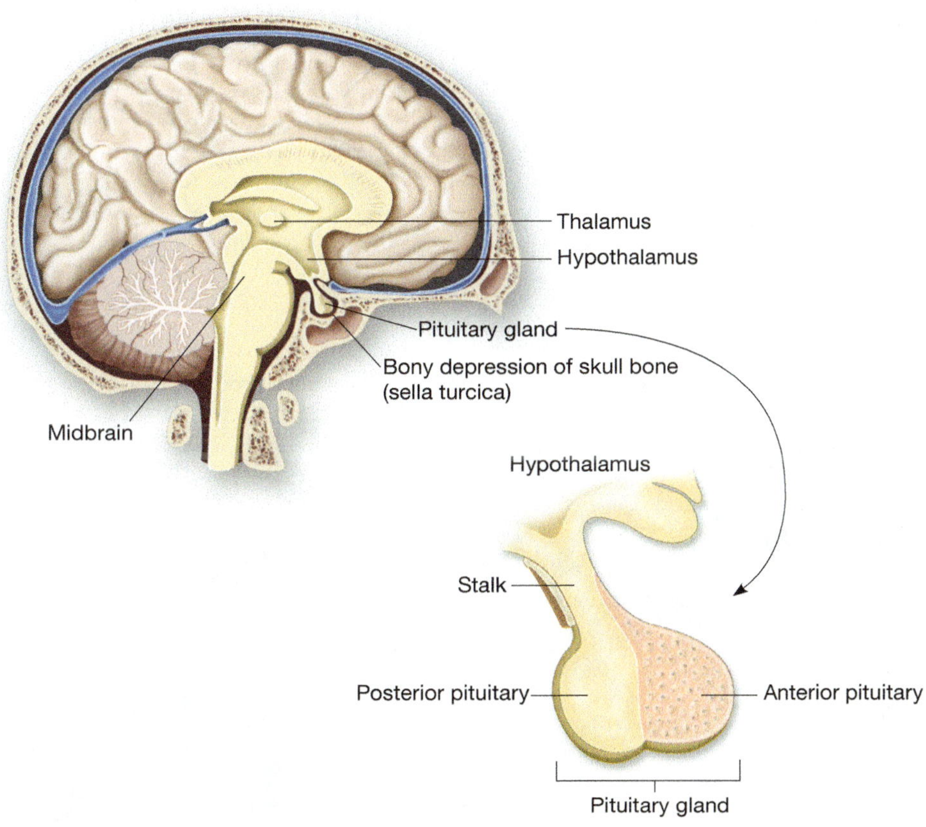

■ **Figure 11.6**
The pituitary gland lies just underneath the brain. It is subdivided into anterior and posterior lobes. Each lobe secretes different hormones.

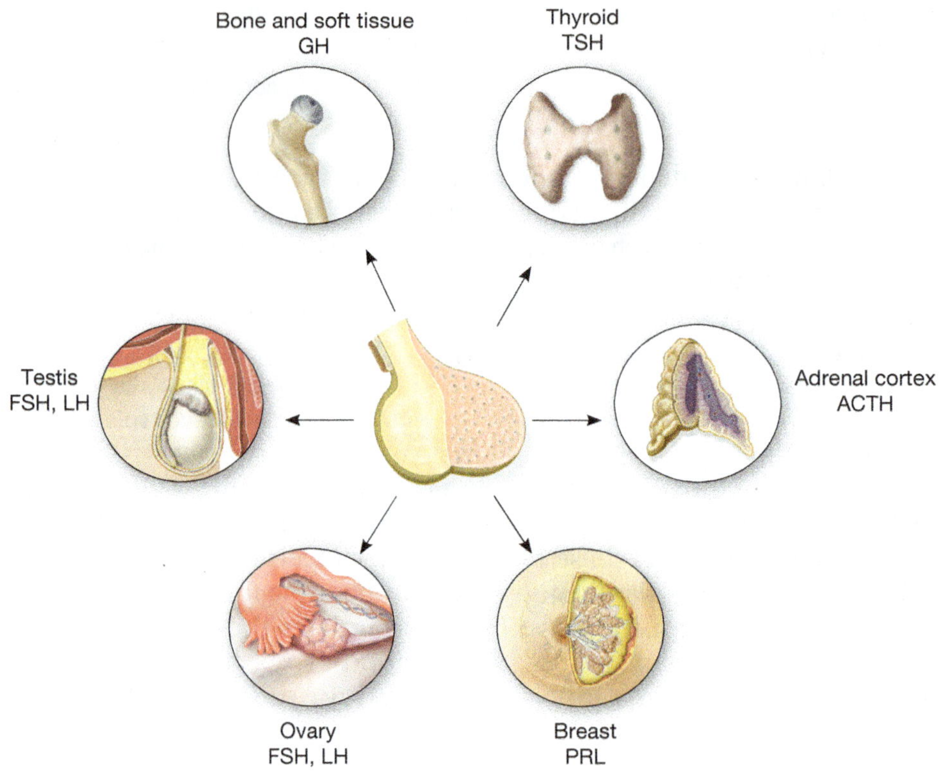

Figure 11.7
The anterior pituitary is sometimes called the master gland because it secretes many hormones that regulate other glands. This figure illustrates the different hormones and target tissues for the anterior pituitary.

Testes

sperm

testosterone (tess-TAHSS-ter-own)

The testes are two oval glands located in the scrotal sac of the male (see Figure 11.8 ■). They are the male gonads, which produce the male gametes, **sperm,** and the male sex hormone, **testosterone.** Testosterone produces the male secondary sexual characteristics and regulates sperm production.

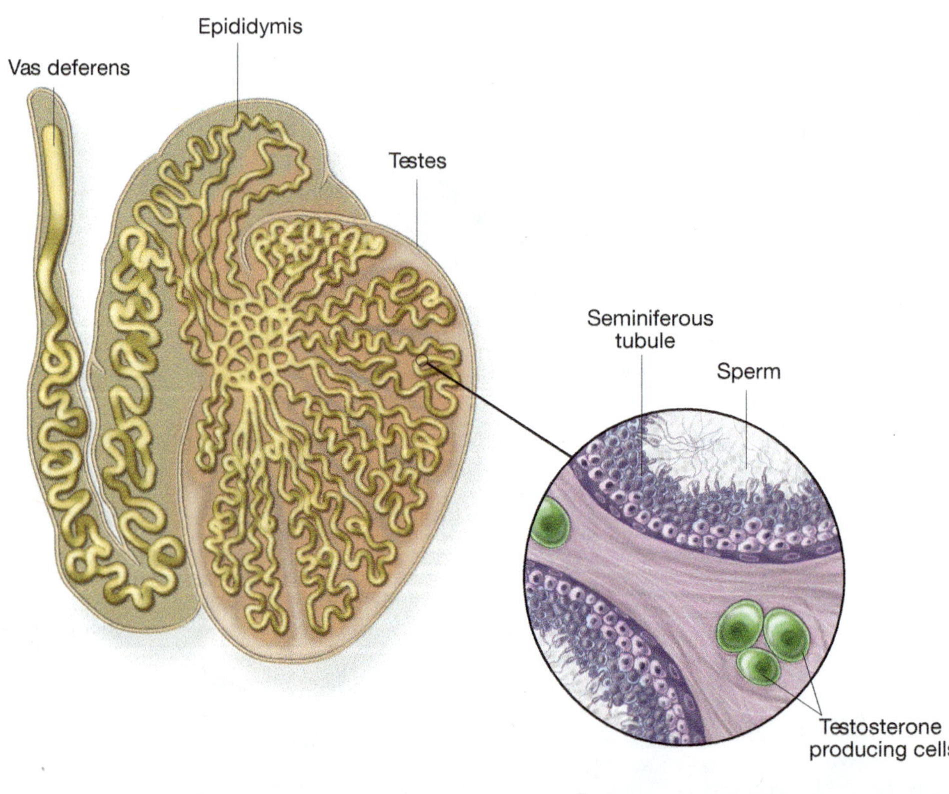

Figure 11.8
The testes. In addition to producing sperm, the testes secrete the male sex hormones, primarily testosterone.

Thymus Gland

T cells | **thymosin** (thigh-MOH-sin)

In addition to its role as part of the immune system, the thymus is also one of the endocrine glands because it secretes the hormone **thymosin.** Thymosin, like the rest of the thymus gland, is important for proper development of the immune system. The thymus gland is located in the mediastinal cavity anterior and superior to the heart (see Figure 11.9 ■). The thymus is present at birth and grows to its largest size during puberty. At puberty it begins to shrink and eventually is replaced with connective and adipose tissue.

The most important function of the thymus is the development of the immune system in the newborn. It is essential to the growth and development of thymic lymphocytes or **T cells,** which are critical for the body's immune system.

Thyroid Gland

calcitonin (kal-sih-TOH-nin)
iodine (EYE-oh-dine)
thyroxine (thigh-ROKS-in)
triiodothyronine (try-eye-oh-doh-THIGH-roh-neen)

The thyroid gland, which resembles a butterfly in shape, has right and left lobes (see Figure 11.10 ■). It is located on either side of the trachea and larynx. The thyroid cartilage, or Adam's apple, is located just above the thyroid gland. This gland produces the hormones **thyroxine** (T_4) and **triiodothyronine** (T_3). These hormones are produced in the thyroid gland from the mineral **iodine.** Thyroxine and triiodothyronine help to regulate the production of energy and heat in the body to adjust the body's metabolic rate.

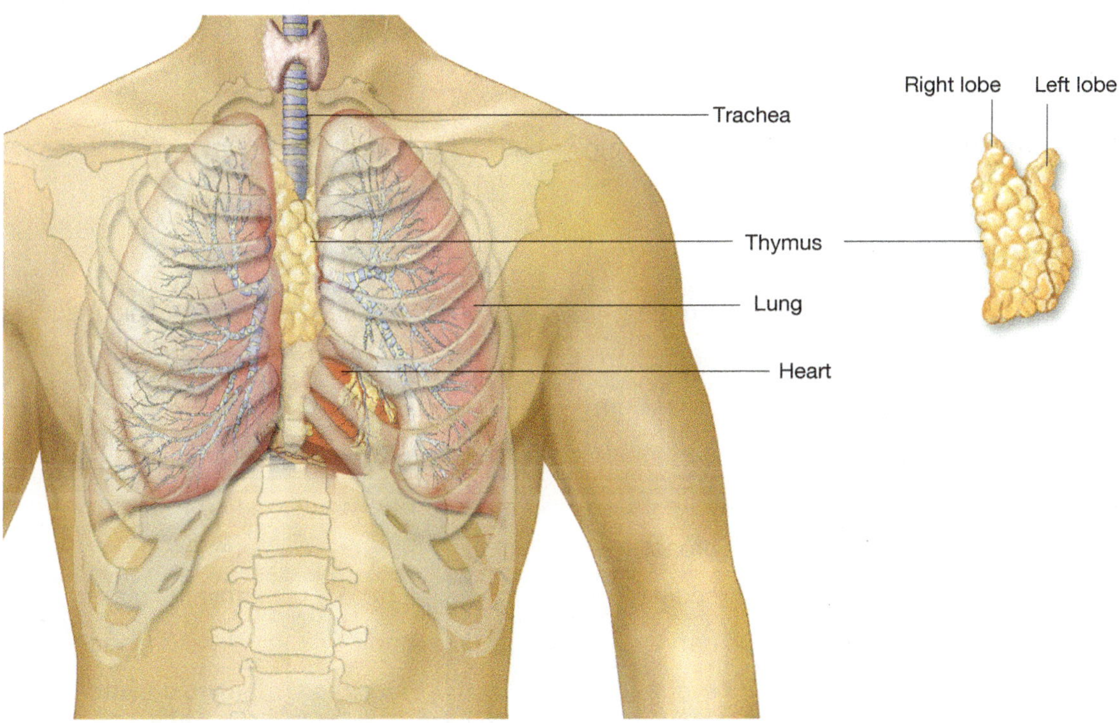

■ **Figure 11.9** The thymus gland. This gland lies in the mediastinum of the thoracic cavity, just above the heart. It secretes thymosin.

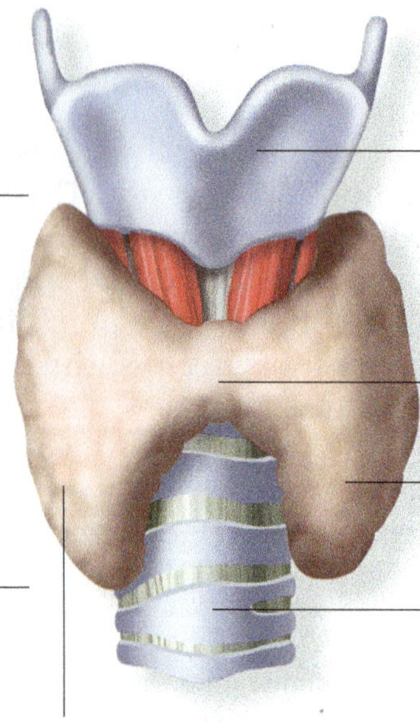

Figure 11.10 The thyroid gland is subdivided into two lobes, one on each side of the trachea.

MED TERM TIP

Iodine is found in many foods, including vegetables and seafood. It is also present in iodized salt, which is one of the best sources of iodine for people living in the Goiter Belt, composed of states located away from saltwater. A lack of iodine in the diet can lead to thyroid disorders, including *goiter.*

The thyroid gland also secretes **calcitonin** (CT) in response to hypercalcemia (too high blood calcium level). Its action is the opposite of parathyroid hormone and stimulates the increased deposition of calcium into bone, thereby lowering blood levels of calcium.

Terminology

Word Parts Used to Build Endocrine System Terms

The following lists contain the combining forms, suffixes, and prefixes used to build terms in the remaining sections of this chapter.

Combining Forms

acr/o	extremities
aden/o	gland
adren/o	adrenal gland
adrenal/o	adrenal gland
calc/o	calcium
carcin/o	cancer
chem/o	drug
cortic/o	outer portion
crin/o	to secrete
cyt/o	cell
glyc/o	sugar
glycos/o	sugar

gynec/o	female
immun/o	protection
kal/i	potassium
lapar/o	abdomen
lob/o	lobe
mast/o	breast
natr/o	sodium
neur/o	nerve
ophthalm/o	eye
or/o	mouth
ovari/o	ovary
pancreat/o	pancreas

parathyroid/o	parathyroid gland
pineal/o	pineal gland
pituitar/o	pituitary gland
radi/o	ray
retin/o	retina
testicul/o	testes
thym/o	thymus gland
thyr/o	thyroid gland
thyroid/o	thyroid gland
toxic/o	poison
vas/o	vessel

Suffixes

-al	pertaining to
-ary	pertaining to
-dipsia	thirst
-ectomy	surgical removal
-emia	blood condition
-emic	relating to a blood condition
-graphy	process of recording
-ia	condition
-ic	pertaining to
-ism	state of
-itis	inflammation
-logy	study of
-megaly	enlarged
-meter	instrument to measure
-oma	tumor
-osis	abnormal condition
-pathy	disease
-prandial	relating to a meal
-pressin	to press down
-scopy	procedure to visually examine
-tic	pertaining to
-uria	urine condition

Prefixes

anti-	against
endo-	within
ex-	outward
hyper-	excessive
hypo-	insufficient
pan-	all
poly-	many
post-	after

Anatomical Terms

TERM	WORD PARTS	DEFINITION
adrenal (ah-DREE-nall)	adren/o = adrenal gland -al = pertaining to	Pertaining to the adrenal glands.
ovarian (oh-VAIR-ee-an)	ovari/o = ovary -ian = pertaining to	Pertaining to the ovary.
pancreatic (pan-kree-AT-ik)	pancreat/o = pancreas -ic = pertaining to	Pertaining to the pancreas.
parathyroidal (pair-ah-THIGH-roy-dall)	parathyroid/o = parathyroid gland -al = pertaining to	Pertaining to the parathyroid gland.
pituitary (pih-TOO-ih-tair-ee)	pituitar/o = pituitary gland -ary = pertaining to	Pertaining to the pituitary gland.
testicular (tes-TIK-yoo-lar)	testicul/o = testes -ar = pertaining to	Pertaining to the testes.
thymic (THIGH-mik)	thym/o = thymus gland -ic = pertaining to	Pertaining to the thymus gland.
thyroidal (thigh-ROYD-all)	thyroid/o = thyroid gland -al = pertaining to	Pertaining to the thyroid gland.

Pathology

TERM	WORD PARTS	DEFINITION
Medical Specialties		
endocrinology (en-doh-krin-ALL-oh-jee)	endo- = within crin/o = to secrete -logy = study of	Branch of medicine involving diagnosis and treatment of conditions and diseases of endocrine glands. Physician is an *endocrinologist.*
Signs and Symptoms		
adrenomegaly (ad-ree-noh-MEG-ah-lee)	adren/o = adrenal gland -megaly = enlarged	Having one or both adrenal glands enlarged.
adrenopathy (ad-ren-OP-ah-thee)	adren/o = adrenal gland -pathy = disease	General term for adrenal gland disease.
edema (eh-DEE-mah)		Condition in which the body tissues contain excessive amounts of fluid.
endocrinopathy (en-doh-krin-OP-ah-thee)	endo- = within crin/o = to secrete -pathy = disease	General term for diseases of the endocrine system.
exophthalmos (eks-off-THAL-mohs)	ex- = outward ophthalm/o = eye	Condition in which the eyeballs protrude, such as in Graves' disease. This is generally caused by an overproduction of thyroid hormone.

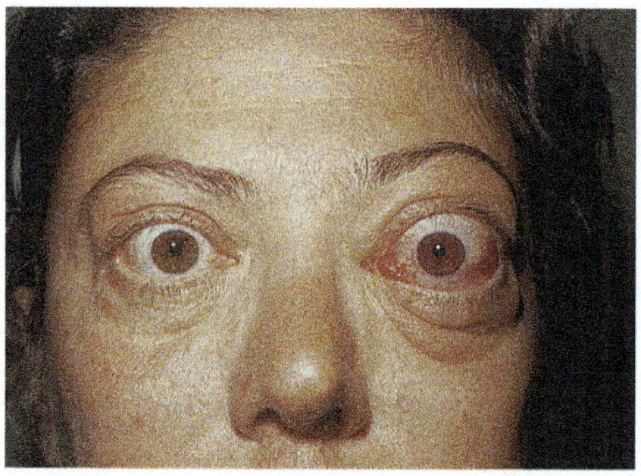

Figure 11.11 A photograph of a woman with exophthalmos. This condition is associated with hypersecretion of the thyroid gland. *(Custom Medical Stock Photo, Inc.)*

TERM	WORD PARTS	DEFINITION
glycosuria (glye-kohs-YOO-ree-ah)	glycos/o = sugar -uria = urine condition	Having a high level of sugar excreted in the urine.
gynecomastia (gigh-neh-koh-MAST-ee-ah)	gynec/o = female mast/o = breast -ia = condition	Development of breast tissue in males. May be a symptom of adrenal feminization.
hirsutism (HER-soot-izm)	-ism = state of	Condition of having an excessive amount of hair. Term generally used to describe females who have the adult male pattern of hair growth. Can be the result of a hormonal imbalance.
hypercalcemia (high-per-kal-SEE-mee-ah)	hyper- = excessive calc/o = calcium -emia = blood condition	Condition of having a high level of calcium in the blood; associated with hypersecretion of parathyroid hormone.
hyperglycemia (high-per-glye-SEE-mee-ah)	hyper- = excessive glyc/o = sugar -emia = blood condition	Condition of having a high level of sugar in the blood; associated with diabetes mellitus.

Pathology *(continued)*

TERM	WORD PARTS	DEFINITION
hyperkalemia (high-per-kal-EE-mee-ah)	hyper- = excessive kal/i = potassium -emia = blood condition	The condition of having a high level of potassium in the blood.
hypersecretion	hyper- = excessive	Excessive hormone production by an endocrine gland.
hypocalcemia (high-poh-kal-SEE-mee-ah)	hypo- = insufficient calc/o = calcium -emia = blood condition	The condition of having a low level of calcium in the blood; associated with hyposecretion of parathyroid hormone. Hypocalcemia may result in tetany.
hypoglycemia (high-poh-glye-SEE-mee-ah)	hypo- = insufficient glyc/o = sugar -emia = blood condition	Condition of having a low level of sugar in the blood.
hyponatremia (high-poh-nah-TREE-mee-ah)	hypo- = insufficient natr/o = sodium -emia = blood condition	Condition of having a low level of sodium in the blood.
hyposecretion	hypo- = insufficient	Deficient hormone production by an endocrine gland.
obesity (oh-BEE-sih-tee)		Having an abnormal amount of fat in the body.
polydipsia (pall-ee-DIP-see-ah)	poly- = many -dipsia = thirst	Excessive feeling of thirst.
polyuria (pall-ee-YOO-ree-ah)	poly- = many -uria = urine condition	Condition of producing an excessive amount of urine.
syndrome (SIN-drohm)		Group of symptoms and signs that, when combined, present a clinical picture of a disease or condition.
thyromegaly (thigh-roh-MEG-ah-lee)	thyr/o = thyroid gland -megaly = enlarged	Having an enlarged thyroid gland.
Adrenal Glands		
Addison's disease (AD-ih-sons)		Disease named for British physician Thomas Addison; results from a deficiency in adrenocortical hormones. There may be an increased pigmentation of the skin, generalized weakness, and weight loss.
adrenal feminization (ad-REE-nal / fem-ih-nigh-ZAY-shun)	adren/o = adrenal gland -al = pertaining to	Development of female secondary sexual characteristics (such as breasts) in a male. Often as a result of increased estrogen secretion by the adrenal cortex.
adrenal virilism (ad-REE-nal / VIR-ill-izm)	adren/o = adrenal gland -al = pertaining to -ism = state of	Development of male secondary sexual characteristics (such as deeper voice and facial hair) in a female. Often as a result of increased androgen secretion by the adrenal cortex.
adrenalitis (ad-ree-nal-EYE-tis)	adrenal/o = adrenal gland -itis = inflammation	Inflammation of one or both adrenal glands.

Pathology *(continued)*

TERM	WORD PARTS	DEFINITION
Cushing's syndrome (CUSH-ings / SIN-drohm) ■ **Figure 11.12** Cushing's syndrome. A photograph of a woman with the characteristic facial features of Cushing's syndrome. *(Biophoto Photo Associates/Photo Researchers, Inc.)*	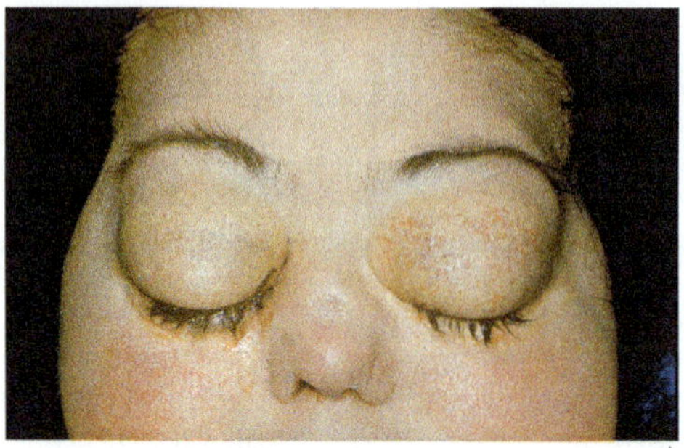	Set of symptoms caused by excessive levels of cortisol due to high doses of corticosteroid drugs and adrenal tumors. The syndrome may present symptoms of weakness, edema, excess hair growth, skin discoloration, and osteoporosis.
pheochromocytoma (fee-oh-kroh-moh-sigh-TOH-ma)	cyt/o = cell -oma = tumor	Usually benign tumor of the adrenal medulla that secretes epinephrine. Symptoms include anxiety, heart palpitations, dyspnea, profuse sweating, headache, and nausea.
Pancreas		
diabetes mellitus (DM) (dye-ah-BEE-teez / MELL-ih-tus)		Chronic disorder of carbohydrate metabolism resulting in hyperglycemia and glycosuria. There are two distinct forms of diabetes mellitus: *insulin-dependent diabetes mellitus* (IDDM) or *type 1,* and *non-insulin-dependent diabetes mellitus* (NIDDM) or *type 2.*
diabetic retinopathy (dye-ah-BET-ik / ret-in-OP-ah-thee)	-tic = pertaining to retin/o = retina -pathy = disease	Secondary complication of diabetes that affects the blood vessels of the retina, resulting in visual changes and even blindness.
insulin-dependent diabetes mellitus (IDDM) (dye-ah-BEE-teez / MELL-ih-tus)		Also called *type 1 diabetes mellitus.* It develops early in life when the pancreas stops insulin production. Patient must take daily insulin injections.
insulinoma (in-sue-lin-OH-mah)	-oma = tumor	Tumor of the islets of Langerhans cells of the pancreas that secretes an excessive amount of insulin.
ketoacidosis (KEE-toh-ass-ih-DOH-sis)	ket/o = ketones -osis = abnormal condition	Acidosis due to an excess of acidic ketone bodies (waste products). A serious condition requiring immediate treatment that can result in death for the diabetic patient if not reversed. Also called *diabetic acidosis.*
non-insulin-dependent diabetes mellitus (dye-ah-BEE-teez / MELL-ih-tus)		Also called *type 2 diabetes mellitus.* It typically develops later in life. The pancreas produces normal to high levels of insulin, but the cells fail to respond to it. Patients may take oral hypoglycemics to improve insulin function, or may eventually have to take insulin.
peripheral neuropathy (per-IF-eh-rall / new-ROP-ah-thee)	-al = pertaining to neur/o = nerve -pathy = disease	Damage to the nerves in the lower legs and hands as a result of diabetes mellitus. Symptoms include either extreme sensitivity or numbness and tingling.

Pathology *(continued)*

TERM	WORD PARTS	DEFINITION
Parathyroid Glands		
hyperparathyroidism (HIGH-per-pair-ah-THIGH-royd-izm)	hyper- = excessive parathyroid/o = parathyroid gland -ism = state of	Hypersecretion of parathyroid hormone; may result in hypercalcemia and Recklinghausen disease.
hypoparathyroidism (HIGH-poh-pair-ah-THIGH-royd-izm)	hypo- = insufficient parathyroid/o = parathyroid gland -ism = state of	Hyposecretion of parathyroid hormone; may result in hypocalcemia and tetany.
Recklinghausen disease (REK-ling-how-zenz)		Excessive production of parathyroid hormone resulting in degeneration of the bones.
tetany (TET-ah-nee)		Nerve irritability and painful muscle cramps resulting from hypocalcemia. Hypoparathyroidism is one cause of tetany.
Pituitary Gland		
acromegaly (ak-roh-MEG-ah-lee)	acr/o = extremities -megaly = enlarged	Chronic disease of adults that results in an elongation and enlargement of the bones of the head and extremities. There can also be mood changes. Due to an excessive amount of growth hormone in an adult.

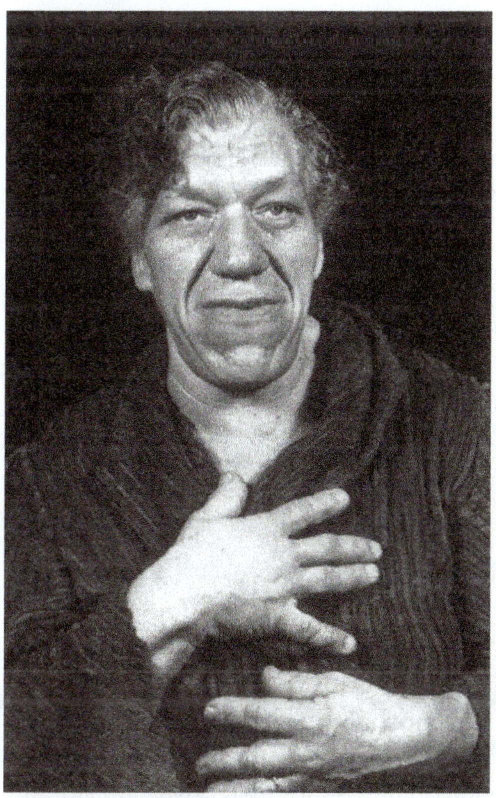

Figure 11.13 Acromegaly. Photo of a woman illustrating the enlarged skull, jaw, and hands typical of acromegaly. *(Reprinted from American Journal of Medicine, Vol 20, Dr. William H. Daughaday, University of California/Irvine, ©1956. With permission from Excerpta Medica Inc.)*

TERM	WORD PARTS	DEFINITION
diabetes insipidus (DI) (dye-ah-BEE-teez / in-SIP-ih-dus)		Disorder caused by the inadequate secretion of antidiuretic hormone by the posterior lobe of the pituitary gland. There may be polyuria and polydipsia.
dwarfism (DWARF-izm)	-ism = state of	Condition of being abnormally short in height. It may be the result of a hereditary condition or a lack of growth hormone.

Pathology *(continued)*

TERM	WORD PARTS	DEFINITION
gigantism (JYE-gan-tizm)	-ism = state of	Excessive development of the body due to the overproduction of the growth hormone by the pituitary gland in a child or teenager. The opposite of *dwarfism.*
hyperpituitarism (HIGH-per-pih-TOO-ih-tuh-rizm)	hyper- = excessive pituitar/o = pituitary gland -ism = state of	Hypersecretion of one or more pituitary gland hormones.
hypopituitarism (HIGH-poh-pih-TOO-ih-tuh-rizm)	hypo- = insufficient pituitar/o = pituitary gland -ism = state of	Hyposecretion of one or more pituitary gland hormones.
panhypopituitarism (pan-high-poh-pih-TOO-ih-tair-izm)	pan- = all hypo- = insufficient pituitar/o = pituitary gland -ism = state of	Deficiency in all the hormones secreted by the pituitary gland. Often recognized because of problems with the glands regulated by the pituitary–adrenal cortex, thyroid, ovaries, and testes.
Thymus Gland		
thymitis (thigh-MY-tis)	thym/o = thymus gland -itis = inflammation	Inflammation of the thymus gland.
thymoma (thigh-MOH-mah)	thym/o = thymus gland -oma = tumor	A tumor in the thymus gland.
Thyroid Gland		
cretinism (KREE-tin-izm)	-ism = state of	Congenital condition in which a lack of thyroid hormones may result in arrested physical and mental development.
goiter (GOY-ter)		Enlargement of the thyroid gland.

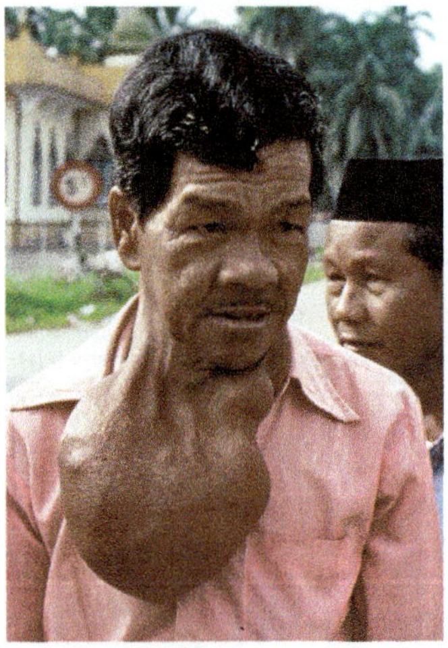

■ **Figure 11.14** Goiter. A photograph of a male with an extreme goiter or enlarged thyroid gland.

TERM	WORD PARTS	DEFINITION
Graves' disease		Condition named for Irish physician Robert Graves that results in overactivity of the thyroid gland and can cause a crisis situation. Symptoms include exophthalmos and goiter. A type of *hyperthyroidism.*
Hashimoto's thyroiditis (hash-ee-MOH-tohz / thigh-roy-DYE-tis)	thyroid/o = thyroid gland -itis = inflammation	Chronic autoimmune form of thyroiditis; results in hyposecretion of thyroid hormones.

Pathology *(continued)*

TERM	WORD PARTS	DEFINITION
hyperthyroidism (hi-per-THIGH-royd-izm)	hyper- = excessive thyroid/o = thyroid gland -ism = state of	Hypersecretion of thyroid gland hormones.
hypothyroidism (high-poh-THIGH-royd-izm)	hypo- = insufficient thyroid/o = thyroid gland -ism = state of	Hyposecretion of thyroid gland hormones.
myxedema (miks-eh-DEE-mah)		Condition resulting from a hyposecretion of the thyroid gland in an adult. Symptoms can include anemia, slow speech, swollen facial features, edematous skin, drowsiness, and mental lethargy.
thyrotoxicosis (thigh-roh-toks-ih-KOH-sis)	thyr/o = thyroid gland toxic/o = poison -osis = abnormal condition	Condition resulting from marked overproduction of the thyroid gland. Symptoms include rapid heart action, tremors, enlarged thyroid gland, exophthalmos, and weight loss.
All Glands		
adenocarcinoma (ad-eh-no-car-sih-NO-mah)	aden/o = gland carcin/o = cancer -oma = tumor	Cancerous tumor in a gland that is capable of producing the hormones secreted by that gland. One cause of hypersecretion pathologies.

Diagnostic Procedures

TERM	WORD PARTS	DEFINITION
Clinical Laboratory Tests		
blood serum test		Blood test to measure the level of substances such as calcium, electrolytes, testosterone, insulin, and glucose. Used to assist in determining the function of various endocrine glands.
fasting blood sugar (FBS)		Blood test to measure the amount of sugar circulating throughout the body after a 12-hour fast.
glucose tolerance test (GTT) (GLOO-kohs)		Test to determine the blood sugar level. A measured dose of glucose is given to a patient either orally or intravenously. Blood samples are then drawn at certain intervals to determine the ability of the patient to use glucose. Used for diabetic patients to determine their insulin response to glucose.
protein-bound iodine test (PBI)		Blood test to measure the concentration of thyroxine (T_4) circulating in the bloodstream. The iodine becomes bound to the protein in the blood and can be measured. Useful in establishing thyroid function.

Diagnostic Procedures *(continued)*

TERM	WORD PARTS	DEFINITION
radioimmunoassay (RIA) (ray-dee-oh-im-yoo-noh-ASS-ay)	radi/o = ray immun/o = protection	Blood test that uses radioactively tagged hormones and antibodies to measure the quantity of hormone in the plasma.
thyroid function test (TFT) (THIGH-royd)		Blood test used to measure the levels of thyroxine, triiodothyronine, and thyroid-stimulating hormone in the bloodstream to assist in determining thyroid function.
total calcium		Blood test to measure the total amount of calcium to assist in detecting parathyroid and bone disorders.
two-hour postprandial glucose tolerance test (post-PRAN-dee-al)	post- = after -prandial = relating to a meal	Blood test to assist in evaluating glucose metabolism. The patient eats a high carbohydrate diet and then fasts overnight before the test. Then the blood sample is taken 2 hours after a meal.
Diagnostic Imaging		
thyroid echography (THIGH-royd / eh-KOG-rah-fee)	-graphy = process of recording	Ultrasound examination of the thyroid that can assist in distinguishing a thyroid nodule from a cyst.
thyroid scan (THIGH-royd)		Test in which radioactive iodine is administered that localizes in the thyroid gland. The gland can then be visualized with a scanning device to detect pathology such as tumors.

Therapeutic Procedures

TERM	WORD PARTS	DEFINITION
Medical Procedures		
chemical thyroidectomy (thigh-royd-EK-toh-mee)	chem/o = drug -al = pertaining to thyroid/o = thyroid gland -ectomy = surgical removal	Large dose of radioactive iodine is given in order to kill thyroid gland cells without having to actually do surgery.
glucometer	gluc/o = glucose -meter = instrument to measure	Device designed for a diabetic to use at home to measure the level of glucose in the bloodstream.
hormone replacement therapy		Artificial replacement of hormones in patients with hyposecretion disorders. May be oral pills, injections, or adhesive skin patches.
Surgical Procedures		
adrenalectomy (ad-ree-nal-EK-toh-mee)	adrenal/o = adrenal gland -ectomy = surgical removal	Surgical removal of one or both adrenal glands.
laparoscopic adrenalectomy (lap-row-SKOP-ik / ad-ree-nal-EK-toh-mee)	lapar/o = abdomen -scopy = procedure to visually examine -ic = pertaining to adren/o = adrenal gland -ectomy = surgical removal	Removal of the adrenal gland through a small incision in the abdomen and using endoscopic instruments.

Therapeutic Procedures *(continued)*

TERM	WORD PARTS	DEFINITION
lobectomy (lobe-EK-toh-mee)	lob/o = lobe -ectomy = surgical removal	Removal of a lobe from an organ. In this case, one lobe of the thyroid gland.
parathyroidectomy (pair-ah-thigh-royd-EK-toh-mee)	parathyroid/o = parathyroid gland -ectomy = surgical removal	Surgical removal of one or more of the parathyroid glands.
pinealectomy (PIN-ee-ah-LEK-toh-mee)	pineal/o = pineal gland -ectomy = surgical removal	Surgical removal of the pineal gland.
thymectomy (thigh-MEK-toh-mee)	thym/o = thymus gland -ectomy = surgical removal	Surgical removal of the thymus gland.
thyroidectomy (thigh-royd-EK-toh-mee)	thyroid/o = thyroid gland -ectomy = surgical removal	Surgical removal of the thyroid gland.

Pharmacology

CLASSIFICATION	WORD PARTS	ACTION	EXAMPLES
antithyroid agents	anti- = against	Medication given to block production of thyroid hormones in patients with hypersecretion disorders.	methimazole, Tapazole; propylthiouracil
corticosteroids (kor-tih-koh-STAIR-oydz)	cortic/o = outer portion	Although the function of these hormones in the body is to regulate carbohydrate metabolism, they also have a strong anti-inflammatory action. Therefore they are used to treat severe chronic inflammatory diseases such as rheumatoid arthritis. Long-term use of corticosteroids has adverse side effects such as osteoporosis and the symptoms of Cushing's disease. Also used to treat adrenal cortex hyposecretion disorders such as Addison's disease.	prednisone, Deltasone
human growth hormone therapy		Hormone replacement therapy with human growth hormone in order to stimulate skeletal growth. Used to treat children with abnormally short stature.	somatropin, Genotropin; somatrem, Protropin
insulin (IN-suh-lin)		Administered to replace insulin for type 1 diabetics or to treat severe type 2 diabetics.	human insulin, Humulin L
oral hypoglycemic agents (high-poh-glye-SEE-mik)	or/o = mouth -al = pertaining to hypo- = insufficient glyc/o = sugar -emic = relating to a blood condition	Medications taken by mouth that cause a decrease in blood sugar; not used for insulin-dependent patients.	metformin, Glucophage; glipizide, Glucotrol

Pharmacology *(continued)*

CLASSIFICATION	WORD PARTS	ACTION	EXAMPLES
thyroid replacement hormone		Hormone replacement therapy for patients with hypothyroidism or who have had a thyroidectomy.	levothyroxine, Levo-T; liothyronine, Cytomel
vasopressin (vaz-oh-PRESS-in)	vas/o = vessel -pressin = to press down	Given to control diabetes insipidus and promote reabsorption of water in the kidney tubules.	desmopressin acetate, Desmopressin; conivaptan, Vaprisol

Abbreviations

α	alpha
ACTH	adrenocorticotropic hormone
ADH	antidiuretic hormone
β	beta
BMR	basal metabolic rate
CT	calcitonin
DI	diabetes insipidus
DM	diabetes mellitus
FBS	fasting blood sugar
FSH	follicle-stimulating hormone
GH	growth hormone
GTT	glucose tolerance test
IDDM	insulin-dependent diabetes mellitus
K^+	potassium
LH	luteinizing hormone
MSH	melanocyte-stimulating hormone
Na^+	sodium
NIDDM	non-insulin-dependent diabetes mellitus
NPH	neutral protamine Hagedorn (insulin)
PBI	protein-bound iodine
PRL	prolactin
PTH	parathyroid hormone
RAI	radioactive iodine
RIA	radioimmunoassay
T_3	triiodothyronine
T_4	thyroxine
TFT	thyroid function test
TSH	thyroid-stimulating hormone

Chapter Review

Real-World Applications

Medical Record Analysis

This Discharge Summary below contains 10 medical terms. Underline each term and write it in the list below the report. Then define each term.

Discharge Summary

Admitting Diagnosis:	Hyperglycemia, ketoacidosis, glycosuria
Final Diagnosis:	New-onset type 1 diabetes mellitus
History of Present Illness:	A 12-year-old female patient presented to her physician's office with a 2-month history of weight loss, fatigue, polyuria, and polydipsia. Her family history is significant for a grandfather, mother, and older brother with type 1 diabetes mellitus. The pediatrician found hyperglycemia with a fasting blood sugar and glycosuria with a urine dipstick. She is being admitted at this time for management of new-onset diabetes mellitus.
Summary of Hospital Course:	At the time of admission, the FBS was 300 mg/100 mL and she was in ketoacidosis. She rapidly improved after receiving insulin; her blood glucose level normalized. The next day a glucose tolerance test confirmed the diagnosis of diabetes mellitus. The patient was started on insulin injections. Patient and family were instructed on diabetes mellitus, insulin, diet, exercise, and long-term complications.
Discharge Plans:	Patient was discharged to home with her parents. Her parents are to check her blood glucose levels twice daily and call the office for insulin dosage. She is to return to the office in 2 weeks.

	Term	Definition
1	______________	______________________________
2	______________	______________________________
3	______________	______________________________
4	______________	______________________________
5	______________	______________________________
6	______________	______________________________
7	______________	______________________________
8	______________	______________________________
9	______________	______________________________
10	______________	______________________________

Chart Note Transcription

The chart note below contains 11 phrases that can be reworded with a medical term that you learned in this chapter. Each phrase is identified with an underline. Determine the medical term and write your answers in the space provided.

Current Complaint:	A 56-year-old female was referred to the <u>specialist in the treatment of diseases of the endocrine glands</u> ❶ for evaluation of weakness, edema, <u>an abnormal amount of fat in the body,</u> ❷ and <u>an excessive amount of hair for a female.</u> ❸
Past History:	Patient reports she has been overweight most of her life in spite of a healthy diet and regular exercise. She was diagnosed with osteoporosis after incurring a pathological rib fracture following a coughing attack.
Signs and Symptoms:	Patient has moderate edema in bilateral feet and lower legs as well as a puffy face and an upper lip moustache. She is 100 lbs. over normal body weight for her age and height. She moves slowly and appears generally lethargic. A test to <u>measure the hormone levels in the blood plasma</u> ❹ reports increased <u>steroid hormone that regulates carbohydrates in the body.</u> ❺ A CT scan demonstrates a <u>gland tumor</u> ❻ in the right <u>outer layer of the adrenal gland.</u> ❼
Diagnosis:	<u>A group of symptoms associated with hypersecretion of the adrenal cortex</u> ❽ secondary to a <u>gland tumor</u> ❾ in the right <u>outer layer of the adrenal gland.</u> ❿
Treatment:	<u>Surgical removal of the right adrenal gland.</u> ⓫

❶ ____________________

❷ ____________________

❸ ____________________

❹ ____________________

❺ ____________________

❻ ____________________

❼ ____________________

❽ ____________________

❾ ____________________

❿ ____________________

⓫ ____________________

Case Study

Below is a case study presentation of a patient with a condition covered in this chapter. Read the case study and answer the questions below. Some questions will ask for information not included within this chapter. Use your text, a medical dictionary, or any other reference material you choose to answer these questions.

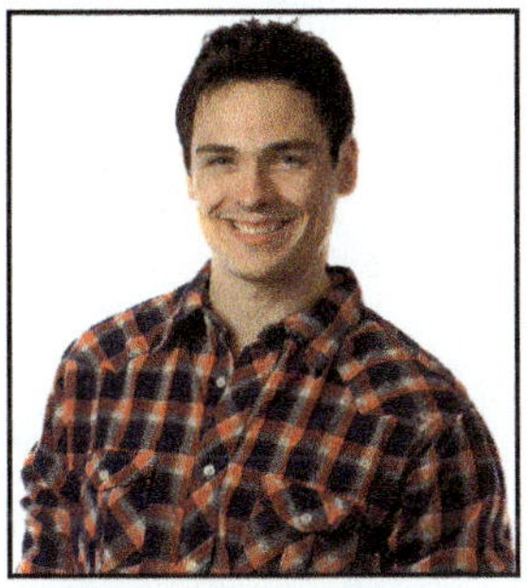

(Flashon Studio/Shutterstock)

A 22-year-old college student was admitted to the emergency room after his friends called an ambulance when he passed out in a bar. He had become confused, developed slurred speech, and had difficulty walking after having only one beer to drink. In the ER he was noted to have diaphoresis, rapid respirations and pulse, and was disoriented. Upon examination, needle marks were found on his abdomen and outer thighs. The physician ordered blood serum tests that revealed hyperglycemia and ketoacidosis. Unknown to his friends, this young man has had diabetes mellitus since early childhood. The patient quickly recovered following an insulin injection.

1. What pathological condition has this patient had since childhood? Look this condition up in a reference source and include a short description of it.

 ____

 ____

2. List and define each symptom noted in the ER in your own words.

 ____

 ____

3. What diagnostic test was performed? Describe it in your own words.

 ____

 ____

4. Explain the results of the test.

 ____

 ____

5. What specific type of diabetes does this young man probably have? Justify your answer.

 ____

 ____

6. Describe the other type of diabetes mellitus that this young man did not have.

 ____

 ____

Practice Exercises

A. Complete the Statement

1. The study of the endocrine system is called ____________________.

2. The master endocrine gland is the ____________________.

3. ____________________ is a general term for the sexual organs that produce gametes.

4. The term for the hormones produced by the outer portion of the adrenal cortex is ____________________.

5. The hormone produced by the testes is ____________________.

6. The two hormones produced by the ovaries are ____________________ and ____________________.

7. An inadequate supply of the hormone ____________________ causes diabetes insipidus.

8. The endocrine gland associated with the immune system is the ____________________.

9. The term for a protrusion of the eyeballs in Graves' disease is ____________________.

10. A general medical term for a hormone-secreting cancerous tumor is ____________________.

B. Combining Form Practice

The combining form **thyroid/o** refers to the thyroid. Use it to write a term that means:

1. removal of the thyroid ____________________
2. pertaining to the thyroid ____________________
3. state of excessive thyroid ____________________

The combining form **pancreat/o** refers to the pancreas. Use it to write a term that means:

4. pertaining to the pancreas ____________________
5. inflammation of the pancreas ____________________
6. removal of the pancreas ____________________
7. cutting into the pancreas ____________________

The combining form **adren/o** refers to the adrenal glands. Use it to write a term that means:

8. pertaining to the adrenal gland ____________________
9. enlargement of the adrenal glands ____________________
10. adrenal gland disease ____________________

The combining form **thym/o** refers to the thymus glands. Use it to write a term that means:

11. tumor of the thymus gland ____________________
12. removal of the thymus gland ____________________
13. pertaining to the thymus gland ____________________
14. inflammation of the thymus gland ____________________

C. Define the Combining Form

	Definition	Example from Chapter
1. natr/o	________________	________________
2. estr/o	________________	________________
3. pineal/o	________________	________________
4. pituitar/o	________________	________________
5. kal/i	________________	________________
6. calc/o	________________	________________
7. parathyroid/o	________________	________________
8. acr/o	________________	________________
9. glyc/o	________________	________________
10. gonad/o	________________	________________

D. Terminology Matching

Match the term to its definition.

1. ________ protein-bound iodine test
2. ________ fasting blood sugar
3. ________ radioimmunoassay
4. ________ thyroid scan
5. ________ 2-hour postprandial glucose tolerance test
6. ________ glucose tolerance test

a. measures levels of hormones in the blood
b. determines glucose metabolism after patient receives a measured dose of glucose
c. test of glucose metabolism 2 hours after eating a meal
d. measures blood sugar level after 12-hour fast
e. measures T4 concentration in the blood
f. uses radioactive iodine

E. What's the Abbreviation?

1. non-insulin-dependent diabetes mellitus ________________
2. insulin-dependent diabetes mellitus ________________
3. adrenocorticotropic hormone ________________
4. parathyroid hormone ________________
5. triiodothyronine ________________
6. thyroid-stimulating hormone ________________
7. fasting blood sugar ________________
8. prolactin ________________

F. Terminology Matching

Match each term to its definition.

1.	_______ Cushing's disease	a.	enlarged thyroid
2.	_______ goiter	b.	overactive adrenal cortex
3.	_______ acromegaly	c.	hyperthyroidism
4.	_______ gigantism	d.	underactive adrenal cortex
5.	_______ cretinism	e.	enlarged bones of head and extremities
6.	_______ myxedema	f.	may cause polyuria and polydipsia
7.	_______ diabetes mellitus	g.	an autoimmune disease
8.	_______ diabetes insipidus	h.	arrested physical and mental development
9.	_______ Hashimoto's thyroiditis	i.	disorder of carbohydrate metabolism
10.	_______ Graves' disease	j.	insufficient thyroid hormone in an adult
11.	_______ Addison's disease	k.	excessive growth hormone in a child

G. What Does it Stand For?

1. PBI ______________________________
2. K^+ ______________________________
3. T_4 ______________________________
4. GTT ______________________________
5. DM ______________________________
6. BMR ______________________________
7. Na^+ ______________________________
8. ADH ______________________________

H. Suffix Practice

Use the following suffixes to create medical terms for the following definitions.

-pressin	-uria	-tropin
-dipsia	-emia	-prandial

1. the presence of sugar or glucose in the urine ______________________________
2. to press down a vessel ______________________________

3. excessive urination ____________________

4. condition of excessive calcium in the blood ____________________

5. excessive thirst ____________________

6. stimulate adrenal cortex ____________________

7. after a meal ____________________

I. Define the Term

1. corticosteroid ____________________
2. hirsutism ____________________
3. tetany ____________________
4. diabetic retinopathy ____________________
5. hyperglycemia ____________________
6. hypoglycemia ____________________
7. adrenaline ____________________
8. insulin ____________________
9. thyrotoxicosis ____________________
10. hypersecretion ____________________

J. Fill in the Blank

insulinoma	ketoacidosis	pheochromocytoma
gynecomastia	panhypopituitarinism	Hashimoto's thyroiditis

1. The doctor found that Marsha's high level of insulin and hypoglycemia was caused by a(n) ____________________.
2. Kevin developed ____________________ as a result of his diabetes mellitus and required emergency treatment.
3. It was determined that Karen had ____________________ when doctors realized she had problems with her thyroid gland, adrenal cortex, and ovaries.
4. Luke's high epinephrine level was caused by a(n) ____________________.
5. When it was determined that Carl's thyroiditis was an autoimmune condition, it became obvious that he had ____________________.
6. Excessive sex hormones caused Jack to develop ____________________.

K. Pharmacology Challenge

Fill in the classification for each drug description, then match the brand name.

	Drug Description	Classification	Brand Name
1.	________ strong anti-inflammatory	______________________	a. genotropin
2.	________ stimulates skeletal growth	______________________	b. Desmopressin
3.	________ treats type 1 diabetes mellitus	______________________	c. Tapazole
4.	________ blocks production of thyroid hormone	______________________	d. glucophage
5.	________ treats type 1 diabetes mellitus	______________________	e. Deltasone
6.	________ controls diabetes insipidus	______________________	f. Humulin

Labeling Exercise

Image A

Write the labels for this figure on the numbered lines provided.

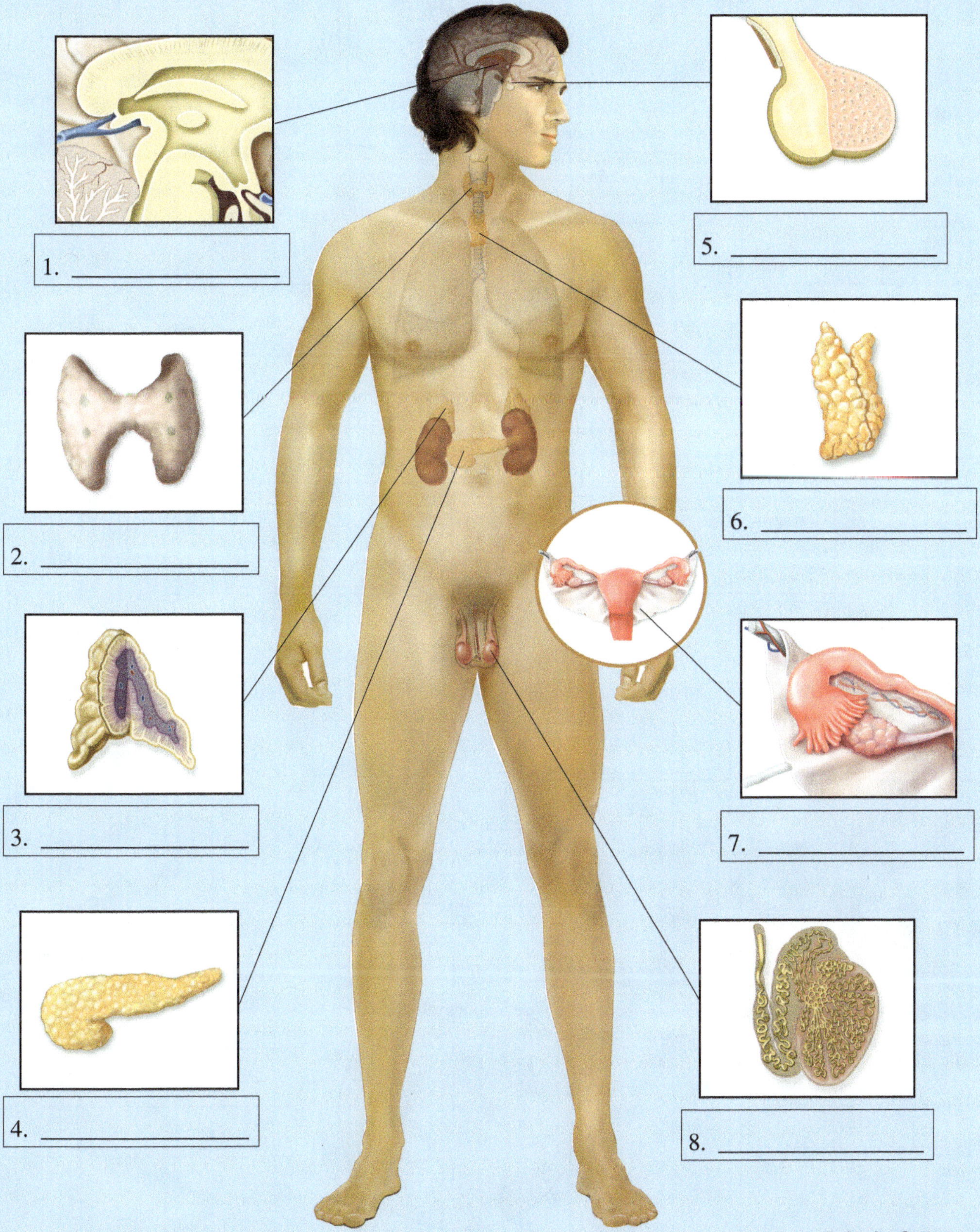

Image B

Write the labels for this figure on the numbered lines provided.

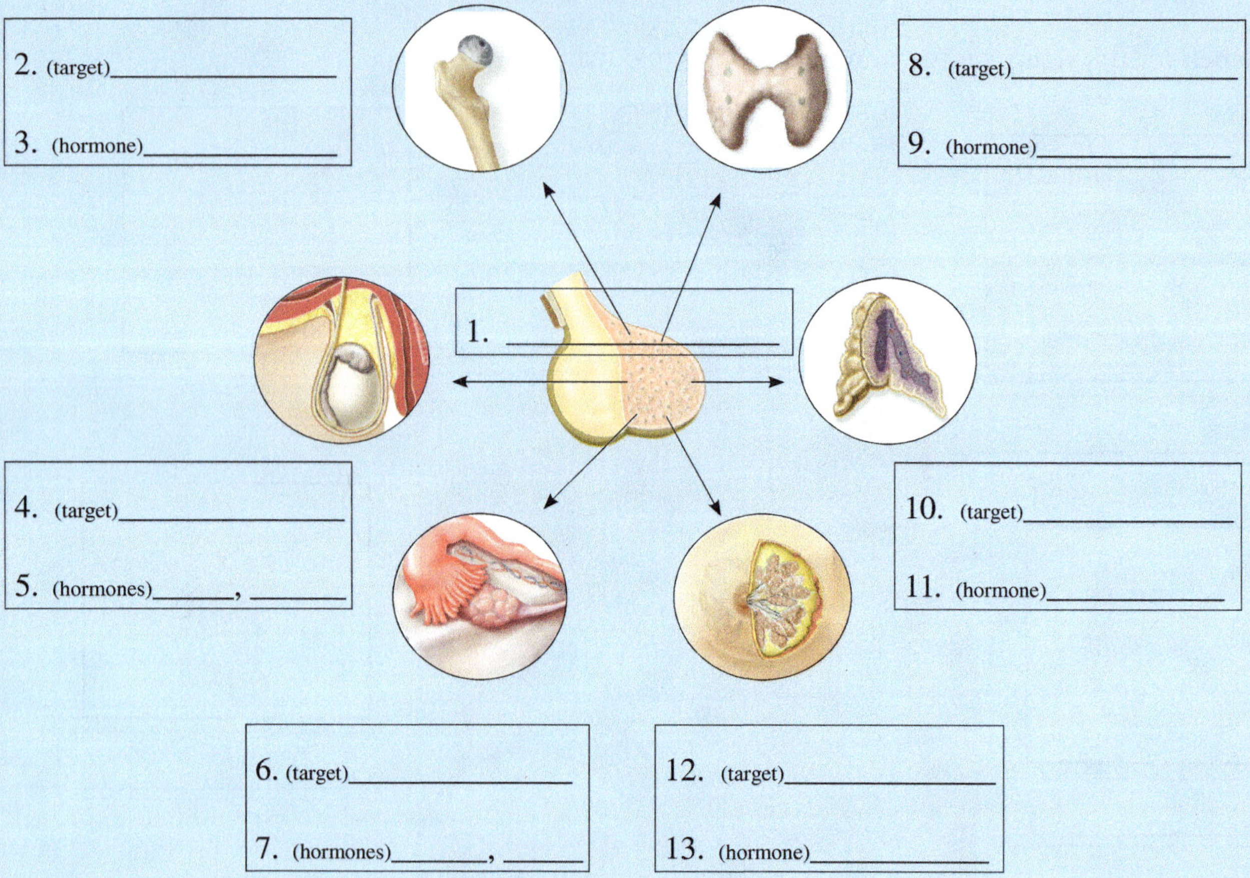

Image C

Write the labels for this figure on the numbered lines provided.

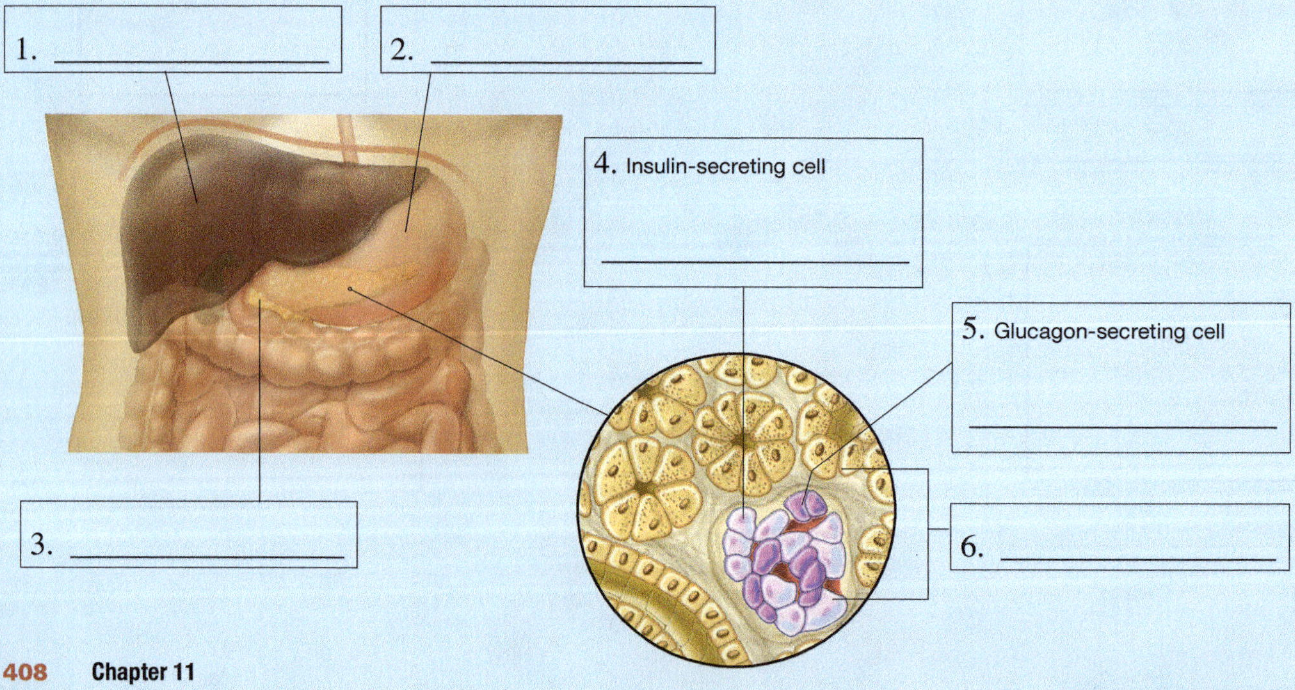

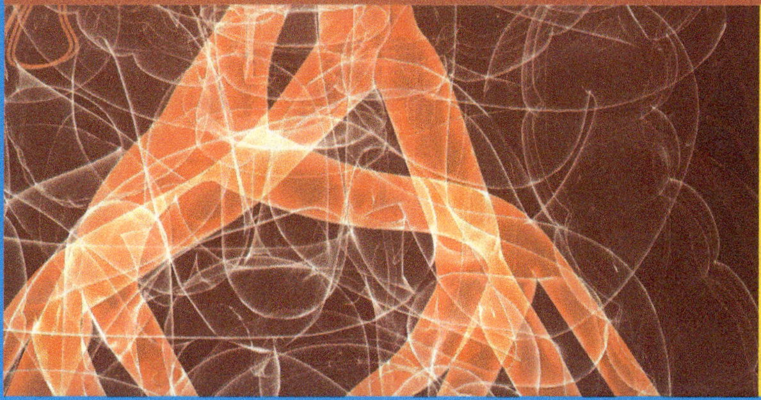

12

NERVOUS SYSTEM

Learning Objectives

Upon completion of this chapter, you will be able to

- Identify and define the combining forms and suffixes introduced in this chapter.
- Correctly spell and pronounce medical terms and major anatomical structures relating to the nervous system.
- Locate and describe the major organs of the nervous system and their functions.
- Describe the components of a neuron.
- Distinguish between the central nervous system, peripheral nervous system, and autonomic nervous system.
- Identify and define nervous system anatomical terms.
- Identify and define selected nervous system pathology terms.
- Identify and define selected nervous system diagnostic procedures.
- Identify and define selected nervous system therapeutic procedures.
- Identify and define selected medications relating to the nervous system.
- Define selected abbreviations associated with the nervous system.

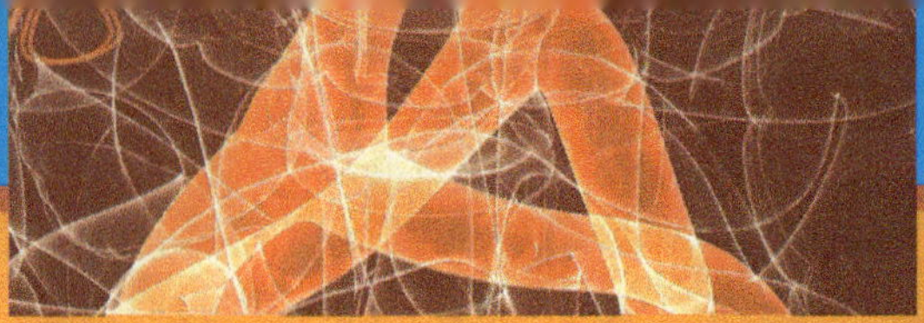

Nervous System at a Glance

Function

The nervous system coordinates and controls body function. It receives sensory input, makes decisions, and then orders body responses.

Structures

Here are the primary structures that comprise the nervous system.

brain
nerves
spinal cord

Word Parts

Here are the most common word parts (with their meanings) used to build nervous system terms. For a more comprehensive list, refer to the Terminology section of this chapter.

Combining Forms

Combining Form	Meaning
alges/o	sense of pain
astr/o	star
cephal/o	head
cerebell/o	cerebellum
cerebr/o	cerebrum
clon/o	rapid contracting and relaxing
dur/o	dura mater
encephal/o	brain
esthes/o	sensation, feeling
gli/o	glue
medull/o	medulla oblongata
mening/o	meninges
meningi/o	meninges
myel/o	spinal cord
neur/o	nerve
poli/o	gray matter
pont/o	pons
radicul/o	nerve root
thalam/o	thalamus
thec/o	sheath (meninges)
ton/o	tone
ventricul/o	ventricle

Suffixes

Suffix	Meaning
-paresis	weakness
-phasia	speech
-plegia	paralysis
-taxia	muscle coordination
-trophic	pertaining to development

Nervous System Illustrated

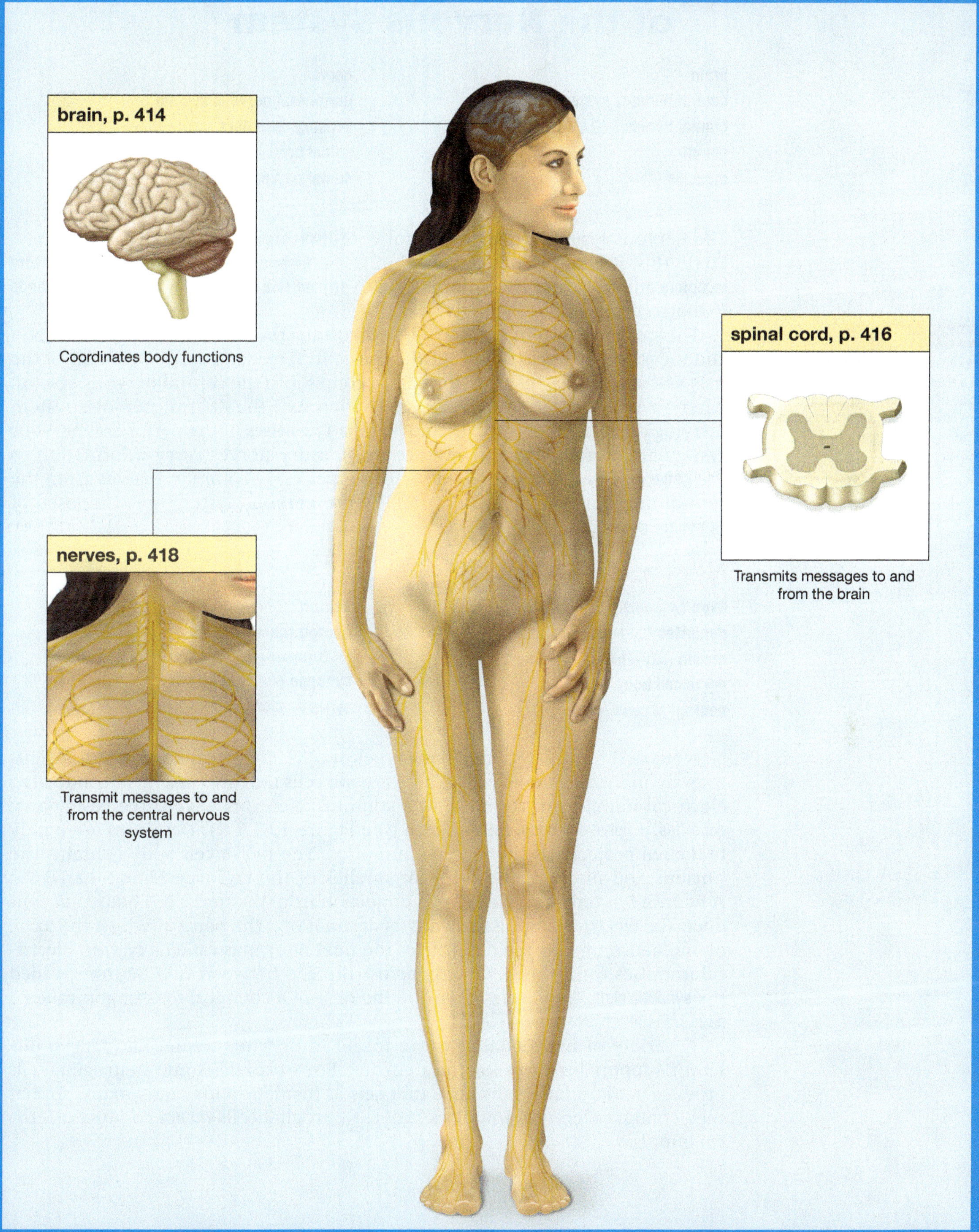

Anatomy and Physiology of the Nervous System

brain
central nervous system
cranial nerves (KRAY-nee-al)
glands
muscles
nerves
peripheral nervous system (per-IF-er-al)
sensory receptors
spinal cord
spinal nerves

The nervous system is responsible for coordinating all the activity of the body. To do this, it first receives information from both external and internal **sensory receptors** and then uses that information to adjust the activity of **muscles** and **glands** to match the needs of the body.

The nervous system can be subdivided into the **central nervous system** (CNS) and the **peripheral nervous system** (PNS). The central nervous system consists of the **brain** and **spinal cord.** Sensory information comes into the central nervous system, where it is processed. Motor messages then exit the central nervous system carrying commands to muscles and glands. The **nerves** of the peripheral nervous system are **cranial nerves** and **spinal nerves.** Sensory nerves carry information to the central nervous system, and motor nerves carry commands away from the central nervous system. All portions of the nervous system are composed of nervous tissue.

MED TERM TIP

Neuroglial tissue received its name as a result of its function. This tissue holds neurons together. Therefore, it was called *neuroglial*, a term literally meaning "nerve glue."

Nervous Tissue

axon (AK-son)
dendrites (DEN-drights)
myelin (MY-eh-lin)
nerve cell body
neuroglial cells (noo-ROH-glee-all)
neuron (NOO-ron)
neurotransmitter (noo-roh-TRANS-mit-ter)
synapse (sih-NAPSE)
synaptic cleft (sih-NAP-tik)

Nervous tissue consists of two basic types of cells: **neurons** and **neuroglial cells.** Neurons are individual nerve cells. These are the cells that are capable of conducting electrical impulses in response to a stimulus. Neurons have three basic parts: **dendrites,** a **nerve cell body,** and an **axon** (see Figure 12.1A ■). Dendrites are highly branched projections that receive impulses. The nerve cell body contains the nucleus and many of the other organelles of the cell (see Figure 12.1B ■). A neuron has only a single axon, a projection from the nerve cell body that conducts the electrical impulse toward its destination. The point at which the axon of one neuron meets the dendrite of the next neuron is called a **synapse.** Electrical impulses cannot pass directly across the gap between two neurons, called the **synaptic cleft.** They instead require the help of a chemical messenger, called a **neurotransmitter.**

A variety of neuroglial cells are found in nervous tissue. Each has a different support function for the neurons. For example, some neuroglial cells produce **myelin,** a fatty substance that acts as insulation for many axons so that they conduct electrical impulses faster. Neuroglial cells *do not* conduct electrical impulses.

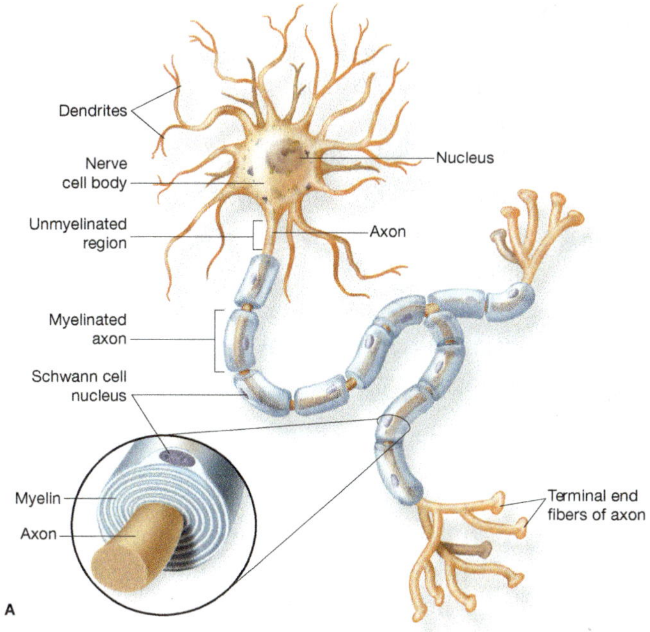

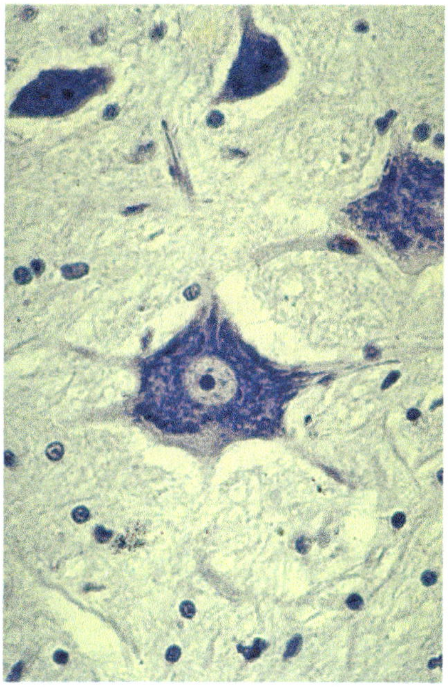

■ **Figure 12.1** (A) The structure of a neuron, showing the dendrites, nerve cell body, and axon. (B) Photomicrograph of typical neuron showing the nerve cell body, nucleus, and dendrites.

Central Nervous System

gray matter
meninges (men-IN-jeez)
myelinated (MY-eh-lih-nayt-ed)
tract
white matter

Because the central nervous system is a combination of the brain and spinal cord, it is able to receive impulses from all over the body, process this information, and then respond with an action. This system consists of both **gray** and **white matter.** Gray matter is comprised of unsheathed or uncovered cell bodies and dendrites. White matter is **myelinated** nerve fibers (see Figure 12.2 ■). The myelin sheath makes the nervous tissue appear white. Bundles of nerve fibers interconnecting different parts of the central nervous system are called **tracts.** The central nervous system is encased and protected by three membranes known as the **meninges.**

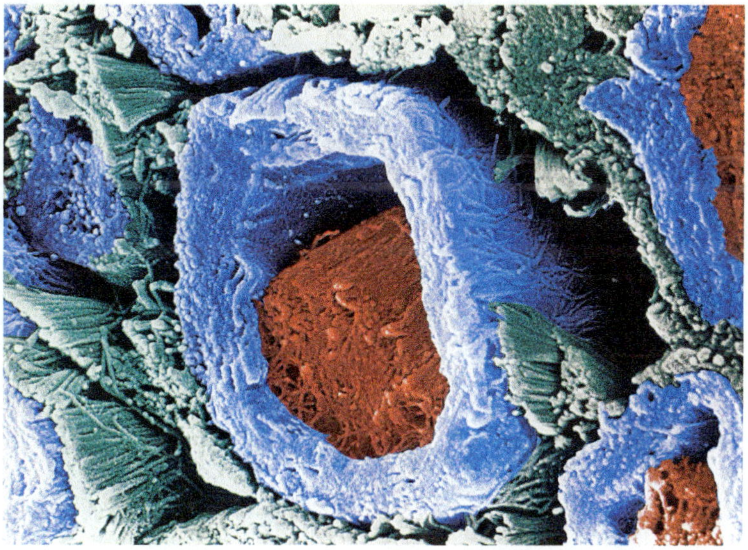

■ **Figure 12.2** Electronmicrograph illustrating an axon (red) wrapped in its myelin sheath (blue). *(Quest/Science Photo Library/Photo Researchers, Inc.)*

MED TERM TIP

Myelin is a lipid and a very white molecule. This is why myelinated neurons are called *white matter.*

The Brain

brain stem
cerebellum (ser-eh-BELL-um)
cerebral cortex (seh-REE-bral / KOR-teks)
cerebral hemisphere
cerebrospinal fluid (ser-eh-broh-SPY-nal)
cerebrum (SER-eh-brum)
diencephalon (dye-en-SEFF-ah-lon)
frontal lobe
gyri (JYE-rye)
hypothalamus (high-poh-THAL-ah-mus)
medulla oblongata (meh-DULL-ah / ob-long-GAH-tah)
midbrain
occipital lobe (ock-SIP-ih-tal)
parietal lobe (pah-RYE-eh-tal)
pons (PONZ)
sulci (SULL-kye)
temporal lobe (TEM-por-al)
thalamus (THAL-ah-mus)
ventricles (VEN-trik-lz)

The brain is one of the largest organs in the body and coordinates most body activities. It is the center for all thought, memory, judgment, and emotion. Each part of the brain is responsible for controlling different body functions, such as temperature regulation, blood pressure, and breathing. There are four sections to the brain: the **cerebrum, cerebellum, diencephalon,** and **brain stem** (see Figure 12.3 ■).

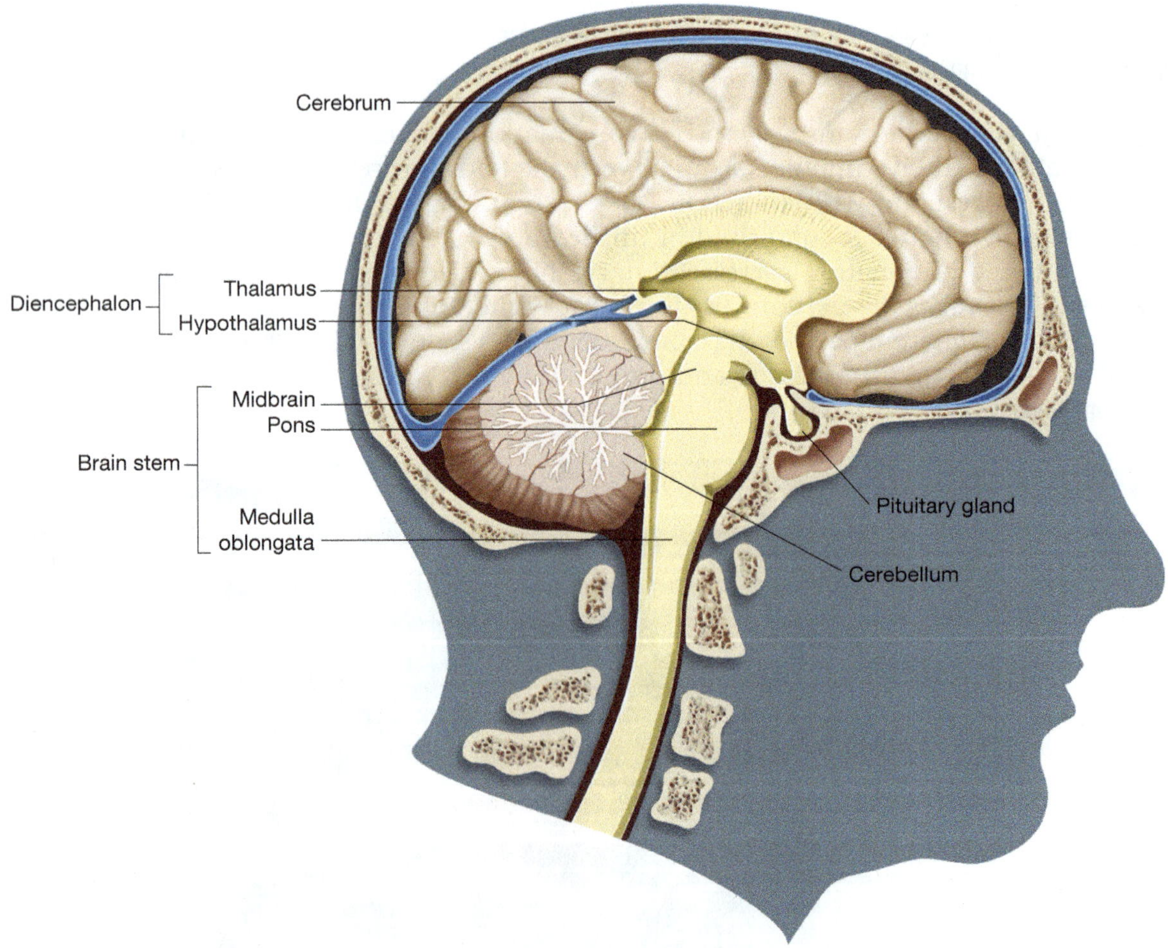

■ **Figure 12.3** The regions of the brain.

The largest section of the brain is the cerebrum. It is located in the upper portion of the brain and is the area that processes thoughts, judgment, memory, problem solving, and language. The outer layer of the cerebrum is the **cerebral cortex,** which is composed of folds of gray matter. The elevated portions of the cerebrum, or convolutions, are called **gyri** and are separated by fissures, or valleys, called **sulci.** The cerebrum is subdivided into left and right halves called **cerebral hemispheres.** Each hemisphere has four lobes. The lobes and their locations and functions are as follows (see Figure 12.4 ■):

1. **Frontal lobe:** Most anterior portion of the cerebrum; controls motor function, personality, and speech
2. **Parietal lobe:** Most superior portion of the cerebrum; receives and interprets nerve impulses from sensory receptors and interprets language
3. **Occipital lobe:** Most posterior portion of the cerebrum; controls vision
4. **Temporal lobe:** Left and right lateral portion of the cerebrum; controls hearing and smell

The diencephalon, located below the cerebrum, contains two of the most critical areas of the brain, the **thalamus** and the **hypothalamus.** The thalamus is composed of gray matter and acts as a center for relaying impulses from the eyes, ears, and skin to the cerebrum. Our pain perception is controlled by the thalamus. The hypothalamus located just below the thalamus controls body temperature, appetite, sleep, sexual desire, and emotions. The hypothalamus is actually responsible for controlling the autonomic nervous system, cardiovascular system, digestive system, and the release of hormones from the pituitary gland.

The cerebellum, the second largest portion of the brain, is located beneath the posterior part of the cerebrum. This part of the brain aids in coordinating voluntary body movements and maintaining balance and equilibrium. The cerebellum refines the muscular movement that is initiated in the cerebrum.

The final portion of the brain is the brain stem. This area has three components: **midbrain, pons,** and **medulla oblongata.** The midbrain acts as a pathway for

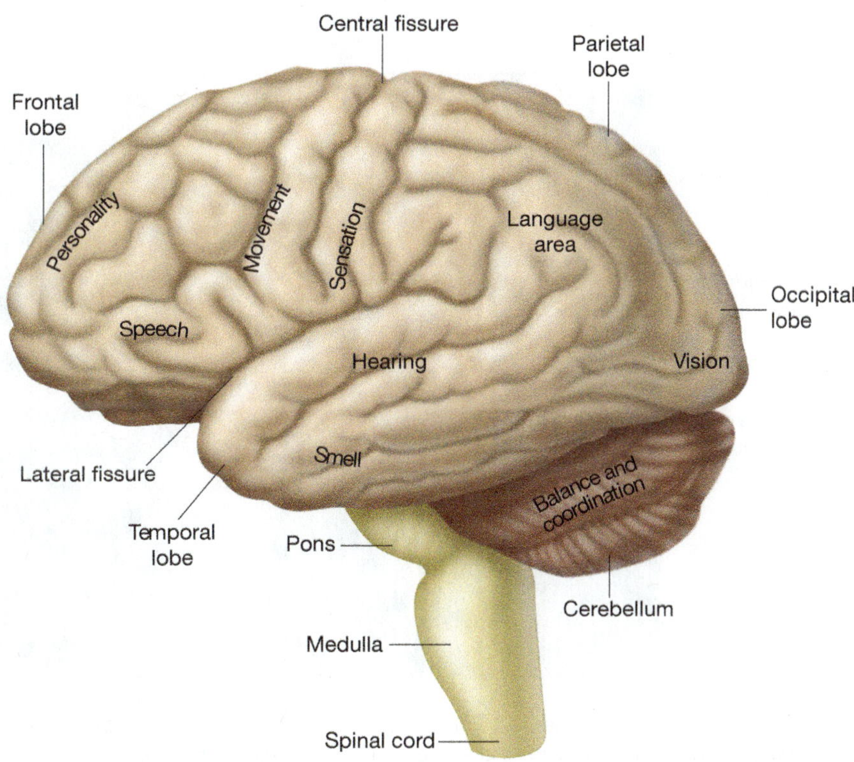

■ **Figure 12.4** The functional regions of the cerebrum.

impulses to be conducted between the brain and the spinal cord. The pons—a term meaning bridge—connects the cerebellum to the rest of the brain. The medulla oblongata is the most inferior positioned portion of the brain; it connects the brain to the spinal cord. However, this vital area contains the centers that control respiration, heart rate, temperature, and blood pressure. Additionally, this is the site where nerve tracts cross from one side of the brain to control functions and movement on the other side of the body. In other words, with few exceptions, the left side of the brain controls the right side of the body and vice versa.

The brain has four interconnected cavities called **ventricles:** one in each cerebral hemisphere, one in the thalamus, and one in front of the cerebellum. These contain **cerebrospinal fluid** (CSF), which is the watery, clear fluid that provides protection from shock or sudden motion to the brain and spinal cord.

Spinal Cord

ascending tracts
central canal
descending tracts
spinal cavity
vertebral canal
vertebral column

The function of the spinal cord is to provide a pathway for impulses traveling to and from the brain. The spinal cord is actually a column of nervous tissue extending from the medulla oblongata of the brain down to the level of the second lumbar vertebra within the **vertebral column.** The 33 vertebrae of the backbone line up to form a continuous canal for the spinal cord called the **spinal cavity** or **vertebral canal** (see Figure 12.5 ■).

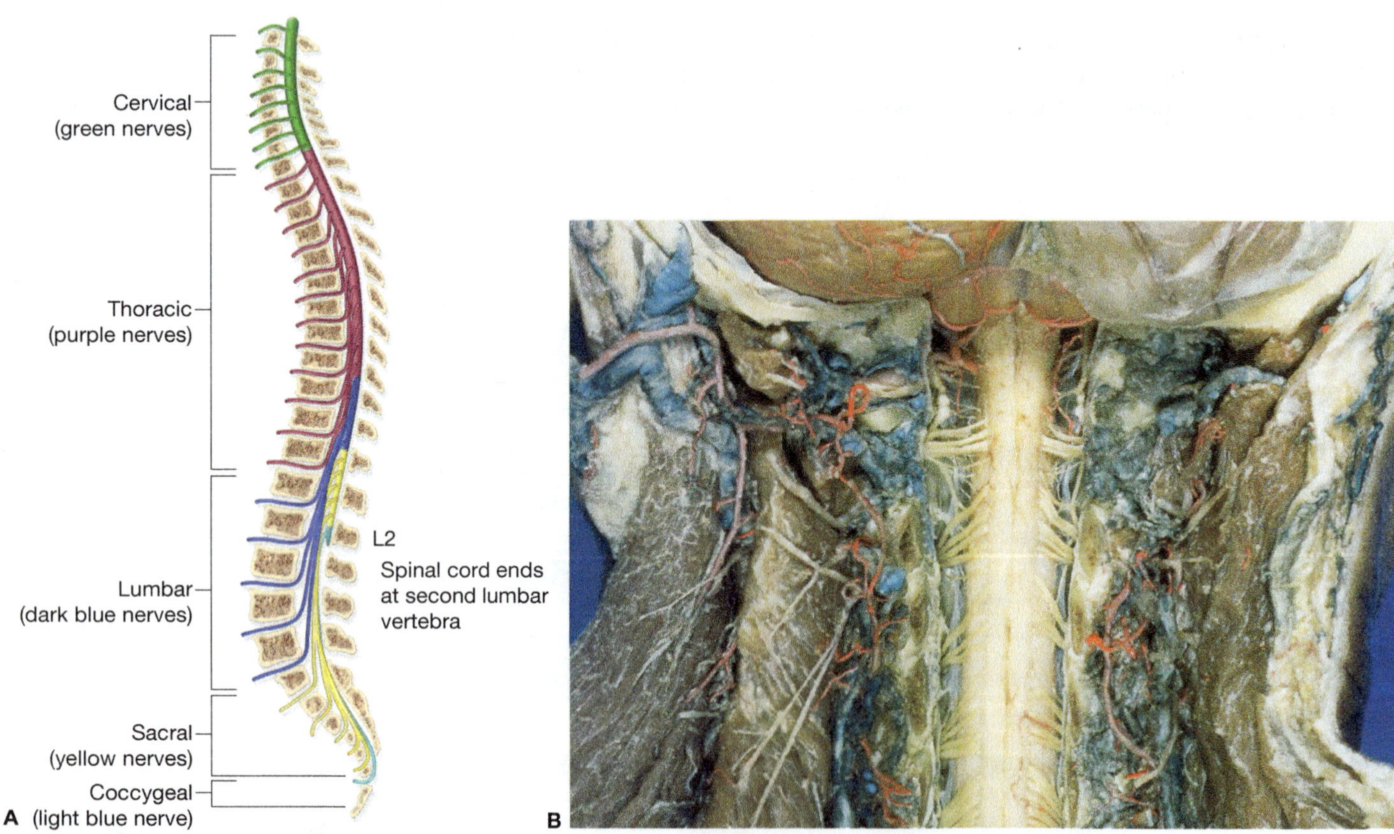

■ **Figure 12.5** (A) The levels of the spinal cord and spinal nerves. (B) Photograph of the spinal cord as it descends from the brain. The spinal nerve roots are clearly visible branching off from the spinal cord. *(Photo Researchers, Inc.)*

Similar to the brain, the spinal cord is also protected by cerebrospinal fluid. It flows down the center of the spinal cord within the **central canal.** The inner core of the spinal cord consists of cell bodies and dendrites of peripheral nerves and therefore is gray matter. The outer portion of the spinal cord is myelinated white matter. The white matter is either **ascending tracts** carrying sensory information up to the brain or **descending tracts** carrying motor commands down from the brain to a peripheral nerve.

Meninges

arachnoid layer (ah-RAK-noyd)
dura mater (DOO-rah / MATE-er)
pia mater (PEE-ah / MATE-er)
subarachnoid space (sub-ah-RAK-noyd)
subdural space (sub-DOO-ral)

The meninges are three layers of connective tissue membranes surrounding the brain and spinal cord (see Figure 12.6 ■). Moving from external to internal, the meninges are:

1. **Dura mater:** Meaning *tough mother;* it forms a tough, fibrous sac around the central nervous system
2. **Subdural space:** Actual space between the dura mater and arachnoid layers
3. **Arachnoid layer:** Meaning *spiderlike;* it is a thin, delicate layer attached to the pia mater by weblike filaments
4. **Subarachnoid space:** Space between the arachnoid layer and the pia mater; it contains cerebrospinal fluid that cushions the brain from the outside
5. **Pia mater:** Meaning *soft mother;* it is the innermost membrane layer and is applied directly to the surface of the brain and spinal cord

MED TERM TIP

Certain disease processes attack the gray matter and the white matter of the central nervous system. For instance, *poliomyelitis* is a viral infection of the gray matter of the spinal cord. The combining term *poli/o* means "gray matter." This disease has almost been eradicated, due to the polio vaccine.

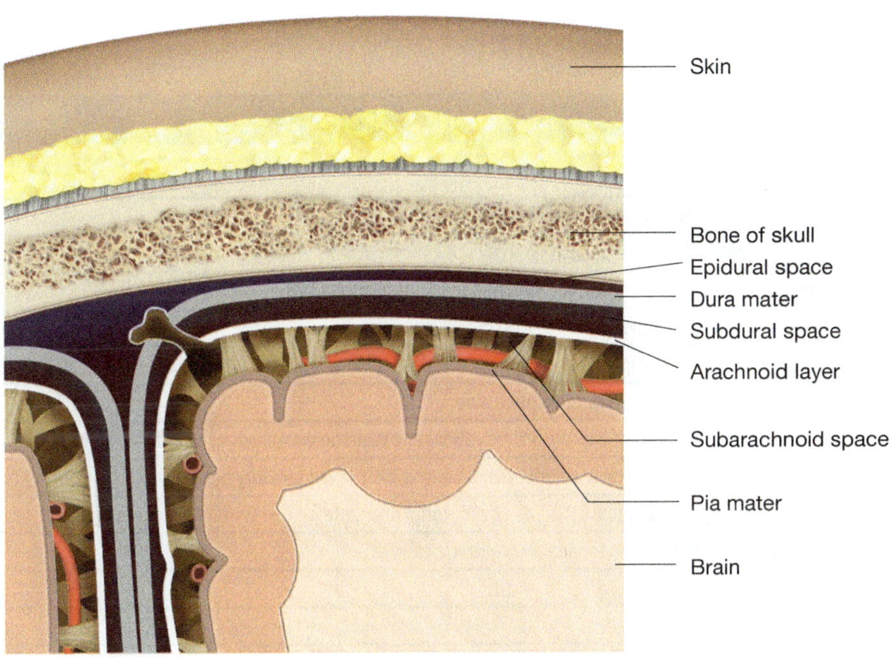

■ **Figure 12.6** The meninges. This figure illustrates the location and structure of each layer of the meninges and their relationship to the skull and brain.

Peripheral Nervous System

afferent neurons (AFF-er-ent)
autonomic nervous system (aw-toh-NOM-ik)
efferent neurons (EFF-er-ent)
ganglion (GANG-lee-on)
motor neurons
nerve root
sensory neurons
somatic nerves

The peripheral nervous system (PNS) includes both the 12 pairs of cranial nerves and the 31 pairs of spinal nerves. A nerve is a group or bundle of axon fibers located outside the central nervous system that carries messages between the central nervous system and the various parts of the body. Whether a nerve is cranial or spinal is determined by where the nerve originates. Cranial nerves arise from the brain, mainly at the medulla oblongata. Spinal nerves split off from the spinal cord, and one pair (a left and a right) exits between each pair of vertebrae. The point where either type of nerve is attached to the central nervous system is called the **nerve root.** The names of most nerves reflect either the organ the nerve serves or the portion of the body the nerve is traveling through. The entire list of cranial nerves is found in Table 12.1 ■. Figure 12.7 ■ illustrates some of the major spinal nerves in the human body.

Although most nerves carry information to and from the central nervous system, individual neurons carry information in only one direction. **Afferent neurons,** also called **sensory neurons,** carry sensory information from a sensory receptor to the central nervous system. **Efferent neurons,** also called **motor neurons,** carry activity instructions from the central nervous system to muscles or glands out in the body (see Figure 12.8 ■). The nerve cell bodies of the neurons forming the nerve are grouped together in a knot-like mass, called a **ganglion,** located outside the central nervous system.

The nerves of the peripheral nervous system are subdivided into two divisions, the **autonomic nervous system** (ANS) and **somatic nerves,** each serving a different area of the body.

MED TERM TIP

Because nerve tracts cross from one side of the body to the other side of the brain, damage to one side of the brain results in symptoms appearing on the opposite side of the body. Since nerve cells that control the movement of the right side of the body are located in the left side of the medulla oblongata, a stroke that paralyzed the right side of the body would actually have occurred in the left side of the brain.

Table 12.1 Cranial Nerves

NUMBER	NAME	FUNCTION
I	Olfactory	Transports impulses for sense of smell
II	Optic	Carries impulses for sense of sight
III	Oculomotor	Motor impulses for eye muscle movement and the pupil of the eye
IV	Trochlear	Controls superior oblique muscle of eye on each side
V	Trigeminal	Carries sensory facial impulses and controls muscles for chewing; branches into eyes, forehead, upper and lower jaw
VI	Abducens	Controls an eyeball muscle to turn eye to side
VII	Facial	Controls facial muscles for expression, salivation, and taste on two-thirds of tongue (anterior)
VIII	Vestibulocochlear	Responsible for impulses of equilibrium and hearing; also called auditory nerve
IX	Glossopharyngeal	Carries sensory impulses from pharynx (swallowing) and taste on one-third of tongue
X	Vagus	Supplies most organs in abdominal and thoracic cavities
XI	Accessory	Controls the neck and shoulder muscles
XII	Hypoglossal	Controls tongue muscles

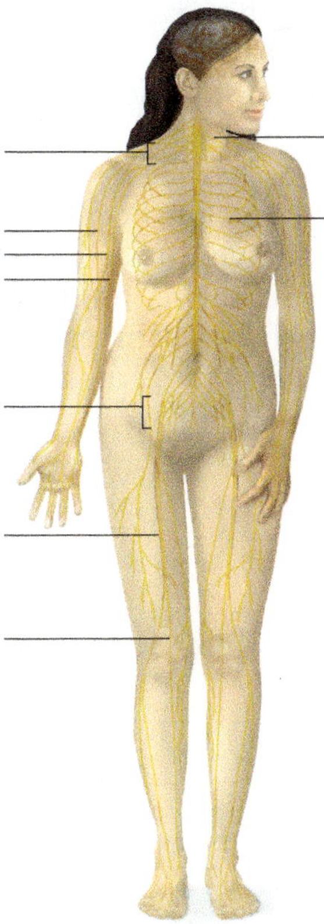

Figure 12.7 The major spinal nerves.

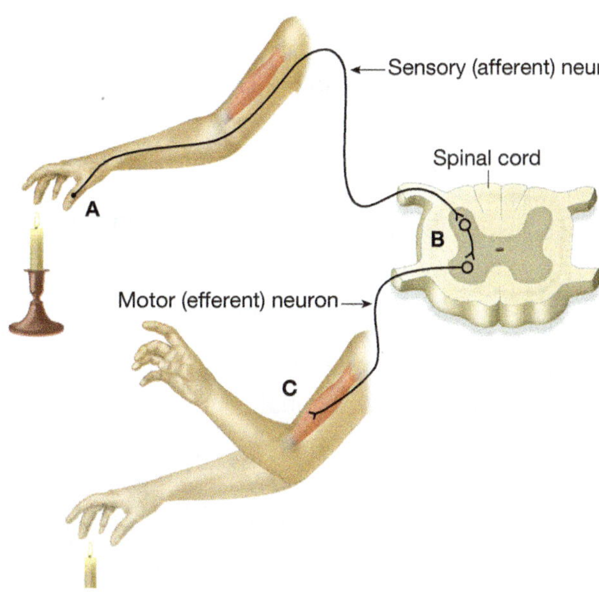

Figure 12.8 The functional structure of the peripheral nervous system. (A) Afferent or sensory neurons carry sensory information to the spinal cord; (B) the spinal cord receives incoming sensory information and delivers motor messages; (C) efferent or motor neurons deliver motor commands to muscles and glands.

Autonomic Nervous System

parasympathetic branch (pair-ah-sim-pah-THET-ik)

sympathetic branch (sim-pah-THET-ik)

The autonomic nervous system is involved with the control of involuntary or unconscious bodily functions. It may increase or decrease the activity of the smooth muscle found in viscera and blood vessels, cardiac muscle, and glands. The autonomic nervous system is divided into two branches: **sympathetic branch** and **parasympathetic branch.** The sympathetic nerves control the "fight or flight" reaction during times of stress and crisis. These nerves increase heart rate, dilate airways, increase blood pressure, inhibit digestion, and stimulate the production of adrenaline during a crisis. The parasympathetic nerves serve as a counterbalance for the sympathetic nerves, the "rest and digest" reaction. Therefore, they cause heart rate to slow down, lower blood pressure, and stimulate digestion.

Somatic Nerves

Somatic nerves serve the skin and skeletal muscles and are mainly involved with the conscious and voluntary activities of the body. The large variety of sensory receptors found in the dermis layer of the skin use somatic nerves to send their information, such as touch, temperature, pressure, and pain, to the brain. These are also the nerves that carry motor commands to skeletal muscles.

Terminology

Word Parts Used to Build Nervous System Terms

The following lists contain the combining forms, suffixes, and prefixes used to build terms in the remaining sections of this chapter.

Combining Forms

alges/o	sense of pain
angi/o	vessel
arteri/o	artery
astr/o	star
cephal/o	head
cerebell/o	cerebellum
cerebr/o	cerebrum
clon/o	rapid contracting and relaxing
cyt/o	cell
dur/o	dura mater
electr/o	electricity

encephal/o	brain
esthes/o	sensation, feeling
gli/o	glue
hemat/o	blood
isch/o	to hold back
later/o	side
lumb/o	low back
medull/o	medulla oblongata
mening/o	meninges
meningi/o	meninges
my/o	muscle
myel/o	spinal cord

neur/o	nerve
poli/o	gray matter
pont/o	pons
radicul/o	nerve root
scler/o	hard
spin/o	spine
thalam/o	thalamus
thec/o	sheath
tom/o	to cut
ton/o	muscle tone
vascul/o	blood vessel
ventricul/o	ventricle

Suffixes

-al	pertaining to
-algia	pain
-ar	pertaining to
-ary	pertaining to
-asthenia	weakness
-cele	protrusion
-eal	pertaining to
-ectomy	surgical removal
-gram	record
-graphy	process of recording

-ia	condition, state
-ic	pertaining to
-ine	pertaining to
-itis	inflammation
-logy	study of
-nic	pertaining to
-oma	tumor, swelling
-osis	abnormal condition
-otomy	cutting into
-paresis	weakness

-pathy	disease
-phasia	speech
-plasty	surgical repair
-plegia	paralysis
-rrhaphy	suture
-taxia	muscle coordination
-tic	pertaining to
-trophic	pertaining to development

Prefixes

a-	without
an-	without
anti-	against
bi-	two
dys-	abnormal, difficult
endo-	within
epi-	above
hemi-	half
hydro-	water
hyper-	excessive
intra-	within
mono-	one
para-	abnormal, two like parts of a pair
poly-	many
quadri-	four
semi-	partial
sub-	below
un-	not

Anatomical Terms

TERM	WORD PARTS	DEFINITION
cerebellar (ser-eh-BELL-ar)	cerebell/o = cerebellum -ar = pertaining to	Pertaining to the cerebellum.
cerebral (seh-REE-bral)	cerebr/o = cerebrum -al = pertaining to	Pertaining to the cerebrum.
cerebrospinal (ser-eh-broh-SPY-nal)	cerebr/o = cerebrum spin/o = spine -al = pertaining to	Pertaining to the cerebrum and spine.
encephalic (IN-seh-FAL-ik)	encephal/o = brain -ic = pertaining to	Pertaining to the brain.
intrathecal (in-tra-THEE-kal)	intra- = within thec/o = sheath -al = pertaining to	Pertaining to within the meninges, specifically the subdural or subarachnoid space.
medullary (MED-yoo-lair-ee)	medull/o = medulla oblongata -ary = pertaining to	Pertaining to the medulla oblongata.
meningeal (meh-NIN-jee-all)	mening/o = meninges -eal = pertaining to	Pertaining to the meninges.
myelonic (MY-eh-LON-ik)	myel/o = spinal cord -nic = pertaining to	Pertaining to the spinal cord.
neural (NOO-rall)	neur/o = nerve -al = pertaining to	Pertaining to nerves.
neuroglial (noo-RIG-lee-al)	neur/o = nerve gli/o = glue -al = pertaining to	Pertaining to the support cells, glial cells, of nerves.
pontine (pon-TEEN)	pont/o = pons -ine = pertaining to	Pertaining to the pons.
thalamic (tha-LAM-ik)	thalam/o = thalamus -ic = pertaining to	Pertaining to the thalamus.
ventricular (ven-TRIK-yoo-lar)	ventricul/o = ventricle -ar = pertaining to	Pertaining to the ventricles.

Pathology

TERM	WORD PARTS	DEFINITION
Medical Specialties		
anesthesiology (an-es-thee-zee-ol-oh-jee)	an- = without esthes/o = sensation, feeling -logy = study of	Branch of medicine specializing in all aspects of anesthesia, including for surgical procedures, resuscitation measures, and the management of acute and chronic pain. Physician is an *anesthesiologist.*
neurology (noo-rol-oh-jee)	neur/o = nerve -logy = study of	Branch of medicine concerned with diagnosis and treatment of diseases and conditions of the nervous system. Physician is a *neurologist.*
neurosurgery (noo-roh-SIR-jury)	neur/o = nerve	Branch of medicine concerned with treating conditions and diseases of the nervous systems by surgical means. Physician is a *neurosurgeon.*
Signs and Symptoms		
absence seizure		Type of epileptic seizure that lasts only a few seconds to half a minute, characterized by a loss of awareness and an absence of activity. It is formerly known as a *petite mal seizure.*
analgesia (an-al-JEE-zee-ah)	an- = without alges/o = sense of pain -ia = state	Absence of pain.
anesthesia (an-ess-THEE-zee-ah)	an- = without esthes/o = feeling, sensations -ia = condition	Lack of feeling or sensation.
aphasia (ah-FAY-zee-ah)	a- = without -phasia = speech	Inability to communicate verbally or in writing due to damage of the speech or language centers in the brain.
ataxia (ah-TAK-see-ah)	a- = without -taxia = muscle coordination	Lack of muscle coordination.
aura (AW-ruh)		Sensations, such as seeing colors or smelling an unusual odor, that occur just prior to an epileptic seizure or migraine headache.
cephalalgia (seff-al-AL-jee-ah)	cephal/o = head -algia = pain	Headache.
coma (COH-mah)		Profound unconsciousness resulting from an illness or injury.
conscious (KON-shus)		Condition of being awake and aware of surroundings.
convulsion (kon-VULL-shun)		Severe involuntary muscle contractions and relaxations. These have a variety of causes, such as epilepsy, fever, and toxic conditions.

Pathology *(continued)*

TERM	WORD PARTS	DEFINITION
delirium (dee-LEER-ee-um)		Abnormal mental state characterized by confusion, disorientation, and agitation.
dementia (dee-MEN-she-ah)		Progressive impairment of intellectual function that interferes with performing activities of daily living. Patients have little awareness of their condition. Found in disorders such as Alzheimer's.
dysphasia (dis-FAY-zee-ah)	dys- = abnormal, difficult -phasia = speech	Difficulty communicating verbally or in writing due to damage of the speech or language centers in the brain.
focal seizure (FOE-kal)	-al = pertaining to	Localized seizure often affecting one limb.
hemiparesis (hem-ee-par-EE-sis)	hemi- = half -paresis = weakness	Weakness or loss of motion on one side of the body.
hemiplegia (hem-ee-PLEE-jee-ah)	hemi- = half -plegia = paralysis	Paralysis on only one side of the body.
hyperesthesia (high-per-ess-THEE-zee-ah)	hyper- = excessive esthes/o = feeling, sensations -ia = condition	Abnormally heightened sense of feeling, sense of pain, or sensitivity to touch.
monoparesis (mon-oh-pah-REE-sis)	mono- = one -paresis = weakness	Muscle weakness in one limb.
monoplegia (mon-oh-PLEE-jee-ah)	mono- = one -plegia = paralysis	Paralysis of one limb.
neuralgia (noo-RAL-jee-ah)	neur/o = nerve -algia = pain	Nerve pain.
palsy (PAWL-zee)		Temporary or permanent loss of the ability to control movement.
paralysis (pah-RAL-ih-sis)		Temporary or permanent loss of function or voluntary movement.
paraplegia (pair-ah-PLEE-jee-ah)	para- = two like parts of a pair -plegia = paralysis	Paralysis of the lower portion of the body and both legs.
paresthesia (par-es-THEE-zee-ah)	para- = abnormal esthes/o = sensation, feeling -ia = condition	Abnormal sensation such as burning or tingling.
quadriplegia (kwod-rih-PLEE-jee-ah)	quadri- = four -plegia = paralysis	Paralysis of all four limbs.
seizure (SEE-zyoor)		Sudden, uncontrollable onset of symptoms, such as in an epileptic seizure.
semiconscious (sem-ee-KON-shus)	semi- = partial	State of being aware of surroundings and responding to stimuli only part of the time.

Pathology *(continued)*

TERM	WORD PARTS	DEFINITION
syncope (SIN-koh-pee)		Fainting.
tonic-clonic seizure	ton/o = muscle tone clon/o = rapid contracting and relaxing -ic = pertaining to	Type of severe epileptic seizure characterized by a loss of consciousness and convulsions. The seizure alternates between strong continuous muscle spasms (tonic) and rhythmic muscle contraction and relaxation (clonic). It is also called a *grand mal seizure.*
tremor (TREM-or)		Involuntary repetitive alternating movement of a part of the body.
unconscious (un-KON-shus)	un- = not	State of being unaware of surroundings, with the inability to respond to stimuli.
Brain		
Alzheimer's disease (ALTS-high-merz)		Chronic, organic mental disorder consisting of dementia, which is more prevalent in adults after 65 years of age. Involves progressive disorientation, apathy, speech and gait disturbances, and loss of memory. Named for German neurologist Alois Alzheimer.
astrocytoma (ass-troh-sigh-TOH-mah)	astr/o = star cyt/o = cell -oma = tumor	Tumor of the brain or spinal cord composed of astrocytes, one type of neuroglial cells.
brain tumor		Intracranial mass, either benign or malignant. A benign tumor of the brain can still be fatal since it will grow and cause pressure on normal brain tissue.

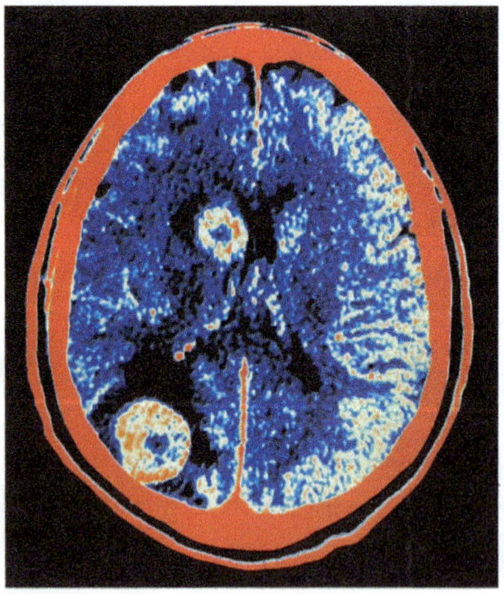

Figure 12.9 Color-enhanced CT scan showing two malignant tumors in the brain. *(Scott Camazine/Photo Researchers, Inc.)*

TERM	WORD PARTS	DEFINITION
cerebellitis (ser-eh-bell-EYE-tis)	cerebell/o = cerebellum -itis = inflammation	Inflammation of the cerebellum.

Pathology *(continued)*

TERM	WORD PARTS	DEFINITION
cerebral aneurysm (AN-yoo-rizm)	cerebr/o = cerebrum -al = pertaining to	Localized abnormal dilation of a blood vessel, usually an artery; the result of a congenital defect or weakness in the wall of the vessel. A ruptured aneurysm is a common cause of a hemorrhagic cerebrovascular accident.

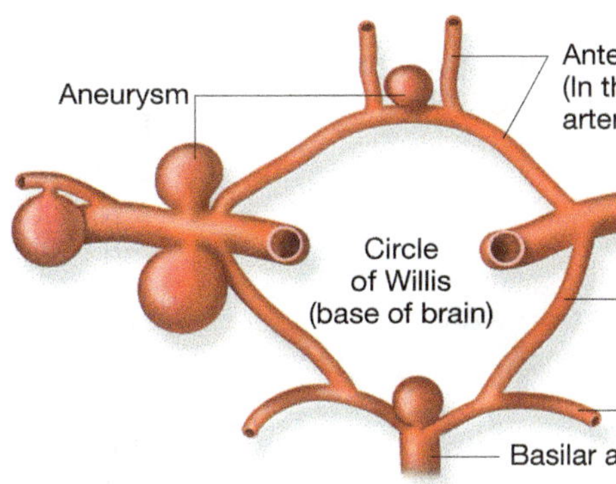

■ **Figure 12.10** Common locations for cerebral artery aneurysms in the Circle of Willis.

TERM	WORD PARTS	DEFINITION
cerebral contusion (kon-TOO-shun)	cerebr/o = cerebrum -al = pertaining to	Bruising of the brain from a blow or impact.
cerebral palsy (CP) (ser-REE-bral / PAWL-zee)	cerebr/o = cerebrum -al = pertaining to	Brain damage resulting from a defect, trauma, infection, or lack of oxygen before, during, or shortly after birth.
cerebrovascular accident (CVA) (ser-eh-broh-VASS-kyoo-lar)	cerebr/o = cerebrum vascul/o = blood vessel -ar = pertaining to	Development of an infarct due to loss in the blood supply to an area of the brain. Blood flow can be interrupted by a ruptured blood vessel (hemorrhage), a floating clot (embolus), a stationary clot (thrombosis), or compression. The extent of damage depends on the size and location of the infarct and often includes dysphasia and hemiplegia. Commonly called a *stroke.*

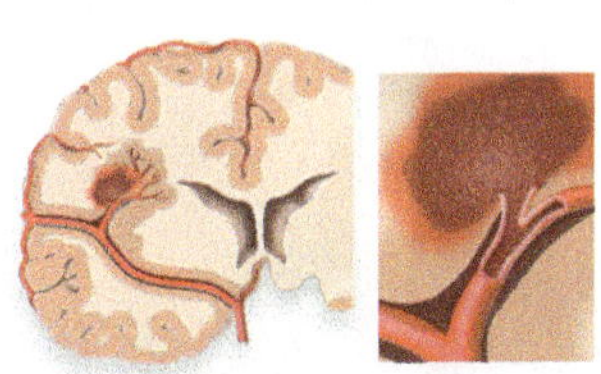

Cerebral hemorrhage: Cerebral artery ruptures and bleeds into brain tissue.

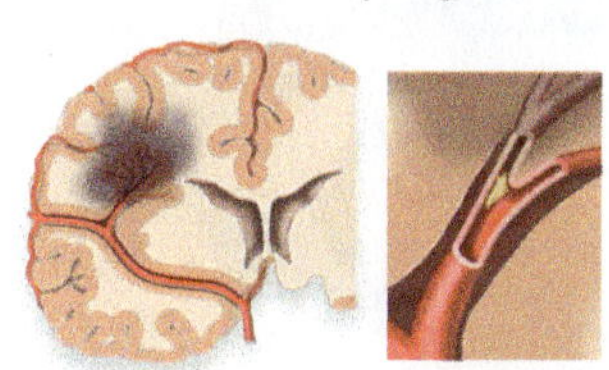

Cerebral embolism: Embolus from another area lodges in cerebral artery and blocks blood flow.

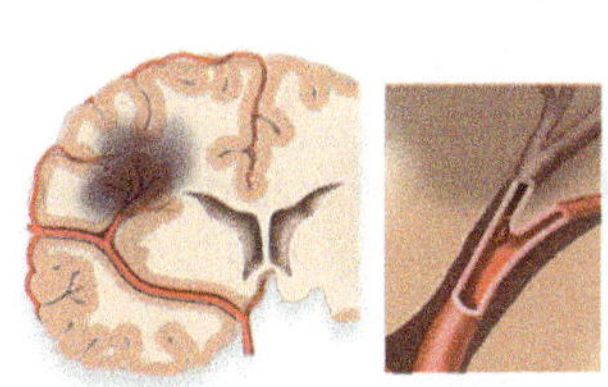

Cerebral thrombosis: Blood clot forms in cerebral artery and blocks blood flow.

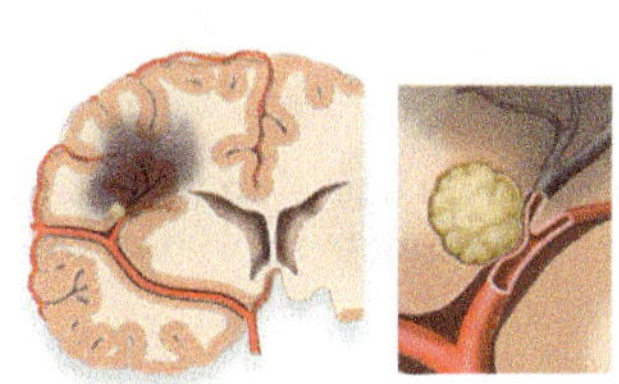

Compression: Pressure from tumor squeezes adjacent blood vessel and blocks blood flow.

■ **Figure 12.11** The four common causes for cerebrovascular accidents.

Pathology (continued)

TERM	WORD PARTS	DEFINITION
concussion (kon-KUSH-un)		Injury to the brain resulting from the brain being shaken inside the skull from a blow or impact. Symptoms vary and may include: headache, blurred vision, nausea or vomiting, dizziness, and balance problems. Also called *mild traumatic brain injury* (TBI).
encephalitis (en-seff-ah-LYE-tis)	encephal/o = brain -itis = inflammation	Inflammation of the brain.
epilepsy (EP-ih-lep-see)		Recurrent disorder of the brain in which seizures and loss of consciousness occur as a result of uncontrolled electrical activity of the neurons in the brain.
hydrocephalus (high-droh-SEFF-ah-lus)	hydro- = water cephal/o = head	Accumulation of cerebrospinal fluid within the ventricles of the brain, causing the head to be enlarged. It is treated by creating an artificial shunt for the fluid to leave the brain. If left untreated, it may lead to seizures and mental retardation.

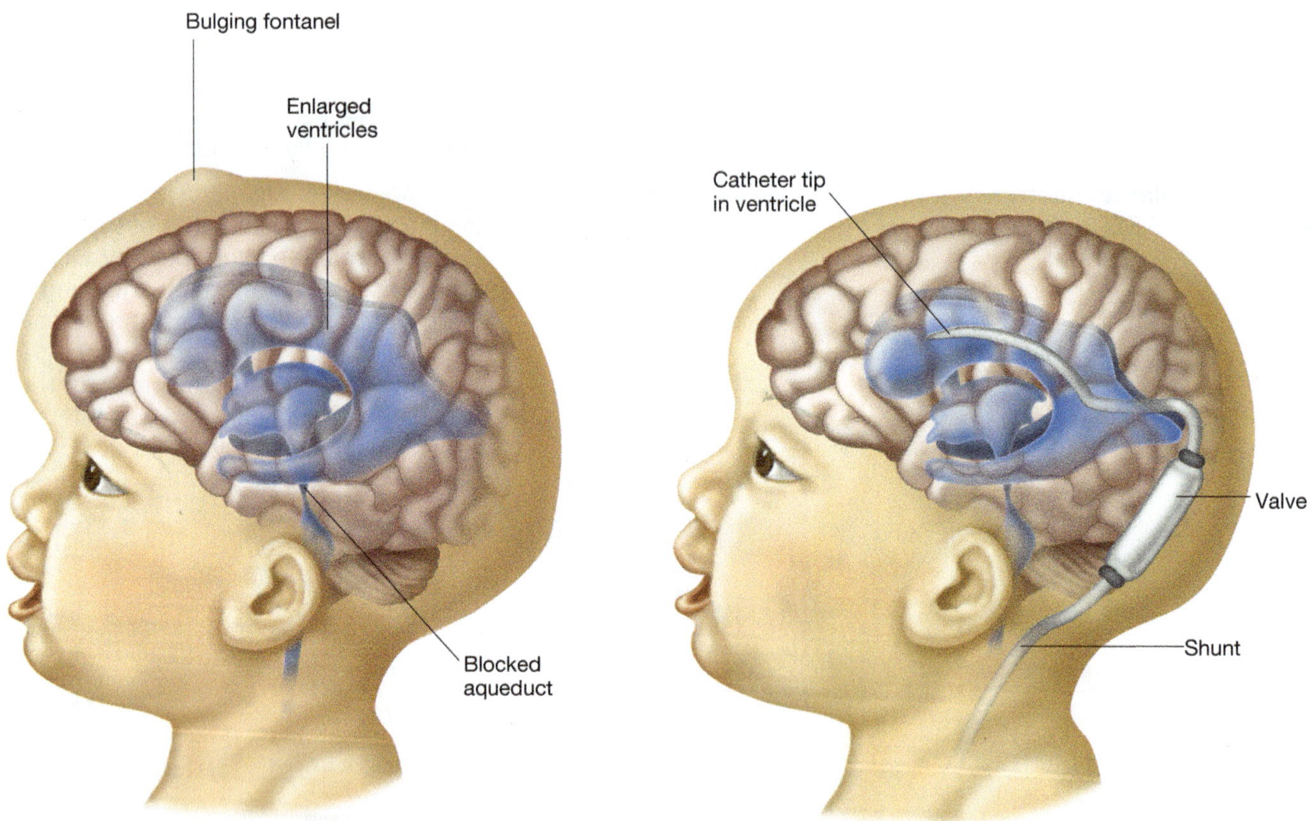

■ **Figure 12.12** Hydrocephalus. The figure on the left is a child with the enlarged ventricles of hydrocephalus. The figure on the right is the same child with a shunt to send the excess cerebrospinal fluid to the abdominal cavity.

Pathology *(continued)*

TERM	WORD PARTS	DEFINITION
migraine (MY-grain)		Specific type of headache characterized by severe head pain, sensitivity to light, dizziness, and nausea.
Parkinson's disease (PARK-in-sons)		Chronic disorder of the nervous system with fine tremors, muscular weakness, rigidity, and a shuffling gait. Named for British physician Sir James Parkinson.
Reye syndrome (RISE / SIN-drohm)		Combination of symptoms first recognized by Australian pathologist R. D. K. Reye that includes acute encephalopathy and damage to various organs, especially the liver. This occurs in children under age 15 who have had a viral infection. It is also associated with taking aspirin. For this reason, it's not recommended for children to use aspirin.
transient ischemic attack (TIA) (TRAN-shent / iss-KEM-ik)	isch/o = to hold back hem/o = blood -ic = pertaining to	Temporary interference with blood supply to the brain, causing neurological symptoms such as dizziness, numbness, and hemiparesis. May eventually lead to a full-blown stroke (cerebrovascular accident).
Spinal Cord		
amyotrophic lateral sclerosis (ALS) (ah-my-oh-TROFF-ik / LAT-er-al / skleh-ROH-sis)	a- = without my/o = muscle -trophic = pertaining to development later/o = side -al = pertaining to scler/o = hard -osis = abnormal condition	Disease with muscular weakness and atrophy due to degeneration of motor neurons of the spinal cord. Also called *Lou Gehrig's disease,* after the New York Yankees baseball player who died from the disease.
meningocele (men-IN-goh-seel)	mening/o = meninges -cele = protrusion	Congenital condition in which the meninges protrude through an opening in the vertebral column (see Figure 12.13B ■). See *spina bifida.*
myelitis (my-eh-LYE-tis)	myel/o = spinal cord -itis = inflammation	Inflammation of the spinal cord.
myelomeningocele (my-eh-loh-meh-NIN-goh-seel)	myel/o = spinal cord mening/o = meninges -cele = protrusion	Congenital condition in which the meninges and spinal cord protrude through an opening in the vertebral column (see Figure 12.13C ■). See *spina bifida.*
poliomyelitis (poh-lee-oh-my-eh-lye-tis)	poli/o = gray matter myel/o = spinal cord -itis = inflammation	Viral inflammation of the gray matter of the spinal cord. Results in varying degrees of paralysis; may be mild and reversible or may be severe and permanent. This disease has been almost eliminated due to the discovery of a vaccine in the 1950s.

Pathology *(continued)*

TERM	WORD PARTS	DEFINITION
spina bifida (SPY-nah / BIFF-ih-dah)	spin/o = spine bi- = two	Congenital defect in the walls of the spinal canal in which the laminae of the vertebra do not meet or close (see Figure 12.13A ■). May result in a meningocele or a myelomeningocele—meninges or the spinal cord being pushed through the opening.

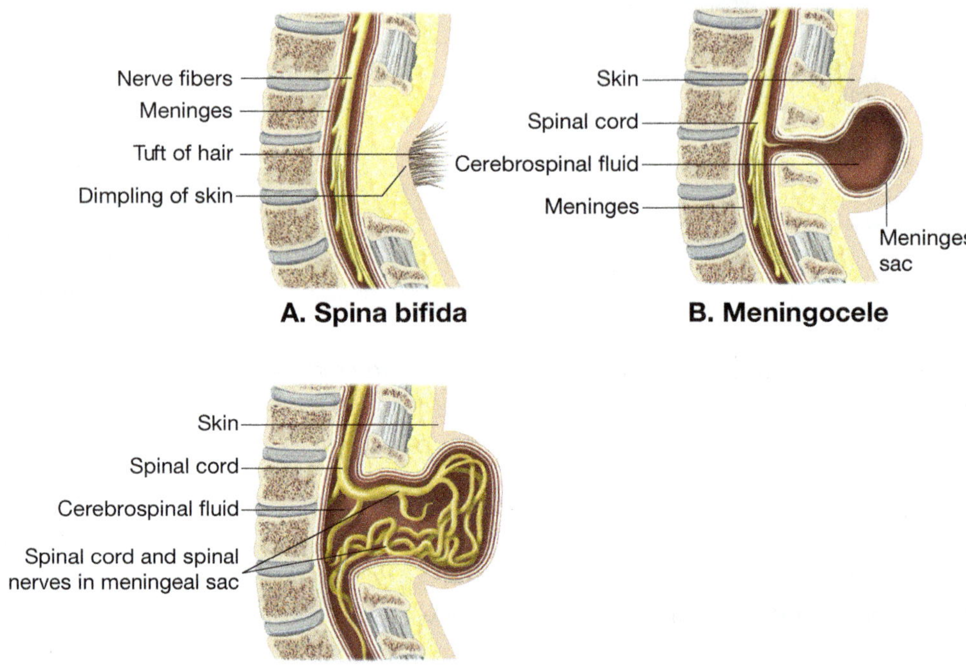

■ **Figure 12.13** Spina bifida. (A) Spina bifica occulta; the vertebra is not complete, but there is no protrusion of nervous system structures. (B) Meningocele; the meninges sac protrudes through the opening in the vertebra. (C) Myelomeningocele; the meninges sac and spinal cord protrude through the opening in the vertebra.

TERM	WORD PARTS	DEFINITION
spinal cord injury (SCI)	spin/o = spine -al = pertaining to	Damage to the spinal cord as a result of trauma. Spinal cord may be bruised or completely severed.
Nerves		
Bell's palsy (BELLZ / PAWL-zee)		One-sided facial paralysis due to inflammation of the facial nerve, probably viral in nature. The patient cannot control salivation, tearing of the eyes, or expression, but most will eventually recover.
Guillain-Barré syndrome (GHEE-yan / bah-RAY)		Disease of the nervous system in which nerves lose their myelin covering. May be caused by an autoimmune reaction. Characterized by loss of sensation and/or muscle control starting in the legs. Symptoms then move toward the trunk and may even result in paralysis of the diaphragm.
multiple sclerosis (MS) (MULL-tih-pl / skleh-ROH-sis)	scler/o = hard -osis = abnormal condition	Inflammatory disease of the central nervous system in which there is extreme weakness and numbness due to loss of myelin insulation from nerves.
myasthenia gravis (my-ass-THEE-nee-ah / GRAV-iss)	my/o = muscle -asthenia = weakness	Disease with severe muscular weakness and fatigue due to insufficient neurotransmitter at a synapse.

Pathology *(continued)*

TERM	WORD PARTS	DEFINITION
neuroma (noo-ROH-mah)	neur/o = nerve -oma = tumor	Nerve tumor or tumor of the connective tissue sheath around a nerve.
neuropathy (noo-ROP-ah-thee)	neur/o = nerve -pathy = disease	General term for disease or damage to a nerve.
polyneuritis (pol-ee-noo-RYE-tis)	poly- = many neur/o = nerve -itis = inflammation	Inflammation of two or more nerves.
radiculitis (rah-dick-yoo-LYE-tis)	radicul/o = nerve root -itis = inflammation	Inflammation of a nerve root; may be caused by a herniated nucleus pulposus.
radiculopathy (rah-dick-yoo-LOP-ah-thee)	radicul/o = nerve root -pathy = disease	Refers to the condition that occurs when a herniated nucleus pulposus puts pressure on a nerve root. Symptoms include pain and numbness along the path of the affected nerve.
shingles (SHING-lz)		Eruption of painful blisters on the body along a nerve path. Thought to be caused by a *Herpes zoster* virus infection of the nerve root.

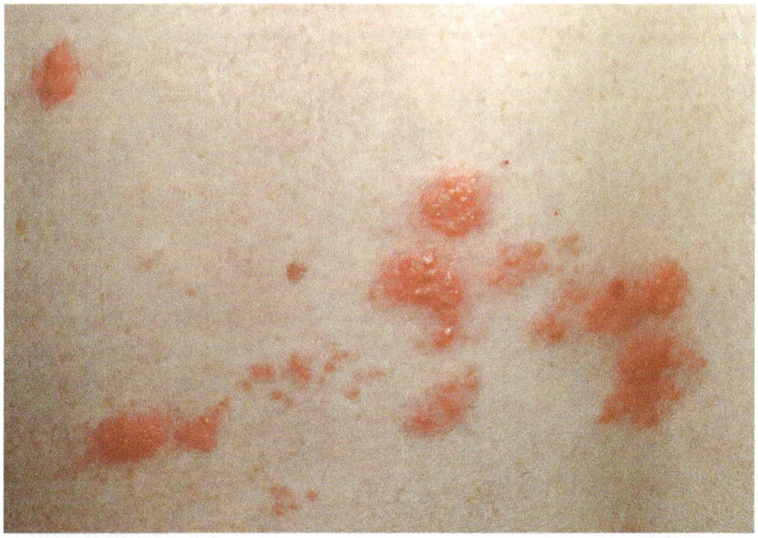

Figure 12.14 Photograph of the skin eruptions associated with shingles. *(Stephen VanHorn/Shutterstock)*

TERM	WORD PARTS	DEFINITION
Meninges		
epidural hematoma (ep-ih-DOO-ral / hee-mah-TOH-mah)	epi- = above dur/o = dura mater -al = pertaining to hemat/o = blood -oma = swelling	Mass of blood in the space outside the dura mater of the brain and spinal cord.
meningioma (meh-nin-jee-OH-mah)	meningi/o = meninges -oma = tumor	A tumor in the meninges.
meningitis (men-in-JYE-tis)	mening/o = meninges -itis = inflammation	Inflammation of the meninges around the brain or spinal cord caused by bacterial or viral infection. Symptoms include fever, headache, neck stiffness, lethargy, vomiting, irritability, and photophobia.

Pathology *(continued)*

TERM	WORD PARTS	DEFINITION
subdural hematoma (sub-DOO-ral / hee-mah-TOH-mah)	sub- = below dur/o = dura mater -al = pertaining to hemat/o = blood -oma = swelling	Mass of blood forming beneath the dura mater if the meninges are torn by trauma. May exert fatal pressure on the brain if the hematoma is not drained by surgery.

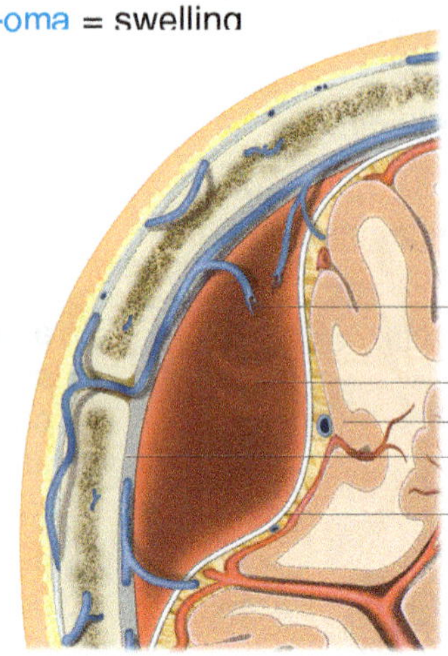

■ **Figure 12.15** A subdural hematoma. A meningeal vein is ruptured and blood has accumulated in the subdural space, producing pressure on the brain.

Diagnostic Procedures

TERM	WORD PARTS	DEFINITION
Clinical Laboratory Tests		
cerebrospinal fluid analysis (ser-eh-broh-SPY-nal / an-NAL-ih-sis)	cerebr/o = cerebrum spin/o = spine -al = pertaining to	Laboratory examination of the clear, watery, colorless fluid from within the brain and spinal cord. Infections and the abnormal presence of blood can be detected in this test.
Diagnostic Imaging		
brain scan		Image of the brain taken after injection of radioactive isotopes into the circulation.
cerebral angiography (seh-REE-bral / an-jee-OG-rah-fee)	cerebr/o = cerebrum -al = pertaining to angi/o = vessel -graphy = process of recording	X-ray of the blood vessels of the brain after the injection of radiopaque dye.
echoencephalography (ek-oh-en-SEFF-ah-log-rah-fee)	encephal/o = brain -graphy = process of recording	Recording of the ultrasonic echoes of the brain. Useful in determining abnormal patterns of shifting in the brain.
myelogram (MY-eh-loh-gram)	myel/o = spinal cord -gram = record	X-ray record of the spinal cord.

MED TERM TIP

The combining form *myel/o* means "marrow" and is used for both the spinal cord and bone marrow. To the ancient Greek philosophers and physicians, the spinal cord appeared to be much like the marrow found in the medullary cavity of a long bone.

Diagnostic Procedures *(continued)*

TERM	WORD PARTS	DEFINITION
myelography (my-eh-LOG-rah-fee)	myel/o = spinal cord -graphy = process of recording	Injection of radiopaque dye into the spinal canal. An X-ray is then taken to examine the normal and abnormal outlines made by the dye.
positron emission tomography (PET) (PAHZ-ih-tron / ee-MISH-un / toh-MOG-rah-fee)	tom/o = to cut -graphy = process of recording	Image of the brain produced by measuring gamma rays emitted from the brain after injecting glucose tagged with positively charged isotopes. Measurement of glucose uptake by the brain tissue indicates how metabolically active the tissue is.
Additional Diagnostic Tests		
Babinski reflex (bah-BIN-skeez)		Reflex test developed by French neurologist Joseph Babinski to determine lesions and abnormalities in the nervous system. The Babinski reflex is present if the great toe extends instead of flexes when the lateral sole of the foot is stroked. The normal response to this stimulation is flexion of the toe.
electroencephalogram (EEG) (ee-lek-troh-en-SEFF-ah-loh-gram)	electr/o = electricity encephal/o = brain -gram = record	Record of the brain's electrical patterns.
electroencephalography (EEG) (ee-lek-troh-en-SEFF-ah-LOG-rah-fee)	electr/o = electricity encephal/o = brain -graphy = process of recording	Recording the electrical activity of the brain by placing electrodes at various positions on the scalp. Also used in sleep studies to determine if there is a normal pattern of activity during sleep.
lumbar puncture (LP) (LUM-bar / PUNK-chur)	lumb/o = low back -ar = pertaining to	Puncture with a needle into the lumbar area (usually the fourth intervertebral space) to withdraw fluid for examination and for the injection of anesthesia. Also called *spinal puncture* or *spinal tap.*
nerve conduction velocity		Test that measures how fast an impulse travels along a nerve. Can pinpoint an area of nerve damage.

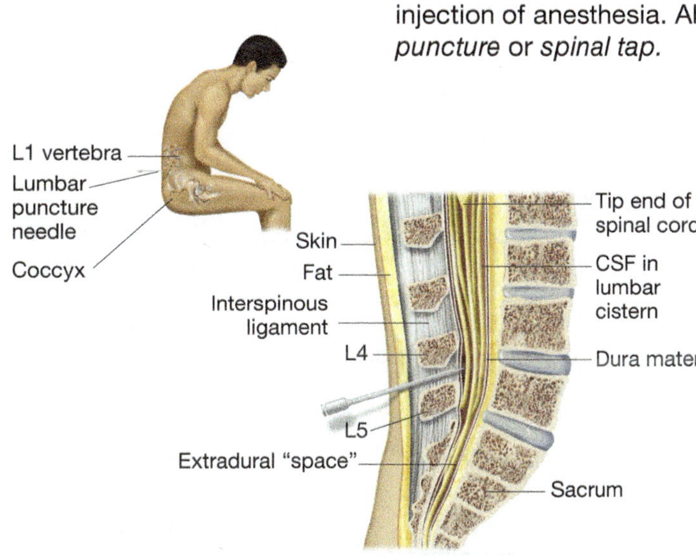

Figure 12.16 A lumbar puncture. The needle is inserted between the lumbar vertebrae and into the spinal canal.

Therapeutic Procedures

TERM	WORD PARTS	DEFINITION
Medical Procedures		
nerve block		Injection of regional anesthetic to stop the passage of sensory or pain impulses along a nerve path.
Surgical Procedures		
carotid endarterectomy (kah-ROT-id / end-ar-ter-EK-toh-mee)	endo- = within arteri/o = artery -ectomy = surgical removal	Surgical procedure for removing an obstruction within the carotid artery, a major artery in the neck that carries oxygenated blood to the brain. Developed to prevent strokes, but is found to be useful only in severe stenosis with transient ischemic attack.
cerebrospinal fluid shunts (ser-eh-bro-SPY-nal)	cerebr/o = cerebrum spin/o = spine -al = pertaining to	Surgical procedure in which a bypass is created to drain cerebrospinal fluid. It is used to treat hydrocephalus by draining the excess cerebrospinal fluid from the brain and diverting it to the abdominal cavity.
laminectomy (lam-ih-NEK-toh-mee)	-ectomy = surgical removal	Removal of a portion of a vertebra, called the lamina, in order to relieve pressure on the spinal nerve.
neurectomy (noo-REK-toh-mee)	neur/o = nerve -ectomy = surgical removal	Surgical removal of a nerve.
neuroplasty (NOOR-oh-plas-tee)	neur/o = nerve -plasty = surgical repair	Surgical repair of a nerve.
neurorrhaphy (noo-ROR-ah-fee)	neur/o = nerve -rrhaphy = suture	To suture a nerve back together. Actually refers to suturing the connective tissue sheath around the nerve.
tractotomy (track-OT-oh-mee)	-otomy = cutting into	Surgical interruption of a nerve tract in the spinal cord. Used to treat intractable pain or muscle spasms.

Pharmacology

CLASSIFICATION	WORD PARTS	ACTION	EXAMPLES
analgesic (an-al-JEE-zik)	an- = without alges/o = sense of pain -ic = pertaining to	Medication to treat minor to moderate pain without loss of consciousness.	aspirin, Bayer, Ecotrin; acetaminophen, Tylenol; ibuprofen, Motrin
anesthetic (an-ess-THET-ik)	an- = without esthes/o = feeling, sensation -tic = pertaining to	Drug that produces a loss of sensation or a loss of consciousness.	lidocaine, Xylocaine; pentobarbital, Nembutal; propofol, Diprivan; procaine, Novocain

Pharmacology *(continued)*

CLASSIFICATION	WORD PARTS	ACTION	EXAMPLES
anticonvulsant (an-tye-kon-VULL-sant)	anti- = against	Substance that reduces the excitability of neurons and therefore prevents the uncontrolled neuron activity associated with seizures.	carbamazepine, Tegretol; phenobarbital, Nembutal
dopaminergic drugs (dope-ah-men-ER-gik)	-ic = pertaining to	Group of medications to treat Parkinson's disease by either replacing the dopamine that is lacking or increasing the strength of the dopamine that is present.	levodopa; L-dopa, Larodopa; levodopa/carbidopa, Sinemet
hypnotic (hip-NOT-tik)	-ic = pertaining to	Drug that promotes sleep.	secobarbital, Seconal; temazepam, Restoril
narcotic analgesic (nar-KOT-tik)	-ic = pertaining to an- = without alges/o = sense of pain -ic = pertaining to	Drug used to treat severe pain; has the potential to be habit forming if taken for a prolonged time. Also called *opiates*.	morphine, MS Contin; oxycodone, OxyContin; meperidine, Demerol
sedative (SED-ah-tiv)		Drug that has a relaxing or calming effect.	amobarbital, Amytal; butabarbital, Butisol

Abbreviations

ALS	amyotrophic lateral sclerosis	**HA**	headache
ANS	autonomic nervous system	**ICP**	intracranial pressure
CNS	central nervous system	**LP**	lumbar puncture
CP	cerebral palsy	**MS**	multiple sclerosis
CSF	cerebrospinal fluid	**PET**	positron emission tomography
CVA	cerebrovascular accident	**PNS**	peripheral nervous system
CVD	cerebrovascular disease	**SCI**	spinal cord injury
EEG	electroencephalogram, electroencephalography	**TBI**	traumatic brain injury
		TIA	transient ischemic attack

Chapter Review

Real-World Applications

Medical Record Analysis

This Discharge Summary contains 12 medical terms. Underline each term and write it in the list below the report. Then define each term.

Discharge Summary

Admitting Diagnosis:	Paraplegia following motorcycle accident.
Final Diagnosis:	Comminuted L2 fracture with epidural hematoma and spinal cord injury resulting in complete paraplegia at the L2 level.
History of Present Illness:	Patient is a 23-year-old male who was involved in a motorcycle accident. He was unconscious for 35 minutes but was fully aware of his surroundings upon regaining consciousness. He was immediately aware of total anesthesia and paralysis below the waist.
Summary of Hospital Course:	CT scan revealed extensive bone destruction at the fracture site and that the spinal cord was severed. Patient was unable to voluntarily contract any lower extremity muscles and was not able to feel touch or pinpricks. Lumbar laminectomy with spinal fusion was performed to stabilize the fracture and remove the epidural hematoma. The immediate postoperative recovery period proceeded normally. Patient began physical therapy and occupational therapy. After 2 months, X-rays indicated full healing of the spinal fusion and patient was transferred to a rehabilitation institute.
Discharge Plans:	Patient was transferred to a rehabilitation institute to continue intensive PT and OT.

	Term	Definition
1	____________	____________________________
2	____________	____________________________
3	____________	____________________________
4	____________	____________________________
5	____________	____________________________
6	____________	____________________________
7	____________	____________________________
8	____________	____________________________
9	____________	____________________________
10	____________	____________________________
11	____________	____________________________
12	____________	____________________________

Chart Note Transcription

The chart note below contains 11 phrases that can be reworded with a medical term that you learned in this chapter. Each phrase is identified with an underline. Determine the medical term and write your answers in the space provided.

Current Complaint:	Patient is a 38-year-old female referred to the specialist in the treatment of diseases of the nervous system ❶ by her family physician with complaints of difficulty with speech, ❷ loss of motion on one side of the body, ❸ and severe involuntary muscle contractions. ❹
Past History:	Patient is married and nulliparous. Has been well prior to current symptoms.
Signs and Symptoms:	Her husband reports he first noted loss of motion on one side of the body when she began to drag her left foot. It has progressed to involve both left upper and lower extremities, with approximately a 50% loss in control of left lower extremity and a 25% loss of control in left upper extremity. Difficulty with speech is mild and mainly with recalling the names of common objects. Severe involuntary muscle contractions appear to be triggered by stress and last approximately 2 minutes. Results of a recording of the electrical activity of the brain ❺ and a puncture with a needle into the low back to withdraw fluid for examination ❻ were normal. However, an injection with radioactive isotopes ❼ revealed the presence of a mass in the right outer layer of the largest section of the brain. ❽
Diagnosis:	Astrocyte tumor ❾ in the right outer layer of the largest section of the brain. ❽
Treatment:	A right skull incision ❿ was performed to permit the surgical use of extreme cold ⓫ to destroy the tumor. Patient experienced moderate improvement in loss of motion on one side of the body ❸ and severe involuntary muscle contractions, ❹ but difficulty with speech ❷ was unchanged.

❶ ____________________

❷ ____________________

❸ ____________________

❹ ____________________

❺ ____________________

❻ ____________________

❼ ____________________

❽ ____________________

❾ ____________________

❿ ____________________

⓫ ____________________

Case Study

Below is a case study presentation of a patient with a condition covered in this chapter. Read the case study and answer the questions below. Some questions will ask for information not included within this chapter. Use your text, a medical dictionary, or any other reference material you choose to answer these questions.

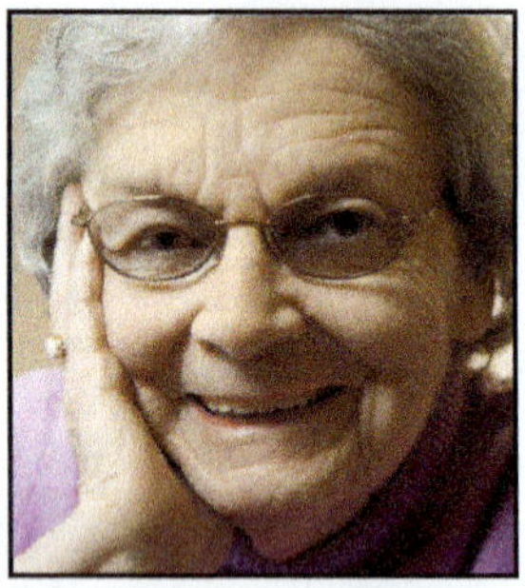

(iofoto/Shutterstock)

Anna Moore, an 83-year-old female, is admitted to the ER with aphasia, hemiparesis on her left side, syncope, and delirium. Her daughter called the ambulance after discovering her mother in this condition at home. Mrs. Moore has a history of hypertension, atherosclerosis, and diabetes mellitus. She was admitted to the hospital after a brain scan revealed an infarct in the right cerebral hemisphere leading to a diagnosis of CVA of the middle cerebral artery.

1. What pathological condition does Ms. Moore have? Look this condition up in a reference source and include a short description of it.

   ____

   ____

2. List and define each of the patient's presenting symptoms in the ER.

   ____

   ____

3. The patient has a history of three significant conditions. Describe each in your own words.

   ____

   ____

4. What diagnostic test did the physician perform? Describe this test and the results in your own words.

   ____

   ____

5. What is an infarct and what causes it?

   ____

   ____

6. List and describe the four common causes of a CVA.

   ____

   ____

Practice Exercises

A. Complete the Statement

1. The study of the nervous system is called ________________.
2. The organs of the nervous system are the ________________, ________________, and ________________.
3. The two divisions of the nervous system are the ________________ and ________________.
4. The neurons that carry impulses away from the brain and spinal cord are called ________________ neurons.
5. The neurons that carry impulses to the brain and spinal cord are called ________________ neurons.
6. The largest portion of the brain is the ________________.
7. The second largest portion of the brain is the ________________.
8. The occipital lobe controls ________________.
9. The temporal lobe controls ________________ and ________________.
10. The two divisions of the autonomic nervous system are the ________________ and ________________.

B. Terminology Matching

Match each term to its definition.

1. ________ olfactory	a. carries facial sensory impulses
2. ________ optic	b. turns eye to side
3. ________ oculomotor	c. controls tongue muscles
4. ________ trochlear	d. controls eye muscles and pupils
5. ________ trigeminal	e. swallowing
6. ________ abducens	f. controls facial muscles
7. ________ facial	g. controls oblique eye muscles
8. ________ vestibulocochlear	h. smell
9. ________ glossopharyngeal	i. controls neck and shoulder muscles
10. ________ vagus	j. hearing and equilibrium
11. ________ accessory	k. vision
12. ________ hypoglossal	l. organs in lower body cavities

C. Combining Form Practice

The combining form **neur/o** refers to the nerve. Use it to write a term that means:

1. inflammation of the nerve ______
2. specialist in nerves ______
3. pain in the nerve ______
4. inflammation of many nerves ______
5. removal of a nerve ______
6. surgical repair of a nerve ______
7. nerve tumor ______
8. suture of a nerve ______

The combining form **mening/o** refers to the meninges or membranes. Use it to write a term that means:

9. inflammation of the meninges ______
10. protrusion of the meninges ______
11. protrusion of the spinal cord and the meninges ______

The combining form **encephal/o** refers to the brain. Use it to write a term that means:

12. X-ray record of the brain ______
13. disease of the brain ______
14. inflammation of the brain ______
15. protrusion of the brain ______

The combining form **cerebr/o** refers to the cerebrum. Use it to write a term that means:

16. pertaining to the cerebrum and spinal cord ______
17. pertaining to the cerebrum ______

D. What Does it Stand For?

1. TIA ______
2. MS ______
3. SCI ______
4. CNS ______
5. PNS ______
6. HA ______

7. CP ______________________________

8. LP ______________________________

9. ALS ______________________________

E. Terminology Matching

Match each term to its definition.

1.	_______ aura	a.	loss of ability to control movement
2.	_______ meningitis	b.	sensations before a seizure
3.	_______ coma	c.	seizure with convulsions
4.	_______ shingles	d.	congenital hernia of meninges
5.	_______ syncope	e.	seizure without convulsion
6.	_______ palsy	f.	inflammation of meninges
7.	_______ absence seizure	g.	profound unconsciousness
8.	_______ tonic-clonic seizure	h.	*Herpes zoster* infection
9.	_______ meningocele	i.	fainting

F. What's the Abbreviation?

1. cerebrospinal fluid ______________________________
2. cerebrovascular disease ______________________________
3. electroencephalogram ______________________________
4. intracranial pressure ______________________________
5. positron emission tomography ______________________________
6. cerebrovascular accident ______________________________
7. subarachnoid hemorrhage ______________________________
8. autonomic nervous system ______________________________

G. Define the Procedures and Tests

1. myelography ____________________
2. cerebral angiography ____________________
3. Babinski's reflex ____________________
4. nerve conduction velocity ____________________
5. cerebrospinal fluid analysis ____________________
6. PET scan ____________________
7. echoencephalography ____________________
8. lumbar puncture ____________________

H. Define the Suffix

	Definition	Example from Chapter
1. **-plegia**	____________________	____________________
2. **-taxia**	____________________	____________________
3. **-trophic**	____________________	____________________
4. **-paresis**	____________________	____________________
5. **-phasia**	____________________	____________________

I. Define the Combining Form

	Definition	Example from Chapter Term
1. **mening/o**	____________________	____________________
2. **encephal/o**	____________________	____________________
3. **cerebell/o**	____________________	____________________
4. **myel/o**	____________________	____________________
5. **cephal/o**	____________________	____________________
6. **thalam/o**	____________________	____________________
7. **neur/o**	____________________	____________________
8. **radicul/o**	____________________	____________________
9. **cerebr/o**	____________________	____________________
10. **pont/o**	____________________	____________________

J. Define the Term

1. astrocytoma ______________________________
2. epilepsy ______________________________
3. anesthesia ______________________________
4. hemiparesis ______________________________
5. neurosurgeon ______________________________
6. analgesia ______________________________
7. focal seizure ______________________________
8. quadriplegia ______________________________
9. subdural hematoma ______________________________
10. intrathecal ______________________________

K. Terminology Matching

Match each term to its definition.

1.	_______ neurologist	a.	sudden attack
2.	_______ cerebrovascular accident	b.	a type of severe headache
3.	_______ concussion	c.	loss of intellectual ability
4.	_______ aphasia	d.	physician who treats nervous problem
5.	_______ migraine	e.	stroke
6.	_______ seizure	f.	mild traumatic brain injury
7.	_______ dementia	g.	loss of ability to speak
8.	_______ ataxia	h.	congenital anomaly
9.	_______ spina bifida	i.	state of being unaware
10.	_______ unconscious	j.	lack of muscle coordination

L. Fill in the Blank

Parkinson's disease	transient ischemic attack	cerebral palsy	cerebrospinal fluid shunt
Bell's palsy	subdural hematoma	amyotrophic lateral sclerosis	nerve conduction velocity
delirium	cerebral aneurysm		

1. Dr. Martin noted that the 96-year-old patient suffered from ______________________ when she determined that he was confused, disoriented, and agitated.
2. Lucinda's ______________________ resulted in increasing muscle weakness as the motor neurons in her spinal cord degenerated.
3. The diagnosis of ______________________ was correct because the weakness affected only one side of Charles's face.
4. A cerebral angiogram was ordered because Dr. Larson suspected Mrs. Constantine had a(n) ______________________.
5. Roberta's symptoms included fine tremors, muscular weakness, rigidity, and a shuffling gait, leading to a diagnosis of ______________________.
6. Matthew's hydrocephalus required the placement of a(n) ______________________.
7. Because Mae's hemiparesis was temporary, the final diagnosis was ______________________.
8. Following the car accident, a CT scan showed a(n) ______________________ was putting pressure on the brain, necessitating immediate neurosurgery.
9. Birth trauma resulted in the newborn developing ______________________.
10. A(n) ______________________ test was performed in order to pinpoint the exact position of the nerve damage.

M. Pharmacology Challenge

Fill in the classification for each drug description, then match the brand name.

	Drug Description	Classification	Brand Name
1.	_______ produces loss of sensation	______________________	a. L-Dopa
2.	_______ treats Parkinson's disease	______________________	b. Amytal
3.	_______ promotes sleep	______________________	c. OxyContin
4.	_______ medication for mild pain	______________________	d. Seconal
5.	_______ produces a calming effect	______________________	e. Xylocaine
6.	_______ treats severe pain	______________________	f. Tegretol
7.	_______ treats seizures	______________________	g. Motrin

Labeling Exercise

Image A

Write the labels for this figure on the numbered lines provided.

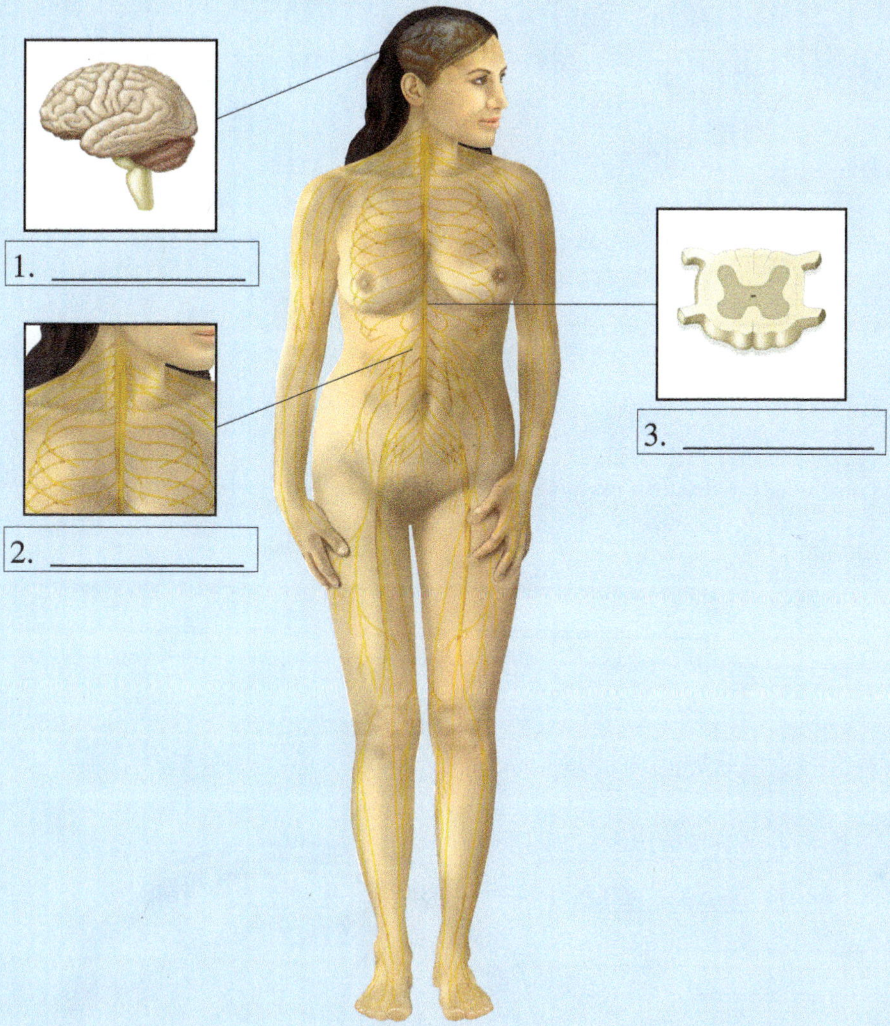

Image B

Write the labels for this figure on the numbered lines provided.

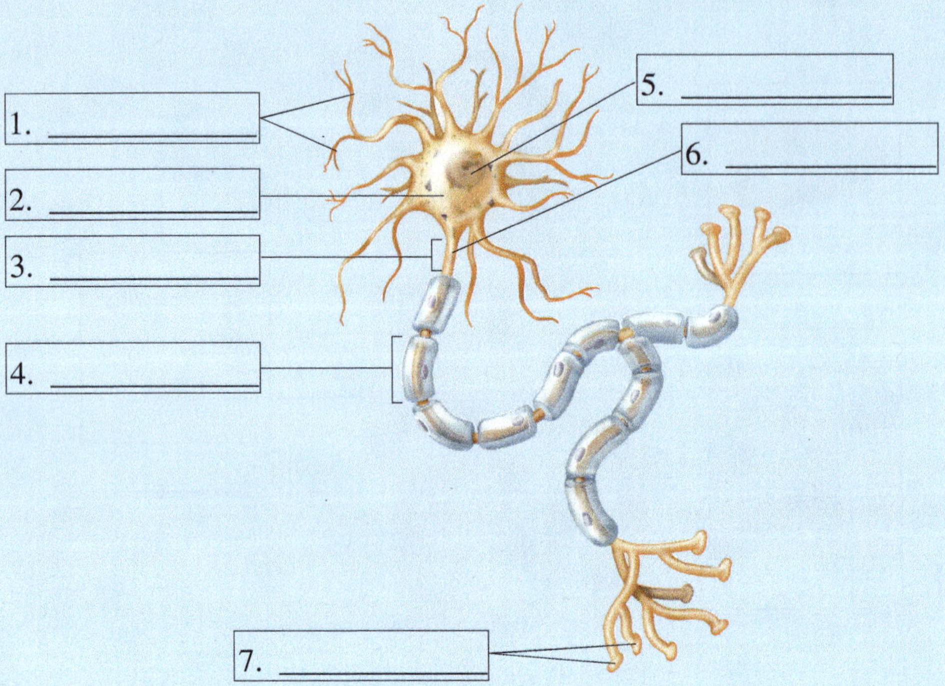

Image C

Write the labels for this figure on the numbered lines provided.

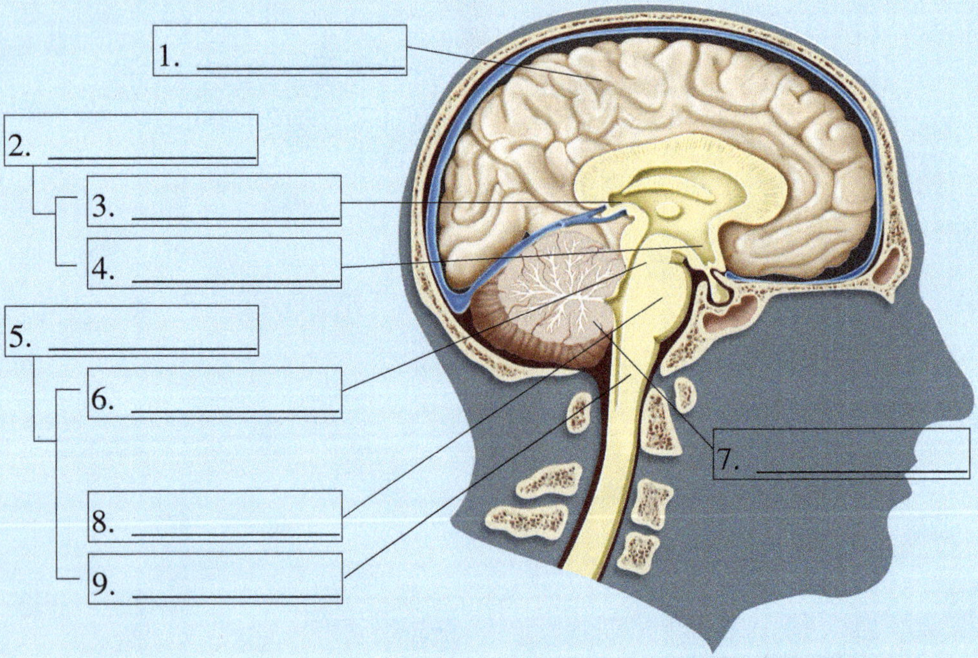

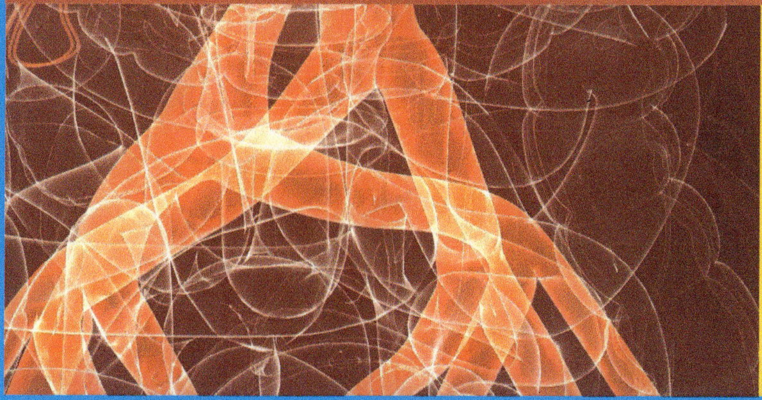

13

SPECIAL SENSES: THE EYE AND EAR

Learning Objectives

Upon completion of this chapter, you will be able to

- Identify and define the combining forms and suffixes introduced in this chapter.
- Correctly spell and pronounce medical terms and major anatomical structures relating to the eye and ear.
- Locate and describe the major structures of the eye and ear and their functions.
- Describe how we see.
- Describe the path of sound vibration.
- Identify and define eye and ear anatomical terms.
- Identify and define selected eye and ear pathology terms.
- Identify and define selected eye and ear diagnostic procedures.
- Identify and define selected eye and ear therapeutic procedures.
- Identify and define selected medications relating to the eye and ear.
- Define selected abbreviations associated with the eye and ear.

Section I: The Eye at a Glance

Function

The eye contains the sensory receptor cells for vision.

Structures

Here are the primary structures that comprise the eye.

choroid
conjunctiva
eye muscles
eyeball
eyelids
lacrimal apparatus
retina
sclera

Word Parts

Here are the most common word parts (with their meanings) used to build eye terms. For a more comprehensive list, refer to the Terminology section of this chapter.

Combining Forms

ambly/o	dull, dim
aque/o	water
blast/o	immature, embryonic
blephar/o	eyelid
chromat/o	color
conjunctiv/o	conjunctiva
corne/o	cornea
cycl/o	ciliary muscle
dacry/o	tear, tear duct
dipl/o	double
emmetr/o	correct, proper
glauc/o	gray
ir/o	iris
irid/o	iris
kerat/o	cornea
lacrim/o	tears
macul/o	macula lutea
mi/o	lessening
mydr/i	widening
nyctal/o	night
ocul/o	eye
ophthalm/o	eye
opt/o	eye, vision
optic/o	eye, vision
papill/o	optic disk
phac/o	lens
phot/o	light
presby/o	old age
pupill/o	pupil
retin/o	retina
scler/o	sclera
stigmat/o	point
uve/o	choroid
vitre/o	glassy

Suffixes

-ician	specialist
-metrist	specialist in measuring
-opia	vision condition
-opsia	vision condition
-tropia	turned condition

The Eye Illustrated

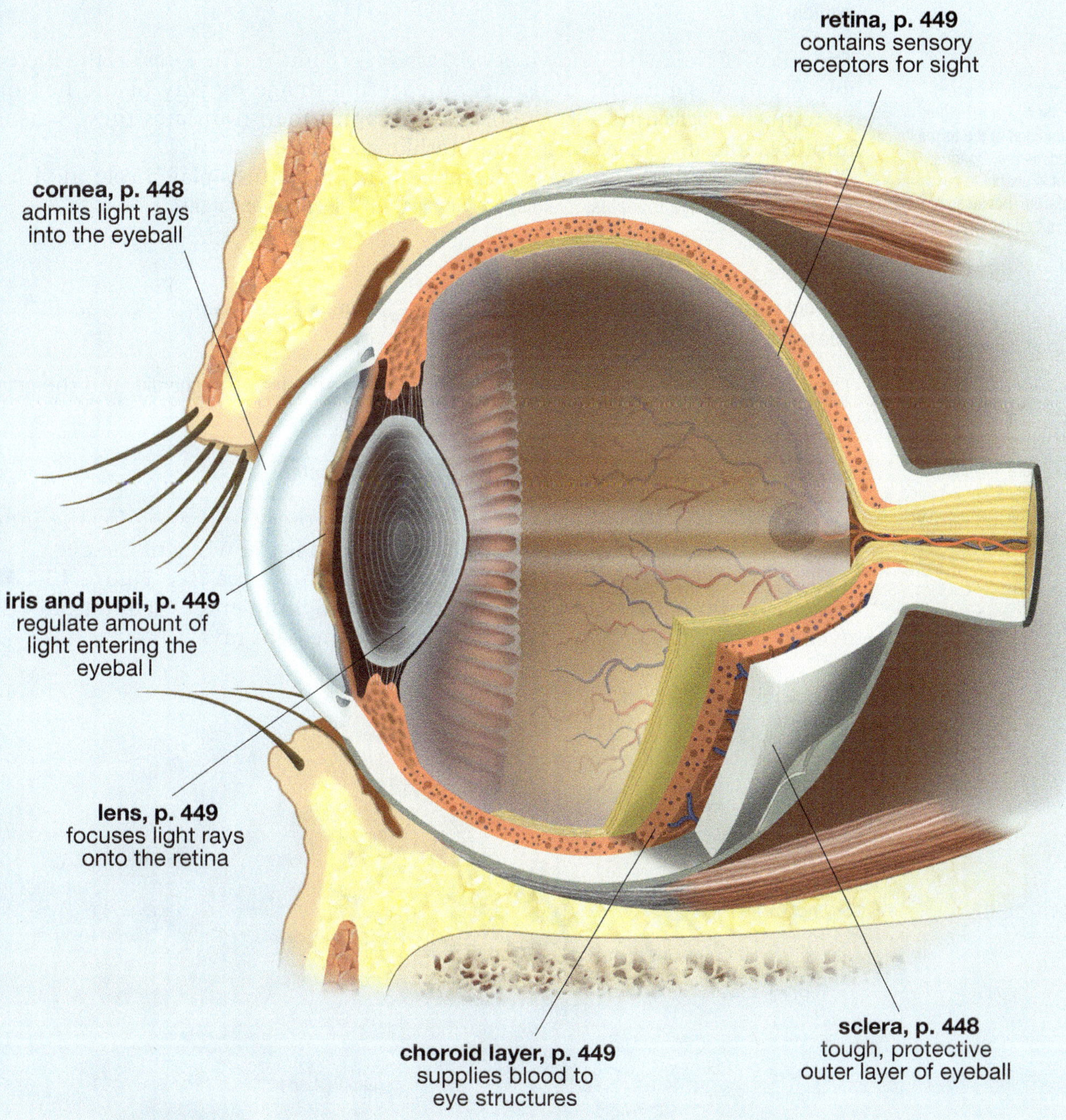

Anatomy and Physiology of the Eye

conjunctiva (kon-JUNK-tih-vah)
eye muscles
eyeball
eyelids
lacrimal apparatus (LAK-rim-al)
ophthalmology (off-thal-MALL-oh-gee)
optic nerve (OP-tik)

MED TERM TIP

When studying the functions and terminology of the eye, it is helpful to know the meanings of the terms *opaque* and *transparent*. Opaque means that light is unable to pass through. Transparent, however, means that light is permitted through.

The study of the eye is known as **ophthalmology** (Ophth). The **eyeball** is the incredible organ of sight that transmits an external image by way of the nervous system—the **optic nerve**—to the brain. The brain then translates these sensory impulses into an image with computerlike accuracy.

In addition to the eyeball, several external structures play a role in vision. These are the **eye muscles, eyelids, conjunctiva,** and **lacrimal apparatus.**

The Eyeball

choroid (KOR-oyd)
sclera (SKLAIR-ah)
retina (RET-in-ah)

The actual eyeball is composed of three layers: the **sclera,** the **choroid,** and the **retina.**

MED TERM TIP

The color of the sclera may indicate the presence of disease. For instance, a yellowish cast to the sclera can be present in liver disease and certain anemias.

Sclera

cornea (COR-nee-ah)
refracts

The outer layer, the sclera, provides a tough protective coating for the inner structures of the eye. Another term for the sclera is the white of the eye.

The anterior portion of the sclera is called the **cornea** (see Figure 13.1 ■). This clear, transparent area of the sclera allows light to enter the interior of the eyeball. The cornea actually bends, or **refracts,** the light rays.

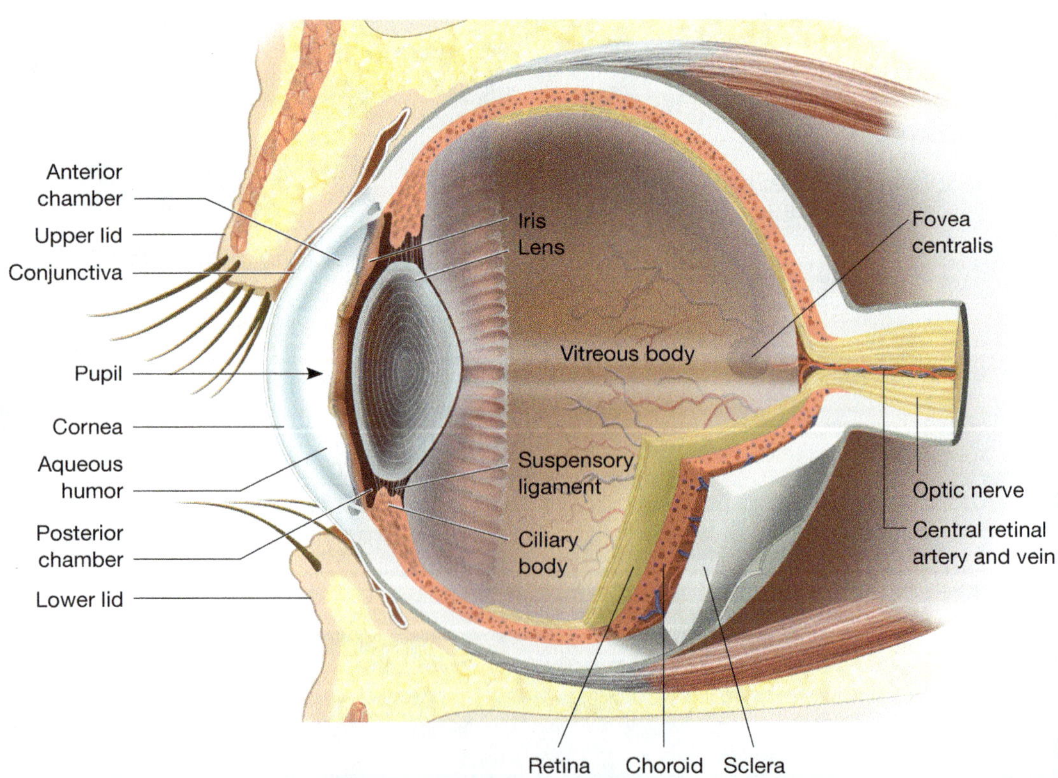

■ **Figure 13.1**
The internal structures of the eye.

Choroid

ciliary body (SIL-ee-ar-ee)
iris
lens
pupil

The second or middle layer of the eyeball is called the choroid. This opaque layer provides the blood supply for the eye.

The anterior portion of the choroid layer consists of the **iris, pupil,** and **ciliary body** (see again Figure 13.1). The iris is the colored portion of the eye and contains smooth muscle. The pupil is the opening in the center of the iris that allows light rays to enter the eyeball. The iris muscle contracts or relaxes to change the size of the pupil, thereby controlling how much light enters the interior of the eyeball. Behind the iris is the **lens.** The lens is not actually part of the choroid layer, but it is attached to the muscular ciliary body. By pulling on the edge of the lens, these muscles change the shape of the lens so it can focus incoming light onto the retina.

MED TERM TIP
The function of the choroid, to provide the rest of the eyeball with blood, is responsible for an alternate name for this layer—*uvea.* The combining form *uve/o* means "vascular."

Retina

aqueous humor (AY-kwee-us)
cones
fovea centralis (FOH-vee-ah / sen-TRAH-lis)
macula lutea (MAK-yoo-lah / loo-TEE-ah)
optic disk
retinal blood vessels (RET-in-al)
rods
vitreous humor (VIT-ree-us)

The third and innermost layer of the eyeball is the retina. It contains the sensory receptor cells (**rods** and **cones**) that respond to light rays. Rods are active in dim light and help us to see in gray tones. Cones are active only in bright light and are responsible for color vision. When one looks directly at an object, the image falls on an area called the **macula lutea,** or yellow spot (see Figure 13.1). In the center of the macula lutea is a depression called the **fovea centralis,** meaning central pit. This pit contains a high concentration of sensory receptor cells and, therefore, is the point of clearest vision. Also visible on the retina is the **optic disk.** This is the point where the **retinal blood vessels** enter and exit the eyeball and where the optic nerve leaves the eyeball (see Figure 13.2 ■). There are no sensory receptor cells in the optic disk and therefore it causes a blind spot in each eye's field of vision. The interior spaces of the eyeball are not empty. The spaces between the cornea and lens are filled with **aqueous humor,** a watery fluid, and the large open area between the lens and retina contains **vitreous humor,** a semisolid gel.

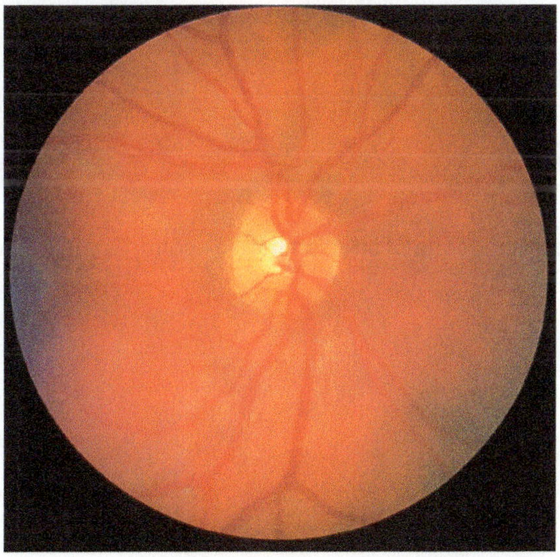

■ **Figure 13.2** Photograph of the retina of the eye. The optic disk appears yellow and the retinal arteries radiate out from it. *(Photo Researchers, Inc.)*

Muscles of the Eye

oblique muscles (oh-BLEEK)

rectus muscles (REK-tus)

MED TERM TIP

Like many other muscles, the names *rectus* and *oblique* provide clues regarding the direction of their fibers, or their *line of pull.* Rectus means straight and oblique means slanted. Rectus muscles have a straight line of pull. Since the fibers of an oblique muscle are slanted on an angle, they produce rotation.

Six muscles connect the actual eyeball to the skull (see Figure 13.3 ■). These muscles allow for change in the direction of each eye's sightline. In addition, they provide support for the eyeball in the eye socket. Children may be born with a weakness in some of these muscles and may require treatments such as eye exercises or even surgery to correct this problem commonly referred to as crossed eyes or *strabismus* (see Figure 13.4 ■). The muscles involved are the four **rectus** and two **oblique muscles.** Rectus muscles (meaning straight) pull the eye up, down, left, or right in a straight line. Oblique muscles are on an angle and produce diagonal eye movement.

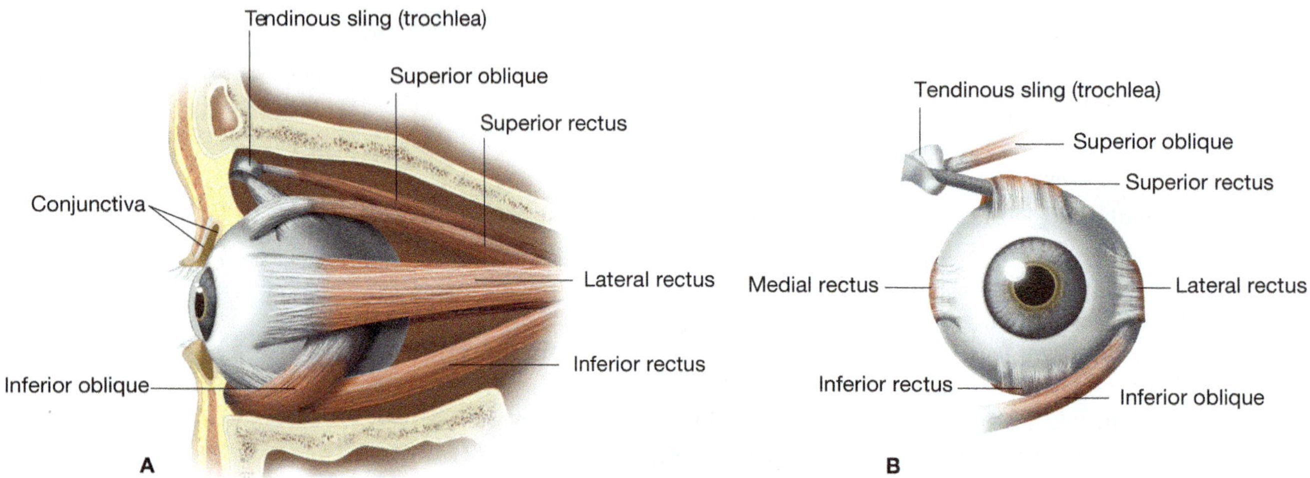

■ **Figure 13.3** The arrangement of the external eye muscles: (A) lateral and (B) anterior views.

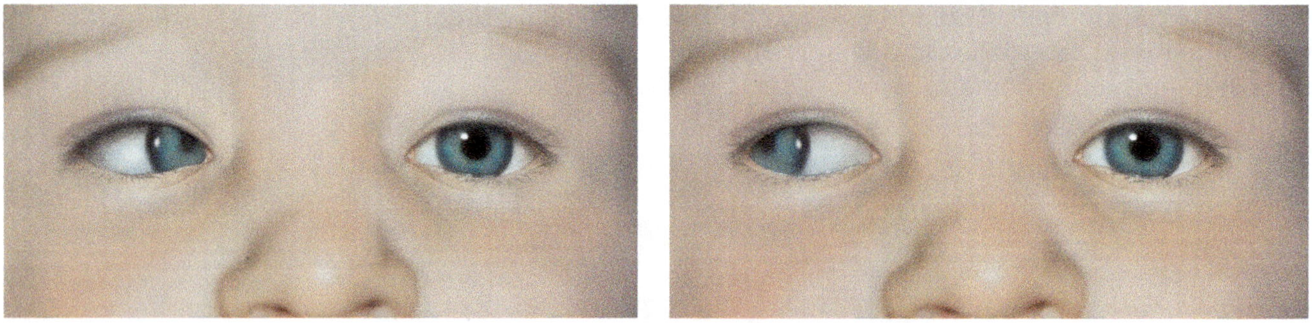

■ **Figure 13.4** Examples of common forms of strabismus: (A) esotropia with the right eye turning inward and (B) exotropia with the right eye turning outward.

The Eyelids

cilia (SIL-ee-ah) — **eyelashes**

sebaceous glands (see-BAY-shus)

A pair of eyelids over each eyeball provides protection from foreign particles, injury from the sun and intense light, and trauma (see Figure 13.1). Both the upper and lower edges of the eyelids have **eyelashes** or **cilia** that protect the eye from foreign particles. In addition, **sebaceous glands** located in the eyelids secrete lubricating oil onto the eyeball.

Conjunctiva

mucous membrane

The conjunctiva of the eye is a **mucous membrane** lining. It forms a continuous covering on the underside of each eyelid and across the anterior surface of each eyeball (see again Figure 13.1). This serves as protection for the eye by sealing off the eyeball in the socket.

Lacrimal Apparatus

lacrimal ducts

nasal cavity

tears

lacrimal gland

nasolacrimal duct (naz-oh-LAK-rim-al)

The **lacrimal gland** is located under the outer upper corner of each eyelid. These glands produce **tears.** Tears serve the important function of washing and lubricating the anterior surface of the eyeball. **Lacrimal ducts** located in the inner corner of the eye socket then collect the tears and drain them into the **nasolacrimal duct.** This duct ultimately drains the tears into the **nasal cavity** (see Figure 13.5 ■).

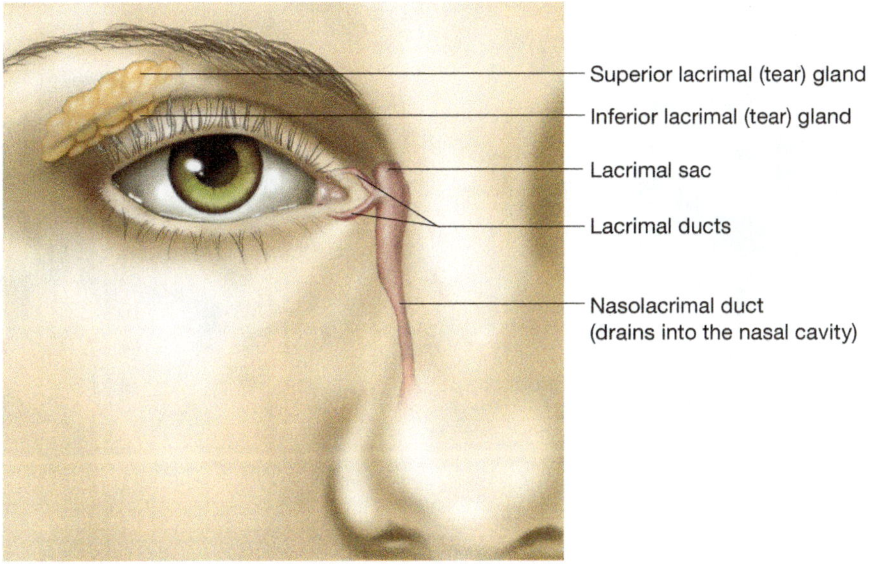

■ **Figure 13.5**
The structure of the lacrimal apparatus.

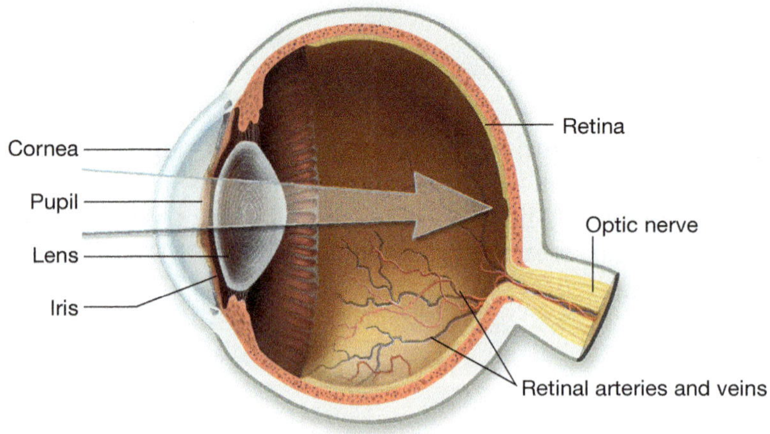

■ **Figure 13.6** The path of light through the cornea, iris, lens, and striking the retina.

How We See

When light rays strike the eye, they first pass through the cornea, pupil, aqueous humor, lens, and vitreous humor (see Figure 13.6 ■). They then strike the retina and stimulate the rods and cones. When the light rays hit the retina, an upside-down image is sent along nerve impulses to the optic nerve (see Figure 13.7 ■). The optic nerve transmits these impulses to the brain, where the upside-down image is translated into the right-side-up image we are looking at.

Vision requires proper functioning of four mechanisms:

1. Coordination of the external eye muscles so that both eyes move together.
2. The correct amount of light admitted by the pupil.
3. The correct focus of light on the retina by the lens.
4. The optic nerve transmitting sensory images to the brain.

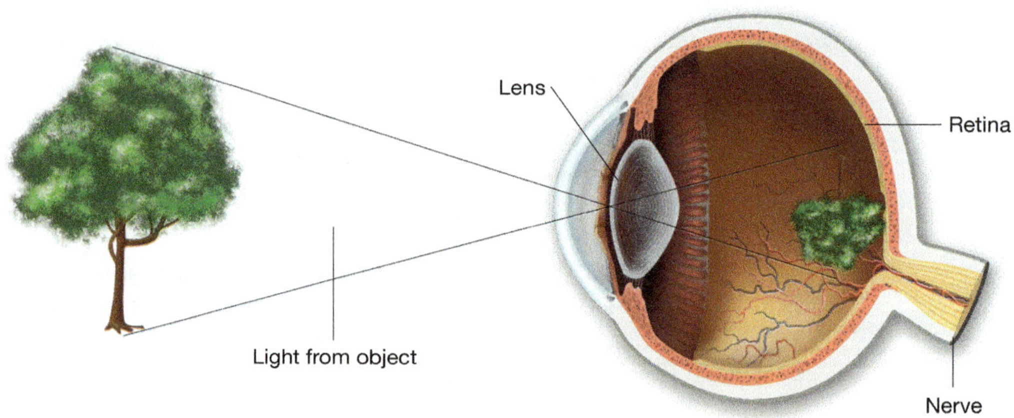

■ **Figure 13.7** The image formed on the retina is inverted. The brain rights the image as part of the interpretation process.

Terminology

Word Parts Used to Build Eye Terms

The following lists contain the combining forms, suffixes, and prefixes used to build terms in the remaining sections of this chapter.

Combining Forms

aden/o	gland
ambly/o	dull, dim
angi/o	vessel
aque/o	water
bi/o	life
blast/o	immature, embryonic
blephar/o	eyelid
chromat/o	color
conjuctiv/o	conjunctiva
corne/o	cornea
cry/o	cold
cycl/o	ciliary body
cyst/o	sac
dacry/o	tears
dipl/o	double
emmetr/o	correct, proper
esthes/o	sensation, feeling
glauc/o	gray
ir/o	iris
irid/o	iris
kerat/o	cornea
lacrim/o	tears
macul/o	macula lutea
mi/o	lessening
myc/o	fungus
mydr/i	widening
nyctal/o	night
ocul/o	eye
ophthalm/o	eye
opt/o	eye, vision
optic/o	eye, vision
papill/o	optic disc
phac/o	lens
phot/o	light
presby/o	old age
pupill/o	pupil
retin/o	retina
scler/o	sclera
stigmat/o	point
ton/o	tone
uve/o	choroid
vitre/o	glassy
xer/o	dry

Suffixes

-al	pertaining to
-algia	pain
-ar	pertaining to
-ary	pertaining to
-atic	pertaining to
-ectomy	surgical removal
-edema	swelling
-graphy	process of recording
-ia	condition
-ic	pertaining to
-ician	specialist
-ism	state of
-itis	inflammation
-logist	one who studies
-logy	study of
-malacia	softening
-meter	instrument to measure
-metrist	specialist in measuring
-metry	process of measuring
-oma	tumor
-opia	vision condition
-opsia	vision condition
-osis	abnormal condition
-otomy	cutting into
-ous	pertaining to
-pathy	disease
-pexy	surgical fixation
-phobia	fear
-plasty	surgical repair
-plegia	paralysis
-ptosis	drooping
-rrhagia	abnormal flow condition
-scope	instrument for viewing
-scopy	process of visually examining
-tic	pertaining to
-tropia	turned condition

Prefixes

a-	without
an-	without
anti-	against
de-	without
eso-	inward

exo-	outward
extra-	outside of
hemi-	half
hyper-	excessive

intra-	within
micro-	small
mono-	one
myo-	to shut

Anatomical Terms

TERM	WORD PARTS	DEFINITION
aqueous (AK-wee-us)	aque/o = water -ous = pertaining to	Pertaining to water or being water-like.
conjunctival (kon-JUNK-tih-vall)	conjuctiv/o = conjunctiva -al = pertaining to	Pertaining to the conjunctiva.
corneal (KOR-nee-all)	corne/o = cornea -al = pertaining to	Pertaining to the cornea. **MED TERM TIP** Word Watch: Be careful using the combining forms *core/o* meaning "pupil" and *corne/o* meaning "cornea."
extraocular (EKS-truh-OK-yoo-lar)	extra- = outside of ocul/o = eye -ar = pertaining to	Pertaining to being outside the eyeball; for example, the extraocular eye muscles.
iridal (ir-id-al)	irid/o = iris -al = pertaining to	Pertaining to the iris.
lacrimal (LAK-rim-al)	lacrim/o = tears -al = pertaining to	Pertaining to tears.
macular (MACK-uoo-lar)	macul/o = macula lutea -ar = pertaining to	Pertaining to the macula lutea.
ocular (OCK-yoo-lar)	ocul/o = eye -ar = pertaining to	Pertaining to the eye.
intraocular (in-trah-OCK-yoo-lar)	intra- = within ocul/o = eye -ar = pertaining to	Pertaining to within the eye.
ophthalmic (off-THAL-mik)	ophthalm/o = eye -ic = pertaining to	Pertaining to the eye.
optic (OP-tik)	opt/o = eye, vision -ic = pertaining to	Pertaining to the eye or vision.
optical (OP-tih-kal)	optic/o = eye, vision -al = pertaining to	Pertaining to the eye or vision.
pupillary (PYOO-pih-lair-ee)	pupill/o = pupil -ary = pertaining to	Pertaining to the pupil.
retinal (RET-in-al)	retin/o = retina -al = pertaining to	Pertaining to the retina.
scleral (SKLAIR-all)	scler/o = sclera -al = pertaining to	Pertaining to the sclera.
uveal (YOO-vee-al)	uve/o = choroid -al = pertaining to	Pertaining to the choroid layer of the eye.
vitreous (VIT-ree-us)	vitre/o = glass -ous = pertaining to	Pertaining to the vitreous humor.

Pathology

TERM	WORD PARTS	DEFINITION
Medical Specialties		
ophthalmologist (opf-thal-MOLL-oh-jist)	ophthalm/o = eye -logist = one who studies	Medical doctor who has specialized in the diagnosis and treatment of eye conditions and diseases.
ophthalmology (opf-thal-MOLL-oh-jee)	ophthalm/o = eye -logy = study of	Branch of medicine involving the diagnosis and treatment of conditions and diseases of the eye and surrounding structures.
optician (op-TISH-an)	opt/o = vision -ician = specialist	Person trained in grinding and fitting corrective lenses.
optometrist (op-TOM-eh-trist)	opt/o = vision -metrist = specialist in measuring	Doctor of optometry.
optometry (op-TOM-eh-tree)	opt/o = vision -metry = process of measuring	Medical profession specializing in examining the eyes, testing visual acuity, and prescribing corrective lenses.
Signs and Symptoms		
blepharoptosis (blef-ah-rop-TOH-sis)	blephar/o = eyelid -ptosis = drooping	Drooping eyelid.
cycloplegia (sigh-kloh-PLEE-jee-ah)	cycl/o = ciliary body -plegia = paralysis	Paralysis of the ciliary body. This affects changing the shape of the lens to bring images into focus.
diplopia (dip-LOH-pee-ah)	dipl/o = double -opia = vision condition	Condition of seeing double.
emmetropia (EM) (em-eh-TROH-pee-ah)	emmetr/o = correct, proper -opia = vision condition	State of normal vision.
iridoplegia (ir-id-oh-PLEE-jee-ah)	irid/o = iris -plegia = paralysis	Paralysis of the iris. This affects changing the size of the pupil to regulate the amount of light entering the eye.
nyctalopia (nik-tah-LOH-pee-ah)	nyctal/o = night -opia = vision condition	Difficulty seeing in dim light; also called *night blindness.* Usually due to damaged rods. **MED TERM TIP** The simple translation of *nyctalopia* is "night vision." However, it is used to mean "night blindness."
ophthalmalgia (off-thal-MAL-jee-ah)	ophthalm/o = eye -algia = pain	Eye pain.
ophthalmoplegia (off-thal-moh-PLEE-jee-ah)	ophthalm/o = eye -plegia = paralysis	Paralysis of one or more of the extraocular eye muscles.
ophthalmorrhagia (off-thal-moh-RAH-jee-ah)	ophthalm/o = eye -rrhagia = abnormal flow condition	Bleeding from the eye.
papilledema (pah-pill-eh-DEEM-ah)	papill/o = optic disc -edema = swelling	Swelling of the optic disk. Often as a result of increased intraocular pressure. Also called *choked disk.*

Pathology *(continued)*

TERM	WORD PARTS	DEFINITION
photophobia (foh-toh-FOH-bee-ah)	phot/o = light -phobia = fear	Although the term translates into *fear of light,* it actually means a strong sensitivity to bright light.
presbyopia (prez-bee-OH-pee-ah)	presby/o = old age -opia = vision condition	Visual loss due to old age, resulting in difficulty in focusing for near vision (such as reading).
scleromalacia (sklair-oh-mah-LAY-she-ah)	scler/o = sclera -malacia = softening	Softening of the sclera.
xerophthalmia (zee-ROP-thal-mee-ah)	xer/o = dry ophthalm/o = eye -ia = condition	Dry eyes.
Eyeball		
achromatopsia (ah-kroh-mah-TOP-see-ah)	a- = without chromat/o = color -opsia = vision condition	Condition of color blindness—unable to perceive one or more colors; more common in males.
amblyopia (am-blee-OH-pee-ah)	ambly/o = dull, dim -opia = vision condition	Loss of vision not as a result of eye pathology. Usually occurs in patients who see two images. In order to see only one image, the brain will no longer recognize the image being sent to it by one of the eyes. May occur if strabismus is not corrected. This condition is not treatable with a prescription lens. Commonly referred to as *lazy eye.*
astigmatism (Astigm) (ah-STIG-mah-tizm)	a- = without stigmat/o = point -ism = state of	Condition in which light rays are focused unevenly on the retina, causing a distorted image, due to an abnormal curvature of the cornea.
cataract (KAT-ah-rakt)		Damage to the lens causing it to become opaque or cloudy, resulting in diminished vision. Treatment is usually surgical removal of the cataract or replacement of the lens.
corneal abrasion	corne/o = cornea -al = pertaining to	Scraping injury to the cornea. If it does not heal, it may develop into an ulcer.
glaucoma (glau-KOH-mah)	glauc/o = gray -oma = mass	Increase in intraocular pressure, which, if untreated, may result in atrophy (wasting away) of the optic nerve and blindness. Glaucoma is treated with medication and surgery. There is an increased risk of developing glaucoma in persons over age 60, of African ancestry, who have sustained a serious eye injury, and in anyone with a family history of diabetes or glaucoma.

MED TERM TIP

The term *cataract* comes from the Latin word meaning "waterfall." This refers to how a person with a cataract sees the world—as if looking through a waterfall.

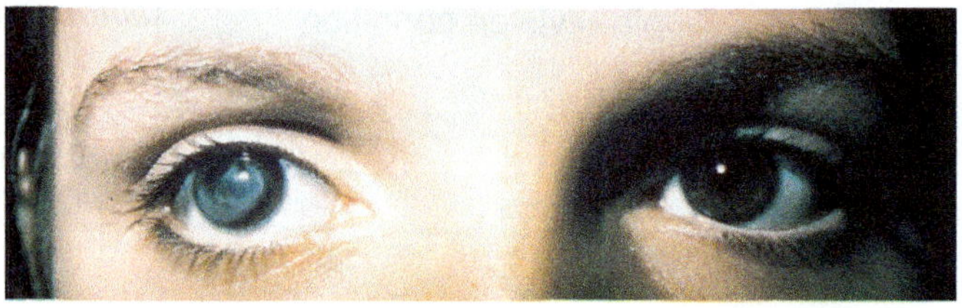

Figure 13.8 Photograph of a person with a cataract in the right eye.

Pathology (continued)

TERM	WORD PARTS	DEFINITION
hyperopia (high-per-OH-pee-ah)	hyper- = excessive -opia = vision condition	With this condition a person can see things in the distance but has trouble reading material at close range. Also known as *farsightedness*. This condition is corrected with converging or biconvex lenses.

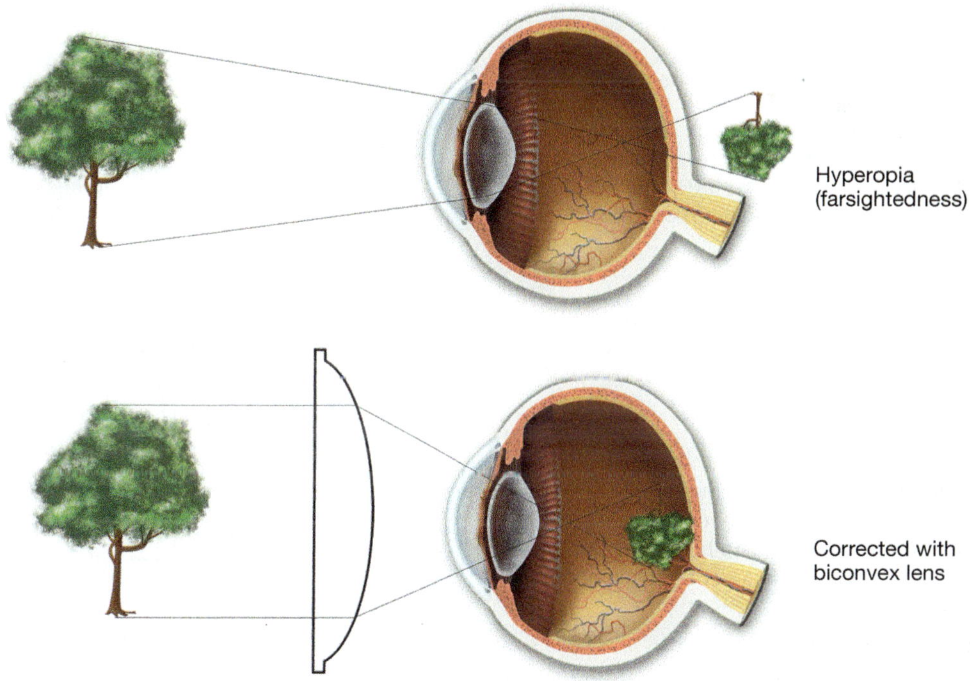

■ **Figure 13.9** Hyperopia (farsightedness). In the uncorrected top figure, the image would come into focus behind the retina, making the image on the retina blurry. The bottom image shows how a biconvex lens corrects this condition.

TERM	WORD PARTS	DEFINITION
iritis (eye-RYE-tis)	ir/o = iris -itis = inflammation	Inflammation of the iris.
keratitis (kair-ah-TYE-tis)	kerat/o = cornea -itis = inflammation	Inflammation of the cornea. **MED TERM TIP** Word Watch: Be careful using the combining form *kerat/o*, which means both "cornea" and "hard protein keratin."
legally blind		Describes a person who has severely impaired vision. Usually defined as having visual acuity of 20/200 that cannot be improved with corrective lenses or having a visual field of less than 20 degrees.
macular degeneration (MAK-yoo-lar)	macul/o = macula lutea -ar = pertaining to	Deterioration of the macular area of the retina of the eye. May be treated with laser surgery to destroy the blood vessels beneath the macula.
monochromatism (mon-oh-KROH-mah-tizm)	mono- = one chromat/o = color -ism = state of	Unable to perceive one color.

Pathology *(continued)*

TERM	WORD PARTS	DEFINITION
myopia (MY) (my-OH-pee-ah)	myo- = to shut -opia = vision condition	With this condition a person can see things close up but distance vision is blurred. Also known as *nearsightedness*. This condition is corrected with diverging or biconcave lenses. Named because persons with myopia often partially shut their eyes, squint, in order to see better.

MED TERM TIP

The term myopia appears to use the combining form, my/o, which means muscle. This combining form comes from the greek word *mys*. But in this case therm uses the prefix myo-, which comes from the Greek word *myo* or *myein,* meaning to shut.

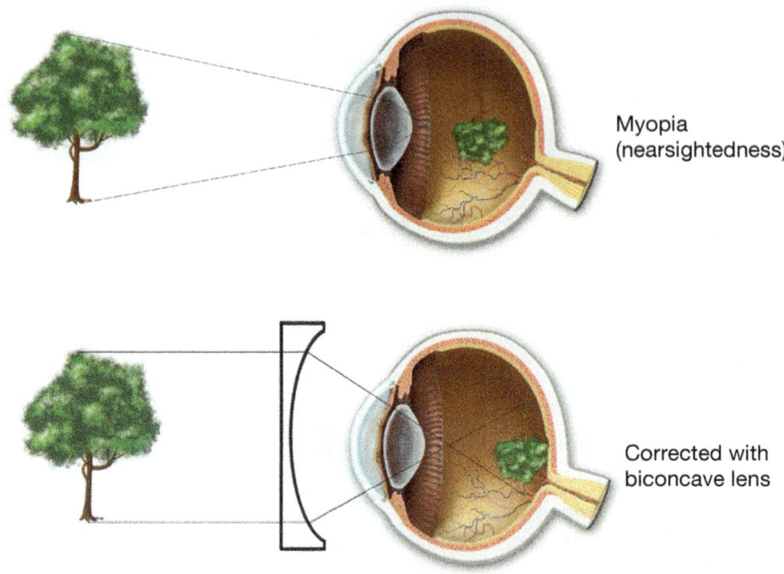

Figure 13.10 Myopia (nearsightedness). In the uncorrected top figure, the image comes into focus in front of the lens, making the image on the retina blurry. The bottom image shows how a biconcave lens corrects this condition.

TERM	WORD PARTS	DEFINITION
oculomycosis (ok-yoo-loh-my-KOH-sis)	ocul/o = eye myc/o = fungus -osis = abnormal condition	Fungus infection of the eye.
retinal detachment (RET-in-al)	retin/o = retina -al = pertaining to	Occurs when the retina becomes separated from the choroid layer. This separation seriously damages blood vessels and nerves, resulting in blindness. May be treated with surgical or medical procedures to stabilize the retina and prevent separation.
retinitis pigmentosa (ret-in-EYE-tis / pig-men-TOH-sah)	retin/o = retina -itis = inflammation	Progressive disease of the eye resulting in the retina becoming hard (sclerosed), pigmented (colored), and atrophying (wasting away). There is no known cure for this condition.
retinoblastoma (RET-in-noh-blast-OH-mah)	retin/o = retina blast/o = immature, embryonic -oma = tumor	Malignant eye tumor occurring in children, usually under the age of 3. Requires enucleation.
retinopathy (ret-in-OP-ah-thee)	retin/o = retina -pathy = disease	General term for disease affecting the retina.
scleritis (skler-EYE-tis)	scler/o = sclera -itis = inflammation	Inflammation of the sclera.

Pathology *(continued)*

TERM	WORD PARTS	DEFINITION
uveitis (yoo-vee-EYE-tis)	uve/o = choroid -itis = inflammation	Inflammation of the choroid layer.
Conjunctiva		
conjunctivitis (kon-junk-tih-VYE-tis)	conjuctiv/o = conjunctiva -itis = inflammation	Inflammation of the conjunctiva usually as the result of a bacterial infection. Commonly called pinkeye.
pterygium (the-RIJ-ee-um)		Hypertrophied conjunctival tissue in the inner corner of the eye.
Eyelids		
blepharitis (blef-ah-RYE-tis)	blephar/o = eyelid -itis = inflammation	Inflammation of the eyelid.
hordeolum (hor-DEE-oh-lum)		Refers to a *stye* (or *sty*), a small purulent inflammatory infection of a sebaceous gland of the eyelid; treated with hot compresses and/or surgical incision.
Lacrimal Apparatus		
dacryoadenitis (dak-ree-oh-ad-eh-NYE-tis)	dacry/o = tears aden/o = gland -itis = inflammation	Inflammation of the lacrimal gland.
dacryocystitis (dak-ree-oh-sis-TYE-tis)	dacry/o = tears cyst/o = sac -itis = inflammation	Inflammation of the lacrimal sac.
Eye Muscles		
esotropia (ST) (ess-oh-TROH-pee-ah)	eso- = inward -tropia = turned condition	Inward turning of the eye; also called *cross-eyed.* An example of a form of strabismus (muscle weakness of the eye).
exotropia (XT) (eks-oh-TROH-pee-ah)	exo- = outward -tropia = turned condition	Outward turning of the eye; also called *wall-eyed.* Also an example of strabismus (muscle weakness of the eye).
strabismus (strah-BIZ-mus)		Eye muscle weakness commonly seen in children resulting in the eyes looking in different directions at the same time. May be corrected with glasses, eye exercises, and/or surgery.
Brain-Related Vision Pathologies		
hemianopia (hem-ee-ah-NOP-ee-ah)	hemi- = half a- = without -opia = vision condition	Loss of vision in half of the visual field. A stroke patient may suffer from this disorder.
nystagmus (niss-TAG-mus)		Jerky-appearing involuntary eye movements, usually left and right. Often an indication of brain injury.

Diagnostic Procedures

TERM	WORD PARTS	DEFINITION
Eye Examination Tests		
color vision tests		Use of polychromic (multicolored) charts to determine the ability of the patient to recognize color.
fluorescein angiography (floo-oh-RESS-ee-in / an-jee-OG-rah-fee)	angi/o = vessel -graphy = process of recording	Process of injecting a dye (fluorescein) to observe the movement of blood and detect lesions in the macular area of the retina. Used to determine if there is a detachment of the retina.
fluorescein staining (floo-oh-RESS-ee-in)		Applying dye eye drops that are a bright green fluorescent color. Used to look for corneal abrasions or ulcers.
keratometer (KAIR-ah-toh-mee-ter)	kerat/o = cornea -meter = instrument to measure	An instrument used to measure the curvature of the cornea.
keratometry (kair-ah-TOM-eh-tree)	kerat/o = cornea -metry = process of measuring	Measurement of the curvature of the cornea using an instrument called a *keratometer.*
ophthalmoscope (off-THAL-moh-scope)	ophthalm/o = eye -scope = instrument for viewing	Instrument used to examine the inside of the eye through the pupil.
ophthalmoscopy (off-thal-MOSS-koh-pee)	ophthalm/o = eye -scopy = process of visually examining	Examination of the interior of the eyes using an instrument called an *ophthalmoscope* (see Figure 13.12 ■). The physician dilates the pupil in order to see the cornea, lens, and retina. Used to identify abnormalities in the blood vessels of the eye and some systemic diseases.

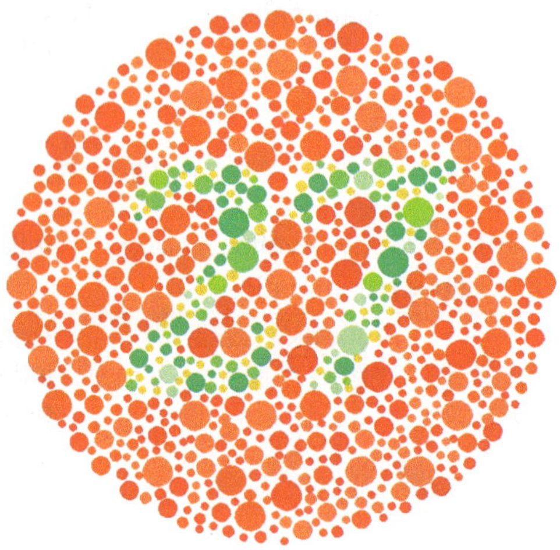

■ **Figure 13.11** An example of color blindness test. A person with red-green color blindness would not be able to distinguish the green 27 from the surrounding red circles.

Diagnostic Procedures *(continued)*

TERM	WORD PARTS	DEFINITION
optometer (op-TOM-eh-ter)	opt/o = vision -meter = instrument to measure	Instrument used to measure how well the eye is able to focus images clearly on the retina.
refractive error test (ree-FRAK-tiv)		Vision test for a defect in the ability of the eye to accurately focus the image that is hitting it. Refractive errors result in myopia and hyperopia.
slit lamp microscopy	micro- = small -scopy = process of visually examining	Examining the conjunctiva, cornea, iris and lens of the eye.
Snellen chart (SNEL-enz)		Chart used for testing distance vision named for Dutch ophthalmologist Hermann Snellen. It contains letters of varying size and is administered from a distance of 20 feet. A person who can read at 20 feet what the average person can read at this distance is said to have 20/20 vision.
tonometry (tohn-OM-eh-tree)	ton/o = tone -metry = process of measuring	Measurement of the intraocular pressure of the eye using a *tonometer* to check for the condition of glaucoma. Generally part of a normal eye exam for adults.
visual acuity (VA) **test** (VIZH-oo-al / ah-KYOO-ih-tee)	-al = pertaining to	Measurement of the sharpness of a patient's vision. Usually, a Snellen chart is used for this test in which the patient identifies letters from a distance of 20 feet.

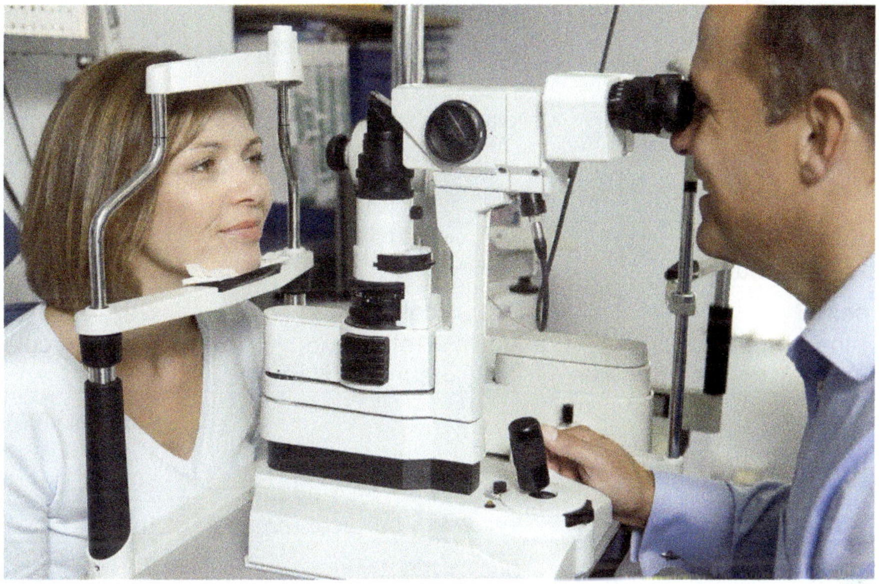

■ **Figure 13.12** Examination of the interior of the eye using an ophthalmoscope. *(Monkey Business Images/Shutterstock)*

Therapeutic Procedures

TERMS	WORD PARTS	DEFINITION
Surgical Procedures		
blepharectomy (blef-ah-REK-toh-mee)	blephar/o = eyelid -ectomy = surgical removal	Surgical removal of all or part of the eyelid.
blepharoplasty (BLEF-ah-roh-plass-tee)	blephar/o = eyelid -plasty = surgical repair	Surgical repair of the eyelid. A common plastic surgery to correct blepharoptosis.
conjunctivoplasty (kon-junk-tih-VOH-plas-tee)	conjuctiv/o = conjunctiva -plasty = surgical repair	Surgical repair of the conjunctiva.
cryoextraction (cry-oh-eks-TRAK-shun)	cry/o = cold	Procedure in which cataract is lifted from the lens with an extremely cold probe.
cryoretinopexy (cry-oh-RET-ih-noh-pek-see)	cry/o = cold retin/o = retina -pexy = surgical fixation	Surgical fixation of the retina by using extreme cold.
enucleation (ee-new-klee-AH-shun)		Surgical removal of an eyeball.
iridectomy (ir-id-EK-toh-mee)	irid/o = iris -ectomy = surgical removal	Surgical removal of a small portion of the iris.
iridosclerotomy (ir-ih-doh-skleh-ROT-oh-mee)	irid/o = iris scler/o = sclera -otomy = cutting into	To cut into the iris and sclera.
keratoplasty (KAIR-ah-toh-plass-tee)	kerat/o = cornea -plasty = surgical repair	Surgical repair of the cornea is the simple translation of this term that is utilized to mean corneal transplant.
laser-assisted insitu keratomileusis (LASIK) (in-SIH-tyoo / kair-ah-toh-mih-LOO-sis)	kerat/o = cornea	Correction of myopia using laser surgery to remove corneal tissue.

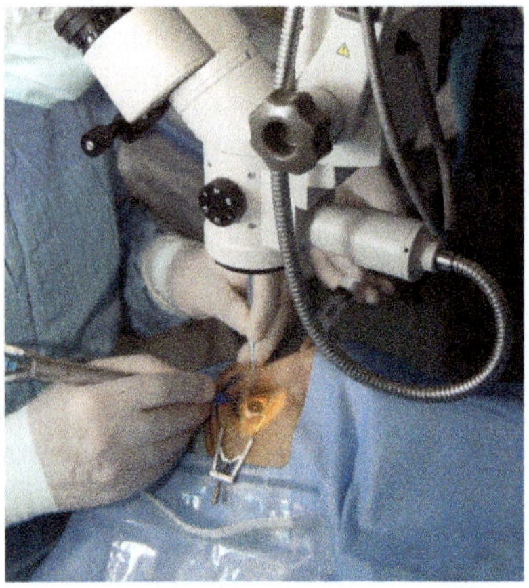

Figure 13.13 LASIK surgery uses a laser to reshape the cornea. *(mehmetcan/Shutterstock)*

TERMS	WORD PARTS	DEFINITION
laser photocoagulation (LAY-zer / foh-toh-koh-ag-yoo-LAY-shun)	phot/o = light	Use of a laser beam to destroy very small precise areas of the retina. May be used to treat retinal detachment or macular degeneration.
phacoemulsification (fak-oh-ee-mull-sih-fih-KAY-shun)	phac/o = lens	Use of high-frequency sound waves to emulsify (liquefy) a lens with a cataract, which is then aspirated (removed by suction) with a needle.
photorefractive keratectomy (PRK) (foh-toh-ree-FRAK-tiv / kair-ah-TEK-toh-mee)	phot/o = light kerat/o = cornea -ectomy = surgical removal	Use of a laser to reshape the cornea and correct errors of refraction.
prosthetic lens implant (pros-THET-ik)		Use of an artificial lens to replace the lens removed during cataract surgery.

Therapeutic Procedures *(continued)*

TERMS	WORD PARTS	DEFINITION
radial keratotomy (RK) (RAY-dee-all / kair-ah-TOT-oh-mee)	-al = pertaining to kerat/o = cornea -otomy = cutting into	Spokelike incisions around the cornea that result in it becoming flatter. A surgical treatment for myopia.
retinopexy (ret-ih-noh-PEX-ee)	retin/o = retina -pexy = surgical fixation	Surgical fixation of the retina. One treatment for a detaching retina.
scleral buckling (SKLAIR-al)	scler/o = sclera -al = pertaining to	Placing a band of silicone around the outside of the sclera that stabilizes a detaching retina.
sclerotomy (skleh-ROT-oh-mee)	scler/o = sclera -otomy = cutting into	To cut into the sclera.
strabotomy (strah-BOT-oh-mee)	-otomy = cutting into	Incision into the eye muscles in order to correct strabismus.

Pharmacology

CLASSIFICATION	WORD PARTS	ACTION	EXAMPLES
anesthetic ophthalmic solution (off-THAL-mik)	an- = without esthes/o = sensation, feeling -ic = pertaining to ophthalm/o = eye -ic = pertaining to	Eye drops for pain relief associated with eye infections, corneal abrasions, or surgery.	proparacain, Ak-Taine, Ocu-Caine; tetracaine, Opticaine, Pontocaine
antibiotic ophthalmic solution (off-THAL-mik)	anti- = against bi/o = life -ic = pertaining to ophthalm/o = eye -ic = pertaining to	Eye drops for the treatment of bacterial eye infections.	erythromycin, Del-Mycin, Ilotycin Ophthalmic
antiglaucoma medications (an-tye-glau-KOH-mah)	anti- = against glauc/o = gray -oma = mass	Group of drugs that reduce intraocular pressure by lowering the amount of aqueous humor in the eyeball. May achieve this by either reducing the production of aqueous humor or increasing its outflow.	timolol, Betimol, Timoptic; acetazolamide, Ak-Zol, Dazamide; prostaglandin analogs, Lumigan, Xalatan
artificial tears		Medications, many of them over the counter, to treat dry eyes.	buffered isotonic solutions, Akwa Tears, Refresh Plus, Moisture Eyes
miotic drops (my-OT-ik)	mi/o = lessening -tic = pertaining to	Any substance that causes the pupil to constrict. These medications may also be used to treat glaucoma.	physostigmine, Eserine Sulfate, Isopto Eserine; carbachol, Carbastat, Miostat
mydriatic drops (mid-ree-AT-ik)	mydr/i = widening -atic = pertaining to	Any substance that causes the pupil to dilate by paralyzing the iris and/or ciliary body muscles. Particularly useful during eye examinations and eye surgery.	atropine sulfate, Atropine-Care Ophthalmic, Atropisol Ophthalmic
ophthalmic decongestants	ophthalm/o = eye -ic = pertaining to de- = without	Over-the-counter medications that constrict the arterioles of the eye and reduce redness and itching of the conjunctiva.	tetrahydrozoline, Visine, Murine

Abbreviations

ARMD	age-related macular degeneration
Astigm	astigmatism
c.gl.	correction with glasses
D	diopter (lens strength)
DVA	distance visual acuity
ECCE	extracapsular cataract extraction
EENT	eye, ear, nose, and throat
EM	emmetropia
EOM	extraocular movement
ICCE	intracapsular cataract extraction
IOP	intraocular pressure
LASIK	laser-assisted insitu keratomileusis
OD	right eye
Ophth.	ophthalmology
OS	left eye
OU	each eye/both eyes
PERRLA	pupils equal, round, react to light and accommodation
PRK	photorefractive keratectomy
REM	rapid eye movement
s.gl.	without correction or glasses
SMD	senile macular degeneration
ST	esotropia
VA	visual acuity
VF	visual field
XT	exotropia

MED TERM TIP

The abbreviations for right eye (OD) and left eye (OS) are easy to remember when we know their origins. OD stands for *oculus* (eye) *dexter* (right). OS has its origin in *oculus* (eye) *sinister* (left). At one time in history it was considered to be sinister if a person looked at another from only the left side. Hence the term *oculus sinister* (OS) means left eye.

Section II: The Ear at a Glance

Function

The ear contains the sensory receptors for hearing and equilibrium (balance).

Structures

Here are the primary structures that comprise the ear.

auricle
external ear
inner ear
middle ear

Word Parts

Here are the most common word parts (with their meanings) used to build ear terms. For a more comprehensive list, refer to the Terminology section of this chapter.

Combining Forms

Combining Form	Meaning
acous/o	hearing
audi/o	hearing
audit/o	hearing
aur/o	ear
auricul/o	ear
cerumin/o	cerumen
cochle/o	cochlea
labyrinth/o	labyrinth (inner ear)
myring/o	tympanic membrane (eardrum)
ot/o	ear
salping/o	auditory tube (eustachian tube)
staped/o	stapes
tympan/o	tympanic membrane (eardrum)

Suffixes

Suffix	Meaning
-cusis	hearing
-otia	ear condition

The Ear Illustrated

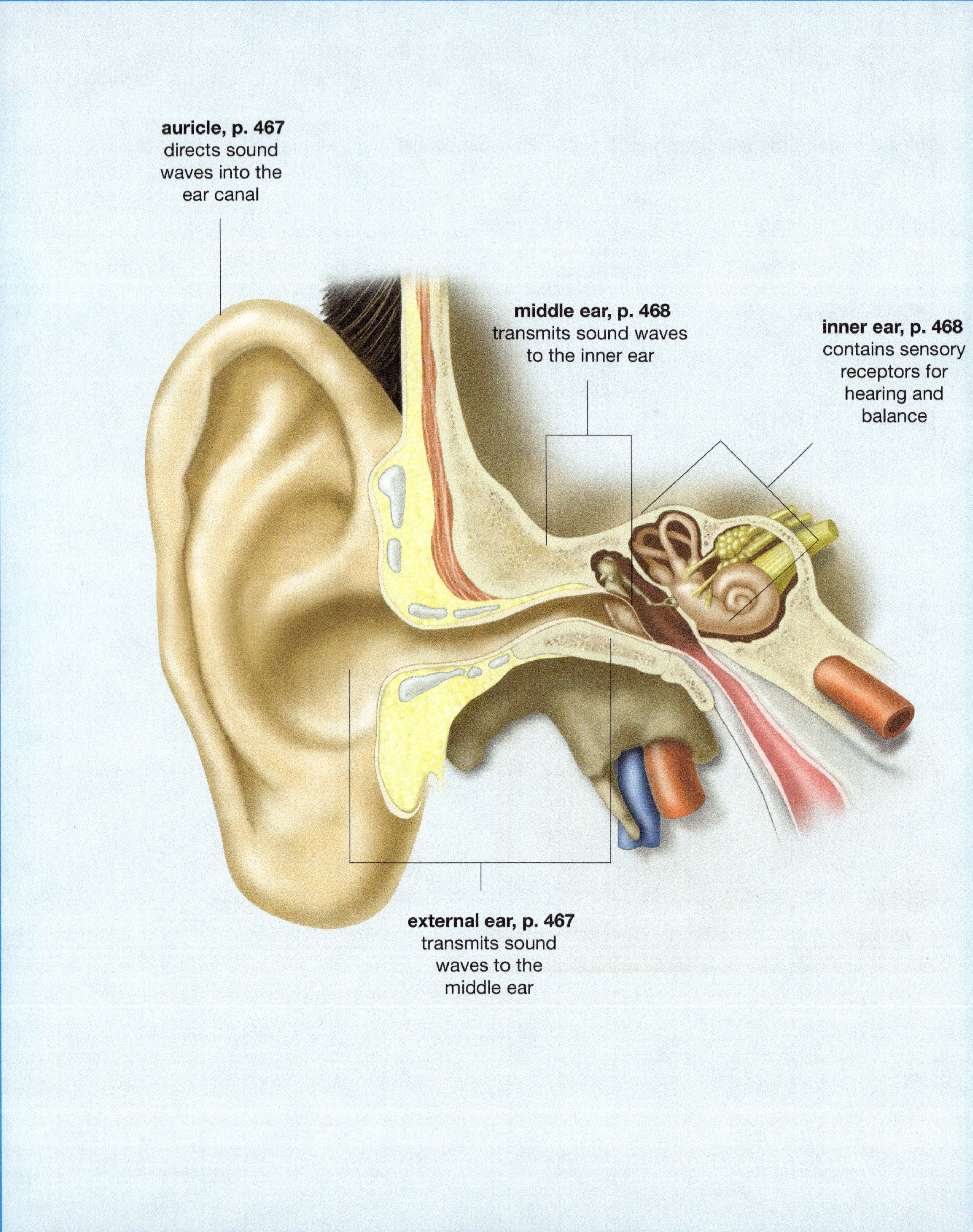

Anatomy and Physiology of the Ear

audiology (aw-dee-OL-oh-jee)
cochlear nerve (KOK-lee-ar)
equilibrium (ee-kwih-LIB-ree-um)
external ear
hearing
inner ear
middle ear
otology (oh-TOL-oh-jee)
vestibular nerve (ves-TIB-yoo-lar)
vestibulocochlear nerve (ves-tib-yoo-loh-KOK-lee-ar)

The study of the ear is referred to as **otology** (Oto), and the study of hearing disorders is called **audiology.** While there is a large amount of overlap between these two areas, there are also examples of ear problems that do not affect hearing. The ear is responsible for two senses: **hearing** and **equilibrium,** or our sense of balance. Hearing and equilibrium sensory information is carried to the brain by cranial nerve VIII, the **vestibulocochlear nerve.** This nerve is divided into two major branches. The **cochlear nerve** carries hearing information, and the **vestibular nerve** carries equilibrium information.

The ear is subdivided into three areas: **external ear, middle ear,** and **inner ear.**

External Ear

auditory canal (AW-dih-tor ee)
auricle (AW-rih-k'l)
cerumen (seh-ROO-men)
external auditory meatus (AW-dih-tor-ee / me-A-tus)
pinna (PIN-ah)
tympanic membrane (tim-PAN-ik)

The external ear consists of three parts: the **auricle,** the **auditory canal,** and the **tympanic membrane** (see Figure 13.14 ■). The auricle or **pinna** is what is commonly referred to as the *ear* because this is the only visible portion. The auricle with its

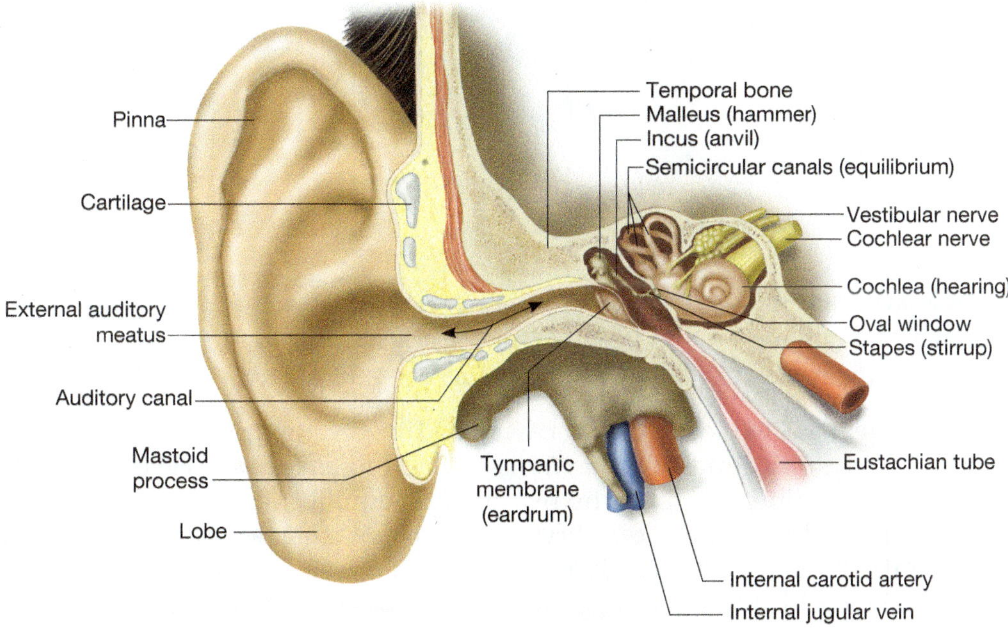

■ **Figure 13.14** The internal structures of the outer, middle, and inner ear.

earlobe has a unique shape in each person and functions like a funnel to capture sound waves as they go past the outer ear and channel them through the **external auditory meatus.** The sound then moves along the auditory canal and causes the tympanic membrane (eardrum) to vibrate. The tympanic membrane actually separates the external ear from the middle ear. Earwax or **cerumen** is produced in oil glands in the auditory canal. This wax helps to protect and lubricate the ear. It is also just barely liquid at body temperature. This causes cerumen to slowly flow out of the auditory canal, carrying dirt and dust with it. Therefore, the auditory canal is self-cleaning.

MED TERM TIP

The term *tympanic membrane* comes from the Greek word for "drumhead." The tympanic membrane or eardrum vibrates to sound waves like a drum head.

Middle Ear

auditory tube (AW-dih-tor-ee)
eustachian tube (yoo-STAY-she-en)
incus (ING-kus)
malleus (MAL-ee-us)
ossicles (OSS-ih-kls)
oval window
stapes (STAY-peez)

The middle ear is located in a small cavity in the temporal bone of the skull. This air-filled cavity contains three tiny bones called **ossicles** (see Figure 13.15 ■). These three bones, the **malleus, incus,** and **stapes,** are vital to the hearing process. They amplify the vibrations in the middle ear and transmit them to the inner ear from the malleus to the incus and finally to the stapes. The stapes, the last of the three ossicles, is attached to a very thin membrane that covers the opening to the inner ear called the **oval window.**

The **eustachian tube** or **auditory tube** connects the nasopharynx with the middle ear (see Figure 13.14). Each time you swallow the eustachian tube opens. This connection allows pressure to equalize between the middle ear cavity and the atmospheric pressure.

MED TERM TIP

The three bones in the middle ear are referred to by terms that are similar to their shape. Thus, the malleus is called the hammer, the incus is the anvil, and the stapes is the stirrup (see Figure 13.15).

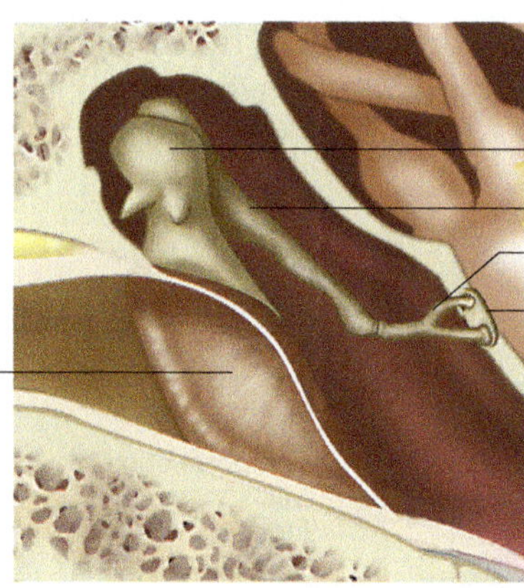

■ **Figure 13.15** Closeup view of the ossicles within the middle ear. These three bones extend from the tympanic membrane to the oval window.

Inner Ear

cochlea (KOK-lee-ah)
labyrinth (LAB-ih-rinth)
organs of Corti (KOR-tee)
saccule (SAK-yool)
semicircular canals
utricle (YOO-trih-k'l)

The inner ear is also located in a cavity within the temporal bone (see again Figure 13.14). This fluid-filled cavity is referred to as the **labyrinth** because of its shape. The labyrinth contains the hearing and equilibrium sensory organs: the **cochlea** for hearing and the **semicircular canals, utricle,** and **saccule** for equilibrium. Each of these organs contains hair cells, which are the actual sensory receptor cells. In the cochlea, the hair cells are referred to as **organs of Corti.**

MED TERM TIP

Frequently, children will twirl in circles and fall or stumble from dizziness when they stop. This is caused from a temporary imbalance in the inner ear.

How We Hear

conductive hearing loss (kon-DUK-tiv)
sensorineural hearing loss (sen-soh-ree-NOO-ral)

Figure 13.16 ■ outlines the path of sound through the outer ear and middle ear and into the cochlea of the inner ear. Sound waves traveling down the external auditory canal strike the eardrum, causing it to vibrate. The ossicles conduct these vibrations across the middle ear from the eardrum to the oval window. Oval window movements initiate vibrations in the fluid that fills the cochlea. As the fluid vibrations strike a hair cell, they bend the small hairs and stimulate the nerve ending. The nerve ending then sends an electrical impulse to the brain on the cochlear portion of the vestibulocochlear nerve.

Hearing loss can be divided into two main categories: **conductive hearing loss** and **sensorineural hearing loss.** Conductive refers to disease or malformation of the outer or middle ear. All sound is weaker and muffled in conductive hearing loss since it is not conducted correctly to the inner ear. Sensorineural hearing loss is the result of damage or malformation of the inner ear (cochlea) or the cochlear nerve. In this hearing loss, some sounds are distorted and heard incorrectly. There can also be a combination of both conductive and sensorineural hearing loss.

MED TERM TIP

Hearing impairment is becoming a greater problem for the general population for several reasons. First, people are living longer. Hearing loss can accompany old age, and there are a greater number of people over 50 years of age requiring hearing assistance. In addition, sound technology has produced music quality that was never available before. However, listening to loud music either naturally or through earphones can cause gradual damage to the hearing mechanism.

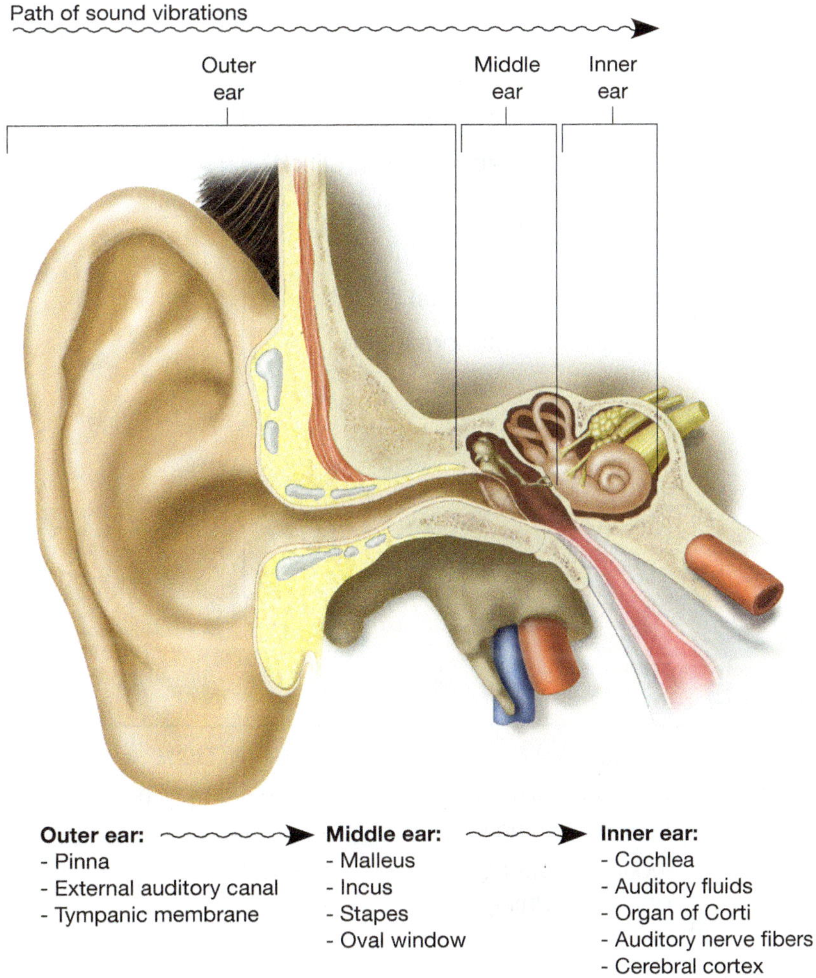

■ **Figure 13.16** The path of sound waves through the outer, middle, and inner ear.

Terminology

Word Parts Used to Build Ear Terms

The following lists contain the combining forms, suffixes, and prefixes used to build terms in the remaining sections of this chapter.

Combining Forms

acous/o	hearing
audi/o	hearing
audit/o	hearing
aur/o	ear
auricul/o	ear
bi/o	life
cerumin/o	cerumen

cochle/o	cochlea
labyrinth/o	labyrinth
laryng/o	larynx
myc/o	fungus
myring/o	tympanic membrane
neur/o	nerve
ot/o	ear

presby/o	old age
py/o	pus
rhin/o	nose
salping/o	auditory tube
staped/o	stapes
tympan/o	tympanic membrane

Suffixes

-al	pertaining to
-algia	pain
-ar	pertaining to
-cusis	hearing
-ectomy	pertaining to
-emesis	vomiting
-gram	record
-ic	pertaining to
-itis	inflammation
-logy	study of

-meter	instrument to measure
-metry	process of measuring
-oma	mass, tumor
-ory	pertaining to
-osis	abnormal condition
-otia	ear condition
-otomy	cutting into
-plasty	surgical repair
-rrhagia	abnormal flow

-rrhea	discharge
-rrhexis	rupture
-sclerosis	hardening
-scope	instrument to visually examine
-scopy	process of visually examining
-tic	pertaining to

Prefixes

an- = without
anti- = against

bi- = two
macro- = large

micro- = small
mono- = one

Anatomical Terms

TERM	WORD PARTS	DEFINITION
acoustic (ah-KOOS-tik)	acous/o = hearing -tic = pertaining to	Pertaining to hearing.
auditory (AW-dih-tor-ee)	audit/o = hearing -ory = pertaining to	Pertaining to hearing.

Anatomical Terms *(continued)*

TERM	WORD PARTS	DEFINITION
aural (AW-ral)	aur/o = ear -al = pertaining to	Pertaining to the ear. **MED TERM TIP** Word Watch: Be careful when using two terms that sound the same—*aural* meaning "pertaining to the ear" and *oral* meaning "pertaining to the mouth."
auricular (aw-RIK-cu-lar)	auricul/o = ear -ar = pertaining to	Pertaining to the ear.
binaural (bin-AW-rall)	bi- = two aur/o = ear -al = pertaining to	Pertaining to both ears.
cochlear (KOK-lee-ar)	cochle/o = cochlea -ar = pertaining to	Pertaining to the cochlea.
monaural (mon-AW-rall)	mono- = one aur/o = ear -al = pertaining to	Pertaining to one ear.
otic (OH-tik)	ot/o = ear -ic = pertaining to	Pertaining to the ear.
tympanic (tim-PAN-ik)	tympan/o = tympanic membrane -ic = pertaining to	Pertaining to the tympanic membrane.

Pathology

TERM	WORD PARTS	DEFINITION
Medical Specialties		
audiology (aw-dee-OL-oh-jee)	audi/o = hearing -logy = study of	Medical specialty involved with measuring hearing function and identifying hearing loss. Specialist is an *audiologist.*
otorhinolaryngology (ENT) (oh-toh-rye-noh-lair-in-GOL-oh-jee)	ot/o = ear rhin/o = nose laryng/o = larynx -logy = study of	Branch of medicine involving the diagnosis and treatment of conditions and diseases of the ear, nose, and throat. Also referred to as *ENT.* Physician is an *otorhinolaryngologist.*
Signs and Symptoms		
macrotia (mah-KROH-she-ah)	macro- = large -otia = ear condition	Condition of having abnormally large ears.
microtia (my-KROH-she-ah)	micro- = small -otia = ear condition	Condition of having abnormally small ears.
otalgia (oh-TAL-jee-ah)	ot/o = ear -algia = pain	Ear pain.
otopyorrhea (oh-toh-pye-oh-REE-ah)	ot/o = ear py/o = pus -rrhea = discharge	Discharge of pus from the ear.
otorrhagia (oh-toh-RAH-jee-ah)	ot/o = ear -rrhagia = abnormal flow	Bleeding from the ear.

Pathology (continued)

TERM	WORD PARTS	DEFINITION
presbycusis (pres-bih-KOO-sis)	presby/o = old age -cusis = hearing condition	Normal loss of hearing that can accompany the aging process.
residual hearing (rih-ZID-yoo-al)	-al = pertaining to	Amount of hearing that is still present after damage has occurred to the auditory mechanism.
tinnitus (tin-EYE-tus)		Ringing in the ears.
tympanorrhexis (tim-pan-oh-REK-sis)	tympan/o = tympanic membrane -rrhexis = rupture	Rupture of the tympanic membrane.
vertigo (VER-tih-goh)		Dizziness caused by the sensation that the room is spinning.
Hearing Loss		
anacusis (an-ah-KOO-sis)	an- = without -cusis = hearing	Total absence of hearing; inability to perceive sound. Also called *deafness.*
deafness		Inability to hear or having some degree of hearing impairment.
External Ear		
ceruminoma (seh-roo-men-oh-ma)	cerumin/o = cerumen -oma = mass	Excessive accumulation of earwax resulting in a hard wax plug. Sound becomes muffled.
otitis externa (OE) (oh-TYE-tis / ex-TERN-ah)	ot/o = ear -itis = inflammation	External ear infection. May be caused by bacteria or fungus. Also called *otomycosis* and commonly referred to as *swimmer's ear.*
otomycosis (oh-toh-my-KOH-sis)	ot/o = ear myc/o = fungus -osis = abnormal condition	Fungal infection of the ear. One type of otitis externa.
Middle Ear		
myringitis (mir-ing-JYE-tis)	myring/o = tympanic membrane -itis = inflammation	Inflammation of the tympanic membrane.
otitis media (OM) (oh-TYE-tis / MEE-dee-ah)	ot/o = ear -itis = inflammation	Seen frequently in children; commonly referred to as a *middle ear infection.* Often preceded by an upper respiratory infection during which pathogens move from the pharynx to the middle ear via the eustachian tube. Fluid accumulates in the middle ear cavity. The fluid may be watery, *serous otitis media,* or full of pus, *purulent otitis media.*
otosclerosis (oh-toh-sklair-OH-sis)	ot/o = ear -sclerosis = hardening	Loss of mobility of the stapes bone, leading to progressive hearing loss.
salpingitis (sal-pin-JIH-tis)	salping/o = auditory tube -itis = inflammation	Inflammation of the auditory tube. **MED TERM TIP** Word Watch: Be careful using the combining form *salping/o,* which can mean either "Eustachian tube" or "fallopian tube."
tympanitis (tim-pan-EYE-tis)	tympan/o = tympanic membrane -itis = inflammation	Inflammation of the tympanic membrane.

Pathology *(continued)*

TERM	WORD PARTS	DEFINITION
Inner Ear		
acoustic neuroma (ah-KOOS-tik / noor-OH-mah)	acous/o = hearing -tic = pertaining to neur/o = nerve -oma = tumor	Benign tumor of the eighth cranial nerve sheath. The pressure causes symptoms such as tinnitus, headache, dizziness, and progressive hearing loss.
labyrinthitis (lab-ih-rin-THIGH-tis)	labyrinth/o = labyrinth -itis = inflammation	May affect both the hearing and equilibrium portions of the inner ear. Also referred to as an *inner ear infection.*
Ménière's disease (may-nee-ARZ)		Abnormal condition within the labyrinth of the inner ear that can lead to a progressive loss of hearing. The symptoms are dizziness or vertigo, hearing loss, and tinnitus (ringing in the ears). Named for French physician Prosper Ménière.

Diagnostic Procedures

TERM	WORD PARTS	DEFINITION
Audiology Tests		
audiogram (AW-dee-oh-gram)	audi/o = hearing -gram = record	Graphic record that illustrates the results of audiometry.
audiometer (aw-dee-OM-eh-ter)	audi/o = hearing -meter = instrument to measure	Instrument to measure hearing.
audiometry (aw-dee-OM-eh-tree)	audi/o = hearing -metry = process of measuring	Test of hearing ability by determining the lowest and highest intensity (decibels) and frequencies (hertz) that a person can distinguish. The patient may sit in a sound-proof booth and receive sounds through earphones as the technician decreases the sound or lowers the tones.

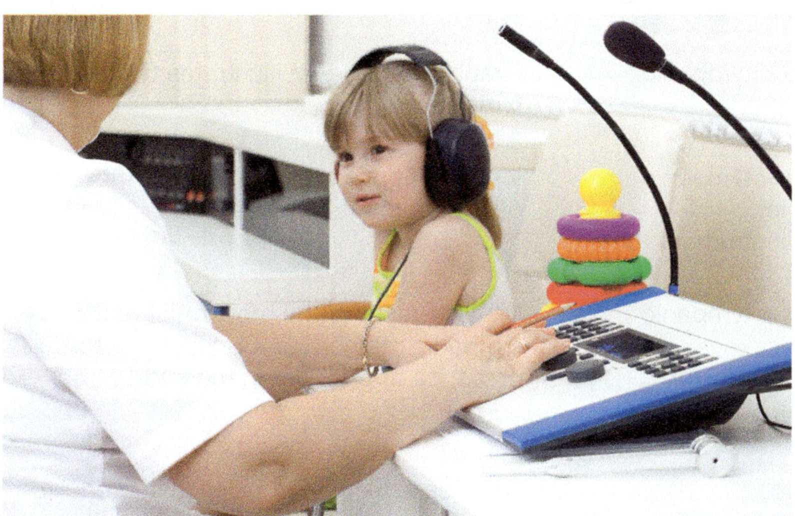

Figure 13.17 Audiometry exam being administered to a young child who is wearing the ear phones through which sounds are given. *(Capifrutta/Shutterstock)*

TERM	WORD PARTS	DEFINITION
decibel (dB) (DES-ih-bel)		Measures the intensity or loudness of a sound. Zero decibels is the quietest sound measured and 120 dB is the loudest sound commonly measured.

Diagnostic Procedures *(continued)*

TERM	WORD PARTS	DEFINITION
hertz (Hz)		Measurement of the frequency or pitch of sound. The lowest pitch on an audiogram is 250 Hz. The measurement can go as high as 8000 Hz, which is the highest pitch measured.
Rinne and Weber tuning-fork tests (RIN-eh)		Tests that assess both nerve and bone conduction of sound. The physician holds a tuning fork, an instrument that produces a constant pitch when it is struck, against or near the bones on the side of the head.
Otology Tests		
otoscope (OH-toh-scope)	ot/o = ear -scope = instrument to visually examine	Instrument to view inside the ear canal.
otoscopy (oh-TOSS-koh-pee)	ot/o = ear -scopy = process of visually examining	Examination of the ear canal, eardrum, and outer ear using an *otoscope*.

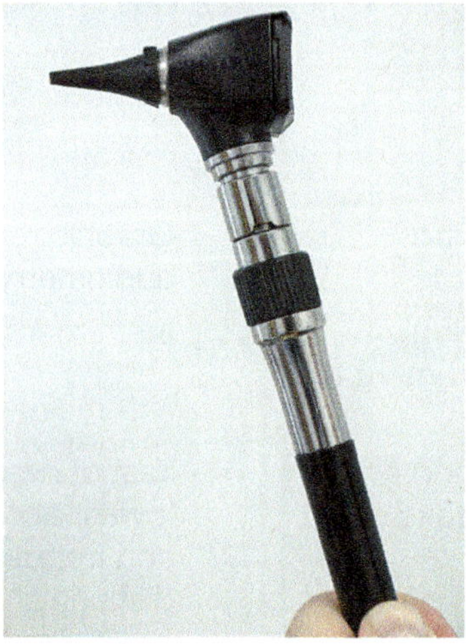

■ **Figure 13.18** An otoscope, used to visually examine the external auditory ear canal and tympanic membrane.

MED TERM TIP

Small children are prone to placing objects in their ears. In some cases, as with peas and beans, these become moist in the ear canal and swell, which makes removal difficult. *Otoscopy,* or the examination of the ear using an *otoscope,* can aid in identifying and removing the cause of hearing loss if it is due to foreign bodies.

TERM	WORD PARTS	DEFINITION
tympanogram (TIM-pah-no-gram)	tympan/o = tympanic membrane -gram = record	Graphic record that illustrates the results of tympanometry.
tympanometer (tim-pah-NOM-eh-ter)	tympan/o = tympanic membrane -meter = instrument to measure	Instrument used to measure the movement of the tympanic membrane.
tympanometry (tim-pah-NOM-eh-tree)	tympan/o = tympanic membrane -metry = process of measuring	Measurement of the movement of the tympanic membrane. Can indicate the presence of pressure in the middle ear.
Balance Tests		
falling test		Test used to observe balance and equilibrium. The patient is observed balancing on one foot, then with one foot in front of the other, and then walking forward with eyes open. The same test is conducted with the patient's eyes closed. Swaying and falling with the eyes closed can indicate an ear and equilibrium malfunction.

Therapeutic Procedures

TERM	WORD PARTS	DEFINITION
Audiology Procedures		
American Sign Language (ASL)		Nonverbal method of communicating in which the hands and fingers are used to indicate words and concepts. Used by both persons who are deaf and persons with speech impairments.
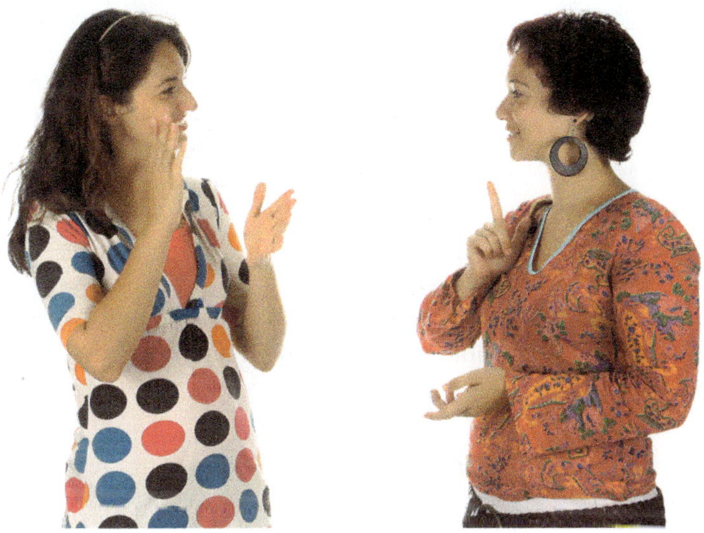		■ **Figure 13.19** Two women having a conversation using American Sign Language. *(Vladimir Mucibabic/ Shutterstock)*
hearing aid		Apparatus or mechanical device used by persons with impaired hearing to amplify sound. Also called an *amplification device.*
Surgical Procedures		
cochlear implant (KOK-lee-ar)	cochle/o = cochlea -ar = pertaining to	Mechanical device surgically placed under the skin behind the outer ear (pinna) that converts sound signals into magnetic impulses to stimulate the auditory nerve. Can be beneficial for those with profound sensorineural hearing loss.
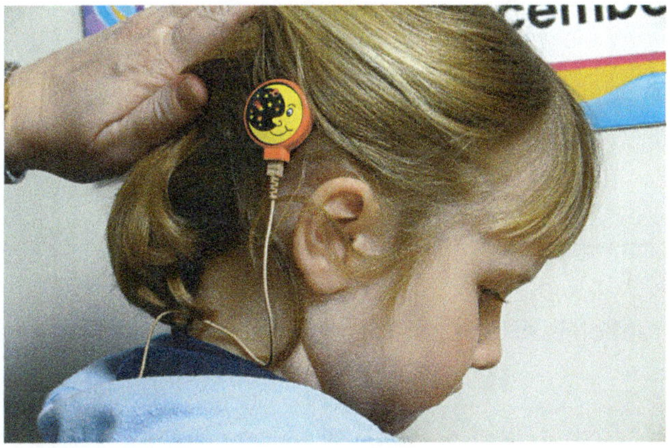		■ **Figure 13.20** Photograph of a child with a cochlear implant. This device sends electrical impulses directly to the brain.
labyrinthectomy (lab-ih-rin-THEK-toh-mee)	labyrinth/o = labyrinth -ectomy = surgical removal	Surgical removal of the labyrinth.
labyrinthotomy (lab-ih-rinth-OT-oh-mee)	labyrinth/o = labyrinth -otomy = cutting into	To cut into the labyrinth.
myringectomy (mir-in-GEK-toh-mee)	myring/o = tympanic membrane -ectomy = surgical removal	Surgical removal of the tympanic membrane.
myringoplasty (mir-IN-goh-plass-tee)	myring/o = tympanic membrane -plasty = surgical repair	Surgical repair of the tympanic membrane.

Therapeutic Procedures *(continued)*

TERM	WORD PARTS	DEFINITION
myringotomy (mir-in-GOT-oh-mee)	myring/o = tympanic membrane -otomy = cutting into	Surgical puncture of the eardrum with removal of fluid and pus from the middle ear to eliminate a persistent ear infection and excessive pressure on the tympanic membrane. A pressure equalizing tube is placed in the tympanic membrane to allow for drainage of the middle ear cavity; this tube typically falls out on its own.
otoplasty (OH-toh-plas-tee)	ot/o = ear -plasty = surgical repair	Surgical repair of the external ear.
pressure equalizing tube (PE tube)		Small tube surgically placed in a child's eardrum to assist in drainage of trapped fluid and to equalize pressure between the middle ear cavity and the atmosphere.
salpingotomy (sal-pin-GOT-oh-mee)	salping/o = auditory tube -otomy = cutting into	To cut into the auditory tube.
stapedectomy (stay-pee-DEK-toh-mee)	staped/o = stapes -ectomy = pertaining to	Removal of the stapes bone to treat otosclerosis (hardening of the bone). A prosthesis or artificial stapes may be implanted.
tympanectomy (tim-pan-EK-toh-mee)	tympan/o = tympanic membrane -ectomy = surgical removal	Surgical removal of the tympanic membrane.
tympanoplasty (tim-pan-oh-PLASS-tee)	tympan/o = tympanic membrane -plasty = surgical repair	Surgical repair of the tympanic membrane.
tympanotomy (tim-pan-OT-oh-mee)	tympan/o = tympanic membrane -otomy = cutting into	To cut into the tympanic membrane.

Pharmacology

CLASSIFICATION	WORD PARTS	ACTION	EXAMPLES
antibiotic otic solution (OH-tik)	anti- = against bi/o = life -tic = pertaining to ot/o = ear -ic = pertaining to	Eardrops to treat otitis externa.	Neomycin, polymyxin B and hydrocortisone solution, Otocort, Cortisporin, Otic Care
antiemetics (an-tye-ee-mit-tiks)	anti- = against -emesis = vomiting -tic = pertaining to	Medications effective in treating the nausea associated with vertigo.	meclizine, Antivert, Meni-D; prochlorperazine, Compazine
anti-inflammatory otic solution (OH-tik)	anti- = against -ory = pertaining to ot/o = ear -ic = pertaining to	Reduces inflammation, itching, and edema associated with otitis externa.	antipyrine and benzoaine, Allergan Ear Drops, A/B Otic
wax emulsifiers		Substances used to soften earwax to prevent buildup within the external ear canal.	carbamide peroxide, Debrox Drops, Murine Ear Drops

Abbreviations

AD	right ear	**HEENT**	head, ears, eyes, nose, throat
AS	left ear	**Hz**	hertz
ASL	American Sign Language	**OM**	otitis media
AU	both ears	**Oto**	otology
BC	bone conduction	**PE tube**	pressure equalizing tube
dB	decibel	**PORP**	partial ossicular replacement prosthesis
EENT	eyes, ears, nose, throat	**SOM**	serous otitis media
ENT	ear, nose, and throat	**TORP**	total ossicular replacement prosthesis

Chapter Review

Real-World Applications

Medical Record Analysis

This Ophthalmology Consultation Report contains 11 medical terms. Underline each term and write it in the list below the report. Then define each term.

Ophthalmology Consultation Report

Reason for Consultation:	Evaluation of progressive loss of vision in right eye.
History of Present Illness:	Patient is a 79-year-old female who has noted gradual deterioration of vision and increasing photophobia during the past year, particularly in the right eye. She states that it feels like there is a film over her right eye. She denies any change in vision in her left eye. Patient has used corrective lenses her entire adult life for hyperopia.
Results of Physical Examination:	Visual acuity test showed no change in this patient's long-standing hyperopia. The pupils react properly to light. Intraocular pressure is normal. Ophthalmoscopy after application of mydriatic drops revealed presence of large opaque cataract in lens of right eye. There is a very small cataract forming in the left eye. There is no evidence of retinopathy, macular degeneration, or keratitis.
Assessment:	Diminished vision in right eye secondary to cataract.
Recommendations:	Phacoemulsification of cataract followed by prosthetic lens implant.

	Term	Definition
1	________________	________________________________
2	________________	________________________________
3	________________	________________________________
4	________________	________________________________
5	________________	________________________________
6	________________	________________________________
7	________________	________________________________
8	________________	________________________________
9	________________	________________________________
10	________________	________________________________
11	________________	________________________________

Chart Note Transcription

The chart note below contains 10 phrases that can be reworded with a medical term that you learned in this chapter. Each phrase is identified with an underline. Determine the medical term and write your answers in the space provided.

Current Complaint:	An 8-year-old female was referred to the specialist in the treatment of diseases of the ear, nose, and throat ❶ by her pediatrician for evaluation of chronic left middle ear infection. ❷
Past History:	Patient's mother reports that her daughter began to experience recurrent ear infections at approximately 6 months of age. Frequency of the infections has increased during the past 2 years, and she is missing school. Mother also reports the child's teacher feels she is having difficulty hearing in the classroom.
Signs and Symptoms:	Both ears ❸ visual examination of the external ear canal and eardrum ❹ revealed that the membrane between the external ear canal and middle ear ❺ is normal on the right and bulging on the left. An excessive amount of earwax ❻ was noted in both ears. ❸ Measurement of the movement of the eardrum ❼ indicates that there is a buildup of fluid in the left middle ear. Tests of hearing ability ❽ report normal hearing on the right and loss of hearing as a result of the blocking of sound transmission in the middle ear ❾ on the left. Patient also noted to have acute pharyngitis with purulent drainage at time of evaluation.
Diagnosis:	Hearing loss secondary to chronic left middle ear infection.
Treatment:	Left eardrum incision ❿ with placement of pressure equalizing tube for drainage.

❶ ______________________________

❷ ______________________________

❸ ______________________________

❹ ______________________________

❺ ______________________________

❻ ______________________________

❼ ______________________________

❽ ______________________________

❾ ______________________________

❿ ______________________________

Case Study

Below is a case study presentation of a patient with a condition covered in this chapter. Read the case study and answer the questions below. Some questions will ask for information not included within this chapter. Use your text, a medical dictionary, or any other reference material you choose to answer these questions.

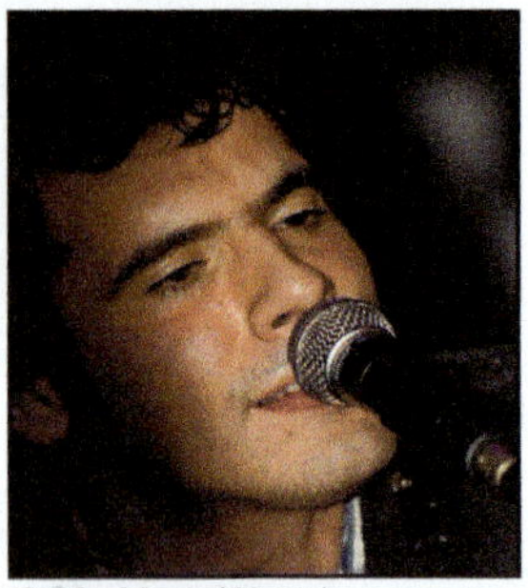

(© My-Music/Alamy)

This 35-year-old male musician was seen in the EENT clinic complaining of a progressive hearing loss over the past 15 years. He is now unable to hear what is being said if there is any environmental noise present. He states that he has played with a group of musicians using amplified instruments and no earplugs for the past 20 years. External ear structures appear normal bilaterally with otoscopy. Tympanometry is normal bilaterally. Audiometry reveals diminished hearing bilaterally. Rinne and Weber tuning-fork tests indicate that the patient has a moderate amount of conductive hearing loss but rule out sensorineural hearing loss. Diagnosis is moderate bilateral conductive hearing loss as a result of prolonged exposure to loud noise. Patient is referred for evaluation for a hearing aid.

1. Which type of hearing loss does this patient appear to have? Look this condition up in a reference source and include a short description of it.

____

____

2. Explain how the other type of hearing loss (the type ruled out by the Rinne and Weber tuning-fork tests) is different from what this patient has.

____

____

3. What diagnostic tests did the physician perform? Describe them in your own words.

____

____

4. Explain the difference between a hearing aid and a cochlear implant.

____

____

5. How do you think this patient could have avoided this hearing loss?

____

____

Practice Exercises

A. Complete the Statement

1. The study of the eye is ____________________.
2. Another term for eyelashes is ____________________.
3. The glands responsible for tears are called ____________________ glands.
4. The clear, transparent portion of the sclera is called the ____________________.
5. The innermost layer of the eye, which is composed of sensory receptors, is the ____________________.
6. The pupil of the eye is actually a hole in the ____________________.
7. The three bones in the middle ear are the ____________________, ____________________, and ____________________.
8. The study of the ear is called ____________________.
9. Another term for the eardrum is ____________________.
10. ____________________ is produced in the oil glands in the auditory canal.
11. The ____________________ tube connects the nasopharynx with the middle ear.
12. The ____________________ is responsible for conducting impulses from the ear to the brain.

B. Pharmacology Challenge

Fill in the classification for each drug description, then match the brand name.

	Drug Description	Classification	Brand Name
1.	_______ treats dry eyes	____________________	a. Atropine-Care
2.	_______ reduces intraocular pressure	____________________	b. Allergan Ear Drops
3.	_______ ear drops for ear infection	____________________	c. Timoptic
4.	_______ dilates pupil	____________________	d. Opticaine
5.	_______ treats nausea from vertigo	____________________	e. Debrox Drops
6.	_______ eye drops for bacterial infection	____________________	f. Eserine Sulfate
7.	_______ treats ear itching	____________________	g. Antivert
8.	_______ constricts pupil	____________________	h. Refresh Plus
9.	_______ softens cerumen	____________________	i. Otocort
10.	_______ eye drops for pain	____________________	j. Del-Mycin

C. Combining Form Practice

The combining form **blephar/o** refers to the eyelid. Use it to write a term that means:

1. inflammation of the eyelid ______________________
2. surgical repair of the eyelid ______________________
3. drooping of the upper eyelid ______________________

The combining form **retin/o** refers to the retina. Use it to write a term that means:

4. a disease of the retina ______________________
5. surgical fixation of the retina ______________________

The combining form **ophthalm/o** refers to the eye. Use it to write a term that means:

6. the study of the eye ______________________
7. pertaining to the eye ______________________
8. an eye examination using a scope ______________________

The combining form **irid/o** refers to the iris. Use it to write a term that means:

9. iris paralysis ______________________
10. removal of the iris ______________________

The combining form **ot/o** refers to the ear. Write a word that means:

11. ear surgical repair ______________________
12. pus flow from the ear ______________________
13. pain in the ear ______________________
14. inflammation of the ear ______________________

The combining form **tympan/o** refers to the eardrum. Write a word that means:

15. eardrum rupture ______________________
16. eardrum incision ______________________
17. eardrum inflammation ______________________

The combining form **audi/o** refers to hearing. Write a word that means:

18. record of hearing ______________________
19. instrument to measure hearing ______________________
20. study of hearing ______________________

D. Name That Suffix

	Suffix	Example from Chapter
1. to turn	______	______
2. vision	______	______
3. inflammation of	______	______
4. the study of	______	______
5. cutting into	______	______
6. surgical repair	______	______
7. surgical fixation	______	______
8. pain	______	______
9. ear condition	______	______
10. hearing	______	______

E. Define the Combining Form

	Definition	Example from Chapter
1. **dacry/o**	______	______
2. **uve/o**	______	______
3. **aque/o**	______	______
4. **phot/o**	______	______
5. **kerat/o**	______	______
6. **vitre/o**	______	______
7. **dipl/o**	______	______
8. **glauc/o**	______	______
9. **presby/o**	______	______
10. **ambly/o**	______	______
11. **aur/o**	______	______
12. **staped/o**	______	______
13. **acous/o**	______	______
14. **salping/o**	______	______
15. **myring/o**	______	______

F. Answer the Question

1. Describe the difference between conductive hearing loss and sensorineural hearing loss. ______________________

____

2. List in order the eyeball structures light rays pass through: ______________, ______________, ______________, ______________

3. Describe the role of the conjunctiva. ______________________

____

4. List the ossicles and what they do. ______________________

____

G. Terminology Matching

Match each term to its definition.

1.	________ emmetropia	a.	opacity of the lens
2.	________ sclera	b.	muscle regulating size of pupil
3.	________ cataract	c.	nearsightedness
4.	________ conjunctiva	d.	protective membrane of eye
5.	________ iris	e.	blind spot
6.	________ xerophthalmia	f.	involuntary movements of eye
7.	________ myopia	g.	white of eye
8.	________ nystagmus	h.	normal vision
9.	________ optic disk	i.	dry eyes
10.	________ vitreous humor	j.	material filling eyeball

H. What Does it Stand For?

1. Oto ______________________
2. OU ______________________
3. REM ______________________
4. Hz ______________________
5. SMD ______________________
6. PERRLA ______________________

7. IOP ____________________

8. dB ____________________

9. OD ____________________

10. VF ____________________

I. Terminology Matching

Match each term to its definition.

1.	________ myringotomy	a.	removal of stapes bone
2.	________ tympanoplasty	b.	reconstruction of eardrum
3.	________ otoplasty	c.	surgical puncture of eardrum
4.	________ stapedectomy	d.	change size of pinna
5.	________ anacusis	e.	absence of hearing
6.	________ falling test	f.	treats sensorineural hearing loss
7.	________ PE tube	g.	tuning fork tests
8.	________ cochlear implant	h.	swimmer's ear
9.	________ otitis externa	i.	drains off fluid
10.	________ Rinne & Weber	j.	balance test

J. What's the Abbreviation?

1. pressure equalizing tube ____________________

2. eye, ear, nose, and throat ____________________

3. bone conduction ____________________

4. both ears ____________________

5. otitis media ____________________

6. emmetropia ____________________

7. exotropia ____________________

8. left eye ____________________

9. extraocular movement ____________________

10. visual acuity ____________________

K. Fill in the Blank

emmetropia	tonometry	Ménière's disease
hyperopia	cataract	hordeolum
acoustic neuroma	strabismus	myopia
otorhinolaryngologist	presbycusis	
conjunctivitis	inner ear	

1. Cheri is having a regular eye checkup. The pressure reading test that the physician will do to detect glaucoma is ____________________.

2. Carlos's ophthalmologist tells him that he has normal vision. This is called ____________________.

3. Ana has been given an antibiotic eye ointment for pinkeye. The medical term for this condition is ____________________.

4. Adrian is nearsighted and cannot read signs in the distance. This is called ____________________.

5. Ivan is scheduled to have surgery to have the opaque lens of his right eye removed. This condition is a(n) ____________________.

6. Roberto has developed a stye on the corner of his left eye. He has been told to treat it with hot compresses. This condition is called a(n) ____________________.

7. Judith has twin boys with crossed eyes that will require surgical correction. The medical term for this condition is ____________________.

8. Beth is farsighted and has difficulty reading textbooks. Her eyeglass correction will be for ____________________.

9. Grace was told by her physician that her hearing loss was a part of the aging process. The term for this is ____________________.

10. Stacey is having frequent middle ear infections and wishes to be treated by a specialist. She would go to a(n) ____________________.

11. Warren was told that his dizziness may be caused by a problem in the ____________________ area.

12. Shantel is suffering from an abnormal condition of the inner ear, vertigo, and tinnitus. She may have ____________________.

13. Keisha was told that her tumor of the eighth cranial nerve was benign, but she still experienced a hearing loss as a result of the tumor. This tumor is called a(n) ____________________.

L. Define the Term

1. amblyopia ______________________________

2. diplopia ______________________________

3. mydriatic ______________________________

4. miotic ______________________________

5. presbyopia ______________________________

6. tinnitus ______________________________

7. stapes ______________________________

8. tympanometry ______________________________

9. eustachian tube ______________________________

10. labyrinth ______________________________

11. audiogram ______________________________

12. otitis media ______________________________

M. Research Project: High Risk Behavior

Teenagers (ages 12-18) are particularly prone to participating in high risk behaviors, often with little thought to the consequences of their actions. Most teens tend to discount their likelihood of experiencing negative life events. These high risk behaviors can include bullying, binge drinking, contact sports, substance abuse, or reckless driving.

Using medical journals and other professional publications, prepare a research report documenting high risk behaviors and resultant injuries, disabling conditions, or illness that may require rehabilitative services. Identify treatments, financial obligations, and the impact on the individual, family members, and society for the care and treatment required. Investigate current debates on how to discourage high risk behaviors and include your personal view on these debates.

Include medical terminology as appropriate when developing the report. Cite all sources accessed using conventional citation methods used in medical literature. Share your article with a peer. Provide feedback and suggestions to each other; then revise your document as necessary.

Labeling Exercise

Image A

Write the labels for this figure on the numbered lines provided.

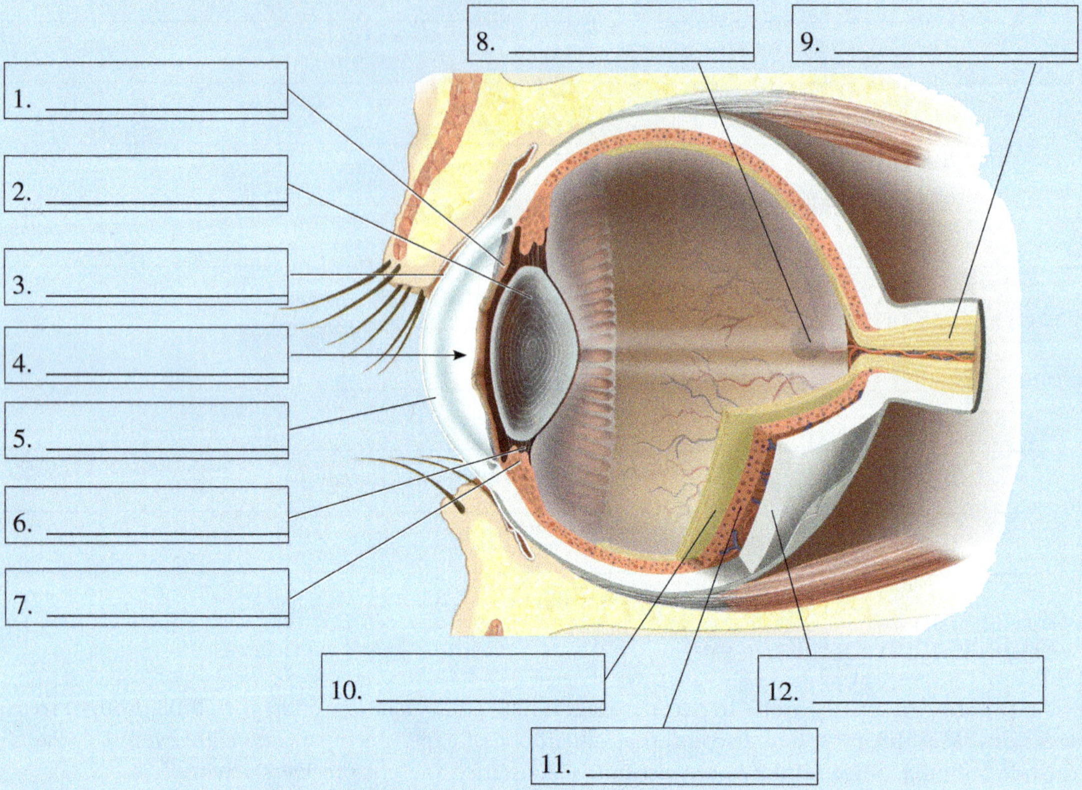

Image B

Write the labels for this figure on the numbered lines provided.

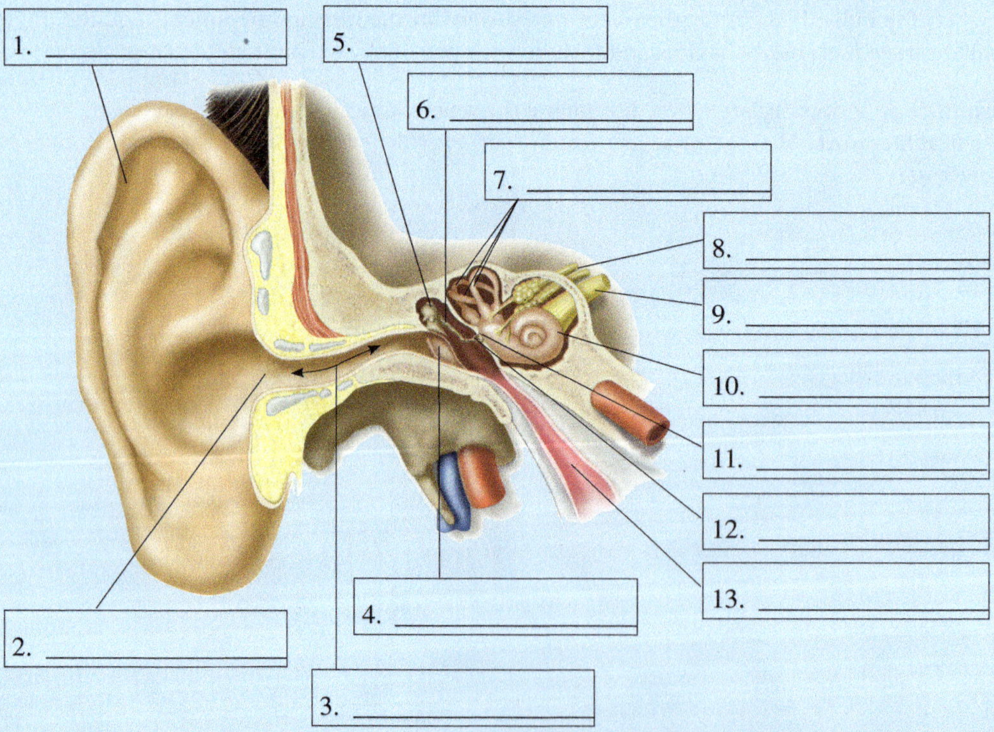

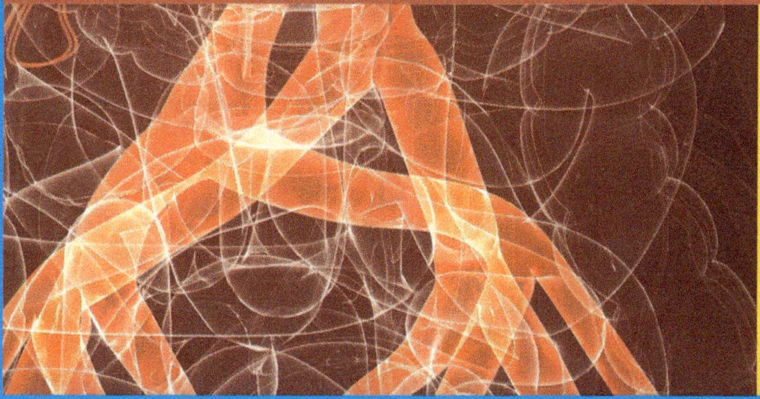

14

SPECIAL TOPICS

Learning Objectives

Upon completion of this chapter, you will be able to

- Identify and define the combining forms and suffixes introduced in this chapter.
- Correctly spell and pronounce medical terms relating to the medical fields introduced in this chapter.
- Describe pertinent information relating to pharmacology.
- Describe pertinent information relating to mental health.
- Describe pertinent information relating to diagnostic imaging.
- Describe pertinent information relating to rehabilitation services.
- Describe pertinent information relating to surgery.
- Describe pertinent information relating to oncology.
- Identify and define vocabulary terms relating to the topics.
- Identify and define selected pathology terms relating to the topics.
- Identify and define selected diagnostic procedures relating to the topics.
- Identify and define selected therapeutic procedures relating to the topics.
- Define selected abbreviations associated with the topics.

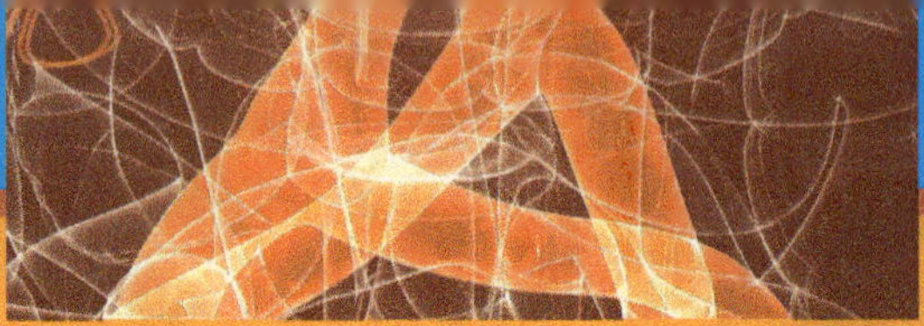

Introduction

There are many specialized areas within medicine, and each has medical terms relating to that field. This chapter presents medical terminology from six of these fields:

1. Pharmacology
2. Mental Health
3. Diagnostic Imaging
4. Rehabilitation Services
5. Surgery
6. Oncology

Section I: Pharmacology at a Glance

Word Parts

Here are the most common word parts (with their meanings) used to build pharmacy terms.

Combining Forms

aer/o	air	**muscul/o**	muscle
bucc/o	cheek	**or/o**	mouth
chem/o	drug	**pharmac/o**	drug
cutane/o	skin	**rect/o**	rectum
derm/o	skin	**thec/o**	sheath (meninges)
enter/o	intestine	**topic/o**	a specific area
hal/o	to breathe	**toxic/o**	poison
iatr/o	physician, medicine, treatment	**vagin/o**	vagina
		ven/o	vein
idi/o	distinctive		
lingu/o	tongue		

Suffixes

-al	pertaining to	**-ical**	pertaining to
-ary	pertaining to	**-ist**	specialist
-genic	produced by	**-logy**	study of
-ic	pertaining to	**-phylaxis**	protection

Prefixes

anti-	against	**para-**	near, beside
contra-	against	**pro-**	before
in-	inward	**sub-**	under
intra-	within	**trans-**	through

Pharmacology

pharmacology (far-ma-KALL-oh-jee)

Pharmacology is the study of the origin, characteristics, and effects of drugs. Drugs are obtained from many different sources. Some drugs, such as vitamins, are found naturally in the foods we eat. Others, such as hormones, are obtained from animals. Penicillin and some of the other antibiotics are developed from mold, which is a fungus. Plants have been the source of many of today's drugs. Many drugs, such as those used in chemotherapy, are synthetic, meaning they are developed by artificial means in a laboratory.

MED TERM TIP

The original Greek and Latin word roots are frequently used in pharmacology. Several most used prefixes used in pharmacology are:

Anti—against, ex., antidote, antibiotic

Hypo—under, ex., hypodermic (under the skin)

Drug Names

brand name
chemical name
generic name
nonproprietary name (non-prah-PRYE-ah-tair-ee)
pharmaceutical (far-mih-SOO-tih-kal)
pharmacist (FAR-mah-sist)
proprietary name (proh-PRYE-ah-tair-ee)
trademark

MED TERM TIP

The terms *drug* and *medication* have the same meaning. However, the general public often uses the term *drug* to refer to a narcotic type of medication. The term can also mean illegal chemical substances. For purposes of medical terminology, use of the word *drug* means medication.

All drugs are chemicals. The **chemical name** describes the chemical formula or molecular structure of a particular drug. For example, the chemical name for ibuprofen, an over-the-counter pain medication, is 2-*p*-isobutylphenyl propionic acid. Just as in this case, chemical names are usually very long, so a shorter name is given to the drug. This name is the **generic** or **nonproprietary name,** and it is recognized and accepted as the official name for a drug.

Each drug has only one generic name, such as ibuprofen, and this name is not subject to copyright protection, so any **pharmaceutical** manufacturer may use it. However, the pharmaceutical company that originally developed the drug has exclusive rights to produce it for 17 years. After that time, any manufacturer may produce and sell the drug. When a company manufactures a drug for sale, it must choose a **brand name,** or **proprietary name** for its product. This is the company's **trademark** for the drug. For example, ibuprofen is known by several brand names, including Motrin™, Advil™, and Nuprin™. All three contain the same ibuprofen; they are just marketed by different pharmaceutical companies. (See Table 14.1 ■ for examples of different drug names.)

Generic drugs are usually priced lower than brand name drugs. A physician can indicate on the prescription if the **pharmacist** may substitute a generic drug for a brand name. The physician may prefer that a particular brand name drug be used if he or she believes it to be more effective than the generic drug.

MED TERM TIP

Look for these word parts:

chem/o = drug
pharmac/o = drug
-al = pertaining to
-ary = pertaining to
-ic = pertaining to
-ical = pertaining to
-ist = specialist
-logy = study of

Table 14.1 Examples of Different Drug Names

CHEMICAL NAME	GENERIC NAME	BRAND NAMES
2-*p*-isobutylphenyl propionic acid	Ibuprofen	Motrin™
		Advil™
		Nuprin™
Acetylsalicylic acid	Aspirin	Anacin™
		Bufferin™
		Excedrin™
S-2-[1-(methylamino) ethyl] benzenemethanol hydrochloride	Pseudoephedrine hydrochloride	Sudafed™
		Actifed™
		Nucofed™

Legal Classification of Drugs

controlled substances
Drug Enforcement Agency
over-the-counter drug
prescription (prih-SKRIP-shun)
prescription drug (prih-SKRIP-shun)

A **prescription drug** can only be ordered by licensed healthcare practitioners such as physicians, dentists, or physician assistants. These drugs must include the words "Caution: Federal law prohibits dispensing without prescription" on their labels. Antibiotics, such as penicillin, and heart medications, such as digoxin, are available only by prescription. A **prescription** is the written explanation to the pharmacist regarding the name of the medication, the dosage, and the times of administration. A licensed practitioner can also give a prescription order orally to a pharmacist.

MED TERM TIP

It is critical that patients receive the correct drug, but it is not possible to list or remember all the drug names. You must acquire the habit of looking up any drug name you do not recognize in the *Physician's Desk Reference (PDR)*. Every medical office or medical facility should have a copy of this book.

A drug that does not require a prescription is referred to as an **over-the-counter** (OTC) **drug.** Many medications or drugs can be purchased without a prescription, for example, aspirin, antacids, and antidiarrheal medications. However, taking aspirin along with an anticoagulant, such as coumadin, can cause internal bleeding in some people, and OTC antacids interfere with the absorption of the prescription drug tetracycline into the body. It is better for the physician or pharmacist to advise the patient on the proper OTC drugs to use with prescription drugs.

Certain drugs are **controlled substances** if they have a potential for being addictive (habit forming) or can be abused. The **Drug Enforcement Agency** (DEA) enforces the control of these drugs. Some of the more commonly prescribed controlled substances are:

- butabarbital
- chloral hydrate
- codeine
- diazepam
- oxycontin
- morphine
- phenobarbital
- secobarbital

Controlled drugs are classified as Schedule I through Schedule V, indicating their potential for abuse. The differences between each schedule are listed in Table 14.2 ■.

Table 14.2 Schedule for Controlled Substances

CLASSIFICATION	MEANING
Schedule I	Drugs with the highest potential for addiction and abuse. They are not accepted for medical use. Examples are heroin and LSD.
Schedule II	Drugs with a high potential for addiction and abuse accepted for medical use in the United States. Examples are codeine, cocaine, morphine, opium, and secobarbital.
Schedule III	Drugs with a moderate to low potential for addiction and abuse. Examples are butabarbital, anabolic steroids, and acetaminophen with codeine.
Schedule IV	Drugs with a lower potential for addiction and abuse than Schedule III drugs. Examples are chloral hydrate, phenobarbital, and diazepam.
Schedule V	Drugs with a low potential for addiction and abuse. An example is low-strength codeine combined with other drugs to suppress coughing.

How to Read a Prescription

A prescription is not difficult to read once you understand the symbols that are used. Symbols and abbreviations based on Latin and Greek words are used to save time for the physician. For example, the abbreviation po, meaning to be taken by mouth, comes from the Latin term *per os,* which means "by mouth."

See Figure 14.1 ■ for an example of a prescription. In this example, the prescribed medication (Rx) is Tagamet (a medication to reduce stomach acid) in the 800 milligram (mg) size. The instructions on the label are to say (Sig) to take 1 ($\dot{\overline{\text{I}}}$) by mouth (po) every (q) bedtime (hs). The pharmacist is to dispense (disp) 30 tablets (#30). The prescription concludes by informing the pharmacist to refill the prescription two times, and he or she may substitute with another medication. Each prescription must contain the date, physician's name, address, and Drug Enforcement Agency number as well as the patient's name and date of birth. The physician must also sign his or her name at the bottom of the prescription. A blank prescription cannot be handed to a patient.

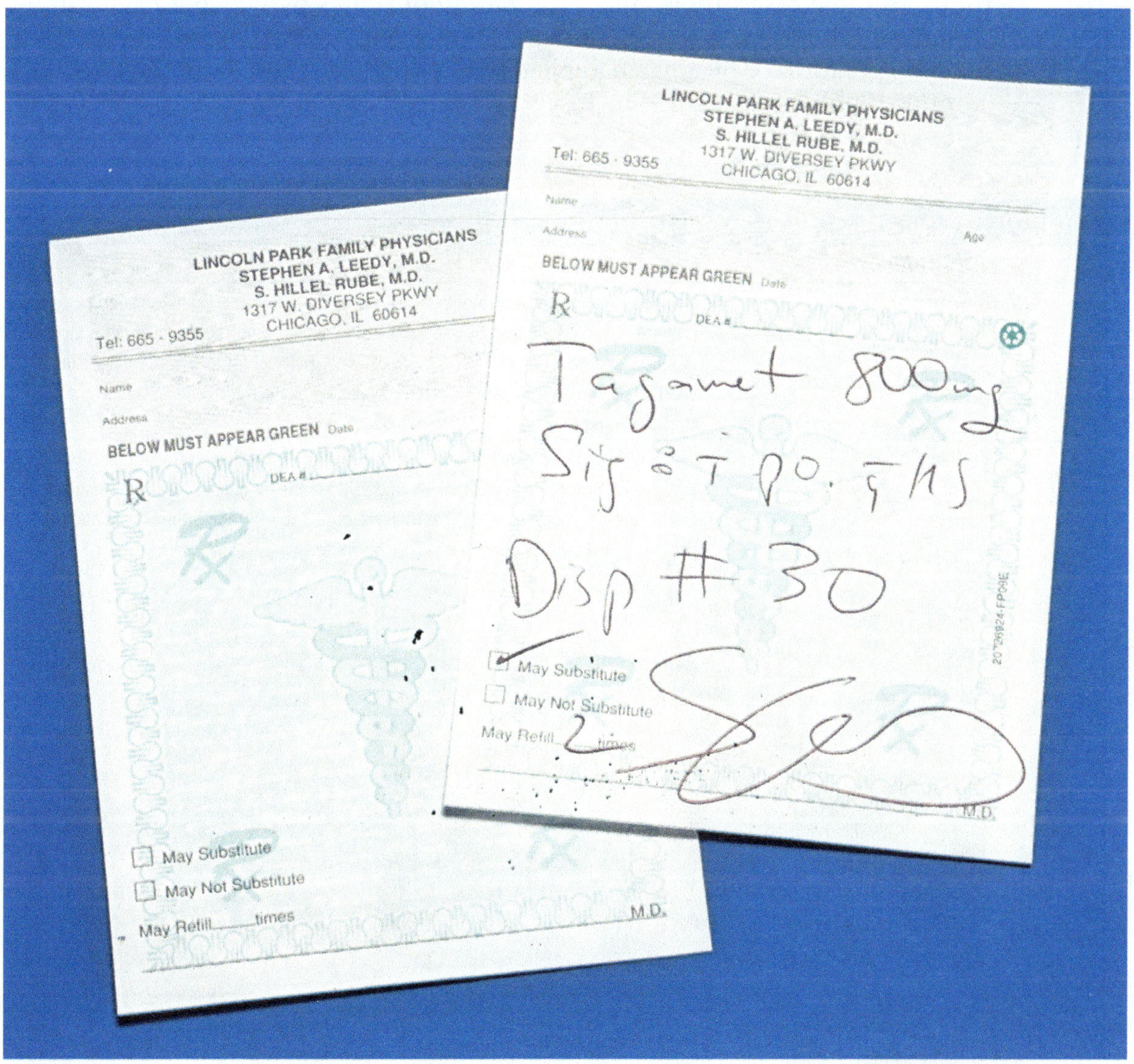

■ **Figure 14.1** A sample prescription written by a physician.

The physician's instruction to the patient will be placed on the label. The pharmacist will also include instructions about the medication and alert the patient to side effects that may need to be reported to the physician. In addition, any special instructions regarding the medication (i.e., take with meals, do not take along with dairy products) will also be supplied by the pharmacist.

Routes and Methods of Drug Administration

aerosol (AIR-oh-sol)
buccal (BUCK-al)
eardrops
eyedrops
inhalation (in-hah-LAY-shun)
oral (OR-al)
parenteral (par-EN-ter-al)
rectal (REK-tal)
sublingual (sub-LING-gwal)
suppositories (suh-POZ-ih-tor-ees)
topical (TOP-ih-kal)
transdermal (tranz-DER-mal)
vaginal (VAJ-in-al)

MED TERM TIP

Many abbreviations have multiple meanings, such as od, which can mean overdose (od) or right eye (OD), depending on whether the letters are lowercase or uppercase. Care must be taken when reading abbreviations since some may be written too quickly, making them difficult to decipher. Never create your own abbreviations.

The method by which a drug is introduced into the body is referred to as the *route of administration*. To be effective, drugs must be administered by a particular route. In some cases, there may be a variety of routes by which a drug can be administered. For instance, the female hormone estrogen can be administered orally in pill form or by a patch applied to the skin. The most common routes of administration are described in Table 14.3 ■.

Table 14.3 Common Routes of Drug Administration

METHOD	WORD PARTS	DESCRIPTION
oral	or/o = mouth -al = pertaining to	Includes all drugs given by mouth. The advantages are ease of administration and a slow rate of absorption via the stomach and intestinal wall. The disadvantages include slowness of absorption and destruction of some chemical compounds by gastric juices. In addition, some medications, such as aspirin, can have a corrosive action on the stomach lining.
sublingual	sub- = under lingu/o = tongue -al = pertaining to	Includes drugs that are held under the tongue and not swallowed. The medication is absorbed by the blood vessels on the underside of the tongue as the saliva dissolves it. The rate of absorption is quicker than the oral route. Nitroglycerin to treat angina pectoris (chest pain) is administered by this route.

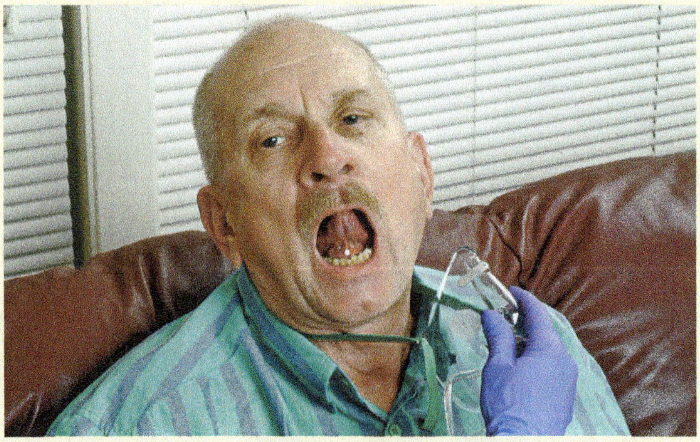

■ **Figure 14.2** Sublingual medication administration. Photograph of a male patient placing a nitroglycerine tablet under his tongue.

METHOD	WORD PARTS	DESCRIPTION
inhalation	in- = inward hal/o = to breathe	Includes drugs inhaled directly into the nose and mouth. **Aerosol** sprays are administered by this route (see Figure 14.3). ■

Table 14.3 Common Routes of Drug Administration (continued)

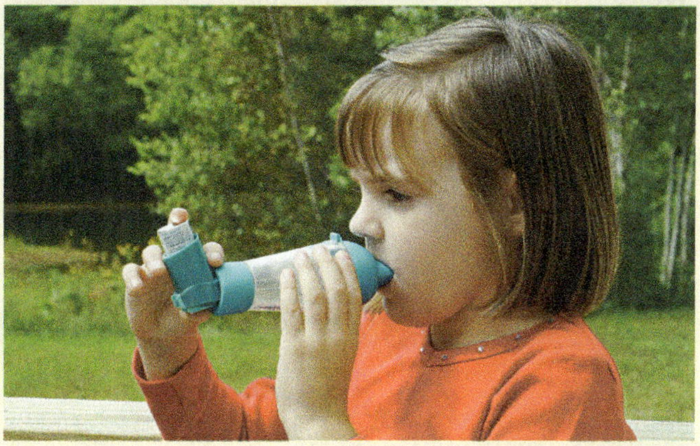

■ **Figure 14.3** Inhalation medication administration. Photograph of a young girl using a metered-dose inhaler.

METHOD	WORD PARTS	DESCRIPTION
parenteral	para- = near, beside enter/o = intestine -al = pertaining to	An invasive method of administering drugs as it requires the skin to be punctured by a needle. The needle with syringe attached is introduced either under the skin or into a muscle, vein, or body cavity.
intracavitary (in-trah-KAV-ih-tair-ee)	intra- = within -ary = pertaining to	Injection into a body cavity such as the peritoneal and chest cavity.
intradermal (ID) (in-trah-DER-mal)	intra- = within derm/o = skin -al = pertaining to	Very shallow injection just under the top layer of skin. Commonly used in skin testing for allergies and tuberculosis testing.

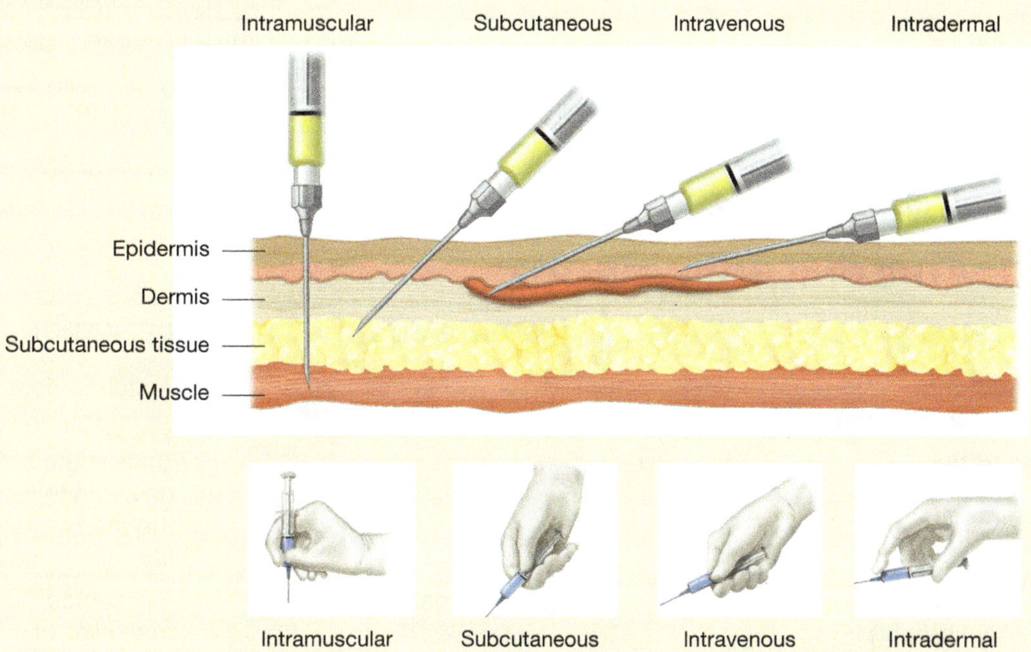

■ **Figure 14.4** Parenteral medication administration. The angle of needle insertion for four different types of parenteral injections.

METHOD	WORD PARTS	DESCRIPTION
intramuscular (IM) (in-trah-MUSS-kyoo-lar)	intra- = within muscul/o = muscle -ar = pertaining to	Injection directly into the muscle of the buttocks, thigh, or upper arm. Used when there is a large amount of medication or it is irritating (see again Figure 14.4).
intrathecal (in-trah-THEE-kal)	intra- = within thec/o = sheath (meninges) -al = pertaining to	Injection into the meningeal space surrounding the brain and spinal cord.

(Continued)

Table 14.3 Common Routes of Drug Administration (continued)

METHOD	WORD PARTS	DESCRIPTION
intravenous (IV) (in-trah-VEE-nus)	intra- = within ven/o = vein -ous = pertaining to	Injection into the veins. This route may be set up to deliver medication very quickly or to deliver a continuous drip of medication (see again Figure 14.4).
subcutaneous (Subc, SubQ) (sub-kyoo-TAY-nee-us)	sub- = under cutane/o = skin -ous = pertaining to	Injection into the subcutaneous layer of the skin, usually the upper, outer arm or abdomen (see again Figure 14.4); for example, insulin injection.
transdermal	trans- = through derm/o = skin -al = pertaining to	Includes medications that coat the underside of a patch, which is applied to the skin where it is then absorbed. Examples include birth control patches, nicotine patches, and sea sickness patches.
rectal	rect/o = rectum -al = pertaining to	Includes medications introduced directly into the rectal cavity in the form of **suppositories** or solution. Drugs may have to be administered by this route if the patient is unable to take them by mouth due to nausea, vomiting, or surgery.
topical	topic/o = a specific area -al = pertaining to	Includes medications applied directly to the skin or mucous membranes. They are distributed in ointment, cream, or lotion form, and are used to treat skin infections and eruptions.
vaginal	vagin/o = vagina -al = pertaining to	Includes tablets and suppositories that may be inserted vaginally to treat vaginal yeast infections and other irritations.
eyedrops		Includes drops used during eye examinations to dilate the pupil of the eye for better examination of the interior of the eye. They are also placed into the eye to control eye pressure in glaucoma and treat infections.
eardrops		Includes drops placed directly into the ear canal for the purpose of relieving pain or treating infection.
buccal	bucc/o = cheek -al = pertaining to	Includes drugs that are placed under the lip or between the cheek and gum.

Pharmacology Terms

TERM	WORD PARTS	DEFINITION
addiction (ah-DICK-shun)		Acquired dependence on a drug.
additive		Sum of the action of two (or more) drugs given. In this case, the total strength of the medications is equal to the sum of the strength of each individual drug.
antidote (AN-tih-doht)	anti- = against	Substance that will neutralize poisons or their side effects.
broad spectrum		Ability of a drug to be effective against a wide range of microorganisms.
contraindication (kon-trah-in-dih-KAY-shun)	contra- = against	Condition in which a particular drug should not be used.
cumulative action		Action that occurs in the body when a drug is allowed to accumulate or stay in the body.

Pharmacology Terms *(continued)*

TERM	WORD PARTS	DEFINITION
drug interaction		Occurs when the effect of one drug is altered because it was taken at the same time as another drug.
drug tolerance		Decrease in susceptibility to a drug after continued use of the drug.
habituation (hah-bich-yoo-AY-shun)		Development of an emotional dependence on a drug due to repeated use.
iatrogenic (eye-ah-troh-JEN-ik)	iatr/o = medicine -genic = produced by	Usually an unfavorable response resulting from taking a medication.
idiosyncrasy (id-ee-oh-SIN-krah-see)	idi/o = distinctive	Unusual or abnormal response to a drug or food.
placebo (plah-SEE-boh)		Inactive, harmless substance used to satisfy a patient's desire for medication. This is also used in research when given to a control group of patients in a study in which another group receives a drug. The effect of the placebo versus the drug is then observed.
potentiation (poe-ten-chee-A-shun)		Giving a patient a second drug to boost (potentiate) the effect of another drug. The total strength of the drugs is greater than the sum of the strength of the individual drugs.
prophylaxis (proh-fih-LAK-sis)	pro- = before -phylaxis = protection	Prevention of disease. For example, an antibiotic can be used to prevent the occurrence of a disease.
side effect		Response to a drug other than the effect desired. Also called an *adverse reaction.*
tolerance (TAHL-er-ans)		Development of a capacity for withstanding a large amount of a substance, such as foods, drugs, or poison, without any adverse effect. A decreased sensitivity to further doses will develop.
toxicity (tok-SISS-ih-tee)	toxic/o = poison	Extent or degree to which a substance is poisonous.
unit dose		Drug dosage system that provides prepackaged, prelabeled, individual medications that are ready for immediate use by the patient.

Abbreviations

@	at
ā	before
ac	before meals
ad lib	as desired
ante	before
APAP	acetaminophen (Tylenol™)
aq	aqueous (water)
ASA	aspirin
bid	twice a day
c̄	with
cap(s)	capsule(s)
d	day
d/c, DISC	discontinue
DC, disc	discontinue
DEA	Drug Enforcement Agency
dil	dilute
disp	dispense
dtd	give of such a dose
Dx	diagnosis
et	and
FDA	Federal Drug Administration
gm	gram
gr	grain
gt	drop
gtt	drops
hs	at bedtime
ī	one
ID	intradermal
īī	two
īīī	three
IM	intramuscular
inj	injection
IV	intravenous
kg	kilogram
L	liter
mcg	microgram
mEq	milliequivalent
mg	milligram
mL	milliliter
no sub	no substitute
noc	night
non rep	do not repeat
NPO	nothing by mouth
NS	normal saline
od	overdose
oint	ointment
OTC	over the counter
oz	ounce
p̄	after
pc	after meals
PCA	patient-controlled administration
PDR	*Physician's Desk Reference*
per	with
po	by mouth
prn	as needed
pt	patient
q	every
qam	every morning
qh	every hour
qhs	at bedtime
qid	four times a day
qs	quantity sufficient
Rx	take
s̄	without
Sig	label as follows/directions
sl	under the tongue
sol	solution
s̄s̄	one-half
stat	at once/immediately
Subc, SubQ	subcutaneous
suppos, supp	suppository
susp	suspension
syr	syrup
T, tbsp	tablespoon
t, tsp	teaspoon
tab	tablet
tid	three times a day
TO	telephone order
top	apply topically
VO	verbal order
wt	weight
x	times

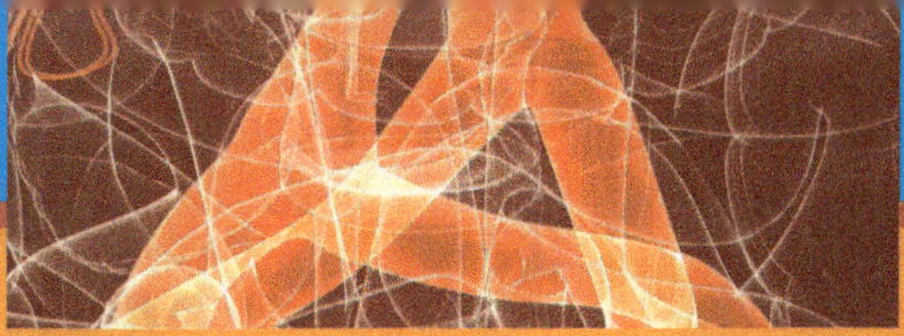

Section II: Mental Health at a Glance

Word Parts

Here are the most common word parts (with their meanings) used to build mental health terms.

Combining Forms

amnes/o	forgetfulness
anxi/o	fear, worry
chondr/o	cartilage
compuls/o	drive, compel
deluss/o	false belief
depress/o	to press down
electr/o	electricity
factiti/o	artificial, contrived
hallucin/o	imagined perception
klept/o	to steal
ment/o	mind
obsess/o	besieged by thoughts
path/o	disease
ped/o	child
pharmac/o	drug
phob/o	irrational fear
phren/o	mind
psych/o	mind
pyr/o	fire
schiz/o	split
soci/o	society
somat/o	body
somn/o	sleep

Suffixes

-al	pertaining to
-ar	pertaining to
-ia	state, condition
-iatrist	physician
-iatry	medical treatment
-ic	pertaining to
-ism	state of
-logical	pertaining to the study of
-logist	one who studies
-logy	study of
-mania	frenzy
-orexia	appetite
-ous	pertaining to
-philia	attracted to
-therapy	treatment
-tic	pertaining to

Prefixes

an-	without
anti-	against
auto-	self
bi-	two
de-	without
dis-	apart
ex-	outward
hyper-	excessive
hypo-	below
in-	not

Mental Health Disciplines

Psychology

abnormal psychology
clinical psychologist (sigh-KALL-oh-jist)
normal psychology
psychology (sigh-KALL-oh-jee)

MED TERM TIP

All social interactions pose some problems for some people. These problems are not necessarily abnormal. One means of judging if behavior is abnormal is to compare one person's behavior with others in the community. Also, if a person's behavior interferes with the activities of daily living, it is often considered abnormal.

Psychology is the study of human behavior and thought processes. This behavioral science is primarily concerned with understanding how human beings interact with their physical environment and with each other. Behavior can be divided into two categories: normal and abnormal. The study of **normal psychology** includes how the personality develops, how people handle stress, and the stages of mental development. In contrast, **abnormal psychology** studies and treats behaviors that are outside of normal and that are detrimental to the person or society. These maladaptive behaviors range from occasional difficulty coping with stress, to bizarre actions and beliefs, to total withdrawal. A **clinical psychologist,** though not a physician, is a specialist in evaluating and treating persons with mental and emotional disorders.

Psychiatry

psychiatric nurse (sigh-kee-AT-rik)
psychiatric social worker
psychiatrist (sigh-KIGH-ah-trist)
psychiatry (sigh-KIGH-ah-tree)

MED TERM TIP

Look for these word parts:

psych/o = mind
-iatrist = physician
-iatry = medical treatment
-logist = one who studies
-logy = study of

Psychiatry is the branch of medicine that deals with the diagnosis, treatment, and prevention of mental disorders. A **psychiatrist** is a medical physician specializing in the care of patients with mental, emotional, and behavioral disorders. Other health professions also have specialty areas in caring for clients with mental illness. Good examples are **psychiatric nurses** and **psychiatric social workers.**

Pathology

The legal definition of mental disorder is "impaired judgment and lack of self-control." The guide for terminology and classifications relating to psychiatric disorders is the *Diagnostic and Statistical Manual of Mental Disorders, Fourth Edition* (Text Revision) (DSM-IV-TR™), which is published by the American Psychiatric Association (2004). The DSM organizes mental disorders into 14 major diagnostic categories of mental disorders.

MED TERM TIP

Mental disorders are sometimes more simply characterized by whether they are a *neurosis* or a *psychosis.* Neuroses are inappropriate coping mechanisms to handle stress, such as phobias and panic attacks. Psychoses involve extreme distortions of reality and disorganization of a person's thinking, including bizarre behaviors, hallucinations, and delusions. Schizophrenia is an example of a psychosis.

TERM	WORD PARTS	DEFINITION
Anxiety disorders	anxi/o = fear, worry	Characterized by persistent worry and apprehension.
panic attacks	-ic = pertaining to	Feeling of intense apprehension, terror, or sense of impending danger.
anxiety (ang-ZY-eh-tee)	anxi/o = fear, worry	Feeling of dread in the absence of a clearly identifiable stress trigger.
phobias (FOH-bee-ahs)	phob/o = irrational fear -ia = state, condition	Irrational fear, such as *arachnophobia,* or fear of spiders.

Pathology *(continued)*

TERM	WORD PARTS	DEFINITION
obsessive–compulsive disorder (OCD) (ob-SESS-iv / kom-PUHL-siv)	obsess/o = besieged by thoughts compuls/o = drive, compel	Performing repetitive rituals to reduce anxiety.
Cognitive disorders		Deterioration of mental functions due to temporary brain or permanent brain dysfunction.
dementia (dee-MEN-she-ah)	de- = without ment/o = mind -ia = state, condition	Progressive confusion and disorientation.
Alzheimer's disease (ALTS-high-merz)		Degenerative brain disorder with gradual loss of cognitive abilities.
Disorders diagnosed in infancy and childhood		Mental disorders associated with childhood; include:
mental retardation	ment/o = mind -al = pertaining to	Subaverage intellectual functioning.
attention-deficit/hyperactivity disorder (ADHD)	hyper- = excessive	Inattention and impulsive behavior.
autism (AW-tizm)	auto- = self -ism = state of	Condition involving deficits in social interaction, communication skills, and restricted patterns of behavior.
Dissociative disorders	dis- = apart soci/o = society	Disorders in which severe emotional conflict is so repressed that a split in the personality may occur or the person may lose memory.
amnesia (am-NEE-zee-ah)	amnes/o = forgetfulness -ia = state, condition	Loss of memory.
dissociative identity disorder		Having two or more distinct personalities.
Eating disorders		Abnormal behaviors related to eating; include:
anorexia nervosa (an-oh-REK-see-ah / ner-VOH-sah)	an- = without -orexia = appetite	Refusal to eat.

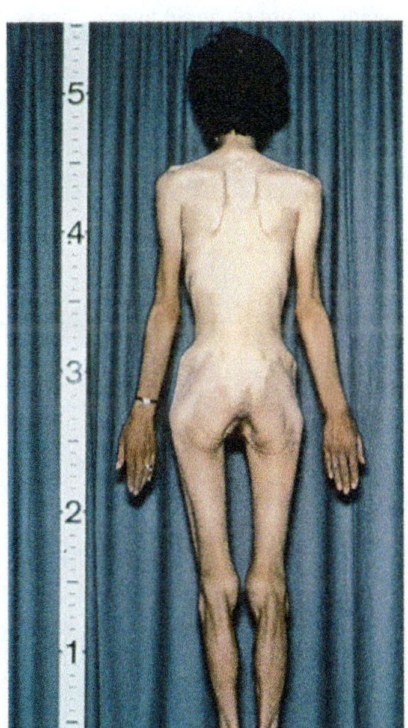

Figure 14.5 Photograph of a young woman suffering from anorexia nervosa, posterior view. *(Custom Medical Stock Photo, Inc.)*

Pathology *(continued)*

TERM	WORD PARTS	DEFINITION
bulimia (boo-LIM-ee-ah)	-ia = state, condition	Binge eating and intentional vomiting.
Factitious disorders	factiti/o = artificial, contrived -ous = pertaining to	Intentionally feigning illness symptoms in order to gain attention.
malingering		Pretending to be ill or injured.
Impulse control disorders		Inability to resist an impulse to perform some act that is harmful to the individual or others; include:
kleptomania (klep-toh-MAY-nee-ah)	klept/o = to steal -mania = frenzy	Stealing.
pyromania (pie-roh-MAY-nee-ah)	pyr/o = fire -mania = frenzy	Setting fires.
explosive disorder	ex- = outward	Violent rages.
pathological gambling (path-ah-LOJ-ih-kal)	path/o = disease -logical = pertaining to the study of	Inability to stop gambling.
Mood disorders		Characterized by instability in mood; include:
major depression	depress/o = to press down	Feelings of hopelessness, helplessness, worthlessness; lack of pleasure in any activity; potential for suicide.
mania (MAY-nee-ah)	-mania = frenzy	Extreme elation.
bipolar disorder (BPD)	bi- = two -ar = pertaining to	Alternation between periods of deep depression and mania.

MED TERM TIP

The healthcare professional must take all threats of suicide from patients seriously. Psychologists tell us that there is no clear suicide type, which means that we cannot predict who will actually take his or her own life. Always tell the physician about any discussion a patient has concerning suicide. If you believe a patient is in danger of suicide, do not be afraid to ask, "Are you thinking about suicide?"

TERM	WORD PARTS	DEFINITION
Personality disorders		Inflexible or maladaptive behavior patterns that affect a person's ability to function in society; include:
paranoid personality disorder		Exaggerated feelings of persecution.
narcissistic personality disorder (nar-sis-SIST-ik)		Abnormal sense of self-importance.
antisocial personality disorder	anti- = against soci/o = society -al = pertaining to	Behaviors that are against legal or social norms.

Pathology *(continued)*

TERM	WORD PARTS	DEFINITION
passive aggressive personality		Indirect expression of hostility or anger.
Schizophrenia	schiz/o = split phren/o = mind -ia = state, condition	Mental disorders characterized by distortions of reality such as:
delusion (dee-LOO-zhun)	deluss/o = false belief	A false belief held even in the face of contrary evidence.
hallucination (hah-loo-sih-NAY-shun)	hallucin/o = imagined perception	Perceiving something that is not there.
Sexual disorders		Disorders include aberrant sexual activity and sexual dysfunction; include:
pedophilia (pee-doh-FILL-ee-ah)	ped/o = child -philia = attracted to	Sexual interest in children.
masochism (MAS-oh-kizm)	-ism = state of	Gratification derived from being hurt or abused.
voyeurism (VOY-er-izm)	-ism = state of	Gratification derived from observing others engaged in sexual acts.
Sleeping disorders		Disorders relating to sleeping; include:
insomnia (in-SOM-nee-ah)	in- = not somn/o = sleep -ia = state, condition	Inability to sleep.
sleepwalking		Getting up and walking around unaware while sleeping.
Somatoform disorders	somat/o = body	Patient has physical symptoms for which no physical disease can be determined; include:
hypochondria (high-poh-KON-dree-ah)	hypo- = below chondr/o = cartilage -ia = state, condition	A preoccupation with health concerns. Named for the location of the liver and spleen, below the rib cartilage. The ancient Greeks thought these organs controlled mood.
conversion reaction		Anxiety is transformed into physical symptoms such as heart palpitations, paralysis, or blindness.
Substance-related disorders		Overindulgence or dependence on chemical substances including alcohol, illegal drugs, and prescription drugs.

Therapeutic Procedures

TERM	WORD PARTS	DEFINITION
Electroconvulsive therapy (ECT) (ee-lek-troh-kon-VULL-siv)	electr/o = electricity	Procedure occasionally used for cases of prolonged major depression. This controversial treatment involves placement of an electrode on one or both sides of the patient's head and a current is turned on briefly causing a convulsive seizure. A low level of voltage is used in modern electroconvulsive therapy, and the patient is administered a muscle relaxant and anesthesia. Advocates of this treatment state that it is a more effective way to treat severe depression than using drugs. It is not effective with disorders other than depression, such as schizophrenia and alcoholism.
Psychopharmacology (sigh-koh-far-mah-KALL-oh-jee)	psych/o = mind pharmac/o = drug -logy = study of	Study of the effects of drugs on the mind and particularly the use of drugs in treating mental disorders. The main classes of drugs for the treatment of mental disorders are:
antipsychotic drugs	anti- = against psych/o = mind -tic = pertaining to	Major tranquilizers include chlorpromazine (Thorazine™), haloperidol (Haldol™), clozapine (Clozaril™), and risperidone. These drugs have transformed the treatment of patients with psychoses and schizophrenia by reducing patient agitation and panic and shortening schizophrenic episodes. One of the side effects of these drugs is involuntary muscle movements, which approximately one-fourth of all adults who take the drugs develop.
antidepressant drugs	anti- = against depress/o = to press down	Classified as stimulants and alter the patient's mood by affecting levels of neurotransmitters in the brain. Antidepressants, such as serotonin norepinephrine reuptake inhibitors, are nonaddictive but they can produce unpleasant side effects such as dry mouth, weight gain, blurred vision, and nausea.
minor tranquilizers		Include Valium™ and Xanax™. These are also classified as central nervous system depressants and are prescribed for anxiety.
lithium		Special category of drug used successfully to calm patients who suffer from bipolar disorder (depression alternating with manic excitement).

Therapeutic Procedures *(continued)*

TERM	WORD PARTS	DEFINITION
Psychotherapy (sigh-koh-THAIR-ah-pee)	psych/o = mind -therapy = treatment	A method of treating mental disorders by mental rather than chemical or physical means. It includes:
psychoanalysis	psych/o = mind	Method of obtaining a detailed account of the past and present emotional and mental experiences from the patient to determine the source of the problem and eliminate the effects. It is a system developed by Sigmund Freud that encourages the patient to discuss repressed, painful, or hidden experiences with the hope of eliminating or minimizing the problem.
humanistic psychotherapy	-tic = pertaining to psych/o = mind -therapy = treatment	Therapist does not delve into the patients' past when using these methods. Instead, it is believed that patients can learn how to use their own internal resources to deal with their problems. The therapist creates a therapeutic atmosphere, which builds patient self-esteem and encourages discussion of problems, thereby gaining insight in how to handle them. Also called *client-centered* or *nondirective psychotherapy.*
family and group psychotherapy	psych/o = mind -therapy = treatment	Often described as solution focused, the therapist places minimal emphasis on patient past history and strong emphasis on having patient state and discuss goals and then find a way to achieve them.

Abbreviations

AD	Alzheimer's disease
ADD	attention-deficit disorder
ADHD	attention-deficit/hyperactivity disorder
BPD	bipolar disorder
CA	chronological age
DSM	*Diagnostic and Statistical Manual of Mental Disorders*
ECT	electroconvulsive therapy
MA	mental age
MMPI	Minnesota Multiphasic Personality Inventory
OCD	obsessive–compulsive disorder
SAD	seasonal affective disorder

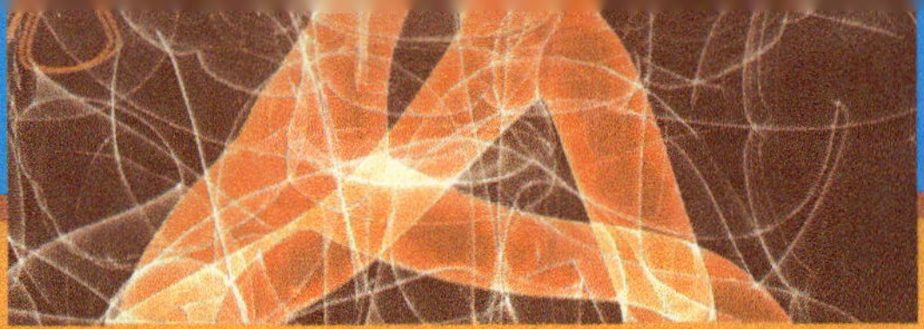

Section III: Diagnostic Imaging at a Glance

Word Parts

Here are the most common word parts (with their meanings) used to build diagnostic imaging terms.

Combining Forms

anter/o	front	**radi/o**	ray (X-ray)
fluor/o	fluorescence, luminous	**roentgen/o**	X-ray
later/o	side	**son/o**	sound
nucle/o	nucleus	**tom/o**	to cut
poster/o	back		

Suffixes

-al	pertaining to	**-logy**	study of
-ar	pertaining to	**-lucent**	to shine through
-graphy	process of recording	**-opaque**	nontransparent
-ic	pertaining to	**-scopy**	process of visually examining
-ior	pertaining to		
-logist	one who studies		

Prefix

ultra-	beyond

Diagnostic Imaging

roentgenology (rent-gen-ALL-oh-jee) **X-rays**

Diagnostic imaging is the medical specialty that uses a variety of methods to produce images of the internal structures of the body. These images are then used to diagnose disease. This area of medicine began as **roentgenology** (**roentgen/o** = X-ray; **-logy** = study of), named after German physicist Wilhelm Roentgen who discovered roentgen rays in 1895. This discovery, now commonly known as **X-rays,** revolutionized the diagnosis of disease.

Diagnostic Imaging Terms

TERM	WORD PARTS	DEFINITION
anteroposterior view (AP view)	anter/o = front poster/o = back -ior = pertaining to	Positioning the patient so that the X-rays pass through the body from the anterior side to the posterior side.
barium (Ba) (BAH-ree-um)		Soft metallic element from the earth used as a radiopaque X-ray dye.
film		Thin sheet of cellulose material coated with a light-sensitive substance that is used in taking photographs. There is a special photographic film that is sensitive to X-rays.
film badge		Badge containing film that is sensitive to X-rays. This is worn by all personnel in radiology to measure the amount of X-rays to which they are exposed.
lateral view	later/o = side -al = pertaining to	Positioning of the patient so that the side of the body faces the X-ray machine.
oblique view (oh-BLEEK)		Positioning of the patient so that the X-rays pass through the body on an angle.
posteroanterior view (PA view)	poster/o = back anter/o = front -ior = pertaining to	Positioning of the patient so that the X-rays pass through the body from the posterior side to the anterior side.
radiography (ray-dee-OG-rah-fee)	radi/o = X-ray -graphy = process of recording	Making of X-ray pictures.
radioisotope (ray-dee-oh-EYE-soh-tohp)	radi/o = X-ray	Radioactive form of an element.
radiologist (ray-dee-ALL-oh-jist)	radi/o = X-ray -logist = one who studies	Physician who uses images to diagnose abnormalities and radiant energy to treat various conditions such as cancer.
radiolucent (ray-dee-oh-LOO-cent)	radi/o = X-ray -lucent = to shine through	Structures that allow X-rays to pass through; expose the photographic plate and appear as black areas on the X-ray.
radiopaque (ray-dee-oh-PAYK)	radi/o = X-ray -opaque = nontransparent	Structures that are impenetrable to X-rays, appearing as a light area on the radiograph (X-ray).

Diagnostic Imaging Terms *(continued)*

TERM	WORD PARTS	DEFINITION
roentgen (RENT-gen)	roentgen/o = X-ray	Unit for describing an exposure dose of radiation.
scan		Recording on a photographic plate the emission of radioactive waves after a substance has been injected into the body.

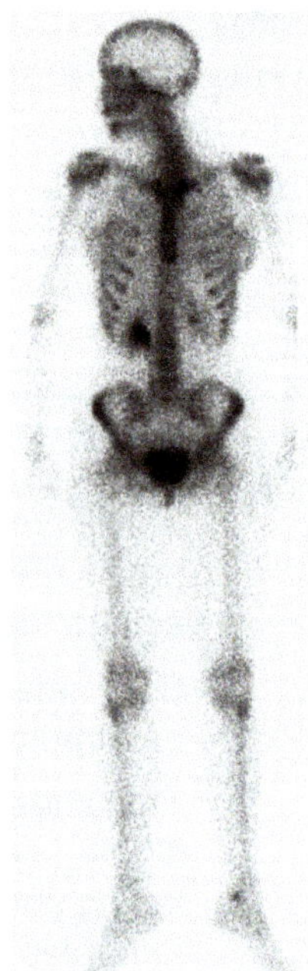

■ **Figure 14.6** Nuclear medicine. Bone scan produced after injection of a radioactive substance into the body. *(Getty Images, Inc/Photodisc)*

TERM	WORD PARTS	DEFINITION
shield		Device used to protect against radiation.
tagging		Attaching a radioactive material to a chemical, and tracing it as it moves through the body.
uptake		Absorption of radioactive material and medicines into an organ or tissue.
X-ray		High-energy wave that can penetrate most solid matter and present the image on photographic film.

Diagnostic Imaging Procedures

TERM	WORD PARTS	DEFINITION
computed tomography scan (CT scan) (toh-MOG-rah-fee)	tom/o = to cut -graphy = process of recording	Imaging technique that is able to produce a cross-sectional view of the body. X-ray pictures are taken at multiple angles through the body. A computer then uses all these images to construct a composite cross-section.

Diagnostic Imaging Procedures *(continued)*

TERM	WORD PARTS	DEFINITION
contrast studies		Radiopaque substance is injected or swallowed. X-rays are then taken that will outline the body structure containing the radiopaque substance. For example, angiograms and myelograms.

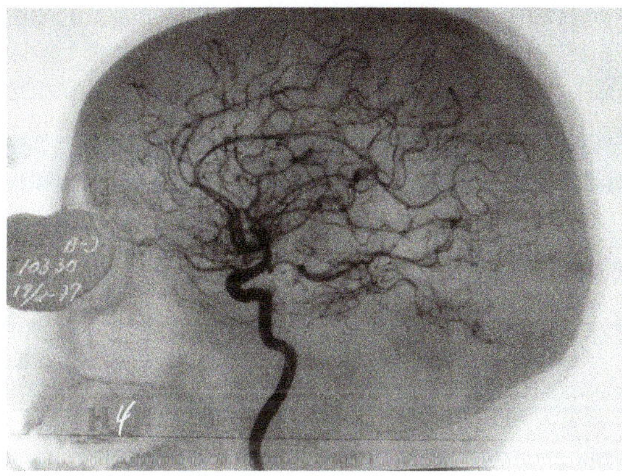

Figure 14.7 Contrast study. X-ray of cerebral blood vessels taken after injection of a radiopaque substance into the bloodstream.

TERM	WORD PARTS	DEFINITION
Doppler ultrasonography	ultra- = beyond son/o = sound -graphy = process of recording	Use of ultrasound to record the velocity of blood flowing through blood vessels. Used to detect blood clots and blood vessel obstructions.
fluoroscopy (floo-or-OS-koh-pee)	fluor/o = luminous -scopy = process of visually examining	X-rays strike a fluorescing screen rather than a photographic plate, causing it to glow. The glowing screen changes from minute to minute; therefore movement, such as the heart beating or the digestive tract moving, can be seen.
magnetic resonance imaging (MRI) (REZ-oh-nence)	-ic = pertaining to	Use of electromagnetic energy to produce an image of soft tissues in any plane of the body. Atoms behave differently when placed in a strong magnetic field. When the body is exposed to this magnetic field the nuclei of the body's atoms emit radio-frequency signals that can be used to create an image.

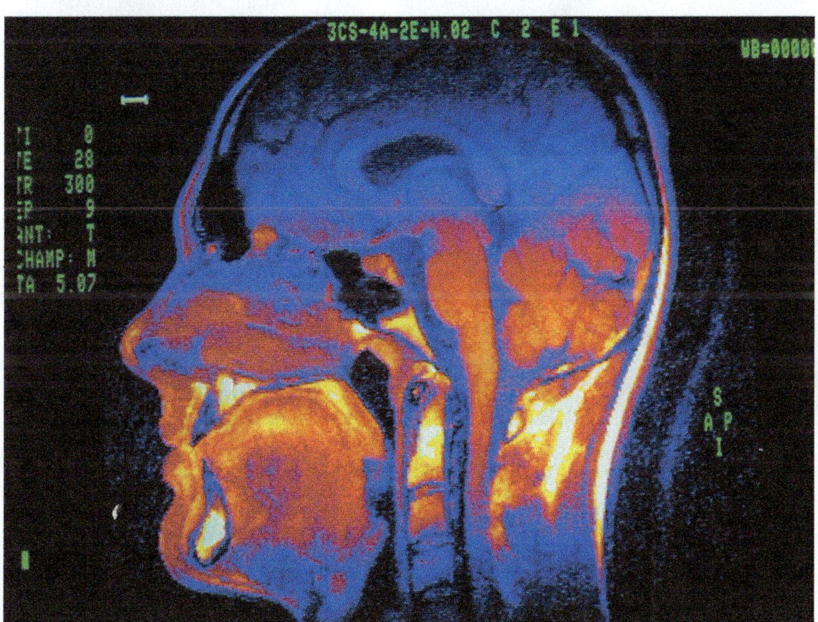

Figure 14.8 Color-enhanced magnetic resonance image (MRI) showing a sagittal view of the head. *(Photo Researchers, Inc.)*

Diagnostic Imaging Procedures *(continued)*

TERM	WORD PARTS	DEFINITION
nuclear medicine	nucle/o = nucleus -ar = pertaining to	Use of radioactive substances to diagnose diseases. A radioactive substance known to accumulate in certain body tissues is injected or inhaled. After waiting for the substance to travel to the body area of interest, the radioactivity level is recorded. Commonly referred to as a *scan* (see again Figure 14.6). See Table 14.4 ■ for examples of the radioactive substances used in nuclear medicine.

Table 14.4 Substances Used to Visualize Various Body Organs in Nuclear Medicine

ORGAN	SUBSTANCE
bone	technetium (^{99m}Tc)–labeled phosphate
tumors	gallium (^{67}Ga)
lungs	xenon (^{133}Xe)
liver	technetium (^{99m}Tc)–labeled sulfur
heart	thallium (^{201}Tl)
thyroid	iodine (^{131}I)

TERM	WORD PARTS	DEFINITION
positron emission tomography (PET) (POS-ih-tron / eh-MIS-shun / toh-MOG-rah-fee)	tom/o = to cut -graphy = process of recording	Image is produced following the injection of radioactive glucose. The glucose will accumulate in areas of high metabolic activity. Therefore, this process will highlight areas that are consuming a large quantity of glucose. This may show an active area of the brain or a tumor.

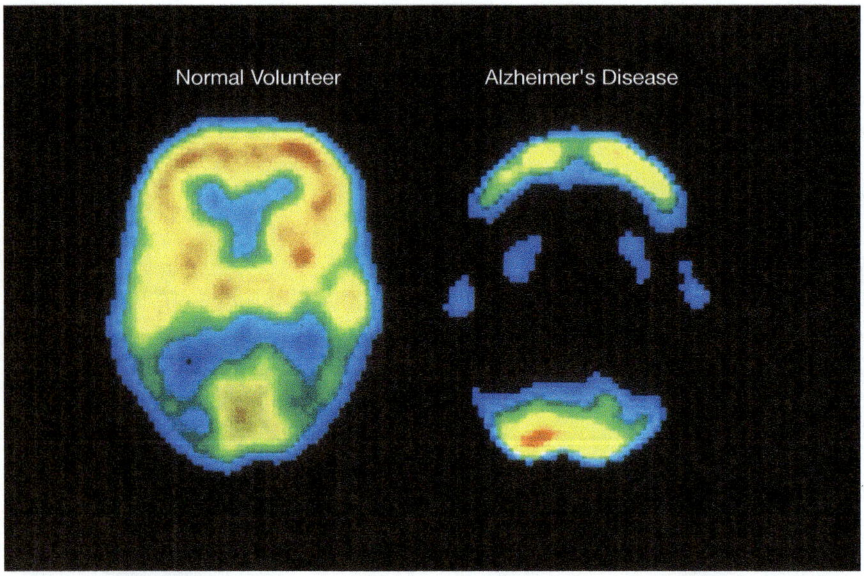

■ **Figure 14.9** Positron emission tomography (PET) image showing the difference in the metabolic activity of the brain of a person with Alzheimer's disease and that of a normal person. *(Science Source/Photo Researchers Inc.)*

TERM	WORD PARTS	DEFINITION
radiology (ray-dee-ALL-oh-jee)	radi/o = X-ray -logy = study of	Use of high-energy radiation, X-rays, to expose a photographic plate. The image is a black-and-white picture with radiopaque structures such as bone appearing white and radiolucent tissue such as muscles appearing dark.

Diagnostic Imaging Procedures *(continued)*

TERM	WORD PARTS	DEFINITION
ultrasound (US) (ULL-trah-sound)	ultra- = beyond	Use of high-frequency sound waves to produce an image. Sound waves directed into the body from a transducer will bounce off internal structures and echo back to the transducer. The speed of the echo is dependent on the density of the tissue. A computer is able to correlate speed of echo with density and produce an image. Used to visualize internal organs, heart valves, and fetuses.

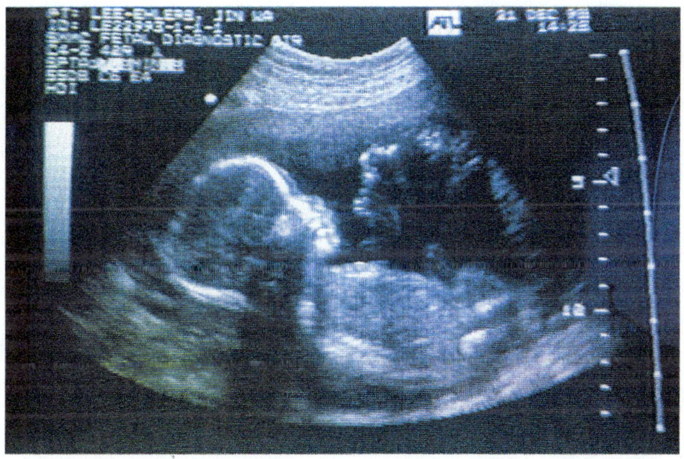

Figure 14.10 Ultrasound showing the outline of a fetus.
(Chad Ehlers/Stock Connection)

Abbreviations

^{67}Ga	radioactive gallium
^{99m}Tc	radioactive technetium
^{131}I	radioactive iodine
^{201}Tl	radioactive thallium
^{133}Xe	radioactive xenon
Angio	angiography
AP	anteroposterior
Ba	barium
BaE	barium enema
CAT	computerized axial tomography
Ci	curie
CT	computerized tomography
CXR	chest X-ray
decub	lying down
DI	diagnostic imaging
DSA	digital subtraction angiography
ERCP	endoscopic retrograde cholangiopancreatography
Fx	fracture
GB	gallbladder X-ray
IVC	intravenous cholangiogram
IVP	intravenous pyelogram
KUB	kidneys, ureters, bladder
LAT	lateral
LGI	lower gastrointestinal series
LL	left lateral
mA	milliampere
mCi	millicurie

Abbreviations *(continued)*

MRA	magnetic resonance angiography
MRI	magnetic resonance imaging
NMR	nuclear magnetic resonance
PA	posteroanterior
PET	positron emission tomography
PTC	percutaneous transhepatic cholangiography
R	roentgen
Ra	radium
rad	radiation-absorbed dose
RL	right lateral
RRT	registered radiologic technologist
UGI	upper gastrointestinal series
US	ultrasound

Section IV: Rehabilitation Services at a Glance

Word Parts

Here are the most common word parts (with their meanings) used to build rehabilitation services terms.

Combining Forms

cry/o	cold	my/o	muscle
cutane/o	skin	orth/o	straight, correct
electr/o	electric current	phon/o	sound
erg/o	work	physic/o	body
habilitat/o	ability	prosthet/o	addition
hydr/o	water	therm/o	heat

Suffixes

-al	pertaining to	-ous	pertaining to
-graphy	process of recording	-phoresis	carrying
-ic	pertaining to	-therapy	treatment
-nomics	pertaining to laws	-tic	pertaining to

Prefixes

re-	again
trans-	across
ultra-	beyond

Rehabilitation Services

occupational therapy | **physical therapy**

The goal of rehabilitation is to prevent disability and restore as much function as possible following disease, illness, or injury. Rehabilitation services include the healthcare specialties of **physical therapy** (PT) and **occupational therapy** (OT).

Physical Therapy

Physical therapy (PT) involves treating disorders using physical means and methods. Physical therapy personnel assess joint motion, muscle strength and endurance, function of heart and lungs, performance of activities required in daily living, and the ability to carry out other responsibilities. Physical therapy treatment includes gait training, therapeutic exercise, massage, joint and soft tissue mobilization, thermotherapy, cryotherapy, electrical stimulation, ultrasound, and hydrotherapy. These methods strengthen muscles, improve motion and circulation, reduce pain, and increase function.

Occupational Therapy

Occupational therapy (OT) assists patients to regain, develop, and improve skills that are important for independent functioning (activities of daily living). Occupational therapy personnel work with people who, because of illness, injury, or developmental or psychological impairments, require specialized training in skills that will enable them to lead independent, productive, and satisfying lives in regard to personal care, work, and leisure. Occupational therapists instruct patients in the use of adaptive equipment and techniques, body mechanics, and energy conservation. They also employ modalities such as heat, cold, and therapeutic exercise.

Rehabilitation Services Terms

TERM	WORD PARTS	DEFINITION
activities of daily living (ADL)		Activities usually performed in the course of a normal day, such as eating, dressing, and washing.

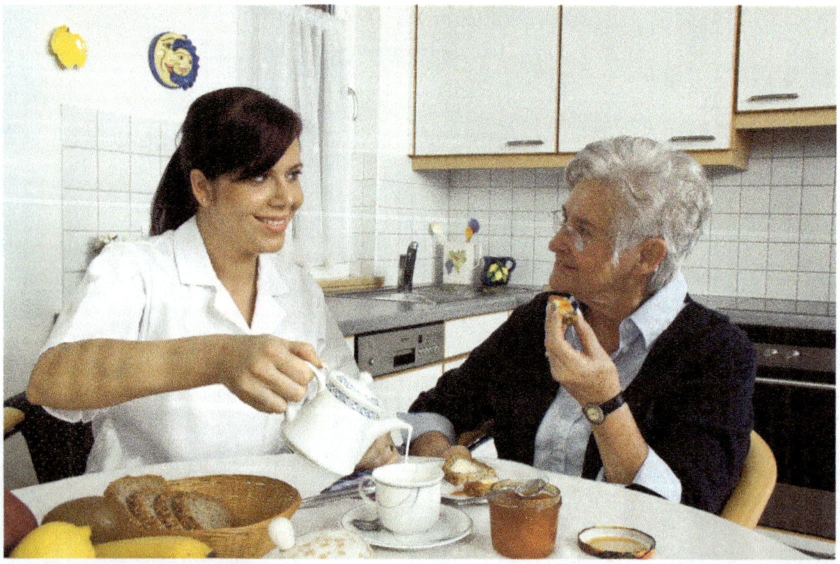

■ **Figure 14.11** Photograph of an occupational therapist assisting a patient with learning independence in activities of daily living (ADLs). *(Gina Sanders/Shutterstock)*

Rehabilitation Services Terms *(continued)*

TERM	WORD PARTS	DEFINITION
adaptive equipment		Modification of equipment or devices to improve the function and independence of a person with a disability.

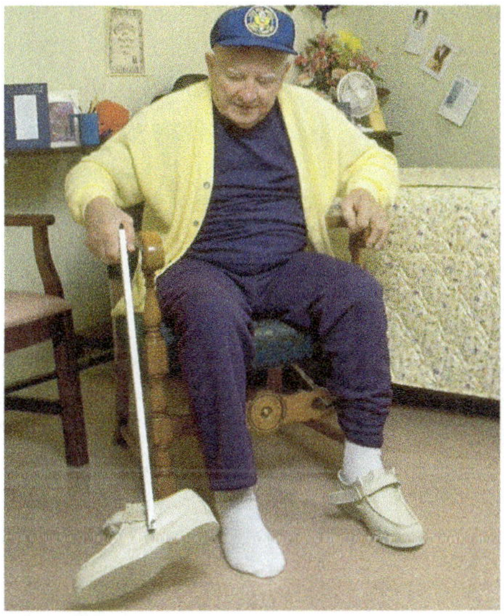

A

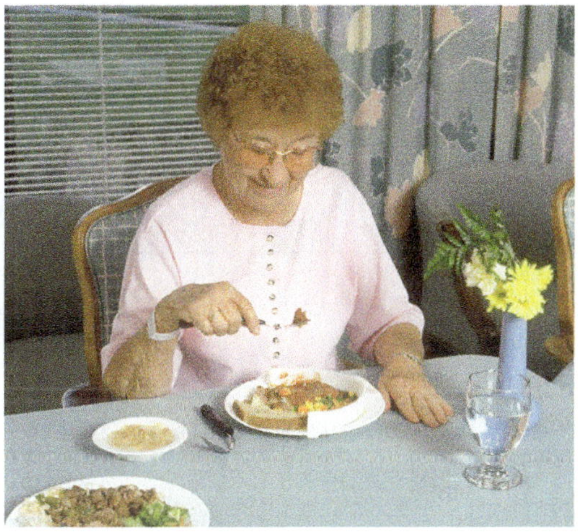

B

Figure 14.12 Using adaptive equipment: (A) male putting on shoe; (B) female eating one handed.

TERM	WORD PARTS	DEFINITION
body mechanics	-ic = pertaining to	Use of good posture and position while performing activities of daily living to prevent injury and stress on body parts.
ergonomics (er-goh-NOM-iks)	erg/o = work -nomics = pertaining to laws	Study of human work including how the requirements for performing work and the work environment affect the musculoskeletal and nervous systems.
fine motor skills		Use of precise and coordinated movements in such activities such as writing, buttoning, and cutting.
gait (GAYT)		Manner of walking.
gross motor skills		Use of large muscle groups that coordinate body movements such as walking, running, jumping, and balance.
lower extremity (LE)		Refers to one of the legs.
mobility		State of having normal movement of all body parts.
orthotics (or-THOT-iks)	orth/o = straight -tic = pertaining to	Use of equipment, such as splints and braces, to support a paralyzed muscle, promote a specific motion, or correct musculoskeletal deformities.
physical medicine	physic/o = body -al = pertaining to	Branch of medicine focused on restoring function. Primarily cares for patients with musculoskeletal and nervous system disorders. Physician is a *physiatrist.*
prosthetics (pros-THET-iks)	prosthet/o = addition -ic = pertaining to	Artificial devices, such as limbs and joints, that replace a missing body part.

Rehabilitation Services Terms *(continued)*

TERM	WORD PARTS	DEFINITION
range of motion (ROM)		Range of movement of a joint, from maximum flexion through maximum extension. It is measured as degrees of a circle.
rehabilitation	re- = again habilitat/o = ability	Process of treatment and exercise that can help a person with a disability attain maximum function and well-being.
upper extremity (UE)		Refers to one of the arms.

Therapeutic Procedures

TERM	WORD PARTS	DEFINITION
active exercises		Exercises that a patient performs without assistance.
active range of motion (AROM)		Range of motion for joints that a patient is able to perform without assistance from someone else.
active-resistive exercises		Exercises in which the patient works against resistance applied to a muscle, such as a weight. Used to increase strength.
cryotherapy (cry-oh-THAIR-ah-pee)	cry/o = cold -therapy = treatment	Using cold for therapeutic purposes.
debridement (day-breed-MON)		Removal of dead or damaged tissue from a wound. Commonly performed for burn therapy.
electromyography (EMG) (ee-LEK-troh-my-OG-rah-fee)	electr/o = electricity my/o = muscle -graphy = process of recording	The recording of a muscle's response to electrical stimulation. The graphic record produced is an *electromyogram.*
gait training		Assisting a patient to learn to walk again or how to use an assistive device to walk.

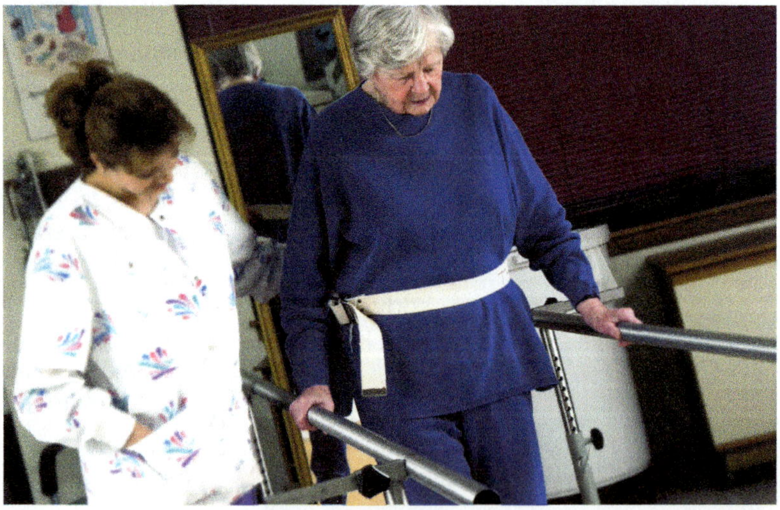

Figure 14.13 Physical therapist assisting a patient to walk in the parallel bars. *(auremar/Shutterstock)*

Therapeutic Procedures *(continued)*

TERM	WORD PARTS	DEFINITION
hydrotherapy (high-droh-THAIR-ah-pee)	hydr/o = water -therapy = treatment	Application of warm water as a therapeutic treatment. Can be done in baths, swimming pools, and whirlpools.
massage		Kneading or applying pressure by hands to a part of the patient's body to promote muscle relaxation and reduce tension.
mobilization		Treatments such as exercise and massage to restore movement to joints and soft tissue.
moist hot packs		Applying moist warmth to a body part to produce the slight dilation of blood vessels in the skin. Causes muscle relaxation in the deeper regions of the body and increases circulation, which aids healing.
nerve conduction velocity		Test to determine if nerves have been damaged by recording the rate at which an electrical impulse travels along a nerve. If the nerve is damaged, the velocity will be decreased.
pain control		Managing pain through a variety of means, including medications, biofeedback, and mechanical devices.
passive range of motion (PROM)		Therapist putting a patient's joints through available range of motion without assistance from the patient.
phonophoresis (foh-noh-foh-REE-sis)	phon/o = sound -phoresis = carrying	Use of ultrasound waves to introduce medication across the skin and into the subcutaneous tissues.
postural drainage with clapping	-al = pertaining to	Draining secretions from the bronchi or a lung cavity by having the patient lie so that gravity allows drainage to occur. Clapping is using the hand in a cupped position to perform percussion on the chest. Assists in loosening secretions and mucus.
therapeutic exercise (thair-ah-PEW-tik)	-ic = pertaining to	Exercise planned and carried out to achieve a specific physical benefit, such as improved range of motion, muscle strength, or cardiovascular function.
thermotherapy (ther-moh-THAIR-ah-pee)	therm/o = heat -therapy = treatment	Applying heat to the body for therapeutic purposes.
traction		Process of pulling or drawing, usually with a mechanical device. Used in treating orthopedic (bone and joint) problems and injuries.
transcutaneous electrical nerve stimulation (TENS) (tranz-kyoo-TAY-nee-us)	trans- = across cutane/o = skin -ous = pertaining to electr/o = electricity -al = pertaining to	Application of an electric current to a peripheral nerve to relieve pain.

Therapeutic Procedures *(continued)*

TERM	WORD PARTS	DEFINITION
ultrasound (US)	ultra- = beyond	Use of high-frequency sound waves to create heat in soft tissues under the skin. It is particularly useful for treating injuries to muscles, tendons, and ligaments, as well as muscle spasms.
whirlpool		Bath in which there are continuous jets of hot water reaching the body surfaces.

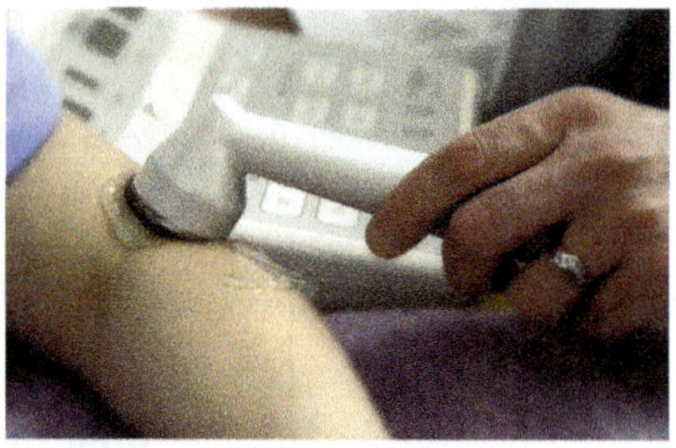

Figure 14.14 Patient receiving ultrasound treatment to the left elbow. *(GWImages/Shutterstock)*

Abbreviations

AAROM	active assistive range of motion	**PROM**	passive range of motion
ADL	activities of daily living	**PT**	physical therapy
AROM	active range of motion	**ROM**	range of motion
EMG	electromyogram	**TENS**	transcutaneous electrical stimulation
e-stim	electrical stimulation	**UE**	upper extremity
LE	lower extremity	**US**	ultrasound
OT	occupational therapy		

Section V: Surgery at a Glance

Word Parts

Here are the most common word parts (with their meanings) used to build surgery terms.

Combining Forms

alges/o	pain	hem/o	blood
aspir/o	to breathe in	later/o	side
cis/o	to cut	lith/o	stone
cry/o	cold	recumb/o	to lie back
cutane/o	skin	sect/o	to cut
dilat/o	to widen	specul/o	to look at
electr/o	electricity	tenacul/o	to hold
esthes/o	sensation, feeling	topic/o	a specific area
hal/o	to breathe	ven/o	vein

Suffixes

-al	pertaining to	-otomy	to cut into
-ia	state, condition	-ous	pertaining to
-ic	pertaining to	-scopic	pertaining to visually examining
-ist	specialist	-stasis	standing still
-logist	one who studies	-stat	standing still
-logy	study of		

Prefixes

an-	without	peri-	around
dis-	apart	post-	after
endo-	within	pre-	before
in-	inward	re-	again
intra-	within	sub-	under

Surgery

operative report
surgeon
surgery

Surgery is the branch of medicine dealing with operative procedures to correct deformities and defects, repair injuries, and diagnose and cure diseases. A **surgeon** is a physician who has completed additional training of 5 years or more in a surgical specialty area. These specialty areas include orthopedics; neurosurgery; gynecology; ophthalmology; urology; and thoracic, vascular, cardiac, plastic, and general surgery. The surgeon must complete an **operative report** for every procedure that he or she performs. This is a detailed description that includes:

- preoperative diagnosis
- indication for the procedure
- name of the procedure
- surgical techniques employed
- findings during surgery
- postoperative diagnosis
- name of the surgeon

This report also includes information pertaining to the patient such as name, address, age, patient number, and date of the procedure.

Surgical terminology includes terms related to anesthesiology, surgical instruments, surgical procedures, incisions, and suture materials. Specific surgical procedures are frequently named by using the combining form for the body part being operated on and adding a suffix that describes the procedure. For example, an incision into the chest is a *thoracotomy*, removal of the stomach is *gastrectomy*, and surgical repair of the skin is *dermatoplasty*.

Anesthesia

anesthesia (an-ess-THEE-zee-ah)
anesthesiologist (an-es-thee-zee-OL-jist)
general anesthesia
inhalation (in-hah-LAY-shun)
intravenous (in-trah-VEE-nus)
local anesthesia
nurse anesthetist (ah-NES-the-tist)
regional anesthesia
subcutaneous (sub-kyoo-TAY-nee-us)
topical anesthesia

An **anesthesiologist** is a physician who specializes in the practice of administering anesthetics. A **nurse anesthetist** is a registered nurse who has received additional training and education in the administration of anesthetic medications. **Anesthesia** results in the loss of feeling or sensation. The most common types of anesthesia are general, regional, local, and topical anesthesia (see Table 14.5 ■).

MED TERM TIP

Look for these word parts:

an- = without
esthesi/o = sensation, feeling
-ist = specialist
-logist = one who studies

Surgical Instruments

Physicians have developed surgical instruments since the time of the early Egyptians. Instruments include surgical knives, saws, clamps, drills, and needles. Some of the more commonly used surgical instruments are listed in Table 14.6 ■ and are shown in Figure 14.15 ■.

Table 14.5 Types of Anesthesia

TYPE	WORD PARTS	DESCRIPTION
general anesthesia (GA)	an- = without esthes/o = sensation, feeling -ia = state, condition	Produces a loss of consciousness including an absence of pain sensation. The patient's vital signs (VS)—heart rate, breathing rate, pulse, and blood pressure—are carefully monitored when using a general anesthetic.
intravenous (IV)	intra- = within ven/o = vein -ous = pertaining to	Route for administering general anesthesia via injection into a vein.
inhalation	in- = inward hal/o = to breath	Route for administering general anesthesia by breathing it in.
regional anesthesia	-al = pertaining to an- = without esthes/o = sensation, feeling -ia = state, condition	Also referred to as a *nerve block*. This anesthetic interrupts a patient's pain sensation in a particular region of the body, such as the arm. The anesthetic is injected near the nerve that will be blocked from sensation. The patient usually remains conscious.
local anesthesia	-al = pertaining to an- = without esthes/o = sensation, feeling -ia = state, condition	Produces a loss of sensation in one localized part of the body. The patient remains conscious.
subcutaneous	sub- = under cutane/o = skin -ous = pertaining to	Method of applying local anesthesia involving injecting the anesthetic under the skin. This type of anesthetic is used to deaden the skin prior to suturing a laceration.
topical	topic/o = a specific area -al = pertaining to	Method of applying local anesthesia involving placing a liquid or gel directly onto a specific area of skin. This type of anesthetic is used on the skin, the cornea, and the mucous membranes in dental work.

Table 14.6 Common Surgical Instruments

INSTRUMENT	WORD PARTS	USE
aspirator (AS-pih-ray-tor)	aspir/o = to breathe in	Suctions fluid
clamp		Grasps tissue; controls bleeding
curette (kyoo-RET)		Scrapes and removes tissue
dilator (dye-LAY-tor)	dilat/o = to widen	Enlarges an opening by stretching
forceps (FOR-seps)		Grasps tissue
hemostat (HEE-moh-stat)	hem/o = blood -stat = standing still	Forceps to grasp blood vessel to control bleeding
probe		Explores tissue
scalpel		Cuts and separates tissue
speculum (SPEK-yoo-lum)	specul/o = to look at	Spreads apart walls of a cavity
tenaculum (the-NAK-yoo-lum)	tenacul/o = to hold	Long-handled clamp
trephine (treh-FINE)		Saw that removes disk-shaped piece of tissue or bone

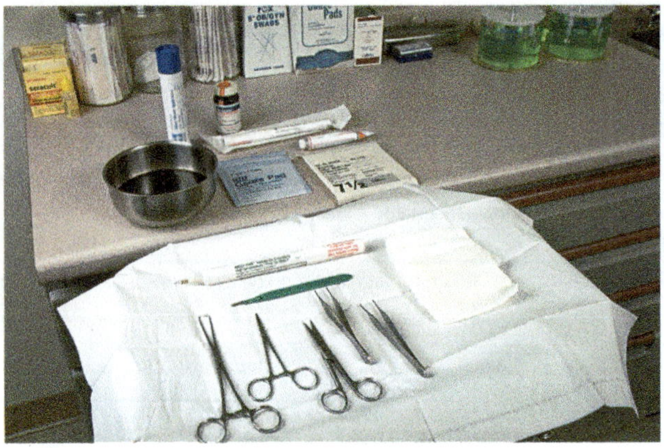

■ **Figure 14.15** Surgical instruments prepared for a procedure.

Surgical Positions

Patients are placed in specific positions so the surgeon is able to reach the area that is to be operated on. Table 14.7 ■ describes and Figure 14.16 ■ illustrates some common surgical positions.

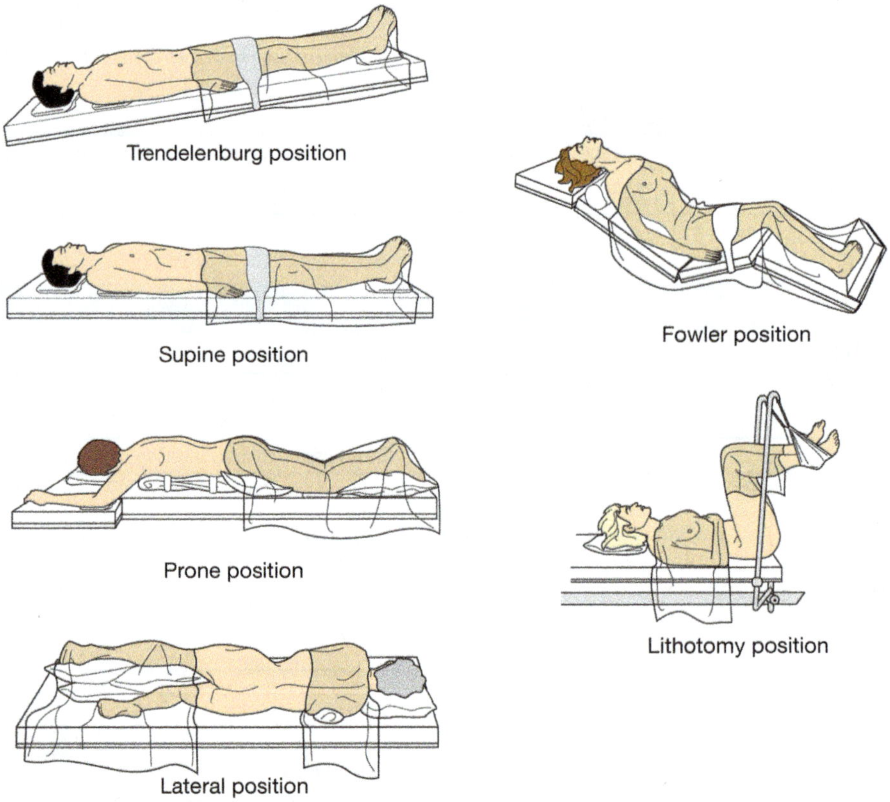

■ **Figure 14.16** Examples of common surgical positions.

Table 14.7 Common Surgical Positions

POSITION	WORD PARTS	DESCRIPTION
Fowler		Sitting with back positioned at a 45° angle
lateral recumbent (ree-KUM-bent)	later/o = side -al = pertaining to recumb/o = to lie back	Lying on either the left or right side
lithotomy (lith-OT-oh-mee)	lith/o = tone -otomy = to cut into	Lying face up with hips and knees bent at 90° angles
prone (PROHN)		Lying horizontal and face down
supine (soo-PINE)		Lying horizontal and face up; also called dorsal recumbent
Trendelenburg (TREN-dee-len-berg)		Lying face up and on an incline with head lower than legs

Surgery Terms

TERM	WORD PARTS	DEFINITION
analgesic (an-al-JEE-zik)	an- = without alges/o = pain -ic = pertaining to	Medication to relieve pain.
anesthetic (an-ess-THET-ik)	an- = without esthes/o = sensation, feeling -ic = pertaining to	Medication to produce partial to complete loss of sensation.
cauterization (kaw-ter-ih-ZAY-shun)		Use of heat, cold, electricity, or chemicals to scar, burn, or cut tissues.
circulating nurse		Nurse who assists the surgeon and scrub nurse by providing needed materials during the procedure and by handling the surgical specimen. This person does not wear sterile clothing and may enter and leave the operating room during the procedure.
cryosurgery (cry-oh-SER-jer-ee)	cry/o = cold	Technique of exposing tissues to extreme cold to produce cell injury and destruction. Used in the treatment of malignant tumors or to control pain and bleeding.
day surgery		Type of outpatient surgery in which the patient is discharged on the same day he or she is admitted; also called *ambulatory surgery*.
dissection (dih-SEK-shun)	dis- = apart sect/o = to cut	Surgical cutting of parts for separation and study.
draping		Process of covering the patient with sterile cloths that allow only the operative site to be exposed to the surgeon.

Surgery Terms *(continued)*

TERM	WORD PARTS	DEFINITION
electrocautery (ee-lek-troh-KAW-ter-ee)	electr/o = electricity	Use of an electric current to stop bleeding by coagulating blood vessels.
endoscopic surgery (en-doh-SKOP-ik)	endo- = within -scopic = pertaining to visually examining	Use of a lighted instrument to examine the interior of a cavity.
hemostasis (hee-moh-STAY-sis)	hem/o = blood -stasis = standing still	Stopping the flow of blood using instruments, pressure, and/or medication.
intraoperative (in-trah-OP-er-ah-tiv)	intra- = within	Period of time during surgery.
laser surgery		Use of a controlled beam of light for cutting, hemostasis, or tissue destruction.
perioperative (per-ee-OP-er-ah-tiv)	peri- = around	Period of time that includes before, during, and after a surgical procedure.
postoperative (post-op) (post-OP-er-ah-tiv)	post- = after	Period of time immediately following the surgery.
preoperative (preop, pre-op) (pree-OP-er-ah-tiv)	pre- = before	Period of time preceding surgery.
resection (ree-SEK-shun)	re- = again sect/o = to cut	To surgically cut out or remove; excision.
scrub nurse		Surgical assistant who hands instruments to the surgeon. This person wears sterile clothing and maintains the sterile operative field.
suture material (SOO-cher)		Used to close a wound or incision. Examples are catgut, silk thread, or staples. They may or may not be removed when the wound heals, depending on the type of material that is used.

Abbreviations

D & C	dilation and curettage
Endo	endoscopy
EUA	exam under anesthesia
GA	general anesthesia
I & D	incision and drainage
MUA	manipulation under anesthesia
OR	operating room
PARR	postanesthetic recovery room
preop, pre-op	preoperative
prep	preparation, prepared
T & A	tonsillectomy and adenoidectomy
TAH	total abdominal hysterectomy
TURP	transurethral resection of prostate

Section VI: Oncology at a Glance

Word Parts

Here are the most common word parts (with their meanings) used to build oncology terms.

Combining Forms

bi/o	life	miss/o	to send back
blast/o	primitive cell	morbid/o	ill
capsul/o	to box	mort/o	death
carcin/o	cancerous	mutat/o	to change
chem/o	drug	onc/o	tumor
cyt/o	cell	path/o	disease
immun/o	protection	radic/o	root
lapar/o	abdomen	radi/o	rays (X-rays)
laps/o	to slide back	tox/o	poison

Suffixes

-al	pertaining to	-oma	tumor
-gen	that which produces	-opsy	to view
-genic	producing	-otomy	to cut into
-logic	pertaining to studying	-plasia	growth, formation
-logist	one who studies	-plasm	growth, formation
-logy	study of	-therapy	treatment

Prefixes

en-	inward	neo-	new
hyper-	excessive	re-	again
in-	within		

Oncology

benign (bee-NINE)
carcinoma (kar-sin-NOH-mah)
malignant (mah-LIG-nant)
oncology (ong-KALL-oh-jee)
protocol (PROH-toh-kall)
tumors

Oncology is the branch of medicine dealing with **tumors.** A tumor can be classified as **benign** or **malignant.** A benign tumor is one that is generally not progressive or recurring. Generally, a benign tumor will have the suffix *-oma* at the end of the term. However, a malignant tumor indicates that there is a cancerous growth present (see Figure 14.17 ■). These terms will usually have the word *carcinoma* added. The medical specialty of oncology primarily treats patients who have cancer.

The treatment for cancer can consist of a variety or a combination of treatments. The **protocol** (prot) for a particular patient will consist of the actual plan of care, including the medications, surgeries, and treatments such as chemotherapy and radiation therapy. Often, the entire healthcare team, including the physician, oncologist, radiologist, nurse, patient, and family, will assist in designing the treatment plan.

MED TERM TIP

Carcinoma or cancer (Ca) can affect almost every organ in the body. The medical term reflects the area of the body affected as well as the type of tumor cell. For example, there can be an esophageal carcinoma, gastric adenocarcinoma, or adenocarcinoma of the uterus.

Staging Tumors

grade
metastases (meh-TASS-tah-seez)
pathologist (path-ALL-oh-jist)
staging

The process of classifying tumors based on their degree of tissue invasion and the potential response to therapy is referred to as **staging.** The TNM staging system is frequently used, with the *T* referring to the tumor's size and invasion, the *N* referring to lymph node involvement, and the *M* referring to the presence of **metastases** (mets) of the tumor cells (see Figure 14.18 ■).

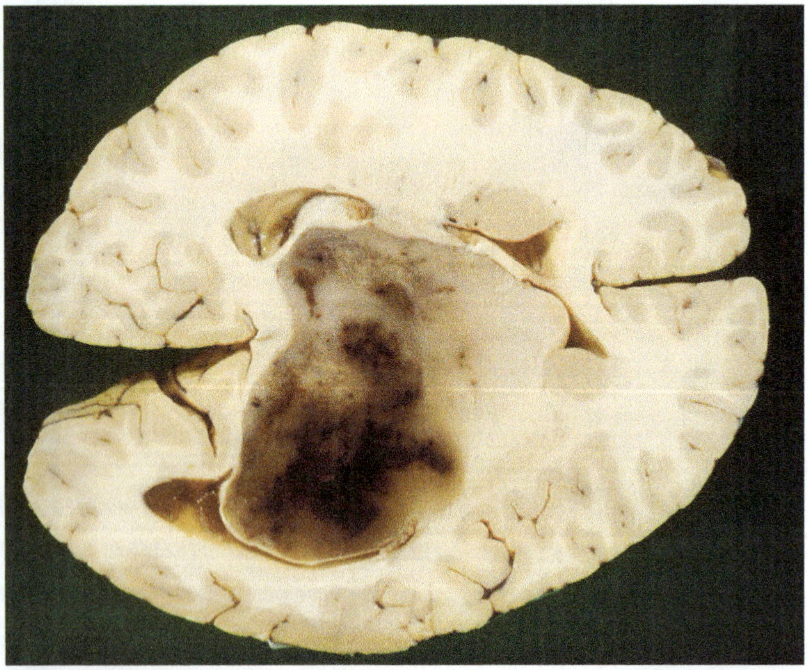

■ **Figure 14.17** Photograph of a brain specimen with a large malignant tumor. *(Biophoto Associates/Photo Researchers, Inc.)*

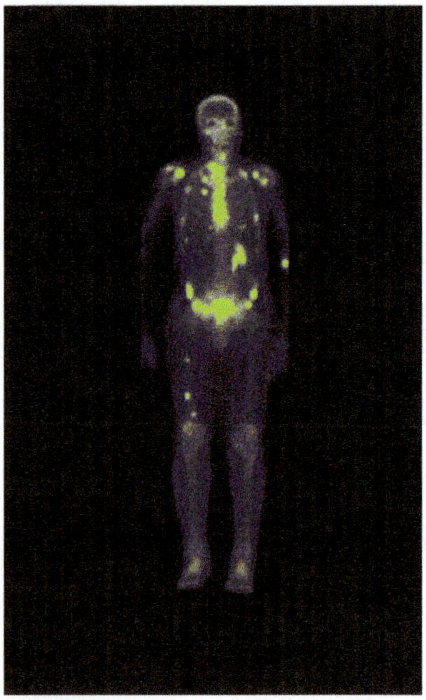

■ **Figure 14.18** Nuclear medicine bone scan showing metastatic tumors in the skeleton. *(Medical Body Scans/Photo Researchers, Inc.)*

In addition, a tumor can be graded from grade I through grade IV. The **grade** is based on the microscopic appearance of the tumor cells. The **pathologist** rates or grades the cells based on whether the tumor resembles the normal tissue. The classification system is illustrated in Table 14.8 ■. The cells in a grade I tumor are well differentiated, which makes it easier to treat than the more advanced grades.

MED TERM TIP

Look for these word parts:

carcin/o = cancer
onc/o = tumor
path/o = disease
-logist = one who studies
-logy = study of
-oma = tumor

Table 14.8 Tumor Grade Classification

GRADE	MEANING
GX	Grade cannot be determined
GI	Cells are well differentiated
GII	Cells are moderately differentiated
GIII	Cells are poorly differentiated
GIV	Cells are undifferentiated

Oncology Terms

TERM	WORD PARTS	DEFINITION
carcinogen (kar-SIN-oh-jen)	carcin/o = cancer -gen = that which produces	Substance or chemical agent that produces or increases the risk of developing cancer. For example, cigarette smoke and insecticides are considered to be carcinogens.
carcinoma in situ (CIS) (kar-sin-NOH-mah)	carcin/o = cancer -oma = tumor	Malignant tumor whose cells have not spread beyond the original site.
encapsulated (en-CAP-soo-lay-ted)	en- = inward capsul/o = to box	Growth enclosed in a sheath of tissue that prevents tumor cells from invading surrounding tissue.
hyperplasia (high-per-PLAY-zee-ah)	hyper- = excessive -plasia = growth	Excessive development of normal cells within an organ.
invasive disease (in-VAY-siv)	in- = within	Tendency of a malignant tumor to spread to immediately surrounding tissue and organs.

MED TERM TIP

The term *benign* comes from the Latin term *bene,* which means "kind or good." On the other hand, the term *malignant* comes from the Latin term *mal,* meaning "bad or malicious."

Oncology Terms *(continued)*

TERM	WORD PARTS	DEFINITION
metastasis (mets) (meh-TASS-tah-sis)		Movement and spread of cancer cells from one part of the body to another. Metastases is plural.

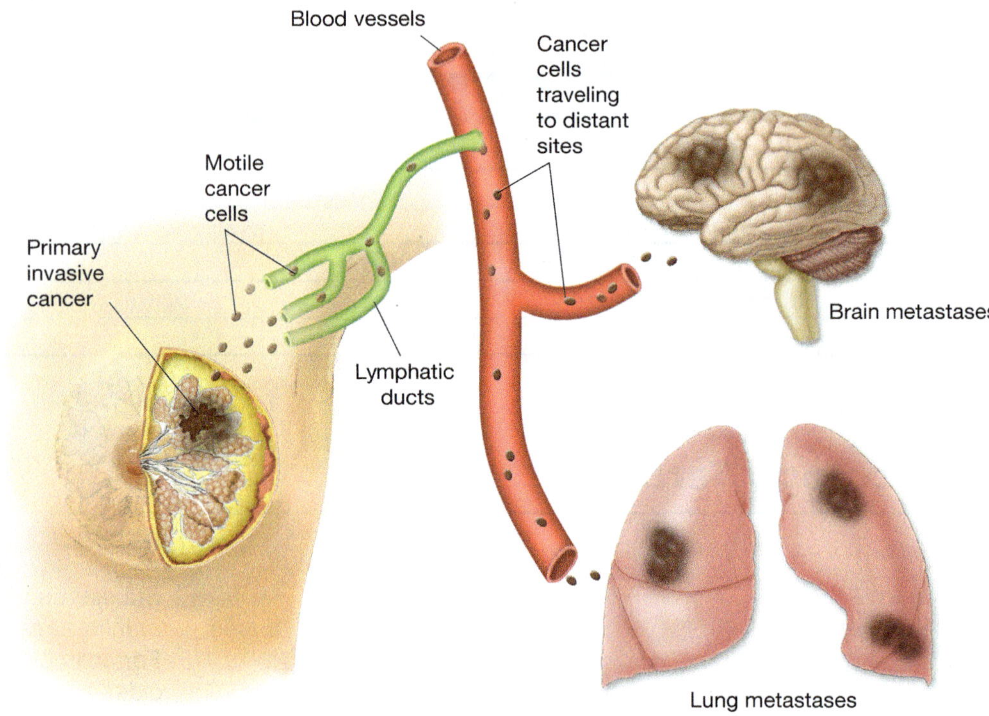

Figure 14.19 Illustration showing how the primary breast tumor metastasized through the lymphatic and blood vessels to secondary sites in the brain and lungs.

TERM	WORD PARTS	DEFINITION
morbidity (mor-BID-ih-tee)	morbid/o = ill	Number representing the sick persons in a particular population.
mortality (mor-TAL-ih-tee)	mort/o = death	Number representing the deaths in a particular population.
mutation (mew-TAY-shun)	mutat/o = to change	Change or transformation from the original.
neoplasm (NEE-oh-plazm)	neo- = new -plasm = growth	New and abnormal growth or tumor. These can be benign or malignant.
oncogenic (ong-koh-JEN-ik)	onc/o = tumor -genic = producing	Cancer causing.
primary site		Term used to designate where a malignant tumor first appeared.
relapse (REE-laps)	re- = again laps/o = to slide back	Return of disease symptoms after a period of improvement.
remission (rih-MISH-un)	re- = again miss/o = to send back	Period during which the symptoms of a disease or disorder leave. Can be temporary.

Diagnostic Procedures

TERM	WORD PARTS	DEFINITION
biopsy (bx) (BYE-op-see)	bi/o = life -opsy = to view	Excision of a small piece of tissue for microscopic examination to assist in determining a diagnosis.
cytologic testing (sigh-toh-LAH-jik)	cyt/o = cell -logic = pertaining to studying	Examination of cells to determine their structure and origin. Pap smears are considered a form of cytologic testing.
exploratory surgery		Surgery performed for the purpose of determining if cancer is present or if a known cancer has spread. Biopsies are generally performed.
staging laparotomy (lap-ah-ROT-oh-mee)	lapar/o = abdomen -otomy = to cut into	Surgical procedure in which the abdomen is entered to determine the extent and staging of a tumor.

Therapeutic Procedures

TERM	WORD PARTS	DEFINITION
chemotherapy (chemo) (kee-moh-THAIR-ah-pee)	chem/o = drug -therapy = treatment	Treating disease by using chemicals that have a toxic effect on the body, especially cancerous tissue.
hormone therapy		Treatment of cancer with natural hormones or with chemicals that produce hormone-like effects.
immunotherapy (im-yoo-noh-THAIR-ah-pee)	immun/o = protection -therapy = treatment	Strengthening the immune system to attack cancerous cells.
palliative therapy (PAL-ee-ah-tiv)		Treatment designed to reduce the intensity of painful symptoms, but does not produce a cure.
radiation therapy	radi/o = X-rays	Exposing tumors and surrounding tissues to X-rays, gamma rays, neutrons, protons, and other sources to kill cancer cells and shrink tumors.
radical surgery	radic/o = root -al = pertaining to	Extensive surgery to remove as much tissue associated with a tumor as possible.
radioactive implant (ray-dee-oh-AK-tiv)	radi/o = rays	Embedding a radioactive source directly into tissue to provide a highly localized radiation dosage to damage nearby cancerous cells. Also called *brachytherapy.*

Abbreviations

bx	biopsy	**mets**	metastases
Ca	cancer	**MTX**	methotrexate
chemo	chemotherapy	**prot**	protocol
CIS	carcinoma in situ	**st**	stage
5-FU	5-fluorouracil	**TNM**	tumor, nodes, metastases
GA	gallium		

Chapter Review

Real-World Applications

Chart Note Transcription

The chart note below contains 11 phrases that can be reworded with a medical term that you learned in this chapter. Each phrase is identified with an underline. Determine the medical term and write your answers in the space provided.

Current Complaint:	A 56-year-old male was referred to a specialist in the treatment of cancer ❶ for treatment of a suspicious right kidney mass discovered by his internist on a CT scan.
Past History:	Patient had been aware of right side pain, difficulty urinating, and weight loss during the past 6 months.
Signs and Symptoms:	Surgery to determine if cancer is present ❷ was performed and small samples of tissue removed for examination under a microscope ❸ were taken from the suspicious right kidney mass. After it was determined to be cancerous with a tendency to grow worse, ❹ a right nephrectomy was performed. Reports indicate that the new and abnormal growth ❺ was graded to be moderately differentiated ❻ and well enclosed in a sheath of tissue ❼ with no signs of spreading to another part of the body. ❽
Diagnosis:	Cancerous tumor of the right kidney. ❾
Treatment:	Post surgery the patient began a plan of treatment ❿ of the use of chemical agents with a specific toxic effect. ⓫

❶ ____________________

❷ ____________________

❸ ____________________

❹ ____________________

❺ ____________________

❻ ____________________

❼ ____________________

❽ ____________________

❾ ____________________

❿ ____________________

⓫ ____________________

Case Study

Below is a case study presentation of a patient with a condition covered by this chapter. Read the case study and answer the questions below. Some questions will ask for information not included within this chapter. Use your text, a medical dictionary, or any other reference material you choose to answer these questions.

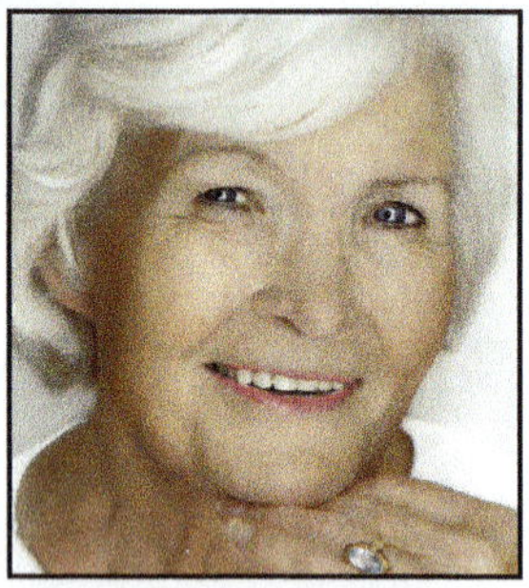

(Martina Ebel/Shuterstock)

Patient is a 72-year-old female complaining of increasing dyspnea with activity during the past 6 months. She now has a frequent harsh cough producing thick sputum and occasional hemoptysis. Patient is thin and short of stature. She is not SOB sitting in examination room. CT scan of the bronchial tree confirmed the presence of a mass in the right lung. Sputum was collected for sputum culture and sensitivity and sputum cytology. Sputum specimen was negative for the presence of bacteria. Sputum cytology revealed bronchogenic carcinoma. Patient will be referred to thoracic surgeon for consultation regarding lobectomy. Following recovery from this surgery she is to return to oncology clinic for chemotherapy and to determine if the tumor has metastasized.

1. What is this patient's diagnosis? Look it up and write a short description.

   ____

   ____

2. The patient had three complaints. List the three complaints and describe each in your own words.

   ____

   ____

3. Describe in your own words the diagnostic imaging procedure used on this patient and the results.

   ____

   ____

4. List and describe in your own words the clinical laboratory diagnostic test run on this patient and the results of each test.

   ____

   ____

5. What surgical procedure will this patient undergo? Describe it in your own words.

   ____

   ____

6. What does the term *metastasized* mean?

   ____

   ____

Practice Exercises

A. Complete the Statement

1. The reference book containing important information regarding medications is the ______________________.
2. A person specializing in the dispensing of medications is a ______________________.
3. The accepted official name for a drug is the ______________________ name.
4. The trade name for a drug is the ______________________ name.
5. What does the chemical name represent? ______________________
6. What federal agency enforces controls over the use of drugs causing dependency? ______________________

B. Drug Administration Practice

Name the route of drug administration for the following descriptions.

1. under the tongue ______________________
2. into the anus or rectum ______________________
3. applied to the skin ______________________
4. injected under the first layer of skin ______________________
5. injected into a muscle ______________________
6. injected into a vein ______________________
7. by mouth ______________________

C. Define the Term

1. idiosyncrasy ______________________
2. parenteral ______________________
3. placebo ______________________
4. toxicity ______________________
5. side effect ______________________
6. unit dose ______________________
7. habituation ______________________
8. antidote ______________________
9. contraindication ______________________
10. prophylaxis ______________________

D. What Does it Stand For?

1. gr ______________________________
2. bid ______________________________
3. tid ______________________________
4. ad lib ______________________________
5. prn ______________________________
6. ante ______________________________
7. OTC ______________________________
8. gt ______________________________
9. Sig ______________________________
10. stat ______________________________
11. mg ______________________________
12. aq ______________________________
13. noc ______________________________
14. NPO ______________________________
15. hs ______________________________
16. IV ______________________________
17. TO ______________________________
18. gtt ______________________________
19. pc ______________________________
20. d/c ______________________________

E. Prescription Practice

Write out the following prescription instructions in the space provided.

1. Pravachol, 20 mg, Sig. ī daily hs, 30, refill 3x, no sub. ______________________________
2. Lanoxin, 0.125 mg, Sig. i̅i̅i̅ stat, then i̅i̅ q AM, 100, refills prn. ______________________________
3. Synthroid, 0.075 mg, Sig. ī daily, 100, refill x4. ______________________________
4. Norvasc, 5 mg, ī q am, 60, refillable. ______________________________

F. Terminology Matching

Match each term to its definition.

1.	_______ cognitive disorder	a.	hypochondria
2.	_______ factitious disorder	b.	kleptomania
3.	_______ dissociative disorder	c.	masochism
4.	_______ eating disorder	d.	narcissistic personality
5.	_______ sleeping disorder	e.	insomnia
6.	_______ mood disorder	f.	bipolar disease
7.	_______ impulse control disorder	g.	panic attacks
8.	_______ somatoform disorder	h.	amnesia
9.	_______ personality disorder	i.	dementia
10.	_______ sexual disorder	j.	anorexia nervosa
11.	_______ anxiety disorder	k.	malingering

G. Name the Treatment

Identify each mental health treatment from its description.

1. depressant drugs prescribed for anxiety _______________
2. client-centered psychotherapy _______________
3. drug used to calm patients with bipolar disorder _______________
4. reduces patient agitation and panic and shortens schizophrenic episodes _______________
5. obtains a detailed account of the past and present emotional and mental experiences _______________
6. stimulants that alter the patient's mood by affecting neurotransmitter levels _______________

H. Name the Anesthesia

Identify the type of anesthesia for each description.

1. produces loss of consciousness and absence of pain _______________
2. produces loss of sensation in one localized part of the body _______________
3. anesthetic applied directly onto a specific skin area _______________
4. also referred to as a nerve block _______________

I. Terminology Matching

Match thet term to its definition.

1. _______ ultrasound	a. radiopaque substances used to outline hollow structures
2. _______ MRI	b. records velocity of blood flowing through vessels
3. _______ Doppler US	c. image created by electromagnetic energy
4. _______ nuclear medicine scan	d. glowing screen shows movement
5. _______ CT scan	e. making an X-ray
6. _______ contrast study	f. multiple-angle X-rays compiled into a cross-section
7. _______ fluoroscopy	g. uses radioactive substances
8. _______ radiography	h. image of internal organs using sound waves
9. _______ PET scan	i. indicates metabolic activity

J. What Does it Stand For?

1. ROM ____________________
2. OT ____________________
3. ADL ____________________
4. LE ____________________
5. EMG ____________________
6. TENS ____________________
7. PT ____________________
8. PROM ____________________
9. e-stim ____________________
10. US ____________________

K. Name the Procedure Described

Identify the rehabilitation procedure described by each phrase.

1. kneading or applying pressure by hands ____________________
2. removal of dead and damaged tissue from a wound ____________________
3. using water for treatment purposes ____________________

4. drainage of secretions from the bronchi ___

5. exercises performed by a patient without resistance ___

6. medication introduced by ultrasound waves ___

7. use of cold for therapeutic purposes ___

8. pulling with a mechanical device ___

L. Terminology Matching

Match each term to its definition.

1.	_______ forceps	a.	scrapes and removes tissue
2.	_______ tenaculum	b.	cuts and separates tissue
3.	_______ Trendelenburg	c.	lying horizontal and face up
4.	_______ lithotomy	d.	lying on either the left or right side
5.	_______ curette	e.	long-handled clamp
6.	_______ aspirator	f.	explores tissue
7.	_______ supine	g.	lying face up with hips and knees bent at 90° angle
8.	_______ probe	h.	grasps tissue
9.	_______ scalpel	i.	suctions fluid
10.	_______ lateral recumbent	j.	lying face up on an incline, head lower than legs

M. What Does it Stand For?

1. MRI ___

2. Ba ___

3. AP ___

4. CT ___

5. RL ___

6. PA ___

7. LL ___

8. PET ___

9. UGI ___

10. KUB ___

N. Terminology Matching

Match each term to its definition.

1. ________ oncogenic
2. ________ benign
3. ________ encapsulated
4. ________ relapse
5. ________ primary site
6. ________ protocol
7. ________ staging laparotomy
8. ________ cytologic testing
9. ________ radioactive implant
10. ________ bx

a. examine cells to determine their structure and origin
b. the plan for care for any individual patient
c. biopsy
d. growth that is not recurrent or progressive
e. placing a radioactive substance directly into the tissue
f. where the malignant tumor first appeared
g. growth is enclosed in a tissue sheath
h. cancer causing
i. abdominal surgery to determine extent of tumor
j. return of disease symptoms

O. Research Project: Mental Health

The increase in diagnosis of mental health conditions has been so significant in recent years that the federal government has assigned multiple agencies to study and prepare reports that address the issue. These include; the National Institute of Mental Health (NIMH), National Ambulatory Medical Care Survey (NAMCS), Diagnostic and Statistical Manual of Mental Disorders (DSM-IV), Center for Disease Control and Prevention (CDC), and Substance Abuse and Mental Health Services Administration (SAMHSA).

Using research based data, prepare an informative report on three mental health diagnosis you find of interest. Include a definition for each diagnosis selected; demographics for the study; age group most affected; education level; and income-poverty ratio. Describe the cause and effect and types of treatment for each diagnosis. Document the rate of increase of each diagnosis and the impact the phenomenon has on the general population.

Use appropriate medical terminology and apply conventional citation methods for all sources including government agency reports, medical journals, and other professional documents. Share your project with a peer for feedback. Revise the publication as necessary.

Sample list of diagnosis: Attention Deficit Hyperactivity Disorder (ADHD), Bipolar Disorder, Alzheimer's, Autism, Illicit Drug Use Disorder, Depression, Eating Disorder, Obsessive-Compulsive Disorder (OCD), Post-Traumatic Stress Disorder (PTSD), Separation Anxiety, Social Phobia.

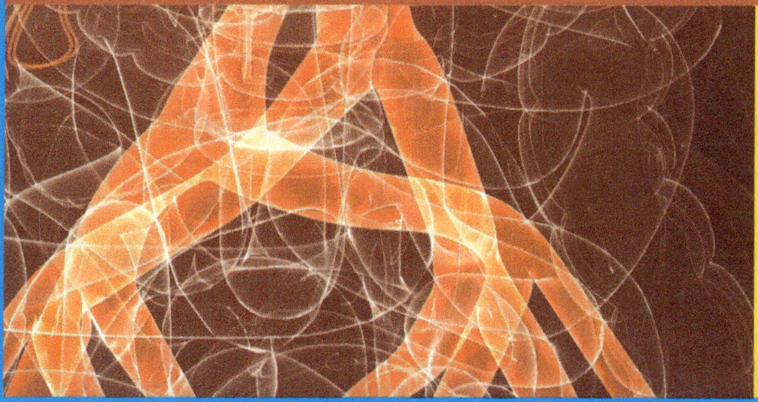

15

HEALTH CARE CAREERS AND CAREER PLANNING

Learning Objectives

Upon completion of this chapter, you will be able to

- Identify interests, values, and abilities.
- Understand health care education and resources.
- Discuss jobs and professions.
- Understand rules and regulations related to certification, licensure, and scope of practice.
- Learn about academic plans.
- List and describe professional and personal characteristics.
- Understand ethical roles and responsibilities of a health care worker.
- Explore job seeking skills, a career plan, and volunteer opportunities.

Choosing the Right Career for You

When you consider an occupation in a health care field, it is important to focus on your interests, values, and abilities. When you understand yourself, it is easier to select the right occupation. There are many different career opportunities in the health care field. Researching several careers will help you choose the right career for you. Learning how to use the resources for researching occupations will make it easier for you to choose a career.

Interests

Your interests tell what you like to do and what you do not like to do. Recognizing your interests helps you make a good career choice. Do you prefer to problem solve as part of a team, or would you prefer to work on your own? For instance, if you like to work alone, a career in direct patient/client care probably is not right for you. Working in one of the lab, medical records or research might be better. When you know your interests early in your career search, you can identify careers that use those interests. If you discover that many of the tasks listed in an occupation are not interesting to you, reconsider your choice, and research careers that match your interests.

Values

A value is the importance that you place on various elements in your life. Money might be more important to you than leisure time. Working with people might be more important to you than what shift you work. Knowing what values you feel most strongly about helps you avoid compromising the things that are most important to you. Recognizing your values also helps you prioritize your work-related values, such as job security, leisure time, wages, recognition, creativity, advancement, working environment, home life, responsibility, and management. Ask yourself the following questions.

- **Job security.** Is it important that you find a job immediately upon the completion of your training program? How important is job availability?
- **Leisure time.** Is it important for you to have extra time for leisure activities?
- **Wages.** Is an average wage acceptable if you like your work, or is a very high wage necessary?
- **Recognition.** Is it important that the job you choose is respected by the people in your community?
- **Creativity.** Do you like to come up with new ideas to solve problems, or do you prefer a job in which there is exactly one way to do things?
- **Advancement.** Do you want a career that provides opportunities for promotion? Working environment. Do you prefer to work indoors or outdoors?
- **Home life.** Do you want to work a daytime schedule (9 to 5) with some overtime and with weekends and holidays off, or are you willing to do shift work (all hours, any day of the week)?

- **Responsibility.** Do you want a job that requires you to make a number of decisions?
- **Management.** Do you want to be responsible for supervising the work of other people or for organizing many tasks at once?

All of these factors affect your job choice. Make a list of these work values and put them in order of their importance to you. When you research an occupation, refer to your list so you do not choose a job that conflicts with many of your values.

Abilities

An ability is something you do well. You have many abilities. For example, you may work well with your hands, or you may be very good at mathematics. It is much more pleasant to work in an occupation that uses your abilities. If you choose an occupation that is too far below your ability level, you will be bored. If it is too far above your ability level, you will be frustrated. It is important to evaluate your abilities during your career search. List your abilities, and use the list when researching an occupation. Match your abilities to the job description.

Health Care Preparation

A majority of those working in health care are required to be certified or licensed to be employed and to perform their assigned responsibilities. Both the certification and licensure preparation is successful completion of a specified program of study at an accredited education agency. Once a licensing law has been passed, it becomes illegal for anyone to engage in that occupation unless he or she has a license.

The certification or licensure also defines the actions and processes that may be performed by the recipient, called a "Scope of Practice." The scope of practice is limited to that for which the individual has received education and clinical experience, and for which he/she has demonstrated competency as defined by the licensing or certifying board.

Technical, community, or four-year colleges in your area may have accredited health care programs. These programs offer a variety of degrees, including:

- **Certification**, where a person is certified as being able to competently complete a job, usually by the passing of an examination.
- **Associates degree**, usually awarded after completion of a two-year program.
- **Bachelor's degree**, usually awarded after completion of a four-year program.
- **Master's degree**, a post-graduate degree awarded after completion of a one- to six-year program.
- **Doctoral degree**, the highest certificate of membership in the academic community.

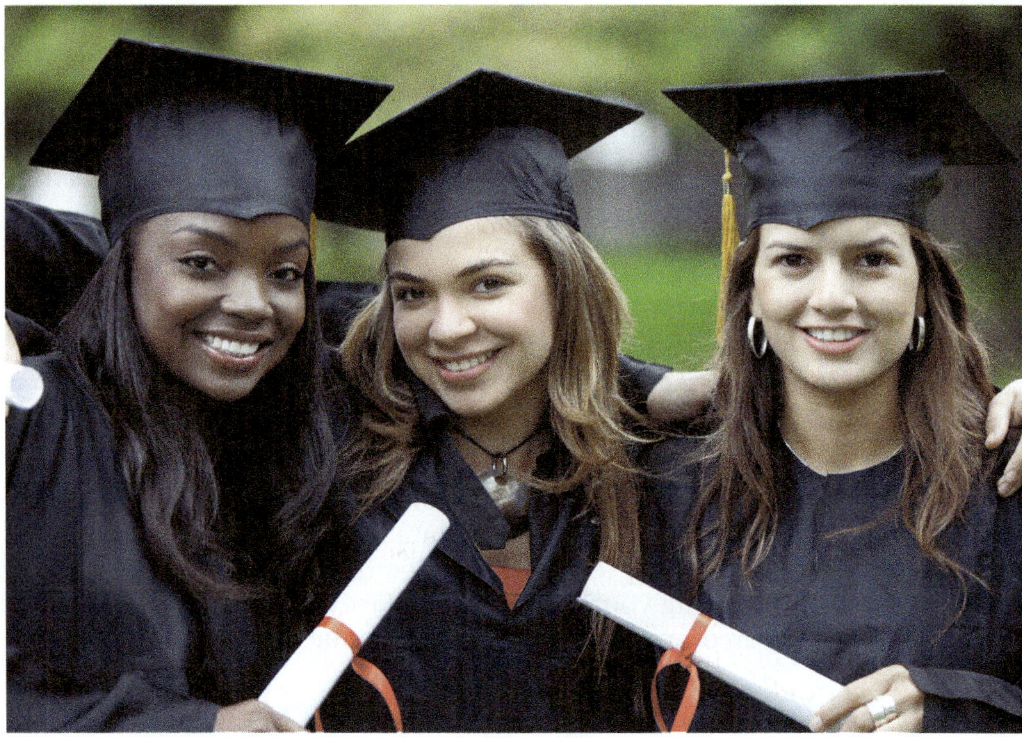

■ **Figure 15.1** When you have decided to become a health care professional, it is important to choose a quality health care education program, such as a technical school, community college, or four-year university, that fits your interests.

Visit the Web sites of different schools to see which program is most appealing to you. Visit each college and talk to students before you enroll. You may also want to talk to health professionals in local clinics or hospitals to see where they received their education.

After enrolling in a health care program, be sure to work hard at your studies. Health care information can be complicated and detailed. It is important for you to learn all procedures correctly, so you can provide the best treatment to patients.

Health care procedures and knowledge change all the time. Even after you are employed as a health care professional, it is important for you to continue your education. Take any training sessions that are provided by your health care facility. Read professional journals to learn about new health breakthroughs. Discuss procedures with other health care professionals in your facility, to make sure you are all providing the most up-to-date treatment. Continuing education credits, or CEUs, are required for maintenance of certification or advancement in many positions. This is to insure that health care professionals stay current on developments in their fields in order to provide the best patient care.

Academic Plan

An academic plan is a document you use to set goals for the things you want to accomplish while you are in school. Your years in school teach you skills and information you need to get and keep a job, and provide an opportunity to prepare for a career. Think about this: Most companies will not hire an employee who has not graduated from high school. A growing number will not hire an employee who does not have a college degree or other post-secondary training.

Developing strong academic skills can help you in any career you choose (see Figure 15.2 ■). An academic plan that is aligned with a selected career or career cluster will help you identify ways to meet the educational and training requirements and build the skills you need for the career of your choice. Start your academic plan by writing a statement that describes your long-term ultimate goal. The goal should be specific and should include career, education, and lifestyle goals. For example, you might write: *I will be an occupational physical therapist living in California by the time I am 30 years old.*

Add short-term goals that define how you will gain the skills, knowledge, and experience that you need to achieve your ultimate goal. Include a timeline for achieving each one. For example, the occupational physical therapist might have the following short-term goals:

- Get an A in health class this semester
- Enroll in advanced science classes next semester
- Volunteer at a physical rehabilitation center this summer
- By the end of the school year, research colleges and universities in California that offer physical therapy degrees Your instructors and school counselor can help you develop an academic plan. Some schools have forms you can use; if not, you can organize your plan in a way that maps your academic achievement and future plans. Most academic plans include goals in four basic areas:
- Career-related planning, skills, and experiences
- Academic preparation and planning
- School and community involvement
- Plans and goals for after high school

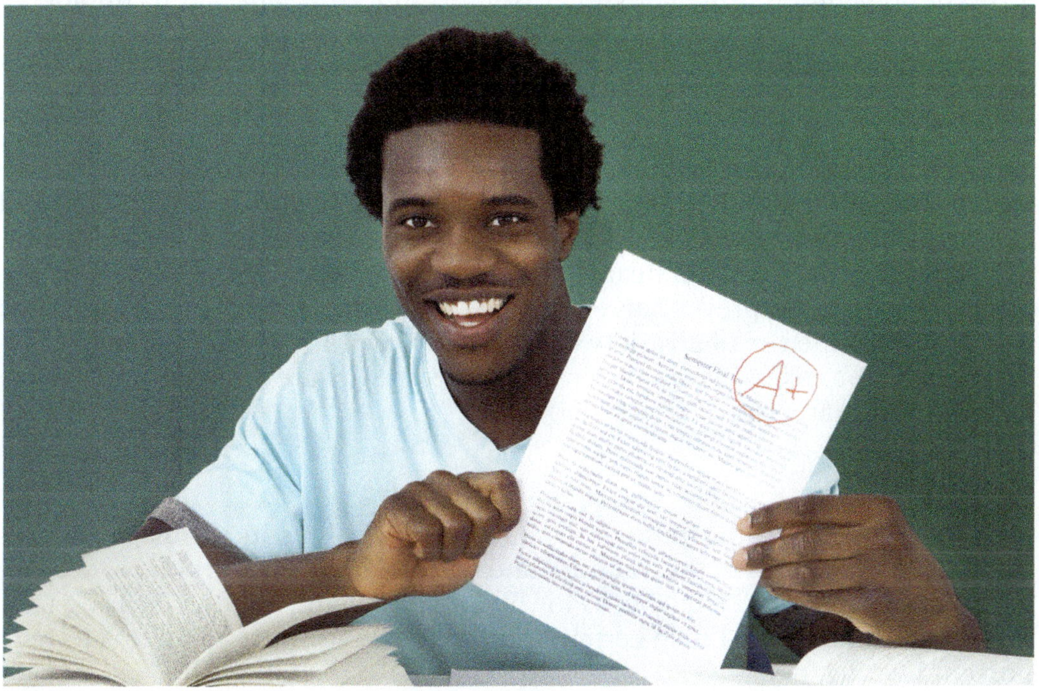

■ **Figure 15.2** Getting an A in your class could be a short-term goal.

Resources for Occupational Research

There are many resources you can use in your research. Two of them are the *Dictionary of Occupational Titles* (http://www.occupationalinfo.org/), which lists job titles, tasks, and duties for 20,000 occupations, and the Occupational Outlook Handbook (http://www.bls.gov/oco/), which discusses the nature of the work, employment outlook, training and qualification requirements, earnings, and working conditions for a variety of occupations. *Work Briefs* by Science Research Associates, the Career Exploratory Kit, the *Encyclopedia of Careers*, and computer programs are also good resources. In addition, check career-related pamphlets, microfilm, and videos. You can find all of these resources in libraries and career centers. Interview individuals who are already working in health care occupations, as well as looking at written materials.

By conducting occupational research, you learn about the tasks performed, the job outlook, the education required, the working environment, and many other things. It requires time and effort to research the occupations that interest you and to prepare for a specific career. If possible, find a mentor who performs this occupation. Spend time following them on the job site. Remember, your efforts allow you to find a job that gives you satisfaction.

Jobs and Professions

There are hundreds of job opportunities in the health care field that span all levels of preparation from aides and assistants to technicians and technologists to highly skilled professionals. Because of the nature of the work at each level, it is critical that all care providers from those involved with research to those that provide direct patient care and support services are prepared to accurately and appropriately communicate and interpret written and oral information, complete computations, possess scientific inquiry and knowledge and behave legally, ethically, and safely. Population growth, the increase of middle-aged and elderly people, new medical technology, and the need for more rehabilitation and long-term care make a health care occupation a very good choice for the future. The focus on preventative medicine and health status maintenance has also promoted the use of a variety of health care workers with different educational backgrounds, skills, and licensing. Listed below are descriptions of some of health care careers.

Audiologist

An audiologist is healthcare professional who specializes in the diagnosis and treatment of disorders of the auditory and vestibular system portions of the ear. Audiologists also screen newborns for hearing problems, conduct hearing tests for school children, and help certain industries design safety programs to help prevent hearing loss.

Audiologists must complete a doctoral degree (Au.D. or Ph.D.) in audiology from an accredited university graduate or professional and a license to practice (see Figure 15.3 ■).

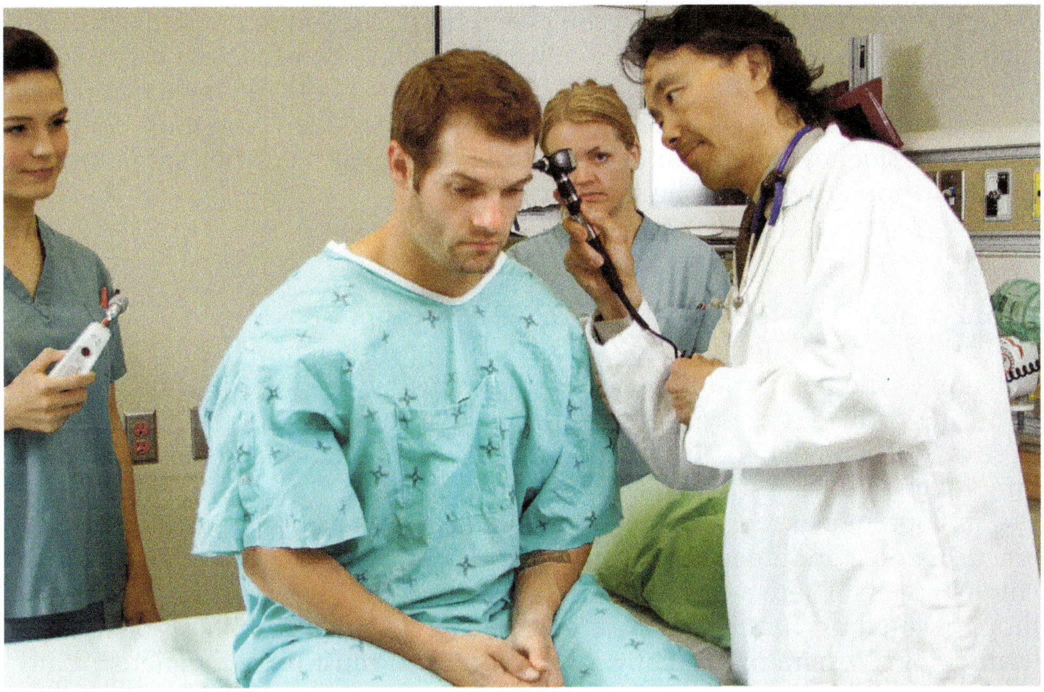

Figure 15.3
What skills and interests do you think might be necessary to become an audiologist?

Anesthesiologist

An anesthesiologist is a doctor trained to administer anesthesia before surgery and other procedures. Anesthesia is used so that patients do not experience pain during surgery and other procedures.

Anesthesiologists must complete a four-year undergraduate college degree, including pre-medical requirements. After the undergraduate degree they must complete four years of medical school. Then they must complete an internship and three years of residency; however, they do get paid during residency.

Biomedical Engineer

A biomedical engineer uses a combination of biology, medicine, and engineering to help solve medical and health-related problems. Biomedical engineers design equipment and supplies, such as MRI machines and microscopes to use in surgery; they develop prostheses; and they evaluate the use of artificial organs. Biomedical engineers must be scientific, technical, and be able to pay close attention to detail. Most biomedical engineers are employed in medical equipment and supplies manufacturing.

You will need at least a four-year degree in order to become a biomedical engineer. Some schools offer undergraduate degrees in biomedical engineering. Most biomedical engineer's hold advanced degrees in this area.

Cardiologist

Cardiologists are medical doctors who diagnose, treat, and try to prevent problems in the cardiovascular system. The cardiovascular system includes the heart and blood vessels. Patients are usually referred to a cardiologist by their primary care physicians. If a problem is suspected, the cardiologist checks the medical records, discusses signs and symptoms, conducts tests, and recommends a course of treatment. This may involve medication, lifestyle changes, or surgery. In the case of surgery, patients are sent to a cardiovascular surgeon.

Cardiologists typically work in clinics and hospitals. Some choose to specialize their practice, such as pediatric or adult cardiology. To become a cardiologist, you must graduate from college and then medical school. You must complete a residency and become certified in internal medicine. Then, you must complete another residency and become certified in cardiology. Further specialization requires another residency and certification.

Cardiopulmonary Technician

A cardiopulmonary technician, also called a perfusionist, is someone who operates a heart-and-lung machine. This life-supporting equipment replaces the function of the heart and lungs when they must be temporarily stopped, such as during cardiac surgery. Cardiopulmonary technicians must pay extremely close attention to detail. They must notice even the slightest change in heart or lung function during surgery, as any change could indicate a problem.

Cardiopulmonary technicians may work for hospitals, surgeons, or in a group practice. Some are independent contractors who work for one or more different employers. There are several different routes to this profession. In general, though, you must have a four-year college degree with an emphasis on medical terminology, respiratory therapy, or nursing. You must then complete a training program that can last anywhere from one to four years. This will result in either a certificate or a master's degree, depending upon the type of program completed. Finally, you pass a test to become certified by the American Board of Cardiovascular Perfusion.

Chiropractor

Chiropractors treat patients with musculoskeletal system problems and the effects these problems may have on the patient's general health. Most chiropractors focus on the spine, using natural, nonsurgical manipulations to realign the spine. Chiropractors may recognize that other factors—such as diet, stress, and exercise—may affect a patient's general health and encourage patients to keep their lifestyles in check.

Chiropractors must complete two to four years of undergraduate education and a four-year chiropractic college course, and pass and state examinations.

Clinical Laboratory Technologists and Technicians

These are the people who examine and analyze body fluids, and they play an important role in detection, diagnosis, and treatment of disease. These technologists and technicians prepare specimens for examinations; look for abnormal cells in blood and body fluids; and look for bacteria, parasites, and other microorganisms. They use microscopes, cell counters, and other sophisticated equipment. Most jobs are in hospitals.

Clinical laboratory technologists usually have a bachelor's degree with a major in medical technology or in one of the life sciences; clinical laboratory technicians generally need either an associate degree or a certificate.

Dental Hygienist

Dental hygienists remove soft and hard deposits from teeth, teach patients how to practice good oral hygiene, and provide other preventive dental care. They examine patients' teeth and gums, recording the presence of diseases or abnormalities.

Dental hygienists must graduate from an accredited dental hygienist program in a two-year community college, a four-year bachelor's degree program, or a five-year master's degree program. They must pass written and clinical exams and be licensed in the state of employment.

Dentist

A dentist is a healthcare professional who specializes in the diagnosis, prevention, and treatment of diseases of the teeth and gums. Other oral health professionals include dental hygienists, dental assistants (see Figure 15.4 ■), and dental technicians.

Dentists must complete at least four years of postgraduate study and have two years of clinical experience working with patients.

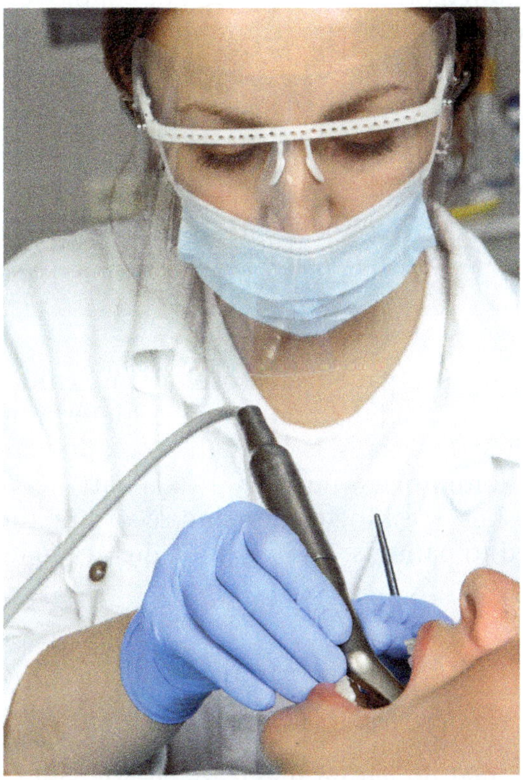

■ **Figure 15.4** The complete oral examination is one of the most important procedures that a dentist performs. What skills might be necessary to become a dentist?

Dermatologist

A dermatologist is a physician trained to treat conditions and diseases of the skin, hair, and nails. This may involve skin allergies, cancer, melanomas, moles, acne, or even some sexually transmitted diseases. Dermatologists must be able to perform various types of dermatologic surgery and be able to analyze and interpret cultures. They must also have a broad base of knowledge that includes things such as allergies and immunology, environmental and industrial medicine, radiology, microbiology, and surgery.

To become a dermatologist, you must complete college and medical school. Following medical school, all dermatologists must complete one year of clinical training. Next, they spend three to four years as a resident specializing in dermatology. Those who choose to specialize must train for one more year in that area.

Dialysis Technician

A dialysis technician is the primary caregiver for patients who are undergoing dialysis, which is a process through which waste products are filtered from the blood when the kidneys are not functioning properly. Although the dialysis technician performs the actual dialysis treatment, a nurse is responsible for overall patient care.

The dialysis technician works under the supervision of that nurse. On-the-job duties include assembling supplies, preparing the machine for use, obtaining patient vital signs, administering local anesthetics and drugs under supervision, and closely monitoring the patient before, during, and after dialysis treatment.

Dialysis technicians work in hospitals, out-patient facilities, and home dialysis programs. To become a dialysis technician, you must have a high school diploma. A dialysis technician may be trained on the job, through an employer-sponsored training program, or at a vocational school or community college.

Diagnostic Services

Diagnostic service workers help with the diagnosis of illness and disease. Some diagnostic service workers have direct contact with the patient/client, whereas others do not. They plan services and prepare and perform tests accurately. They also understand quality control and report results in a timely manner.

Dietary Aide

A dietary aide prepares and delivers food trays to patients in hospitals or facilities such as nursing homes. Duties may include: reading menu cards to determine which items to place on a tray; placing items on trays; helping the cook prepare food items; preparing foods for soft or liquid diets; pushing a food cart; serving meals to patients; collecting dirty dishes; washing dishes; and recording the amount and type of special foods served to patients. To become a dietary aide, you must have a high school diploma.

Dietician

Dieticians plan food and nutrition programs that help treat or prevent disease. They are often part of a medical team in a hospital, private practice, or other health care facility. Dieticians promote healthy eating habits, evaluate clients' diets, and suggest modifications. Some dieticians specialize in the management of overweight or critically ill patients.

Because they help identify and treat health ailments, a detailed knowledge of growth and development, metabolism, and biochemistry of nutrients and food components is required.

To become a registered dietician, you must have at least a bachelor's degree in nutrition or dietetics and complete a six- to twelve-month internship at a health care facility, food service company, or nonprofit agency. You must also pass an exam given by the Commission on Dietetic Registration.

ECG/EKG Technician

ECG/EKG technicians perform tests, such as electrocardiograms (ECGs/EKGs) and stress tests, that help physicians diagnose and treat problems with the heart and blood vessels (see Figure 15.5 ■). These tests record and monitor the

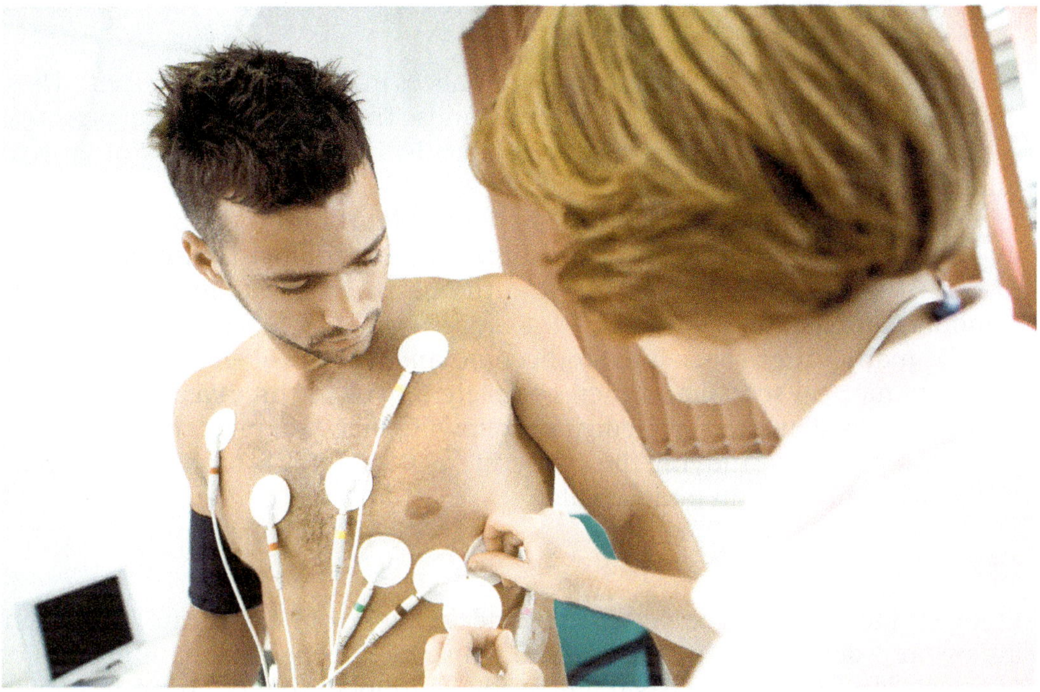

Figure 15.5 An EKG technician performing an electrocardiogram. Why does an EKG technician perform an electrocardiogram?

electrical impulses transmitted by the heart. Tracking these impulses can identify any irregularities and potential problems. ECG/EKG technicians work in hospitals and physicians' offices. Community colleges and vocational/technical schools offer training in this area, but most ECG/EKG technicians are trained on the job by an EKG supervisor or a cardiologist. Not all ECG/EKG technicians are certified, but there is a growing trend in that direction.

Echocardiogram Technician

Echocardiogram technicians use ultrasound equipment to perform specialized tests called echocardiograms. During these tests, high-frequency sounds waves are transmitted into the heart chambers, valves, and blood vessels to create an image. The technician checks the image on screen for any abnormalities, photographs or videotapes the image, and sends the images and a report to the patient's physician for evaluation.

Nearly three-fourths of all echocardiogram technicians work in cardiology departments in hospitals. Others are employed in physicians' offices or diagnostic laboratories. Although some are trained on the job, most have completed a two- or four-year program in this specialty. Professional certification is available.

EMT (Emergency Medical Technician)

EMTs are providers of pre-hospital medical care in an emergency. A heart attack, unscheduled birth, automobile accident, or near drowning all require immediate attention. The EMT administers basic life support and transports sick and injured people to medical facilities. EMT workers have many career opportunities and may work in rescue, police, and fire departments, ski patrols, hospital emergency departments, and private ambulance services.

Training may occur at a career technical school or community college. There are various levels of EMTs. The level of expertise wanted will determine the amount of training needed.

Endocrinologist

An endocrinologist is a physician who specializes in the endocrine system. These doctors treat conditions that affect your glands. This may include diabetes, thyroid diseases, metabolic disorders, osteoporosis, hypertension, lack of growth, infertility, or cancer.

Endocrinologists treat these hormone problems and try to restore a normal balance of hormones in their patients. Endocrinologists also do research to learn how glands work and to find the best treatments for patients with glandular problems.

Like many other specialties, to become an endocrinologist you must first complete medical school and then complete a two- to three-year residency to become certified in internal medicine. Following that, you must then spend two or three more years studying the endocrine system. It takes more than 10 years to become trained as an endocrinologist.

Epidemiologist

Epidemiologists study the occurrence and frequency of disease in large populations and determine the source and cause of infectious disease epidemics. For example, epidemiologists might study childhood obesity, avian influenza, or AIDS.

Most epidemiologists are physicians and work in the community, universities, hospitals, and government agencies such as the Centers for Disease Control.

Family Practitioner

A family practitioner is a doctor who provides primary care, which includes preventative care, diagnosis and treatment of illness, and health education. For many people, the family practitioner is the first point of contact for people seeking health care. The family practitioner will refer patients to a specialist as needed.

A family practitioner must complete four years of undergraduate school, four years of medical school, and three to eight years of internship and residency, depending on the specialty selected. All states require licensing. They must also complete a post-graduate year of training, more commonly called a rotating internship.

Forensic Scientist

Forensic scientists help solve crimes by collecting and analyzing physical evidence and other facts found at the scene of the crime. They analyze evidence such as fingerprints, blood, semen, firearms, and saliva. They may also reconstruct skeletal bones (see Figure 15.6 ■). Very often forensic scientists need to testify in court to help prove a person's guilt or innocence in a crime.

To become a forensic scientist, you must complete a four-year degree in physics, biology, microbiology, chemistry, medical technology, or genetics.

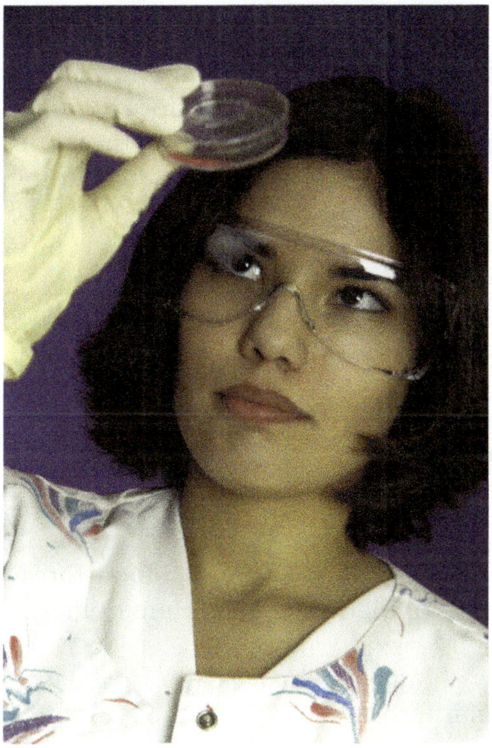

■ **Figure 15.6** Forensic science is the application of science to criminal and civil laws that are enforced by police agencies in a criminal justice system. The dramatization of forensic science in television has made this a popular area of study. What skills and interests do you think might be necessary to become a forensic scientist?

Gastroenterologist

A gastroenterologist is a physician who specializes in the digestive system. A gastroenterologist treats diseases of the gastrointestinal tract, which includes the esophagus, stomach, small intestine, colon and rectum, pancreas, gallbladder, bile ducts, and liver. A gastroenterologist treats conditions including colon polyps, cancer, hepatitis, gastroesophageal reflux (heartburn), and irritable bowel syndrome.

Gastroenterologists are trained in endoscopy, which is the use of narrow, lighted tubes with built-in cameras. By utilizing these instruments, one can see the inside of the intestinal tract.

To become a gastroenterologist, you must complete medical school followed by a three-year residency in internal medicine. Then you must complete additional specialized training in gastroenterology, which lasts two to three years.

Gene Therapist

A gene therapist treats disease by replacing, altering, or supplementing a gene that is absent or abnormal and whose absence or abnormality is responsible for the disease. Gene therapists may use DNA, the genetic material itself, as the means of the treatment.

You must have a graduate degree, such as a Master of Science in Human Genetics or a Ph.D. in Genetics and Complex Diseases, in order to become a gene therapist. Some undergraduate programs are available, including a Bachelor of Science in Genomics and Molecular Genetics, which prepares students for graduate study or entry-level research positions.

Gynecologist

Gynecologists are physicians who specialize in the female organs and reproductive system. They manage hormonal disorders, treat infections, perform routine pap smears, diagnose cancers of the reproductive system, and perform operations such as hysterectomies. Much of a gynecologists work is to perform routine check-ups so that serious problems do not occur. Some gynecologists specialize in a specific area such as critical care medicine, gynecologic oncology, or reproductive endocrinology.

To become a gynecologist, you must graduate from college and medical school. You must then complete a four-year gynecology residency and two years of clinical practice. One to three additional years of training is required if you decide to pursue a specialty area. All gynecologists must pass an exam to become certified before practicing medicine.

Hematologist

A hematologist is a physician that specializes in the study of blood, blood-forming organs, and the treatment and prevention of blood diseases. Hematologists may also run hematology laboratories.

A hematologist must complete four years of undergraduate school, four years of medical school, and three to eight years of internship and residency. All states require licensing.

Hepatologist

A hepatologist is a physician who specializes in treatment of the liver. As a hepatologist, you might deal with hepatitis, cirrhosis, genetic or metabolic liver diseases, liver cancer, liver transplants, or metabolic or immunologic issues related to the liver. To become a hepatologist, you must first be trained as a gastroenterologist.

To become a certified gastroenterologist, you must complete college, medical school, a three-year residency in internal medicine, and a two- to three-year fellowship in gastroenterology. To become a hepatologist, you must complete another one-year fellowship in which you will receive both clinical and research training specific to hepatology. Once this training is complete, you must pass an exam to become certified in this field.

Immunologist

An immunologist is someone who studies and/or treats the immune system. An immunologist may be a research scientist who works in a laboratory. The scientist investigates the components needed for a healthy immune system or the diseases that disrupt the immune system.

An immunologist can also be a doctor who treats people with immune system disorders including allergies or autoimmune disease. Some immunologists perform both duties and combine research with patient care.

Immunologists who conduct independent research usually have an advanced degree such as a Ph.D. or MD, although some jobs only require a master's degree. Training must include a combination of course- work, laboratory research, and a thesis or dissertation, followed by two to four years in a postdoctoral training fellowship. Physicians who work as immunologists typically go to medical school, complete a residency in internal medicine, pediatrics, or a medicine-pediatrics program, and then spend more two years specializing in allergies/immunology.

Internist

An internist is a physician who may provide either primary or long-term comprehensive care. They also may specialize in fields such as cardiology, critical care, infectious disease, or pulmonology. Internists, as the name implies, focus on the health of internal organs. They generally treat illnesses such as high blood pressure or diabetes, which do not require surgery. The majority of an internist's patients are adults.

Internists must complete medical school followed by a three-year residency in which they receive training focused on internal medicine. In order to specialize in a particular area, internists must complete another one to three years of training. Between 20% and 25% of all physicians are internists.

Licensed Practical and Licensed Vocational Nurse

A licensed practical nurse (LPN), or licensed vocational nurse (LVN) as they are called in Texas and California, provides basic bedside care for patients. Responsibilities are limited as all duties are conducted under the direct supervision of a physician or registered nurse (see Figure 15.7 ■).

A common task for a LPN/LVN is to take a patient's vital signs, which includes temperature, blood pressure, pulse, and respiration. LPN/LVNs also give injections and enemas, monitor catheters, collect samples, and conduct routine laboratory tests. LPN/LVNs also apply dressings, treat bedsores, and give alcohol rubs and massages. They observe patients and report any adverse reactions to medications or treatment. They also help patients with personal hygiene and ensure that patients are comfortable.

People wishing to become a LPN/LVN can attend a one-year program at a career technical school or community college. They then must pass a licensing examination regulated by the state. Many LPN/LVNs work in hospitals and nursing-care facilities. Others work in physicians' offices, outpatient-care facilities, or for pubic healthcare agencies.

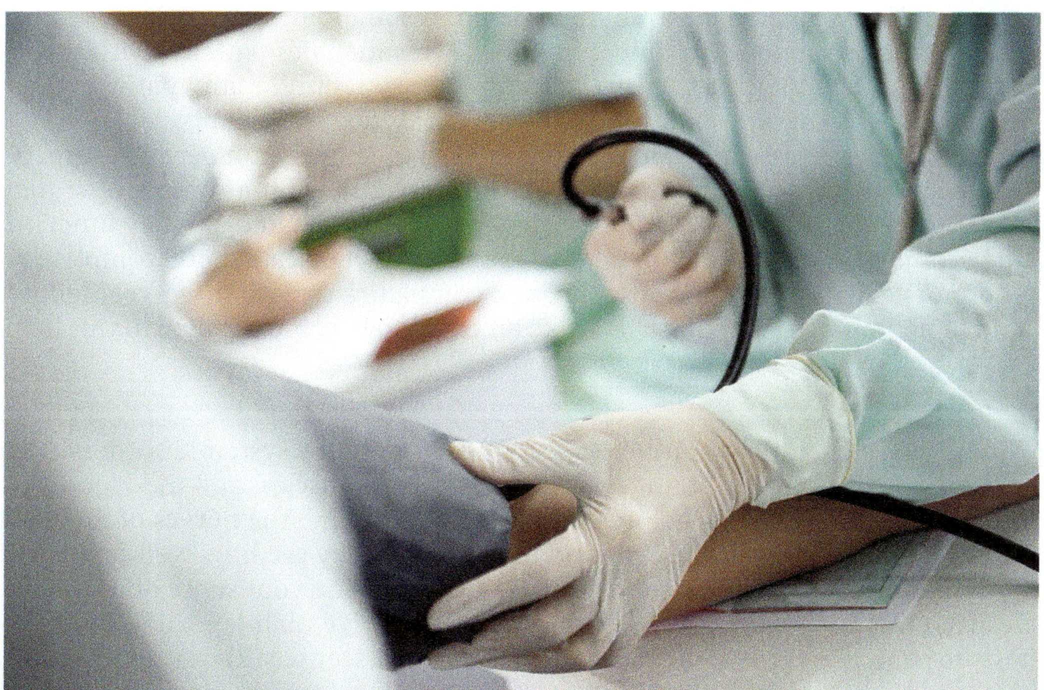

■ **Figure 15.7** Employment of licensed practical and licensed vocational nurses is projected to grow 16 percent from 2016 to 2024, much faster than the average for all occupations. What skills might be required to become an LPN or LVN?

Medical Doctor (MD)

A medical doctor (MD) is a licensed physician who is responsible for comprehensive patient care. An MD promotes, maintains health, and treats both injuries and disease. Duties include, but are not limited to: examining patients; obtaining medical histories; ordering, performing, and interpreting diagnostic tests; counseling patients on health-related issues; and prescribing medicines. Many physicians with an MD go on to specialize in other areas.

In general, MDs complete four years of undergraduate school, four years of medical school, and three to eight years of internship and residency, depending upon the specialty pursued. All candidates must also pass a licensing exam, and they must continue to study throughout their careers to keep up with advances in medical technology.

Midwife

Midwives are trained medical professionals who care for and support women throughout normal pregnancies. This care extends from the onset of pregnancy to just after delivery. Midwives stress communication with the mother and provide individualized health care information, emotional and social support, and continuous hands-on assistance during labor and delivery. If any problems arise, the midwife does not deliver the baby but calls for an obstetrician.

There are two types of midwives in the United States: direct-entry midwives and nurse-midwives. Direct-entry midwives are not nurses. However, they have at least a bachelor's degree, have completed specific health science courses, have graduated from an accredited midwifery education program, and have passed a national exam to become a certified midwife. Nurse-midwives are registered nurses who have completed an accredited midwifery program and passed an exam to become certified in this area.

Nephrologist

A nephrologist, also called a renal physician, is someone who specializes in the treatment of patients with kidney diseases. This includes patients with diabetes, polycystic kidney disease, and chronic kidney failure. Many patients must receive dialysis therapy and some will require kidney transplants.

Nephrologists are trained in internal medicine. They do not perform surgery. However, they may do a kidney biopsy in order to obtain a sample of kidney tissue. Their goal is to find ways to preserve patients' remaining kidney function. To become a nephrologist, you must graduate from medical school, complete an internal medicine residency program, and complete a two- to three-year fellowship in nephrology. You must also take an exam to become certified in this field.

Neurologist

A neurologist is a physician who specializes in nervous system disorders. This includes diseases of the brain, spinal cord, nerves, muscles, and the blood vessels that relate to these structures. Neurologists examine the nerves of the head or neck and test muscle strength and movement. They see how well you move and balance. They test your reflexes. They also examine your sense of sensation, your memory, speech, language, and other cognitive abilities. They do many tests to complete these assessments, including CAT scans, MRIs, and spinal taps.

To become a neurologist, you must complete medical school followed by a one-year internship. At least eight months of that internship must be spent in internal medicine. Then, you must complete a three-year residency in neurology and pass an exam to become a certified neurologist. If you choose to pursue a specialty area, such as child neurology, clinical neurophysiology, or pain medicine, you must complete one to three years of additional training.

Nursing Assistant

Nursing assistants (NAs) work under the direct supervision of a nurse. They have extensive daily contact with patients and are the caregivers who help patients perform day-to-day tasks such as bathing, feeding, and dressing. They help patients walk and go to the bathroom. They transport patients, take vital signs, make beds, and set up equipment. NAs assist patients with activities of daily living and works as part of a collaborative team in the delivery of health care. Because of the physical requirements of the jobs, good physical conditioning is a plus.

NAs work in hospitals, physicians' offices, home health agencies, nursing homes, private homes, and mental health institutions. To become a NA, you need at least a high school diploma followed by 120 hours of training. Some employers offer on-site training. Courses are also offered through high school allied health science programs and community and state colleges. Once training is complete, the NA may have the opportunity to be certified as a nursing assistant.

Nurse Practitioner

A nurse practitioner (NP) is a registered nurse who has received additional education and clinical training in the diagnosis and treatment of illness. Most NPs have completed a two- or three-year master's degree program. Some have a doctorate degree in their specialty. These specialties include acute care; adult or family health; gerontology health; neonatal health; oncology; pediatric/child health; psychiatric/mental health; and women's health. NPs may further specialize in everything from allergy and immunology to urology.

Nurse practitioners work in a variety of settings. They can be found everywhere from clinics, hospitals, and private practices to nursing homes, schools, and public health departments. On the job, they order, perform, and interpret diagnostic tests, diagnose and treat common acute illnesses and injuries, prescribe medications and therapies, perform procedures, and educate patients and their families on living a healthy lifestyle.

Obstetrician

An obstetrician is a physician who cares for women throughout childbirth. Some of their patients are women who are having complications during pregnancy. Obstetricians closely monitor the mother's health and diagnose any abnormalities or health issues in the developing fetus. If an issue does arise, the obstetrician may refer the mother to a specialist for treatment.

Many doctors who become obstetricians also train as gynecologists. To become an obstetrician, you must complete college and medical school. You must also complete a four-year residency specializing in obstetrics and gynecology and two more years of clinical practice. One to three more years of training is required for those who pursue an area of specialization. All obstetricians must also pass a national examination to become certified to practice in this field.

Occupational Therapist

An occupational therapist works with disabled people to help them maximize their abilities to perform the tasks of daily life. These therapists serve people who have mentally, physically, developmentally, or emotionally disabling conditions. OTs help their patients improve their basic motor functions, or, in cases where there is a permanent loss of function, they help the patient physically compensate for that loss.

Occupational therapists must complete a master's degree in occupational therapy, have 6 months of supervised fieldwork, and pass national and State examinations. Occupational therapists must be licensed.

Oncologist

An oncologist is a physician who diagnosis and treats cancer. Oncologists typically specialize in a particular form or cancer. Oncologists work closely with pathologists to assess the biological nature of the tumor being treated. Treatments include chemotherapy and radiotherapy, or surgery to remove the entire tumor.

Oncologists must complete four years of undergraduate school, four years of medical school, and three to eight years of internship and residency, depending upon the specialty pursued. All candidates must also pass a licensing exam, and they must continue to study throughout their careers to keep up with advances in medical technology.

Opthalmologist

An opthalmologist is a medical doctor who specializes in the eye and the visual system. Their job is to diagnose and treat eye disease. They also treat eye injuries. This may entail routine eye exams, diagnosis and treatment of eye disorders or diseases, prescribing eyeglasses or contact lenses, surgery, or managing problems caused by systemic illness.

To become an opthalmologist, you must complete college and medical school. That is followed by a one-year clinical internship and at least three years as a hospital resident in opthalmology. To specialize in a specific area, such as a disease, an eye part, or pediatrics, you must complete one or two years of addition- al training. Once training is complete, opthalmologists must pass an exam to become certified in this profession.

Optometrist

Optometrists provide vision care by examining the eyes for diseases such as glaucoma, nearsightedness and farsightedness, and depth and color perception. Optometrists prescribe eyeglasses and contact lenses. Optometrists do not perform surgery.

Optometrist must complete a four-year program at an accredited optometry school, preceded by at least three years of pre-optometric study at an accredited college or university. All states require optometrists to be licensed.

Orthopedist

An orthopedist, also called an orthopedic surgeon, is a physician who specializes in treating disorders of the musculoskeletal system (see Figure 15.8 ■). The musculoskeletal system is comprised of bones, joints, muscles, tendons, ligaments, nerves, skin, and any of the structures related to these body parts. Orthopedists

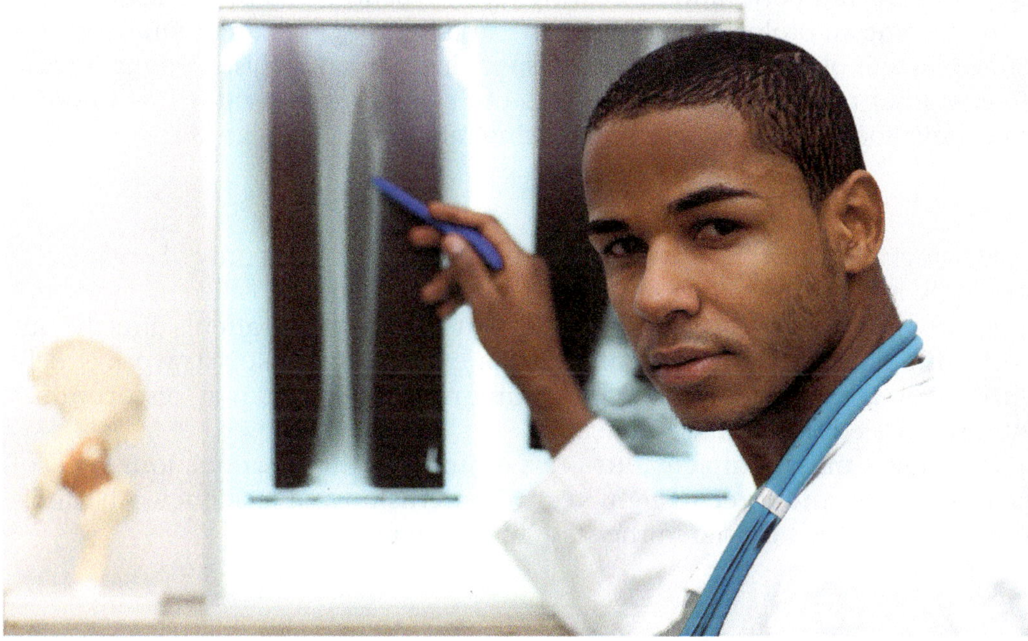

■ **Figure 15.8**
What skills and interests do you think might be necessary to become an orthopedist?

use casts to repair broken bones, prescribe exercise and medication for musculoskeletal injury or disease, and perform surgeries such as implanting artificial joints or reconstructing damaged limbs. Although historically orthopedists primarily worked with children, modern orthopedists have patients of all ages. Some orthopedists specialize in one area, such as sports injuries, but most treat a wide variety of conditions.

To become an orthopedist, you must first become a physician. That means four years of medical school and passing an exam to get a medical license. Then, you must complete one year of general surgery training followed by four years of orthopedic surgery training and two years in clinical practice. At this point, you must take an exam to become certified. Another year of training is needed to practice in a subspecialty area such as pediatric orthopedics or orthopedic sports medicine. Once certified, orthopedic surgeons must continue to take medical courses to keep their knowledge and skills up to date.

Otolaryngologist

An otolaryngologist, also called an ENT (for "ear, nose, and throat" specialist), is a doctor who specializes in the diagnosis and treatment of ear, nose, throat, head, and neck disorders.

Otolaryngologists must complete four years of undergraduate school, four years of medical school, and at least five years of surgical residency training, including one year in general surgical training and four years in otolaryngology and in head and neck surgery. All otolaryngologist must be licensed in the state in which they practice.

Otologist

An otologist, also known as a neurotologist, is a physician who specializes in conditions affecting the ears. These conditions include problems with balance and dizziness, all types of hearing loss, noises in the ear, facial nerve disorders, persistent infections, congenital malformations of the ear, and tumors of the ear. Trained as a surgeon, an otologist performs surgical procedures such as the repair of eardrum perforations, hearing reconstruction, and tumor removal.

To become an otologist, you must attend medical school and then become a trained otorhinolaryngologist. Then to specialize as an otologist, you must complete another residency in that area. All otologists must pass an exam in order to become board certified before practicing medicine.

Pathologist

A pathologist is a doctor who diagnosis disease through the study of organs, tissues, cells, and bodily fluids. Pathologists take tissue samples, called biopsies, and other specimens for analysis. Pathologists don't actually see patients directly, but work with other doctors as consultants. For example, pathologists work closely with oncologists sample and analyze tumors. Pathologists may also conduct autopsies to determine cause of death.

Pathologist must complete four years of undergraduate school, four years of medical school, and three to eight years of internship and residency. All candidates must also be licensed in the state that they practice.

Pediatrician

Pediatricians study and treat the care and health of infants, children, teenagers, and young adults (see Figure 15.9 ■). Like other doctors a pediatrician is a licensed physician who is responsible for comprehensive patient care. Pediatrician promotes, maintains health, and treats both injuries and disease.

Pediatricians must complete four years of undergraduate school, four years of medical school, and three to eight years of internship and residency. All candidates must also pass a licensing exam, and they must continue to study throughout their careers to keep up with advances in medical technology.

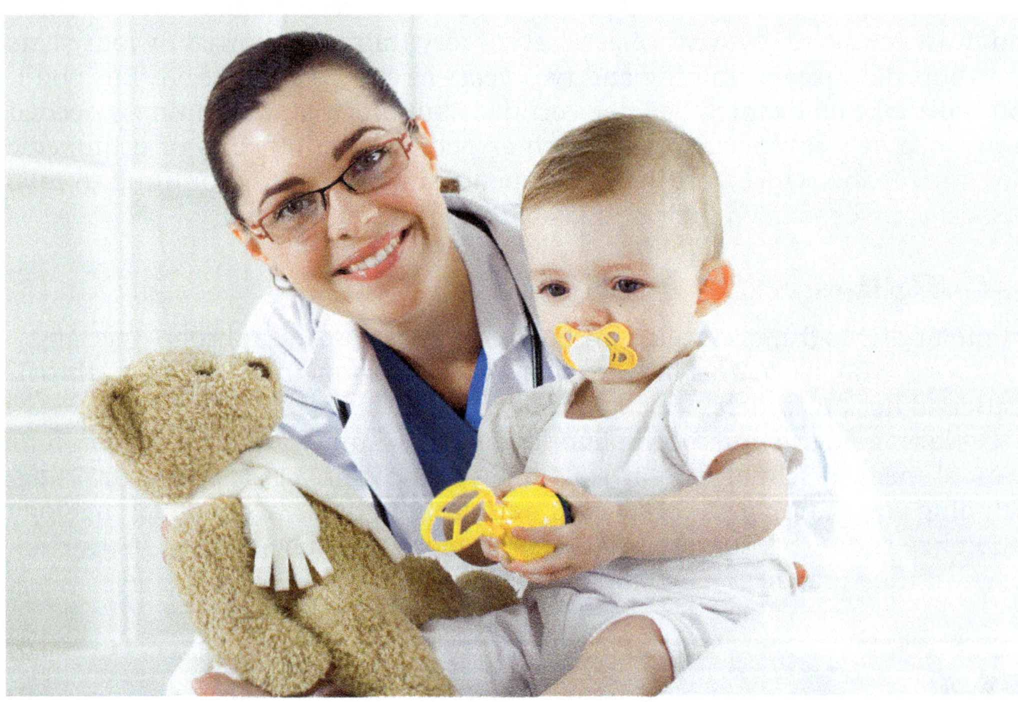

■ **Figure 15.9** What are the education, certification, licensure or degree, and skills needed to prepare for a pediatric career?

Pharmacy Technician

Pharmacy technicians work with licensed Pharmacists to provide medication to patients. Pharmacy technicians have many administrative responsibilities, such as filing, helping customers, answering the phones, stocking the shelves. They may also be responsible for counting tablets and labeling bottles. Technicians who are employed in retail may also work the cash register. Technicians employed in a hospital, may also be responsible for reading the patient's chart and preparing the medication, which would then be checked by the pharmacist. The pharmacy technician always refers any questions or problems to the pharmacist.

Currently, there are few State and no Federal requirements for formal training or certification. Most training is done on-the-job.

Plastic Surgeon

A plastic surgeon is a doctor who uses surgical techniques to correct or enhance the look or function of a person's body. Plastic surgery is used for reconstructive surgery, such as breast reconstruction for women who have had mastectomies, correction of congenital abnormalities, such as cleft palates and cleft palates, and skin grafts for burn victims. The term "cosmetic surgery" is typically used when the procedure is done strictly for cosmetic reasons.

Surgeons are required to complete four years of undergraduate school, four years of medical school, and three to eight years of internship and residency, depending on the specialty selected. All states require licensing.

Pharmacist

A pharmacist prepares and dispenses medications prescribed by physicians, podiatrists, dentists, and other health care professionals. They provide information to health care professionals and to the public about medicines. Another important task is to review the medicines that patients/clients are taking. This reduces the chance that the patient/client will have a drug interaction that can cause illness or an allergic reaction.

A pharmacist must complete five years in an accredited pharmacy program, one year of pharmacy internship, and be licensed in state of employment.

Physician's Assistant

A physician assistant practices medicine under the supervision of a physician or surgeon. Duties include, but are not limited to, providing preventive care services, diagnostic services, and therapeutic services as delegated by the physician. PAs may also be responsible for taking and maintaining the patient's medical history, ordering and reviewing laboratory tests and X-rays, and treating minor injuries.

Physician assistants programs usually last at least two years; physician assistants must complete an accredited education program and pass a national exam in order to obtain a license.

Physical Therapist

Physical therapists (PTs) work with accident victims and people who suffer from disabling conditions such as lower back pain, fractures, heart disease, and cerebral palsy. They help these patients restore function, improve mobility, relieve pain, and prevent or limit permanent physical disabilities. PTs test and measure everything from a patient's strength and range of motion to their balance and coordination. They develop individualized treatment plans that may include things such as electrical stimulation, hot packs and cold compresses, ultrasound, traction, or deep-tissue massage.

To become a physical therapist, you must graduate from an accredited physical therapy program. The minimum requirement is a B.S. degree. Many have a master's or doctoral degree.

Podiatrist

Podiatrists diagnose and treat diseases and injuries of the foot including corns, calluses, bunions, skin and nail infections, and deformities. Podiatrists also create orthotics, which are corrective shoe inserts. Problems with the feet may indicate more a more serious condition, such as arthritis, diabetes, or a heart condition.

Podiatrists must complete three to four years of undergraduate education, a four-year podiatric college program, and passing scores on national and state examinations. All podiatrists need to be licensed.

Proctologist

A proctologist, also referred to as a colorectal surgeon, is a doctor who specializes in diseases of the colon, rectum, and anus. A proctologist diagnosis and treats a variety of conditions, including cancers of the colon and rectum, severe constipation, and hemorrhoids. Proctologists often work closely with urologists, doctors of the urogenital tract in males and urinary tract of women.

Proctologists must complete four years of undergraduate school, four years of medical school, and three to eight years of internship and residency. All candidates must also pass a licensing exam, and they must continue to study throughout their careers to keep up with advances in medical technology.

Psychiatrist

A physiatrist is a doctor who specializes in the diagnosis and treatment of mental illness. Mental health problems may be treated with non-medical treatments (such as psychotherapy and psychoanalysis) in which the doctor helps the patient work through their problems. If necessary, medication is used to correct chemical imbalances. Hospitalization may also be required.

A physiatrist must complete four years of undergraduate school, four years of medical school, and three to eight years of internship and residency, depending on the specialty selected. All states require licensing.

Psychologist

Psychologists study human behavior and the human mind. There are many different fields of psychology including clinical, educational, and research. The majority of psychologists are clinical psychologists (see Figure 15.10 ■). They provide mental and emotional health care for people in crisis. Clinical psychologists are

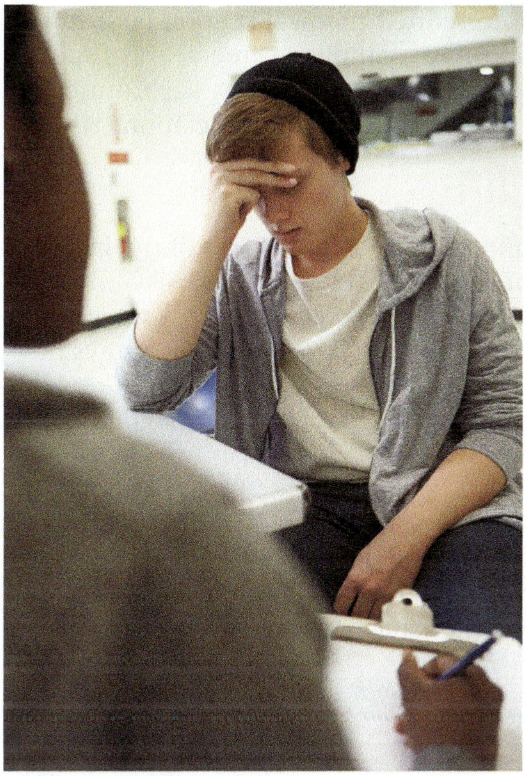

■ **Figure 15.10** School psychologists are mental health experts who help students succeed both in and outside of the classroom. What skills might be required of a school psychologist?

typically not allowed to prescribe medication. They can consult with a psychiatrist when treatment requires medication. Other types of psychologists include school psychologists, who work with students, teachers, and families, and counseling psychologists.

A psychologist must complete a master's or doctoral degree, and a license is required. To have an independent practice, a doctoral degree is required.

Pulmonologist

Pulmonologists are physicians who are specially trained to treat diseases and conditions of the chest. These conditions, which affect the lungs and bronchial tubes, include such things as pneumonia, asthma, tuberculosis, and emphysema. Pulmonologists do not perform major surgical procedures, but they do often obtain samples from the lining of a lung or the chest wall for diagnostic testing.

Pulmonology is a subspecialty of internal medicine. This means that in order to become a pulmonologist, you must first become certified in internal medicine. It takes at least seven years to accomplish this. Once this is completed, you must continue your studies for two or three more years focusing on conditions specifically related to the respiratory system.

Radiologist

A radiologist is a doctor who uses medical imaging techniques to diagnosis and treat disease. A variety of tools are used, including X-rays; fluoroscopy, which provides real-time images of the internal organs; magnetic resonance imaging (MRI); and ultrasound. The radiologic technologist (see below) is typically the person who acquires the images and then the radiologist analysis and evaluates the images.

A radiologist must graduate from an accredited medical school, be licensed to practice medicine in the state of employment, complete three years of special training in radiology, and be recognized and by the board and by the Council on Medical Education and Hospitals of the American Medical Association.

Radiologic Technician/Technologist

Radiologic technicians operate X-ray equipment to take pictures of the internal parts of the body. The X- rays provide information for the diagnosis and treatment of patients. For example, X-rays of the chest help detect lung diseases such as lung cancer and tuberculosis. Some of the diseases or injuries that X-rays help diagnose or treat include ulcers, blood clots, cancer, and fractures. The use of imaging techniques like ultra- sound and magnetic resonance imaging (MRI) is growing. The term diagnostic imaging includes these procedures as well as X-ray techniques.

A radiologic technologist must graduation from an accredited program, have a bachelor's degree in radiologic technology, experience in two or more radiologic disciplines (such as nuclear medicine or radiation therapy), and be registered as a radiologic technologist through the American Registry of Radiologic Technologies (ARRT).

Registered Nurse

Registered nurses (RNs) are involved in every aspect of patient care. Some RNs treat patients. They per- form diagnostic tests and analyze the results. They give treatment and medication, and they closely observe patients and record their progress as well as any reactions. Other medical professionals use this detailed record as a basis for proper patient care. RNs also help with patient follow-up and rehabilitation.

Some RNs work with the public rather than individual patients. They educate the public on warning signs and symptoms of various conditions and tell them where to get help. Some RNs run immunization clinics and blood drives. Some are trained in grief counseling. RNs account for the largest health-care occupation. Although they may work in a variety of settings, roughly three out of every five RNs works in a hospital.

To become an RN, one must graduate from an approved nursing program and pass a national licensing exam. There are three main ways to become an RN. One option is to get a Bachelor of Science degree in nursing (BSN) through a four-year program at a college or university. A second option is an associate's degree in nursing (ADN) through a two- or three-year program at a community or junior college.

The third option is to go through a three-year diploma program at a hospital. Advancement opportunities are usually broader for those who complete a BSN program. A master's degree is usually required to work in administration or teaching.

Respiratory Therapist

Respiratory therapists work with patients who have breathing or other cardiopulmonary disorders. Working under the direction of a physician, these specialists evaluate, treat, and care for patients and are primarily responsible for all respiratory care therapeutic treatments and diagnostic procedures. They also supervise respiratory care technicians, who perform many of these same functions.

Many respiratory therapists work in hospitals. Some work for home health care agencies and travel to patients' homes. Many programs at colleges, universities, medical schools, and vocational/technical schools offer programs in respiratory therapy.

Some programs offer associate's degrees, which would prepare you for an entry-level position. Others offer bachelor's degrees, which would prepare you for an advanced position in this field. Graduates must then pass a test and become either a Registered Respiratory Therapist or a Certified Respiratory Therapist.

Surgeon

A surgeon is a medical doctor who performs surgery. Surgeons also correct physical deformities and repair bone and tissue after injuries (see Figure 15.11 ■). A patient must be under anesthesia before surgery is performed. Most surgeons specialize in a specific type of surgery, such as cardiovascular surgery, neurological surgery, orthopedic surgery, or plastic surgery.

Surgeons are required to complete four years of undergraduate school, four years of medical school, and three to eight years of internship and residency, depending on the specialty selected. All states require licensing.

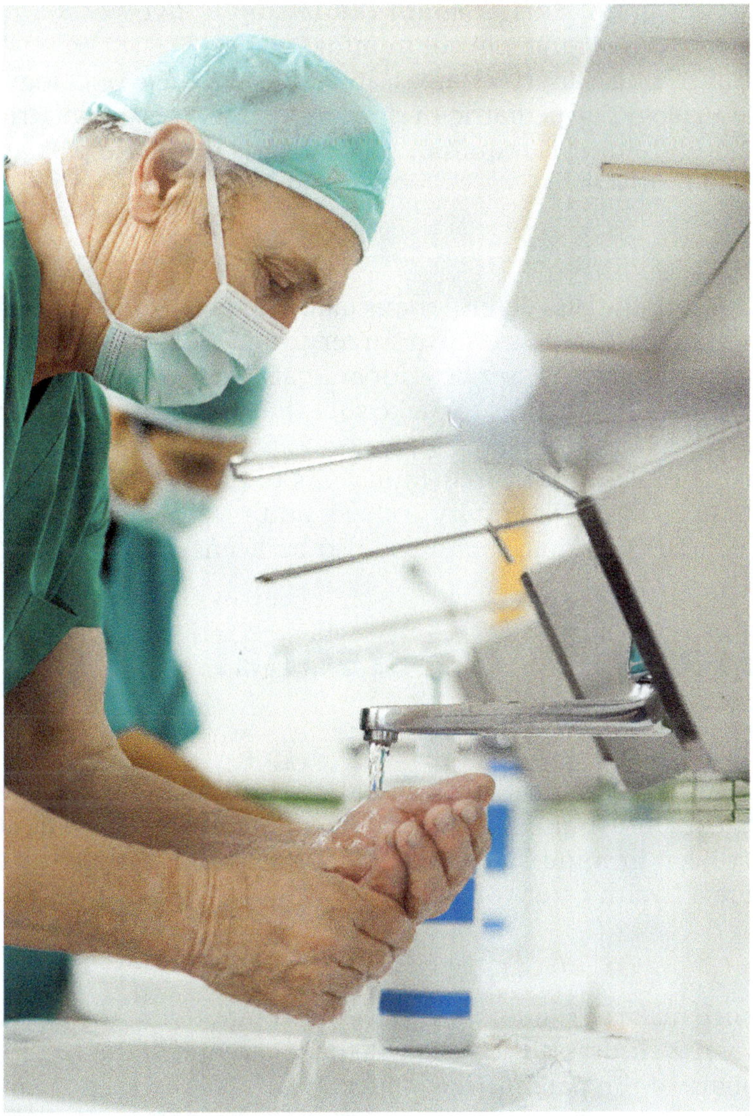

■ **Figure 15.11** What special skills might be required of a surgeon?

Surgical Technologist

These are the people who help prepare the operating room before surgery. Surgical technologists set up the surgical instruments and equipment, sterile drapes, and sterile solutions. They assemble equipment, and check and adjust it to ensure that it is working properly during surgery.

In order to become a surgical technologist, you need an undergraduate degree in this area. You can also obtain certification in this field by attending a CAAHEP-accredited program and passing a national certification examination.

Urologist

Urologists specialize in issues related to the male and female urinary tracts and the male reproductive organs. People see urologists for issues ranging from discomfort while urinating to male infertility. Urologists look for such things as signs of infection, blood in the urine, or excess sugars or protein, which could indicate diabetes or other kidney problems. Because urologists encounter such a wide variety of issues, they must have a broad knowledge of internal medicine, pediatrics, gynecology, and other specialties.

Urologists must graduate from medical school and then complete an accredited urology residency pro- gram. This program can last up to five years and involves a combination of surgical and clinical training.

Urologists can specialize in a variety of areas, including urologic oncology, male infertility, female urology, or pediatric urology. To practice as a pediatric urologist, one more year of training is required. All urologists must also pass an exam to become certified in this field.

Veterinarian

A veterinarian is a doctor for animals. Veterinarians take care of sick and injured animals; provide preventative services; perform surgery as needed; and provide offer all other diagnostic and treatment services for animals. Some veterinarians may focus on animal production practices to make sure that animal diseases are not spread to humans.

A veterinarian must completion of three–four years of pre-veterinary college, graduate from an accredited veterinary college, and receive a Doctor of Veterinary Medicine degree. Veterinarians must also be licensed in the state of employment.

Professional and Personal Characteristics

Health care workers must maintain a professional appearance and practice professional behavior. They must also safeguard the confidentiality of patient information. You must keep in mind all of these standards of appearance and behavior as you become a health care worker.

Standards of Appearance

A professional appearance makes a statement about your commitment to patient care. A well-groomed and well-dressed staff signals that everyone in the facility is interested in the welfare of the patient (see Figure 15.12 ■). A clean appearance reassures patients who may be anxious and sick that the staff is efficient,

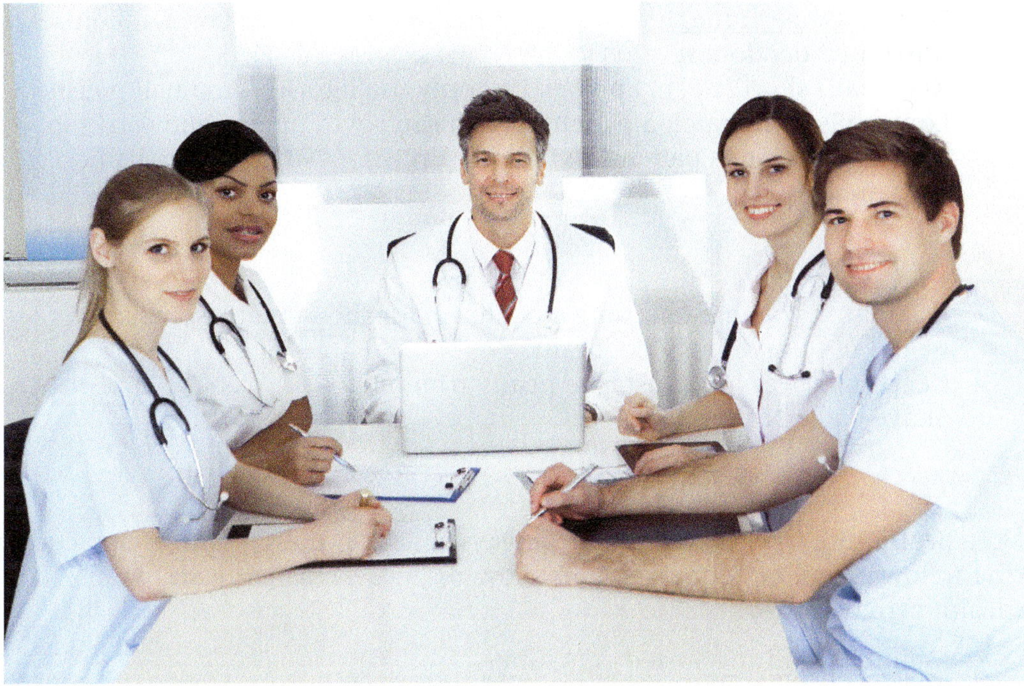

Figure 15.12
Health care workers should be well-groomed and professional. Why do the health care workers in the photograph appear professional?

professional, and capable of providing necessary medical service. The following are recommendations for maintaining a well-groomed, professional appearance.

- Dress according to your facility's dress code. This usually means that clothes will be clean, neat, and in good repair. They should not be of extreme fashion.
- Wear your name badge every day, in view of patients/clients. People need to be able to relate to you, and to call you if they need you. It also helps them identify who is assisting them.
- Wear clean and appropriate shoes every day.
- Keep your hair clean.
- Follow rules of good hygiene:
- Brush your teeth at least twice a day.
- Floss daily.
- Use mouthwash or breath mints.
- Bathe daily.
- Use unscented deodorant. Remember that odors can be offensive to patients that are ill and nauseated and some patients may be allergic to perfumes and scented deodorants.
- Wear your hair up and off your collar. You do not want your hair to fall on a patient when working with them, nor do you want to block their view.

Female

- Undergarments should match the body color, so as not to "show." When wearing a skirt, wear full-length hose without runs.
- Keep makeup conservative (e.g., no dark, heavy makeup).
- Keep jewelry to a minimum (e.g., watch, stud earrings, and a ring). Jewelry can cause injury to the patient and the professional (if the patient grabs on to it), as well as transmit germs. Body piercings do not indicate a professional appearance, and can cause infections.

- Do not use perfume or cologne, for the same reason as you would use unscented deodorant.
- Keep nails short, clean, and bare, or only use light-colored nail polish. Long nails can scratch a patient. Polish can cover up dirt and can chip and contaminate a patient's wound or dressing. No acrylic or artificial nails are allowed.

Male

- Do not use cologne or strong aftershave, for the same reason as you would use unscented deodorant.
- Keep your beard or mustache neatly trimmed.
- Shave daily. No stubble!

Standards of Behavior

As a health care worker, you should always behave professionally. By practicing the following set of behaviors, you show respect for patients and your fellow health care workers.

- Maintain a calm, courteous manner.
- Listen carefully when patients or other health care workers are speaking with you.
- Monitor patients appropriately, in order to ensure their safety.
- Perform tasks efficiently and carefully.
- Do not gossip about patients or other health care workers.
- Do not use coarse or offensive language.
- Do not practice horseplay or other dangerous behaviors.
- Watch for hazardous situations and correct any hazards that you see.
- Follow all safety procedures that are required by your health care facility.

Personal Characteristics

In addition to professional behavior, health care workers who exhibit the following personal characteristics will be more involved and interested in the welfare of their patients and in being a critical part of the medical team.

- **Empathy:** being sensitive to and experiencing the feelings, thoughts, and experiences of another
- **Honesty:** being fair, truthful, and morally upright
- **Dependability:** being reliable or trustworthy
- **Willingness to learn:** having the openness to admit that you don't know the answer or that you can be helped to understand a situation more fully
- **Patience:** having the ability to put up with waiting, delay, or provocation without becoming annoyed or upset, or to act calmly when faced with difficulties
- **Acceptance of criticism:** having the ability to deal with disapproval or a suggestion that something can be improved
- **Enthusiasm:** showing excited interest in or eagerness to do something
- **Self-motivation:** being energetic, ambitious and able to get things done without being directed by others
- **Tact:** avoiding giving offense; having an intuitive sense of what is right or appropriate

- **Competence:** having the ability to do something well, measured against a standard, especially ability acquired through experience or training
- **Responsibility:** accountability; the state of being accountable to somebody or for something
- **Discretion:** showing tact; the good judgment and sensitivity needed to avoid embarrassing or upsetting others
- **Teamwork:** working cooperatively with other people, subordinating personal interests in order to achieve a common goal

Communicating in the Workplace

Knowing how to use communication skills to manage workplace conflict will help you earn the respect of your supervisor and co-workers (see Figure 15.13 ■). It will make you a valuable member of your work team.

The steps for effective communication include:

- **Be clear.** Use words and body language that the other person can understand, and that send a clear message.
- **Be personal.** Address the other person by his or her name or title. Use "I" statements to show that you take responsibility for your role in the conflict.
- **Be positive.** State your message in positive terms directed at how to achieve your common goal.
- **Get to the point.** Explain why you feel or think this way.
- **Use active listening.** Be sure you hear the response.
- **Think before you respond.** Use critical thinking instead of emotions.
- **Recognize any potential communication barriers,** such as language barriers, cultural barriers, or value/belief barriers. Think about ways you can overcome these barriers—both when you listen and when you speak.

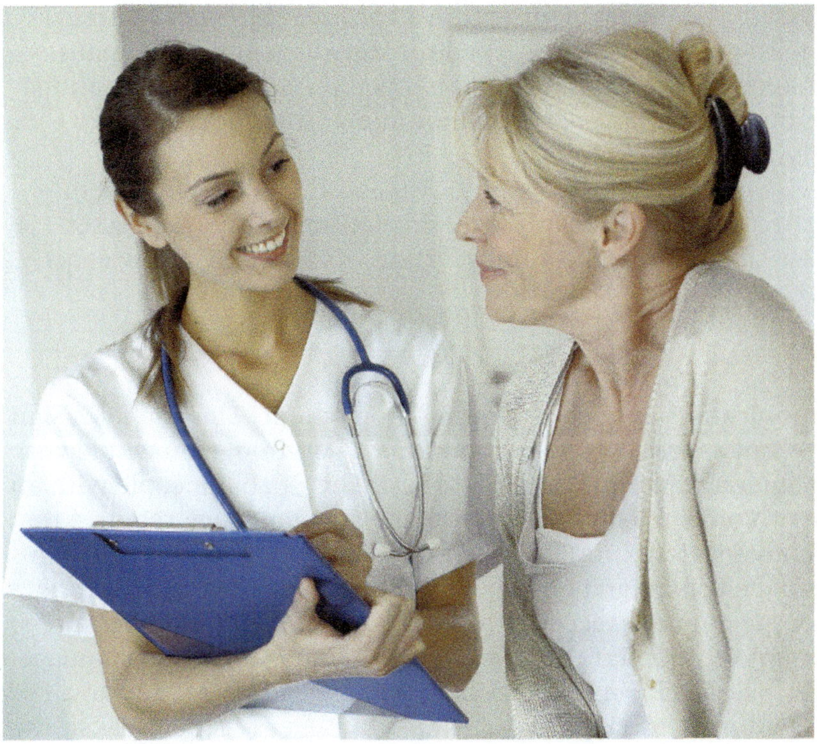

■ **Figure 15.13** Why is communication such an important skill for health care workers?

Good interpersonal relationships are fostered through positive attitudes toward each other. Interpersonal competency comes from being self-aware and using that self-awareness to relate to others. Respecting and valuing the input of your team members creates an environment in which each person gives individually to make a better whole. Practicing positive interactions encourages each team member to focus on team goals and quality outcomes.

Different Types of Verbal Communication

Just as you use different types of verbal communication when speaking to your friends and your parents, you use different types of verbal communication when speaking to people with whom you relate on the job, such as your boss, your co-workers, your customers, and your subordinates—the people you supervise.

- Your boss has a higher rank in the company than you do and has control over your job. When communicating with a boss, you usually use a formal style of verbal communication. You show deference—courteous regard or respect—by using his or her title and refraining from jokes or casual remarks you might use with a friend. You must also recognize that your boss has the final say on most matters, and so you must know when to agree with his or her decisions, even if you disagree with them personally.
- Your co-workers, or colleagues, have the same rank in the company that you do. This does not mean that you should joke around with them as you do with your friends. It also does not mean you should use the same style of verbal communication you would use with your boss. You can speak to them more casually.
- Your customers are the source of your business. When communicating with customers, remember the old saying, "the customer is always right." This means that in order to be successful, you must respect your customers and speak with them positively. You may also interact with "internal customers." If one department within a company supplies another department with goods or services, then the department being supplied is the "internal customer." What would happen if customer expectations for good communication and service are unmet? How should you go about identifying customers?
- If you supervise others in the company, you communicate with them using the respect that is due to any worker. You can also use an assertive or positive style of verbal communication, so that they know exactly what is expected of them.

Different Types of Non-Verbal Communication

Non-verbal communication helps puts words into context. This includes sign language and body language. You can communicate everything you would with speech using sign language, without saying a word. This enables people with an inability to use their voices to communicate. Using sign language requires that all parties in the conversation know how to understand the various signs. This problem is often solved using sign language interpreters who sign as someone is speaking to deliver spoken messages to those who cannot hear them, and translate the signed communication for those who cannot understand sign language.

Body language includes facial expressions, posture, gestures, and tone. A smile indicates friendliness or happiness. Rolling your eyes or slouching shows disrespect. Crossed arms indicate defensiveness. Body language can be either positive or negative. It can show you are confident and prepared or that you are unsure or afraid.

Finally, one other way to communicate without speaking or writing is to use visual aids—pictures, graphs, charts, or anything without words that conveys your ideas. Visual aids can often deliver a clearer or more easily understood message than written or verbal communication.

Be cognizant of the non-verbal communications that you utilize both with patients and with colleagues. By using the above techniques, you can clearly demonstrate non-verbal communication in a clear, concise, and effective manner. This will help you in your overall communications as a health professional.

Maintaining Confidentiality

On April 14, 2003, new federal regulations to protect medical privacy went into effect. The law, known as Health Insurance Portability and Accountability Act (HIPAA), creates a national standard for medical privacy and gives patients greater control over their personal health information. Any oral or recorded information relating to the past, present or future physical or mental health of an individual, including the provision of healthcare to the individual, or the payment for healthcare is by law to be kept confidential. The term covers not only the traditional medical records but also a doctor's personal notes and billing information.

Maintaining the confidentiality of medical records is critical. Medical records contain private information that must not be shared with people who are not involved in the patient's health care. If some private information gets into the wrong hands, it may be used to damage the patient's personal reputation or financial well-being.

Each patient signs a confidentiality form before receiving treatment. This form is a legally binding document that promises that the medical facility will protect patient information. Any health care worker who does not follow procedures to ensure patient confidentiality may be reprimanded.

As a health care worker, you should learn your health care facility's policies and procedures related to confidentiality. Carefully follow these procedures to protect patient privacy.

Ethical Roles and Responsibilities of a Health Care Worker

Many health care facilities have an adopted "Code of Ethics" for their staff. Members of the health care team must be aware of their ethical roles and responsibilities. This awareness protects them, the patients, their co-workers, and the facility where they work. Ethical behavior ensures quality patient care, positive work relationships, and a well-managed workplace environment.

Ethics is a code of conduct representing ideal behavior for a group of people. A health care worker observes the following code of ethics.

Recognizing and Reporting Illegal and Unethical Behavior

Health care workers must be aware of their ethical responsibilities for the protection of their patients/clients, their co-workers, their employers, and themselves. One of a health care worker's main responsibilities is to recognize and report unsafe, illegal, or unethical behaviors occurring in their work environment. How can you recognize reportable incidents? A reportable incident is any event that can adversely affect the health, safety, or welfare of students, clients, or co-workers. There are countless ways someone's behavior can negatively affect the people in the hospital. Here are a few examples:

- A nurse might administer the wrong medicine.
- A cleaning person might unplug important equipment.
- A doctor might harass another employee.
- An administrator might misuse hospital funds.
- An employee might disclose a patient's condition to a reporter.

There is no set list of reportable behaviors. Rather, it is required and expected that every employee will:

- Obey the laws of the city, state, and federal government.
- Fulfill his or her job requirements to the best of his or her ability, including following a code of ethics and respecting others.
- Treat everyone in the hospital environment with care, dignity, and respect.

If you or anyone fails to fulfill these obligations, that behavior must be reported. Reporting an illegal or unethical incident helps ensure the health, safety, and welfare of everyone in the hospital environment. If you even suspect an incident might be illegal or unethical, report it at once. Follow your employer's policy regarding how you report illegal and unethical incidents.

Your employee manual should explain clearly how you should report illegal and unethical conduct. In most cases, your manager should be able to help you report illegal and unethical behavior. If you have any doubt about how to report an incident, contact your human resources department. They will either help you report it, or direct you to those who can.

Meetings in the Workplace

Meetings are important in the workplace. There are different types of meetings: a team meeting for co-workers to communicate about team duties; a staff meeting for supervisors and managers to communicate information to a group about topics such as policies and schedules; a status meeting for team members to report on procedures, schedules, and so forth.

Meetings are a way for teams to communicate. Effective meetings requires specific leadership:

- **Set goals.** These goals are based on topics that need to be covered.
- **Schedule.** Set a time and location for the meeting. Be firm about attendance. Prepare an agenda to share objective(s) before, or at the start of, the meeting.
- **Maintain control.** Begin on time. Assign a note-taker. Introduce each topic, guiding the team to focus and make decisions. If something cannot be resolved, set a time to address the issue. In concluding, all attendees should be aware of resulting duties.
- **Follow up.** After the meeting, send a memo with a brief summary. List action steps and a timeline for the team to achieve required follow-up.

Safety in the Workplace

In 1970, the federal government passed a law called the Occupational Safety and Health Act. This law requires all employers to provide a safe and healthful workplace. Workers must be provided with safe equipment, protective clothing when needed, and education about safety practices. The Occupational Safety and Health Administration (OSHA) was formed to inspect companies and enforce safety laws. Even so, more than 5,000 Americans die from on-the-job accidents every year. As a worker under the Occupational Safety and Health Act, you have the following rights and responsibilities:

- **Right to know.** You have the right to know about hazards in your workplace, as well as the right to training to learn how to identify workplace hazards and what to do if there is an incident.
- **Right to refuse unsafe work.** If you have reasonable grounds to believe the work you do or the piece of equipment you use is unsafe, you can stop work immediately. You cannot be laid off, suspended, or penalized for refusing unsafe work if you follow the proper procedures.
- **Responsibility to follow safety rules.** It is your employer's responsibility to teach you the safety rules; it is your responsibility to follow the rules.
- **Responsibility to ask for training.** If you feel that you need more training than your employer provides, it is your responsibility to ask for it.
- **Responsibility to speak up.** It is your responsibility to report incidents and unsafe work practices as well as unsafe conditions.

Part of your responsibility as a worker is to make sure that you keep your work environment safe for yourself and for others. You have to take some responsibility for your own safety. If you are a new worker, enroll in any safety classes offered by the company. If you work around chemicals, poisons, or dangerous machinery, ask how they can be handled safely. If a company offers you hard hats or other safety equipment, use them. Read your manuals and handbook, and don't take shortcuts if it means endangering your safety or the safety of customers or co-workers. Remember—failure to follow safety guidelines is cause for dis- missal. What are some of the safety issues you might encounter in a selected career?

Job-Seeking Skills

Before you apply the skills you have learned, you must find a job and be hired as an employee. It is important to learn the skills needed to find a job and to keep a job. These skills will enable you to practice the career you worked so hard to learn about.

Developing Your Portfolio

As time approaches to begin your search for a job, review your portfolio notebook. Obtain a new cover and section dividers, so your finished portfolio has a clean, crisp look. A portfolio is a collection of materials that show the knowledge, abilities, skills, and insights you gain in your search for a career. The purpose in developing a portfolio is to show your mastery of vocational requirements to an employer, a college, or a higher-level training program. You also see your own growth and accomplishments over time. Identify the items that best reflect your knowledge level, skills, and personality. When you complete your résumé and other portfolio requirements, place them in the appropriate section of your new portfolio.

Places To Seek Employment

There are many potential sources of job information. Some of them include the following:

- **Newspaper ads.** Jobs in health care careers appear in newspaper ads. When you look for a job in the newspaper, turn to the classified ads and look under "Help Wanted." There are different ways of listing jobs. Some papers list all health care positions under "Medical." Others list them under a particular job. You also need to become familiar with the abbreviations used by newspapers. Table 15.1 ■ provides some of these.

Table 15.1 Common Abbreviations

ABBREVIATION	MEANING
appl.	applicant
asst.	assistant
cert.	certified
exp.	experience
FT	full time
immed.	immediately
incl.	included
lic.	licensed
N.A.	nurse aide
PT	part time

- **Directly to the employer.** If you are looking for a position in a laboratory, you might apply directly to a medical laboratory. If you want to work in a hospital, you go to the Personnel department. The Yellow Pages of your phone book offer an excellent resource of possible employers.
- **Friends and relatives.** You may know of someone working in the health care field who can suggest a place to apply or who can introduce you to a possible employer.
- **School counselors.** Many schools have career counselors and/or work experience counselors. They are a good resource for the types of jobs available in your community.
- **School bulletin boards.** If you have a career center or a bulletin board where jobs are listed, be sure to check it daily.
- **Employment agencies.** There are both public and private employment agencies. Employers call these agencies to list the job openings that they have. A public agency does not charge a fee; however, a private agency charges either the employer or the person seeking a position. The Yellow Pages list employment agencies, and some of them specialize in health care careers. The public agencies are listed in the white pages under "Government Agencies."
- **Internet.** If you have access to a computer that is connected to the Internet, go to Search and type in the words *"job search"* or *"job link."* You can find job referrals, workshops, placement activities, and tips on writing a resume or interviewing.

Your Career Plan

A career plan is a strategy for a person's growth as a professional. Many employers require employees to create a career plan that shows how their career will change and grow over the next few years. The plan shows the responsibilities that the employee should take on and the skills he or she should learn to advance to the next stage of his or her career. Employees should review their career plan annually with a supervisor who can help adjust or revise the plan as needed.

During the annual review and evaluation conference, the employee and the employer will evaluate the employee's success at meeting the goals set up for the past term. If any problems are identified the employee should expect the scheduling of frequent sessions until any problems identified are corrected. This is a joint effort and should reflect the goal of the organization to provide quality care and support the employee's growth in the job role.

As you grow professionally, your career plan needs to be updated annually. With a supervisor or men- tor, review any professional development experiences you have had over the past year, and evaluate those experiences. Next, make a new set of learning goals for the coming year, and find concrete ways to achieve those learning goals. Discuss specific work opportunities that can help you learn and apply what you need to know.

Career Self-Assessment

A career self-assessment is a process by which you learn more about your career-related skills, interests, values, and abilities (see Figure 15.14 ■). To perform a career self-assessment, you examine your strengths and weaknesses honestly and objectively.

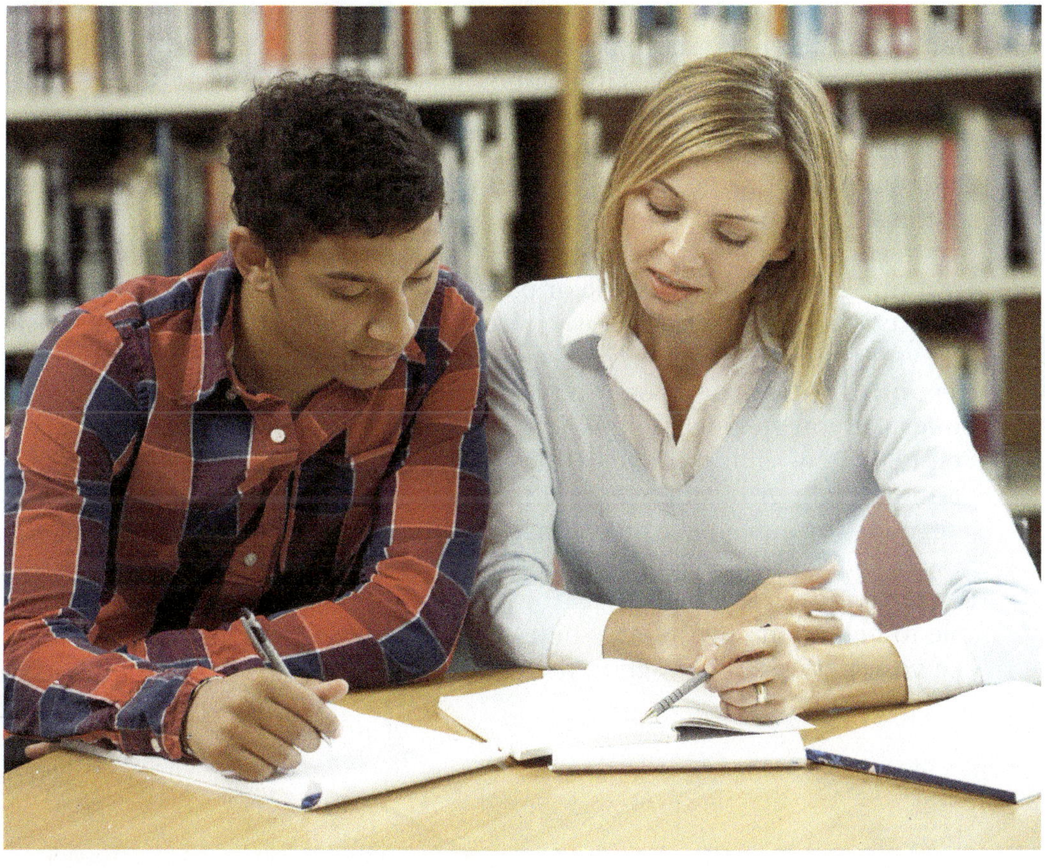

■ **Figure 15.14**
Why is it important to work with someone objective when you develop a career self-assessment?

Changing Careers

When you review your career plan, you might find that you are growing in a different direction than you expected. For example, you might discover that you really enjoyed training people in a new skill, and so make training and teaching a focus of your career.

People change careers for other reasons, too. For example:

- Some people get tired, and simply need a change.
- Some careers become out-dated, and replaced.
- Some people decide that they have a better chance of advancing professionally in another career.

If you decide you would like to change careers, use the same process to investigate your new career that you used to find your first one. You can research on your own, as well as seek the help of career counselors and career centers, such as those at colleges and universities.

Reasons to Grow as a Professional

Why should a health science professional always learn and grow? There are many reasons, such as:

- **Ethical behavior demands it.** If you are to provide the best, and most up-to-date service to your patients and clients, you need to learn the latest developments in your field. It would be unethical to offer out-dated, sub- standard care. In fact, many licensed professionals, such as doctors, nurses, and EMTs, must participate in a specific number of hours of continuing education each year to maintain their license.
- **Technology changes.** Technology in the health science industry changes rapidly. Diagnostic equipment that was unavailable a generation ago is part of routine medical care now. Computers and software programs continue to be more powerful and useful in all aspects of health care. Each of these changes in technology enables professionals to provide new services and better care to patients and clients, but only if professionals learn to use the technology effectively.
- **Client needs change.** The population you serve as a health science professional is dynamic. An increase in the number of older people means you need to learn more about the health care needs of seniors. If you are a nurse, and a new disease or pathogen emerges and affects your patients, you need to learn how to treat patients with the new disease as best you can.
- **Responsibilities increase.** You probably want to advance in your career. As you advance, you will have new responsibilities at every stage. You need new skills to manage these responsibilities. For example, your position might grow and you might need you to know how to make a budget. If you have never have made a budget before, you need to learn how to make one.
- **Become more flexible.** By learning skills outside your own job, you are able to help your coworkers when they need it. You may learn that you like your new skills enough to move your career in a new direction.

Resources for Professional Development

Where can you get professional development? There are many resources available for the professional development of people working in the health sciences:

- **Associations** Many professional associations provide meetings, courses, workshops, and other opportunities for professional development.
- **Employer training courses** Many employers offer training courses that help develop employees. Employer programs often include workshops to improve management and communication skills and courses to help employees use new equipment and software.
- **Colleges and Universities** Many colleges and universities offer classes that can help you learn more about your profession.
- **Journals** Professional journals help alert people to the latest developments in their fields.
- **Job Shadowing** Spending a period of time with a experienced worker, observing everything that he or she does that is related to the job responsibilities.

Career and Technical Student Organizations

Career and technical student organizations (CTSOs) are groups of students who are enrolled in a career and technical education program that engages in career and technical activities as part of the curriculum. There are different CTSOs for different career and technical programs; students join the organization related to the CTE program in which they are enrolled.

CTSOs provide members with a range of individual and group programs and activities. They promote career education and training and provide opportunities for leadership, teamwork, competition, and citizenship. CTSOs offer a unique program of career and leadership development, motivation, and recognition for students in grades 6 through 12.

Members benefit from:

- Belonging to a positive and supportive group of their peers
- Examining firsthand the relationship between academics and the world of work
- Identifying career opportunities
- Building confidence and knowledge through competition
- Exercising leadership and teamwork skills
- Practicing personal skills for success
- Developing employability skills
- Recognizing and developing interests and abilities that align with career goals

The National CTSOs supported by educators in most states include the following:

- Health Occupations Students of America (HOSA) for students in health services programs (www.hosa.org)

Volunteering

Volunteering—in other words, doing work without pay—is a great way to contribute to the communities you care about and gain valuable work experience.

Many types of organizations welcome volunteers, including schools, environmental protection groups, social services organizations, and political action groups. All of these thrive on the work of many volunteers and are likely to have well-established programs set up that make it easy to contribute your time. Some organizations have restrictions on volunteer work because of insurance liability, laws, or medical privacy issues. For example, some medical facilities may require that everyone who provides care to patients be paid employees, so there may be limits on the things you can do for residents there. When you go through volunteer orientation/training at such facilities, the limits will be explained to you. Think of ways that you can get involved in your community.

Chapter Review

Practice Exercises

1. When you want to achieve something quickly, you set short-term goals. Typically you need to accomplish your short-term goals before you accomplish long-term goals—something you want to achieve in the more distant future. Describe self-motivation techniques, and make a list of ways to pursue short-term and long-term goals.
2. Prepare a presentation on a career that interests you. Find out the educational requirements, job responsibilities, average starting salaries, and more. Present your findings to your class.
3. Take turns role playing a job interview with a classmate. Take turns being the interviewer and the interviewee. List specific examples of effective, clear, and concise verbal and non-verbal communication that occurred during the mock interviews.
4. Select and research a business in your community. If possible, obtain an application form from the business. Identify the different parts of the application, and practice completing the form.
5. Managing your time is a key skill. For a week, keep track of how you spend your time—how much time you spend socializing with friends, doing homework, spending time with your family, etc. Write a short paragraph on ways in which you can improve your time-management skills.
6. Select a professional journal and prepare a presentation describing the target audience for the journal, the content, and the format of the journal.
7. Attend a meeting in your community. Report to your class what you learned about meeting procedures and rules. Take turns role-playing meeting skills.
8. Working with a partner, brainstorm the roles and responsibilities of a manager or supervisor.
9. You are working in a clinic that deals with people who have a variety of diseases that carry some "social stigma." What can you do to create an atmosphere of confidence and openness with your clients?
10. You have decided that you want to pursue a career as a health care professional. What does this entail, other than choosing a field and studying hard? What other factors will impact your success as a health care worker?

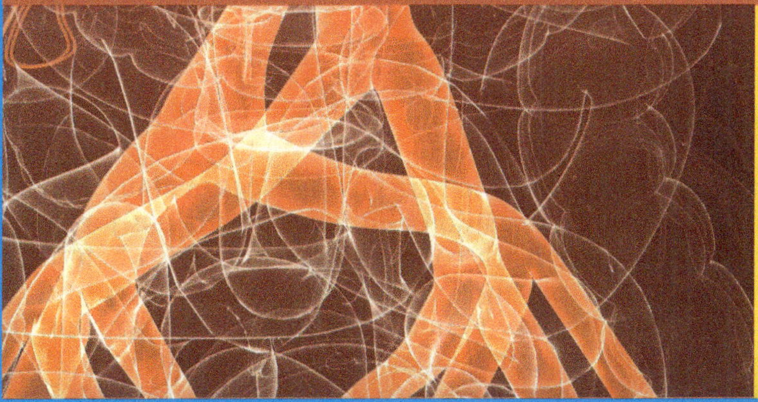

16

MEDICAL MATH

Learning Objectives

Upon completion of this chapter, you will be able to

- Add and subtract whole numbers, decimals, and percentages.
- Multiply and divide whole numbers, fractions, mixed numbers, decimals, and percentages.
- Convert decimals to percentages and percentages to decimals.
- State the metric unit of measure used to determine length, distance, weight, and volume.
- Use metric terms to express 100 and 1,000 units of measure.
- Use metric terms to express 0.1, 0.01, and 0.001 units of measure.
- List four basic rules to follow when using the metric system.
- Identify metric measures of length and volume.
- Convert ounces to cubic centimeters/milliliters, pounds to kilograms, and ounces to grams.
- Match key terms with their correct meanings.
- Recognize time on a 24-hour clock.
- Express 24-hour time/military time verbally and in writing.
- Convert Greenwich time to 24-hour time.

Math Review

Health care workers are required to perform math calculations when doing various tasks, such as dosage calculation and unit conversions for patient weight and height. Knowing basic math concepts and knowing when to apply them are essential skills for all health care workers. To be a successful health care worker, you should know how to add, subtract, convert standard figures into metric figures, calculate percentages, and manipulate fractions. Because math skills are critical to success in all health care jobs, this chapter begins with a math skills review.

Numbers

Numbers are expressed in different forms:

- Whole numbers
- Nonwhole numbers
- Mixed numbers
- Percentages

Numbers that have more than one digit are defined by their place value. For example, the number 7777 is given the following values:

	7	7	7	7
	▲	▲	▲	▲
Place value ⟶	*thousands*	*hundreds*	*tens*	*ones*

This number is described by saying "seven thousand, seven hundred seventy-seven." Numbers are written with a comma placed to the left of every third digit. The number 7777 is properly written "7,777." The number 22222 is given the following place values:

	2	2	2	2
	▲	▲	▲	▲
Place value ⟶	*ten thousands*	*thousands*	*hundreds*	*tens*

It is written "22,222" and described as "twenty-two thousand, two hundred twenty-two."

Numbers indicating less than a whole number are placed to the right of a decimal. The number 7777.255 is given the following place values:

	7	7	7	7	2	5	5
	▲	▲	▲	▲	▲	▲	▲
Place value ⟶	*thousands*	*hundreds*	*tens*	*ones*	*tenths*	*hundredths*	*thousandths*

It is written "7,777.255" and described as "seven thousand, seven hundred seventy-seven and two hundred and fifty-five thousandths."

Whole Numbers

Whole numbers are the counting numbers and zero. Whole numbers do not contain decimals or fractions. *Examples:* 1, 2, 3, 10, 15, 18, 0. Ignore zeros before whole numbers. *Example:* 025 à ∅25 and is written "25."

Nonwhole Numbers

Nonwhole numbers are numbers that have decimals. *Examples:* 7,777.255, 12.25, 5.9.

Mixed Numbers

Mixed numbers are whole numbers and a fraction. *Examples:* $12\frac{1}{4}$ or $45\frac{3}{4}$.

Percentages

The word *percent* means "by the hundred"; 100 percent = the whole or all of something. The symbol for percent is %. (Figure 16.1 ■) *Example:* Four bananas = 100% or all of the bananas present. When one banana is sold, $\frac{1}{4}$ (one-fourth) or 25% of them are gone and $\frac{3}{4}$ (three-fourths) or 75% are left.

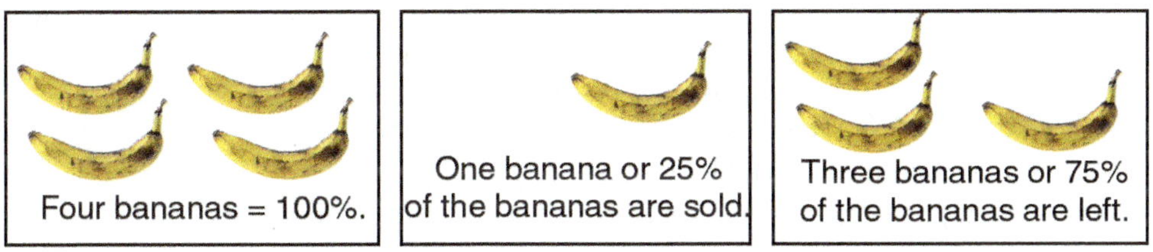
Four bananas = 100%.
One banana or 25% of the bananas are sold.
Three bananas or 75% of the bananas are left.

■ **Figure 16.1 Percentages.** If there were five bananas in the figure, what percentage would one banana represent?

Addition

Addition is the totaling of two or more numbers. For example, 2 computers in the reception area + 3 computers in accounting = a total of 5 computers in the office. To add, place numbers in columns. Put a line under the last number in the column. Add all the numbers above the line and write the total or sum of the numbers below the line.

Examples:

$$\begin{array}{lrr} & 2 & 34 \\ & +\,3 & +\,4 \\ \hline \text{Total} & 5 & 38 \end{array}$$

When adding more than one column of numbers, always keep the numbers in each column in a line under each other. This helps you add the correct numbers together. Always start adding numbers in the right column first.

Example:

11 + 234 + 10 + 4 is written like this:

$$\begin{array}{r} 11 \\ 234 \\ 10 \\ +\ \ 4 \\ \hline \boxed{259} \end{array}$$

When figuring numbers that total more than 10 in a column, it is necessary to carry numbers to the left of the column being added. In the next example, the first column of 1 + 4 + 0 + 9 = 14. In the total, the number to the left of the 4 is 1. Move or carry the 1 to the column at the left and add it to the top number of that column (8), then add the remaining numbers in the column, 1 + 8 + 8 + 1 = 18. The number to the left of the 8 is 1. Move or carry the 1 to the column at the left and add it to the top number of that column (3), then add the remaining numbers in the column, 1 + 3 = 4. The total is 484. (See the examples that follow.)

Example 1:

		$^{1}8$	1
	$^{1}3$	8	4
		1	0
+			9
Total	4	8	4

(carry 1) 81
(carry 1) 384
10
+ 9
484

= 14; leave the 4 in the total row and carry the 1 to the top of column at the left.

= 18; leave the 8 in the total row and carry the 1 to top of the column at the left.

= 4; place the 4 in the total row of the column added.

Example 2:

		$^{1}8$	1
	$^{3}9$	8	4
		9	0
+		9	9
Total 1	2	5	4

(carry 1) 81
(carry 3) 984
90
+ 99
1,254

= 14; leave the 4 in the total row and carry the 1 to the top of column at the left.

= 35; leave the 5 in the total row, carry the 3 to top of the column at the left.

= 12; leave the 2 in the column you're working in at the total row, carry the 1 to the column at the left. (Since there is no number above the total line, write the 1 in the total column.)

Subtraction

Subtraction is the opposite of addition. Subtracting numbers means taking a number away from another number. Simple subtraction problems are written in the following way:

84 − 23 = 61 or 84 − 23 = 61 *136* − 12 = 124 or 136 − 12 = 124

Check your answer by adding the answer to the number subtracted. If your answer is correct, your total will equal the number at the top of your problem.

Examples:

84 check − 23 + 61 = 84 or 23 + 61 = 84

136 check − 12 + 124 = 136 or 12 + 124 = 136

Subtracting by Borrowing Numbers

Borrow a number from the column to the left. This allows a larger number, such as 8, to be subtracted from 5. See the following examples to help you understand.

Examples:

$$\begin{array}{r} {}^{2}\not{3}\ {}^{1}5 \\ -\ 1\ 8 \\ \hline \boxed{1\ 7} \end{array}$$

5 becomes 15 when 1 is borrowed from the 3
3 becomes 2

$$\begin{array}{r} {}^{1}\not{2}\,{}^{16}\not{7}\ {}^{1}\not{2} \\ -\ 1\ 9\ 5 \\ \hline \boxed{\not{0}\ 7\ 7} \end{array}$$

2 becomes 12 when 1 is borrowed from the 7
7 becomes 6 because you borrowed 1; 6 becomes 16
when 1 is borrowed from the 2; 2 becomes 1

Multiplication

Multiplication is a quick, easy way to add. For example, $9 + 9 + 9 = 27$, but an easier process is $3 \times 9 = 27$. Adding large numbers is bulky and takes a lot of time. Multiplication is much easier.

To multiply numbers easily, memorize the multiplication table. (Table 16.1 ■) Memorizing this table allows you to calculate numbers quickly and without difficulty. You probably already know the basics of multiplication.

The following symbols are used to indicate multiplication: ×, ()(), ., or *. These symbols are used in writing problems.

Examples:

$$\begin{array}{r} 8 \\ \times 9 \\ \hline 72 \end{array} \quad \text{or} \quad 8 \times 9 = 72 \quad \text{or} \quad 8\,.\,9 = 72 \quad \text{or} \quad (8)\ (9) = 72 \quad \text{or} \quad 8 * 9 = 72$$

Using calculators is helpful when figuring complicated calculations; however, you are responsible for knowing how to calculate numbers without a calculator. Most of the calculations in your work are simple and easy to figure without the use of a calculator.

Table 16.1 Multiplication Table

	1	2	3	4	5	6	7	8	9	10
1	1	2	3	4	5	6	7	8	9	10
2	2	4	6	8	10	12	14	16	18	20
3	3	6	9	12	15	18	21	24	27	30
4	4	8	12	16	20	24	28	32	36	40
5	5	10	15	20	25	30	35	40	45	50
6	6	12	18	24	30	36	42	48	54	60
7	7	14	21	28	35	42	49	56	63	70
8	8	16	24	32	40	48	56	64	72	80
9	9	18	27	36	45	54	63	72	81	90
10	10	20	30	40	50	60	70	80	90	100

Multiplying Fractions

Like a whole or nonwhole number, fractions can be multiplied. The **numerators**, or top numbers of the fractions, are multiplied; and the **denominators**, or bottom numbers of the fractions, are multiplied. *For example:*

$$\frac{3}{4} \times \frac{12}{15} = \frac{3 \times 12}{4 \times 15} = \frac{36}{60} = \frac{3}{5}$$

Note that the final answer for the example above is simplified, or reduced. To reduce the fraction, you must divide the numerator and denominator by the largest number that goes into both—in this case, 12.

To multiply mixed numbers, convert the number to a fraction first. *For example:*

$$1\frac{3}{4} \times 2\frac{2}{3} = \frac{7}{4} \times \frac{8}{3} = \frac{56}{12} = 4\frac{8}{12} = 4\frac{2}{3}$$

Long Multiplication

When you are multiplying numbers that have more than one digit, it is sometimes necessary to carry and add. See the following examples to review these steps.

The next problem does not require carrying numbers. It does require multiplying and adding.

A.

		5	2
	×	3	2
	1	0	4

2 × 2 = 4; place 4 in the first column, below 2 and 2.
2 × 5 = 10; place 0 in column under the 5 and 3 and place 1 in column at left.

B.

		5	2
	×	3	2
	1	0	4
+ 1	5	6	

3 × 2 = 6; place 6 in column under the 5, 3, and 0.
3 × 5 = 15; place 5 in column under 1 and place 1 in column at left.

C.

		5	2
	×	3	2
	1	0	4
+ 1	5	6	
1	6	6	4

Add together, keeping each number in the correct column.

Answer

This problem requires carrying, adding, and multiplying:

A.

		[1]8	[1]9	8
×	5	6	2	
1	7	9	6	

$2 \times 8 = 16$; place 6 in first column and carry 1 to top of column at left. $2 \times 9 = 18 + 1$ [that was carried] = 19; place 9 in column under 9 and 6 and carry 1 to top of column at left. $2 \times 8 = 16 + 1$ [that was carried] = 17; place 7 in column under 8 and 5 and place 1 in column at left of 7.

B.

		[5]8	[4]9	8
	×	5	6	2
	1	7	9	6
5	3	8	8	

$6 \times 8 = 48$; place 8 in column under 9, 6, and 9 and carry 4 to the top of column at left. $6 \times 9 = 54 + 4$ [that was carried] = 58; place 8 in column under 8, 5, 7 and carry 5 to top of column at left. $6 \times 8 = 48 + 5$ [that was carried] = 53; place 3 in column under 1 and place 5 in column at left next to 3.

C.

			[4]8	[4]9	8
		×	5	6	2
		1	7	9	6
	5	3	8	8	
4	4	9	0		

$5 \times 8 = 40$; place 0 in column under 8, 5, 7 and 8 and carry 4 to the top of column at left. $5 \times 9 = 45 + 4$ [that was carried] = 49; place 9 below 1 and 3. Carry 4 to top of column at left. $5 \times 8 = 40 + 4$ [that was carried] = 44; place 4 below 5 and place 4 next to 4 in column at left.

D.

			8	9	8
		×	5	6	2
		[1]1	[1]7	9	6
	[1]5	3	8	8	
+ [1]4	4	9	0		
5	0	4	6	7	6

Add together, keeping each number in the correct column.

Answer

Division

Division is the opposite of multiplication. Knowing the multiplication table is essential when dividing. As a health care worker, you may divide to determine costs per item or to determine the amount of items used daily. Here is a simple example: A medical office budget allows \$600 a year for magazines. You are responsible for selecting and ordering the magazines. As you survey appropriate magazine subscriptions, you determine that the average annual cost is \$35 per magazine. To determine how many subscriptions you can purchase, you divide \$35 into \$600. This problem is written as follows:

$600 \div 35$, or $35\overline{)600}$

$\begin{array}{r} 17 \\ 35\overline{)600} \end{array}$ magazine subscription

To understand how 17 magazine subscriptions can be purchased for \$600, review the following division skills:

Dividing three-digit numbers by one-digit numbers:

812 ÷ 4 — *Divide hundreds* — *Divide tens* — *Divide ones*

Divide hundreds:

$\begin{array}{r} 2 \\ 4\overline{)812} \\ 8 \\ \hline 0 \end{array}$

Divide tens:

$\begin{array}{r} 20 \\ 4\overline{)812} \\ 8 \\ \hline 01 \\ 00 \\ \hline 1 \end{array}$

4 does not divide into 1. Place a 0 next to the 2 in the answer.

Divide ones:

$\begin{array}{r} 203 \\ 4\overline{)812} \\ 8 \\ \hline 01 \\ 00 \\ \hline 12 \\ 12 \end{array}$

Divide 4 into 12.

Dividing four-digit numbers by one-digit numbers:

7,216 ÷ 9

```
    8          80         801        801 R or 7/9 or 0.8
9)7,216    9)7,216    9)7,216    9)7,216.0   Add 0s to carry answer.
  7 2        7 2↓       7 2 ↓      7 2
               1          16         16
               0           9          9↓
               1           7          70
                                      63
                                       7
```

Answer is $801\frac{7}{9}$ or 801.8

As shown in the example, "R" stands for **remainder**. The remainder is what is left over that is less than a whole number. A remainder is usually expressed as a fraction or a decimal.

Dividing Fractions

To divide fractions, you will need to invert, or turn over, the divisor (dividing number) in the calculation. So, the denominator will be on top and the numerator will be on bottom. Then, you multiply the fractions to find the answer. For example:

Step 1: Invert the divisor.

$$\frac{7}{10} \div \frac{2}{9}$$

So, $\frac{2}{9}$ is converted to $\frac{9}{2}$.

Step 2: Multiply the fractions.

$$\frac{7}{10} \times \frac{9}{2} = \frac{7 \times 9}{10 \times 2} = \frac{63}{20} = 3\frac{3}{20}$$

Note that the answer was converted from a fraction to a mixed number. When dividing mixed numbers, you will need to convert them to fractions first.

So, for example:

$$3\frac{7}{8} \div \frac{21}{4}$$

would convert to

$$\frac{31}{8} \div \frac{9}{4}$$

before you can divide the numbers.

Decimals, Percentages, and Fractions

Numbers to the left of a decimal are whole numbers. Numbers to the right of a decimal are less than one.

Dividing *decimals* by whole numbers:

$24.5 \div 4 = 4\overline{)24.5}$ Place the decimal point in the answer directly above the decimal point in the dividend.

```
   6.           6.1            6.125
4)24.5       4)24.5        4)24.500
  24           24 ↓          24
                  5             5
                  4             4↓
                  1             10
                                 8↓
                                 20
                                 20   Add 0s to carry answer.
```

Numbers to the right of a decimal point indicate less than one whole. For example, 1.5 is the same as 1½.

Examples:

Decimal		Percentage		Fraction(s)
0.10	=	10%	=	$^{10}/_{100}$ or $^{1}/_{10}$
0.25	=	25%	=	$^{25}/_{100}$ or $^{1}/_{4}$
6.25	=	625%	=	$^{625}/_{100}$ or $6^{1}/_{4}$

Change a decimal number into a percentage by moving the decimal two places to the right.

Examples:

0.5 = 0.5 0. = 50%

30.0 = 30.0 0. = 3000%

0.04 = .0 4. = 4%

To change a percentage into a decimal number, replace the percent sign with a decimal and move the decimal two spaces to the left.

To find the percentage of a number, first change the percentage to a decimal. Then multiply that decimal by the number.

Examples:

15% of 63 change 15% to 0.15 then multiply 0.15 × 63 = 9.45

9.45 is 15% of 63

20% of 100 change 20% to 0.20 then multiply 0.20 × 100 = 20

20 is 20% of 100

The Metric System

The health care worker is expected to measure and calculate weights, heights, and volume in metric units of measure. Understanding how to convert standard and metric units of measure is an essential requirement of all health care professionals.

Using the Metric System

The health care industry uses the metric system for measuring. The metric system is used by 90 percent of the world and is known as the International System of Units. Table 16.2 ■ will help you learn the metric terms, their abbreviations, and what they measure. Each metric unit in this table is a single unit of measure. Table 16.3 ■ explains terms used when more than one unit of measure (meter, gram, liter) is being measured. Following are examples of more than one unit:

- Measures of weight:
  1 hectogram = 100 grams
  1.5 hectograms = 150 grams
  1 kilogram = 1,000 grams
  1.5 kilograms = 1,500 grams
- Measures of **length**:
  1 hectometer = 100 meters
  1.5 hectometers = 150 meters
  1 kilometer = 1,000 meters
  1.5 kilometers = 1,500 meters

Table 16.2 Metric Terms, Their Abbreviations, and What They Measure

TERM	ABBREVIATION	MEASURES	IN PLACE OF
meter	m	Length	inch, foot, yard, mile
gram	g	Weight	ounce, pound
liter	L*	Volume	fluid ounce, cup, pint, quart, gallon

*Capital *L* is commonly used to prevent confusion of lowercase letter *l* and the number *1*.

Table 16.3 Metric Terms, Their Abbreviations, and What They Measure

TERM	ABBREVIATION	WHAT IT MEASURES
kilo	k	1,000 units
hecto	h	100 units

Table 16.4 ■ explains terms used when *less than one unit* of measure is being measured. Following are examples of less than one unit:

- Measures of length:
  1 decimeter (dm) = $\frac{1}{10}$ or 0.1 of a meter
  1 centimeter (cm) = $\frac{1}{100}$ or 0.01 of a meter
  1 millimeter (mm) = $\frac{1}{1000}$ or 0.001 of a meter
- Measures of volume:
  1 deciliter (dL) = $\frac{1}{10}$ or 0.1 of a liter
  1 milliliter (mL) = $\frac{1}{1000}$ or 0.001 of a liter

Table 16.4 Metric Terms, Their Abbreviations, and What They Measure

TERM	ABBREVIATION	WHAT IT MEASURES
deci	d	1/10 or 0.1 unit
centi	c	1/100 or 0.01 unit
milli	m	1/1000 or 0.001 unit

There are four basic rules to follow when using the metric system:

- Numbers indicating less than one unit are always written in **decimal** form, not as fractions. *Example:* 1/10 = 0.1 or 1/100 = 0.01 or 1/1000 = 0.001.
- When writing decimals, if there is no number before the decimal, always write a 0. *Example:* .1 is 0.1, .5 is 0.5, .75 is 0.75.
- Abbreviations for metric terms are never plural; they are always written in singular form. *Examples:* grams is *g*, not *gs*, and liters is *L*, not *Ls*. Always capitalize the abbreviation L for liter to reduce confusing the lowercase l with the number 1.
- Leave a space between the number and the abbreviation, as shown in the following examples: 8 g or 0.1 dm.

Using the Metric System to Measure

Meters, Centimeters, and Millimeters

A **meterstick** can be used to measure length in the following units:

- Centimeters (cm) (Figure 16.2 ■)
- Millimeters (mm)
- Meters (m)

One meter is slightly more than 3 feet.

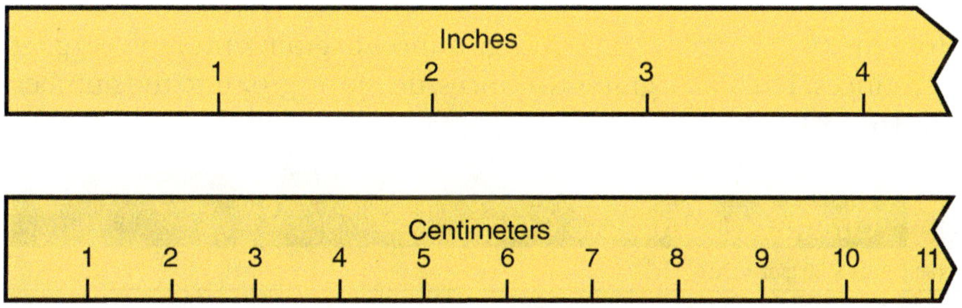

■ **Figure 16.2** Comparison of standard and metric units of length. About how many centimeters are in one inch?

Liters, Milliliters, and Cubic Centimeters

- A liter (L) is slightly larger than a quart.
- A milliliter (mL) is 1/1000 of a liter.
- Cubic centimeters (cc) are interchangeable with mL.

Scales can be used to measure weight in grams, hectograms, and kilograms.

Celsius (C) and Centigrade

The metric measure of heat is Celsius or centigrade, which are the same. Boiling water (at normal pressure) measures 100° in Celsius, but 212° in Fahrenheit, and as water freezes it measures 0° in Celsius, but 32° in Fahrenheit. Most people think of a "normal" body temperature as an oral temperature of 37° Celsius (98.6° Fahrenheit).

Changing Standard Measures to Metric Measures

It is easy to change liquid or volume measurement by multiplying 30 cc/mL times the number of ounces. (Table 16.5 ■)

Table 16.5	Changing Ounces to Milliliters and Cubic Centimeters
1 oz medicine	1 oz × 30 cc/mL = 30 cc = 30 mL
8 oz water	8 oz × 30 cc/mL = 240 cc = 240 mL
6 oz soup	6 oz × 30 cc/mL = 180 cc = 180 mL
4 oz juice	4 oz × 30 cc/mL = 120 cc = 120 mL
12 oz soda	12 oz × 30 cc/mL = 360 cc = 360 mL

Health care workers use various types of measuring devices to measure liquid.

To change measurements of **mass** or weight, compare pounds with kilograms and grams with ounces. One pound equals 0.45 kg; 1 kilogram equals 2.2 lb. (Table 16.6 ■)

Table 16.6 Changing Pounds to Kilograms and Kilograms to Pounds
110 lb changed to kilograms: 110 lb × 0.45 kg/lb = 49.5 kg
200 lb changed to kg: 200 lb × 0.45 kg/lb = 91 kg
50 kg changed to lb: 50 kg × 2.2 lb/kg = 110 lb
91 kg changed to lb: 91 kg × 2.2 lb/kg = 200 lb

- To change pounds to kilograms, multiply the number of pounds by 0.45 lb/kg.
- To change kilograms to pounds, multiply the number of kilograms by 2.2 lb/kg.

One ounce (oz) equals 30 grams (g). To change ounces to grams, multiply 30 g/oz by the number of ounces. To change grams to ounces, divide 30 g/oz into the number of grams. (Table 16.7 ■)

Table 16.7 Changing Ounces to Grams
1 oz changed to grams: 1 oz × 30 g/oz = 30 g
8 oz changed to grams: 8 oz × 30 g/oz = 240 g

The 24-Hour Clock/Military Time

Medical facilities frequently use the 24-hour clock system. The 24-hour clock clearly states time and eliminates confusion when documenting information. A health care worker is required to understand and interpret time in every health care setting.

Introduction to the 24-Hour Clock/ Military Time

In the health care setting, it is important that time be stated in a clear, concise manner. All medical records are legal documents. Time indicates when treatment, medication, and other activities are done and how long procedures or incidents last. A 24-hour clock eliminates the confusion between a.m. (12 midnight to 12 noon) and p.m. (12 noon to 12 midnight) hours. It provides a clear, concise record for recording medical services. The military services were the first to use a 24-hour clock; therefore, the 24-hour system is often referred to as **24-hour time/military time**. Table 16.8 ■ shows you the difference in expressing **Greenwich** and military time. (Figure 16.3 ■)

Table 16.8 Comparison of Greenwich and 24-Hour/Military Time

GREENWICH	MILITARY	GREENWICH	MILITARY
1:00 A.M.	0100	1:00 P.M.	1300
2:00 A.M.	0200	2:00 P.M.	1400
3:00 A.M.	0300	3:00 P.M.	1500
4:00 A.M.	0400	4:00 P.M.	1600
5:00 A.M.	0500	5:00 P.M.	1700
6:00 A.M.	0600	6:00 P.M.	1800
7:00 A.M.	0700	7:00 P.M.	1900
8:00 A.M.	0800	8:00 P.M.	2000
9:00 A.M.	0900	9:00 P.M.	2100
10:00 A.M.	1000	10:00 P.M.	2200
11:00 A.M.	1100	11:00 P.M.	2300
12:00 noon	1200	12:00 P.M./midnight	2400/0000

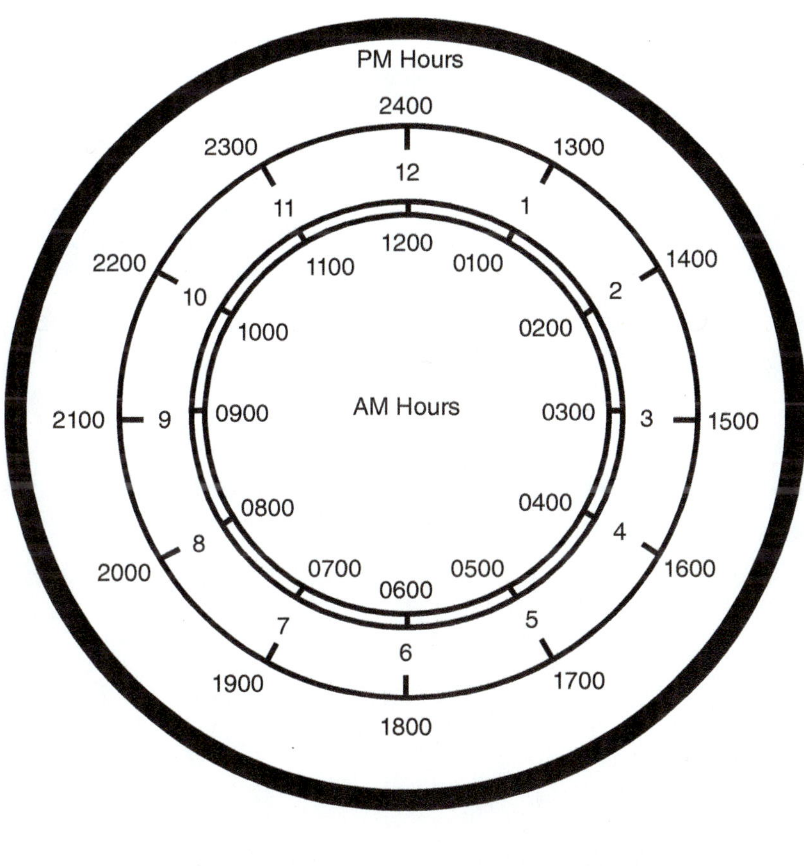

■ **Figure 16.3** 24-hour clock: military time. What is the military time for the following: 8:30 a.m., 7:45 p.m., 3:15 p.m., and 12:10 a.m.?

Military time is always expressed in four digits, and no colons are used to separate hours and minutes. Always use a 0 to complete the four-digit number (for example, for 1:00 a.m., use 0100 instead of 100). When expressing military time, remember to state it in hundreds: for example, zero one hundred hours (0100) is 1:00 a.m.; eleven hundred hours (1100) is 11:00 a.m.; twenty-three hundred hours (2300) is 11:00 p.m.

It is easy to remember that morning hours are 0100 to 1200 hours. The afternoon and nighttime hours can be added to the 1200 hours of noon. For example:

- To determine how 5:00 p.m. is expressed in military time, add 1200 and 0500 (1200 + 0500 = 1700 hours).
- To determine how 12 midnight is expressed in military time, add 1200 and 1200 = 2400 hours.

Chapter Review

Practice Exercises

1. Multiply and divide the following pair of numbers: 13⅘ and 7⅓.
2. Convert the following percentages to decimals: 128.3%, 0.46%, and 32%.
3. Identify the characteristic that each of the following units is used to measure: m, mL, cm, kg, and cc.
4. What do deci, centi, and milli measure?
5. Convert the following ounce measurements to mL: 4 oz, 10 oz, and 32 oz.
6. Convert the following kilograms to pounds: 1 kg, 50 kg, and 75 kg?
7. What is the formula for changing pounds to kilograms?)
8. Describe the 24-hour time system.
9. Express the following time in military time numerically and verbally: 1:00 p.m.
10. A woman goes into labor at 1400. She waits two hours before she goes to the hospital. At what time does she arrive at the hospital?

Suggested Activities

1. You have been given a list of duties and times, but the times are in minutes and fractions: updating records—1 hour; cleaning—2⅓ hours; working with patients—4 hours and 10 minutes; lunch—one-half hour. Assume your scheduled shift starts at 8:00 a.m. Set up a schedule for your day, using Standard Greenwich Time, showing when you are performing each duty. Then, redo the calendar using 24-Hour Military Time.
2. Your teacher will set up a Medical Math Obstacle course. Bring in a favorite recipe. Convert the measurements from household to metric. Use the following basic measurements to start:
    - 3 teaspoons = 1 tablespoon
    - 4 tablespoons = ¼ cup
    - 5⅓ tablespoons = ⅓ cup
    - 8 tablespoons = ½ cup
    - 10⅔ tablespoons = ⅔ cup
    - 12 tablespoons = ¾ cup
    - 16 tablespoons = 1 cup
    - 1 tablespoon = ½ fluid oz.
    - 1 cup = 8 fluid oz.
    - 1 cup = ½ pint
    - 2 cups = 1 pint
    - 4 cups = 1 quart
    - 2 pints = 1 quart
    - 4 quarts = 1 gallon
3. Pick out 10 items in your refrigerator or kitchen cabinet, such as cereal, juice, or household cleaners. Create a chart and convert all of the ingredient measurements on the label to decimals.

Case Studies

1. A new mother arrives for the baby's first well-baby checkup at 1:00 p.m. You know that she should be taken to an examination room within 5 minutes. Your employer uses military time. Explain how 1:05 p.m. is written in military time. You call the patient's name and ask her to follow you to the scales. You weigh the baby and find she weighs 3.84 kilograms. What will you tell the mother her baby's weight is in pounds and ounces?
2. Health care workers are expected to communicate effectively with co-workers, patients, and their families. In the United States, standard units of measure are common, and metric units of measure are less common. Patients or their families may be expected to measure their medicine and fluid intake and convert these measurements to metric units. It is essential to explain how to do this in terms a patient will understand. Write instructions to a 75-year-old patient explaining the difference between ounces and cubic centimeters. Your instructions must describe how to measure and calculate the patient's 24-hour fluid intake.

Thinking Critically

1. **Safety Alert**—Describe two scenarios in which instructions given to patients using a 12-hour clock may be confusing and put patients at risk. Explain how instructions given using a 24-hour clock can prevent problems.
2. **Medical Math**—A mother gets a prescription for her child. The instructions say to give the child 15mL of antibiotic tid. The mother only has teaspoons at home and does not know how much medicine to give her child. Can you help her?
3. **Math Facts**—Use filling prescriptions as the example for determining accurate measures. In a team of three, complete the following exercise. Fill four simulated prescriptions. Each prescription will require mathematical calculations.
   - Medication A is a liquid to be taken as 2 fl. oz., four times a day, until gone. The bottle has 96 oz. How long will it last?
   - Give Medication B as 10mg/kg body weight, 2 times per day for 10 days. The patient weighs 79 lbs. Each pill cannot contain more than 200 mg. of Medication B. How many mg. per day would the patient require, and how many pills per day would that be? What would be the mg. dosage of each pill?
   - The patient requires 50 mg. of medication C every morning, via teaspoon. The medication solution contains 25 mg. /teaspoon. How many teaspoons must your patient take per day?
   - The patient requires 1.25 mg. of Medication D. Medication D comes in a solution of 5 mg. per 5 ml. How many ml of Medication D will the patient receive?

   Teams report on their conclusions and their process for finding the answers.

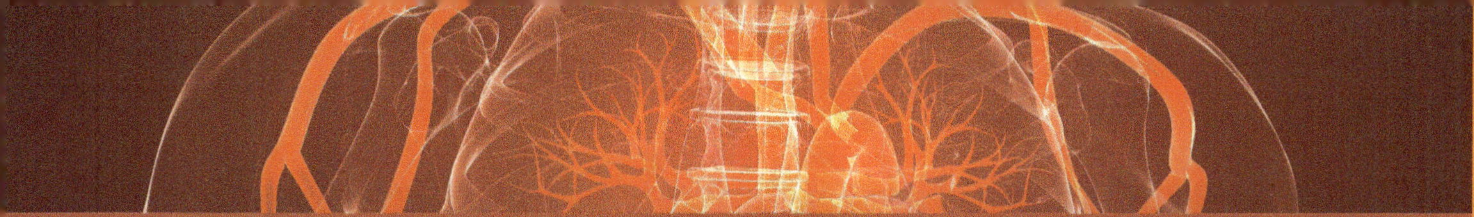

Appendices

Appendix I

Word Parts Arranged Alphabetically and Defined

The word parts that have been presented in this textbook are summarized with their definitions for quick reference. Prefixes are listed first, followed by combining forms and suffixes.

Prefix	Definition
a-	without, away from
ab-	away from
ad-	toward
allo-	other, different from usual
an-	without
ante-	before, in front of
anti-	against
auto-	self
bi-	two
brady-	slow
circum-	around
contra-	against
de-	without
dis-	apart
dys-	abnormal, difficult, painful
e-	outward, without
en-	inward
endo-	inner, within
epi-	upon, over, above
eso-	inward
eu-	normal, good
ex-	external, outward
exo-	outward
extra-	outside of
hemi-	half
hetero-	different
homo-	same
hydro-	water
hyper-	excessive, over, above
hypo-	below, under, insufficient
in-	inward, without, not, within
inter-	among, between
intra-	inside, within
macro-	large
micro-	small
mono-	one
multi-	many
myo-	to shut
neo-	new
nulli-	none
pan-	all
para-	abnormal, two like parts of a pair, beside, near
per-	through
peri-	around
poly-	many
post-	after
pre-	before, in front of
primi-	first
pro-	before
pseudo-	false
quadri-	four
re-	again
retro-	backward, behind
semi-	partial, half
sub-	below, under
supra-	above
tachy-	fast, rapid
tetra-	four
trans-	across, through
tri-	three
ultra-	beyond, excess
un-	not
xeno-	strange, foreign

Combining Form	Definition
abdomin/o	abdomen
acous/o	hearing
acr/o	extremities
aden/o	gland
adenoid/o	adenoids
adip/o	fat
adren/o	adrenal glands

Combining Form	Definition
adrenal/o	adrenal glands
aer/o	air
agglutin/o	clumping
albin/o	white
alges/o	sense of pain
alveol/o	alveolus; air sac
ambly/o	dull, dim
amnes/o	forgetfulness
amni/o	amnion
an/o	anus
andr/o	male
angi/o	vessel
ankyl/o	stiff joint
anter/o	front
anthrac/o	coal
anxi/o	fear, worry
aort/o	aorta
append/o	appendix
appendic/o	appendix
aque/o	water
arteri/o	artery
arthr/o	joint
articul/o	joint
aspir/o	to breathe in
astr/o	star
atel/o	incomplete
ather/o	fatty substance
atri/o	atrium
audi/o	hearing
audit/o	hearing
aur/o	ear
auricul/o	ear
axill/o	axilla, underarm
azot/o	nitrogenous waste
bacteri/o	bacteria
balan/o	glans penis
bar/o	weight
bas/o	base
bi/o	life
blast/o	immature, embryonic
blephar/o	eyelid
brachi/o	arm
bronch/o	bronchus
bronchi/o	bronchus
bronchiol/o	bronchiole
bucc/o	cheek
burs/o	bursa, sac
calc/o	calcium
capsul/o	to box
carcin/o	cancer
cardi/o	heart
carp/o	carpus, wrist
caud/o	tail
cec/o	cecum
cephal/o	head

Combining Form	Definition
cerebell/o	cerebellum
cerebr/o	cerebrum
cerumin/o	cerumen
cervic/o	neck, cervix
chem/o	chemical, drug
chol/e	bile, gall
cholangi/o	bile duct
cholecyst/o	gallbladder
choledoch/o	common bile duct
chondr/o	cartilage
chori/o	chorion
chrom/o	color
chromat/o	color
cirrh/o	yellow
cis/o	to cut
clavicul/o	clavicle
clon/o	rapid contracting and relaxing
coagul/o	clotting
coccyg/o	coccyx
cochle/o	cochlea
col/o	colon
colon/o	colon
colp/o	vagina
compuls/o	drive, compel
coni/o	dust
conjunctiv/o	conjunctiva
corne/o	cornea
coron/o	heart
corpor/o	body
cortic/o	outer portion, cortex
cost/o	rib
crani/o	skull
crin/o	to secrete
crur/o	leg
cry/o	cold
crypt/o	hidden
culd/o	cul-de-sac
cutane/o	skin
cyan/o	blue
cycl/o	ciliary body, ciliary muscle
cyst/o	bladder, pouch, sac
cyt/o	cell
dacry/o	tear duct, tears
deluss/o	false belief
dent/o	tooth
depress/o	to press down
derm/o	skin
dermat/o	skin
diaphor/o	profuse sweating
diaphragmat/o	diaphragm
dilat/o	to widen
dipl/o	double
dist/o	away from
diverticul/o	pouch
dors/o	back of body

Combining Form	Definition
duct/o	to bring
duoden/o	duodenum
dur/o	dura mater
electr/o	electricity
embol/o	plug
embry/o	embryo
emmetr/o	correct, proper
encephal/o	brain
enter/o	small intestine
eosin/o	rosy red
epididym/o	epididymis
epiglott/o	epiglottis
episi/o	vulva
epitheli/o	epithelium
erg/o	work
erythr/o	red
esophag/o	esophagus
esthes/o	sensation, feeling
estr/o	female
extens/o	to stretch out
factiti/o	artificial, contrived
fasci/o	fibrous band
femor/o	femur
fet/o	fetus
fibr/o	fibers
fibrin/o	fibers, fibrous
fibul/o	fibula
flex/o	to bend
fluor/o	fluorescence, luminous
fus/o	pouring
gastr/o	stomach
genit/o	genitals
gingiv/o	gums
glauc/o	gray
gli/o	glue
glomerul/o	glomerulus
gloss/o	tongue
gluc/o	glucose
glute/o	buttock
glyc/o	sugar
glycos/o	sugar, glucose
gonad/o	sex glands
granul/o	granules
gynec/o	female, woman
habilitat/o	ability
hal/o	to breathe
hallucin/o	imagined perception
hem/o	blood
hemat/o	blood
hepat/o	liver
hidr/o	sweat
hist/o	tissue
home/o	sameness
humer/o	humerus
hydr/o	water

Combining Form	Definition
hymen/o	hymen
hyster/o	uterus
iatr/o	physician, medicine, treatment
ichthy/o	scaly, dry
idi/o	distinctive
ile/o	ileum
ili/o	ilium
immun/o	immunity, protection
infer/o	below
inguin/o	groin region
iod/o	iodine
ir/o	iris
irid/o	iris
isch/o	to hold back
ischi/o	ischium
jejun/o	jejunum
kal/i	potassium
kerat/o	cornea, hard, horny
ket/o	ketones
keton/o	ketones
kinesi/o	movement
klept/o	to steal
kyph/o	hump
labi/o	lip
labyrinth/o	labyrinth (inner ear)
lacrim/o	tears
lact/o	milk
lamin/o	lamina, part of vertebra
lapar/o	abdomen
laps/o	to slide back
laryng/o	larynx, voice box
later/o	side
leuk/o	white
lingu/o	tongue
lip/o	fat
lith/o	stone
lob/o	lobe
lord/o	bent backwards
lumb/o	loin, low back
lymph/o	lymph
lymphaden/o	lymph node
lymphangi/o	lymph vessel
macul/o	macula lutea
mamm/o	breast
mandibul/o	mandible
mast/o	breast
maxill/o	maxilla
meat/o	meatus
medi/o	middle
medull/o	inner portion, medulla, oblongata
melan/o	black
men/o	menses, menstruation
mening/o	meninges
meningi/o	meninges

Combining Form	Definition
ment/o	mind
metacarp/o	metacarpals
metatars/o	metatarsals
metr/o	uterus
mi/o	lessening
mineral/o	minerals, electrolytes
miss/o	to send back
morbid/o	ill
morph/o	shape
mort/o	death
muc/o	mucus
muscul/o	muscles
mutat/o	to change
my/o	muscle
myc/o	fungus
mydr/i	widening
myel/o	bone marrow, spinal cord
myocardi/o	heart muscle
myos/o	muscle
myring/o	tympanic membrane (eardrum)
nas/o	nose
nat/o	birth
natr/o	sodium
necr/o	death
nephr/o	kidney
neur/o	nerve
neutr/o	neutral
noct/i	night
nucle/o	nucleus
nyctal/o	night
o/o	egg
obsess/o	besieged by thoughts
ocul/o	eye
odont/o	tooth
olig/o	scanty
onc/o	tumor
onych/o	nail
oophor/o	ovary
ophthalm/o	eye
opt/o	eye, vision
optic/o	eye, vision
or/o	mouth
orch/o	testes
orchi/o	testes
orchid/o	testes
orth/o	straight, correct, upright
oste/o	bone
ot/o	ear
ovari/o	ovary
ox/o, ox/i	oxygen
palat/o	palate
pancreat/o	pancreas
papill/o	optic disc
parathyroid/o	parathyroid gland

Combining Form	Definition
patell/o	patella
path/o	disease
pector/o	chest
ped/o	child, foot
pedicul/o	lice
pelv/o	pelvis
pen/o	penis
perine/o	perineum
peritone/o	peritoneum
phac/o	lens
phag/o	eat, swallow
phalang/o	phalanges
pharmac/o	drug
pharyng/o	pharynx (throat)
phleb/o	vein
phob/o	irrational fear
phon/o	sound
phot/o	light
phren/o	mind
physic/o	body
pineal/o	pineal gland
pituitar/o	pituitary gland
plant/o	sole of foot
pleur/o	pleura
pneum/o	lung, air
pneumon/o	lung, air
pod/o	foot
poli/o	gray matter
polyp/o	polyp
pont/o	pons
poster/o	back
presby/o	old age
proct/o	rectum and anus
prostat/o	prostate gland
prosthet/o	addition
protein/o	protein
proxim/o	near to
psych/o	mind
pub/o	genital region, pubis
pulmon/o	lung
pupill/o	pupil
py/o	pus
pyel/o	renal pelvis
pylor/o	pylorus
pyr/o	fire
radi/o	radius, ray (X-ray)
radic/o	root
radicul/o	nerve root
rect/o	rectum
recumb/o	to lie back
ren/o	kidney
retin/o	retina
rhin/o	nose
rhytid/o	wrinkle
roentgen/o	X-ray

Combining Form	Definition
rotat/o	to revolve
sacr/o	sacrum
salping/o	auditory tube (eustachian tube), uterine tubes, fallopian tubes
sanguin/o	blood
sarc/o	flesh (muscular substance)
scapul/o	scapula
schiz/o	split
scler/o	hard, sclera
scoli/o	crooked, bent
seb/o	oil
sect/o	to cut
sept/o	a wall
septic/o	infection
sialaden/o	salivary gland
sigmoid/o	sigmoid colon
sinus/o	sinus
soci/o	society
somat/o	body
somn/o	sleep
son/o	sound
specul/o	to look at
spermat/o	sperm
sphygm/o	pulse
spin/o	spine
spir/o	breathing
splen/o	spleen
spondyl/o	vertebrae
staped/o	stapes
stern/o	sternum
steth/o	chest
stigmat/o	point
super/o	above
synov/o	synovial membrane
synovi/o	synovial membrane
system/o	systems
tars/o	ankle, tarsus
ten/o	tendon
tenacul/o	to hold
tend/o	tendon
tendin/o	tendon
testicul/o	testes, testicle
thalam/o	thalamus
thec/o	sheath (meninges)
therm/o	heat
thorac/o	chest, thorax
thromb/o	clot
thym/o	thymus gland
thyr/o	thyroid gland
thyroid/o	thyroid gland
tibi/o	tibia
tom/o	to cut
ton/o	tone
tonsill/o	tonsils
topic/o	a specific area
tox/o	poison
toxic/o	poison
trache/o	trachea, windpipe
trich/o	hair
tuss/o	cough
tympan/o	tympanic membrane (eardrum)
uln/o	ulna
ungu/o	nail
ur/o	urine
ureter/o	ureter
urethr/o	urethra
urin/o	urine
uter/o	uterus
uve/o	choroid
vagin/o	vagina
valv/o	valve
valvul/o	valve
varic/o	dilated vein
vas/o	vas deferens, vessel, duct
vascul/o	blood vessel
ven/o	vein
ventr/o	belly
ventricul/o	brain ventricle, ventricle
vers/o	to turn
vertebr/o	vertebra
vesic/o	bladder
vesicul/o	seminal vesicle
viscer/o	internal organ
vitre/o	glassy
vulv/o	vulva
xer/o	dry

Suffix	Definition
-ac	pertaining to
-al	pertaining to
-algia	pain
-an	pertaining to
-apheresis	removal, carry away
-ar	pertaining to
-arche	beginning
-ary	pertaining to
-asthenia	weakness
-atic	pertaining to
-blast	immature, embryonic
-capnia	carbon dioxide
-cele	hernia, protrusion
-centesis	puncture to withdraw fluid
-cide	to kill
-clasia	to surgically break

Suffix	Definition
-crit	separation of
-cusis	hearing
-cyesis	state of pregnancy
-cyte	cell
-cytosis	more than the normal number of cells
-derma	skin condition
-desis	fuse, stabilize
-dipsia	thirst
-dynia	pain
-eal	pertaining to
-ectasis	dilation
-ectomy	surgical removal
-edema	swelling
-emesis	vomit
-emia	blood condition
-gen	that which produces
-genesis	produces, generates
-genic	producing, produced by
-globin	protein
-globulin	protein
-gram	record or picture
-graph	instrument for recording
-graphy	process of recording
-gravida	pregnancy
-ia	condition, state
-iac	pertaining to
-iasis	abnormal condition
-iatrist	physician
-iatry	medical treatment
-ic	pertaining to
-ical	pertaining to
-ician	specialist
-ile	pertaining to
-ine	pertaining to
-ion	action, condition
-ior	pertaining to
-ism	state of
-ist	specialist
-istry	specialty of
-itis	inflammation
-kinesia	movement
-listhesis	slipping
-lith	stone
-lithiasis	condition of stones
-logic	pertaining to studying
-logical	pertaining to the study of
-logist	one who studies
-logy	study of
-lucent	to shine through
-lysis	destruction
-lytic	destruction
-malacia	abnormal softening
-mania	frenzy

Suffix	Definition
-manometer	instrument to measure pressure
-megaly	enlargement, large
-meter	instrument for measuring
-metrist	specialist in measuring
-metry	process of measuring
-nic	pertaining to
-nomics	pertaining to laws
-oid	resembling
-ole	small
-oma	mass, tumor, swelling
-opaque	nontransparent
-opia	vision condition
-opsia	vision condition
-opsy	view of
-orexia	appetite
-ory	pertaining to
-ose	pertaining to
-osis	abnormal condition
-osmia	smell
-ostomy	surgically create an opening,
-otia	ear condition
-otomy	cutting into
-ous	pertaining to
-para	to bear (offspring)
-paresis	weakness
-partum	childbirth
-pathy	disease
-penia	abnormal decrease, too few
-pepsia	digestion
-pexy	surgical fixation
-phagia	eat, swallow
-phasia	speech
-phil	attracted to
-philia	attracted to
-phobia	fear
-phonia	voice
-phoresis	carrying
-phylaxis	protection
-plasia	development, growth, formation
-plasm	formation, development, growth
-plastic	pertaining to development
-plasty	surgical repair
-plegia	paralysis
-pnea	breathing
-poiesis	formation
-porosis	porous
-prandial	pertaining to a meal
-pressin	to press down
-ptosis	drooping
-ptysis	spitting
-rrhage	abnormal flow, excessive

Suffix	Definition
-rrhagia	abnormal flow condition
-rrhagic	pertaining to abnormal flow
-rrhaphy	suture
-rrhea	discharge, flow
-rrhexis	rupture
-salpinx	uterine tube
-sclerosis	hardening
-scope	instrument for viewing
-scopic	pertaining to visually examining
-scopy	process of visually examining
-spasm	involuntary muscle contraction
-spermia	condition of sperm
-stasis	standing still
-stat	standing still
-stenosis	narrowing

Suffix	Definition
-taxia	muscle coordination
-tension	pressure
-therapy	treatment
-thorax	chest
-tic	pertaining to
-tocia	labor, childbirth
-tome	instrument to cut
-tonia	tone
-tonic	pertaining to tone
-tripsy	surgical crushing
-trophic	pertaining to development
-trophy	nourishment, development
-tropia	turned condition
-tropin	to stimulate
-ule	small
-uria	condition of the urine

Appendix II

Word Parts Arranged Alphabetically by Definition

The definitions of the word parts that have been presented in this textbook are presented here and are arranged alphabetically. Prefixes are listed first, followed by combining forms and suffixes.

Definition	Prefix
abnormal	dys-, para-
above	hyper-, epi-, supra-
across	trans-
after	post-
again	re-
against	anti-, contra-
all	pan-
among	inter-
apart	dis-
around	circum-, peri-
away from	a-, ab-
backward	retro-
before	ante-, pre-, pro-
behind	retro-
below	hypo-, sub-
beside	para-
between	inter-
beyond	ultra-
different from usual	allo-
different	hetero-
difficult	dys-
excess	ultra-
excessive	hyper-
external	ex-
false	pseudo-
fast	tachy-
first	primi-
foreign	xeno-
four	quadri-, tetra-
good	eu-
half	semi-, hemi-
in front of	ante-, pre-
inner	endo-
inside	intra-
inward	en-, eso-, in-
large	macro-
many	multi-, poly-
near	para-
new	neo-
none	nulli-
normal	eu-
not	in-, un-
one	mono-
other	allo-
outside of	extra-
outward	ex-, exo-, e-
over	epi-, hyper-
painful	dys-
partial	semi-
same	homo-
self	auto-
to shut	myo-
slow	brady-
small	micro-
strange	xeno-
three	tri-
through	trans-, per-
toward	ad-
two	bi-
two like parts of a pair	para-
under	hypo-, sub-
upon	epi-
water	hydro-
within	endo-, in-, intra-
without	e-, a-, an-, de-, in-

Definition	Combining Form
abdomen	abdomin/o, lapar/o
ability	habilitat/o
above	super/o
addition	prosthet/o
adenoids	adenoid/o
adrenal glands	adren/o, adrenal/o
air	aer/o, pneum/o, pneumon/o
air sac	alveol/o
alveolus	alveol/o
amnion	amni/o
ankle	tars/o

Definition	Combining Form
anus	an/o
aorta	aort/o
appendix	append/o, appendic/o
arm	brachi/o
artery	arteri/o
artificial	factiti/o
atrium	atri/o
auditory tube	salping/o
away from	dist/o
axilla	axill/o
back	poster/o
back of body	dors/o
bacteria	bacteri/o
base	bas/o
belly	ventr/o
below	infer/o
to bend	flex/o
bent	scoli/o
bent backwards	lord/o
besieged by thoughts	obsess/o
bile duct	cholangi/o
bile	chol/e
birth	nat/o
black	melan/o
bladder	vesic/o, cyst/o
blood	hem/o, hemat/o, sanguin/o
blood vessel	vascul/o
blue	cyan/o
body	corpor/o, physic/o, somat/o
bone	oste/o
bone marrow	myel/o
to box	capsul/o
brain	encephal/o
brain ventricle	ventricul/o
breast	mamm/o, mast/o
to breathe	hal/o
to breathe in	aspir/o
breathing	spir/o
to bring	duct/o
bronchiole	bronchiol/o
bronchus	bronch/o, bronchi/o
bursa	burs/o
buttock	glute/o
calcium	calc/o
cancer	carcin/o
carpus	carp/o

Definition	Combining Form
cartilage	chondr/o
cavity	sinus/o
cecum	cec/o
cell	cyt/o
cerebellum	cerebell/o
cerebrum	cerebr/o
cerumen	cerumin/o
cervix	cervic/o
to change	mutat/o
cheek	bucc/o
chemical	chem/o
chest	pect/o, steth/o, thorac/o
child	ped/o
chorion	chori/o
choroid	uve/o
ciliary body	cycl/o
ciliary muscle	cycl/o
clavicle	clavicul/o
clot	thromb/o
clotting	coagul/o
clumping	agglutin/o
coal	anthrac/o
coccyx	coccyg/o
cochlea	cochle/o
cold	cry/o
colon	col/o, colon/o
color	chrom/o, chromat/o
common bile duct	choledoch/o
compel	compuls/o
conjunctiva	conjunctiv/o
contrived	factiti/o
cornea	corne/o, kerat/o
correct	emmetr/o, orth/o
cortex	cortic/o
cough	tuss/o
crooked	scoli/o
cul-de-sac	culd/o
to cut	cis/o, sect/o, tom/o
death	mort/o, necr/o
diaphragm	diaphragmat/o
dilated vein	varic/o
dim	ambly/o
disease	path/o
distinctive	idi/o
double	dipl/o
drive	compuls/o
drug	chem/o, pharmac/o
dry	ichthy/o, xer/o

Definition	Combining Form	Definition	Combining Form
duct	vas/o	glassy	vitre/o
dull	ambly/o	glomerulus	glomerul/o
duodenum	duoden/o	glucose	glycos/o, gluc/o
dura mater	dur/o	glue	gli/o
dust	coni/o	granules	granul/o
ear	aur/o, auricul/o, ot/o	gray	glauc/o
		gray matter	poli/o
eardrum	myring/o, tympan/o	groin region	inguin/o
eat	phag/o	gums	gingiv/o
egg	o/o	hair	trich/o
electricity	electr/o	hard	kerat/o, scler/o
electrolytes	mineral/o	head	cephal/o
embryo	embry/o	hearing	audi/o, audit/o, acous/o
embryonic	blast/o		
epididymis	epididym/o	heart	cardi/o, coron/o
epiglottis	epiglott/o	heart muscle	myocardi/o
epithelium	epitheli/o	heat	therm/o
esophagus	esophag/o	hidden	crypt/o
eustachian tube	salping/o	to hold	tenacul/o
extremities	acr/o	to hold back	isch/o
eye	ocul/o, ophthalm/o, opt/o, optic/o	horny	kerat/o
		humerus	humer/o
eyelid	blephar/o	hump	kyph/o
fallopian tubes	salping/o	hymen	hymen/o
false belief	deluss/o	ileum	ile/o
fat	adip/o, lip/o	ilium	ili/o
fatty substance	ather/o	ill	morbid/o
fear	anxi/o	imagined perception	hallucin/o
feeling	esthes/o	immature	blast/o
female	estr/o, gynec/o	immunity	immun/o
femur	femor/o	incomplete	atel/o
fetus	fet/o	infection	septic/o
fibers	fibr/o, fibrin/o	inner portion	medull/o
fibrous	fibrin/o	internal organ	viscer/o
fibrous band	fasci/o	iodine	iod/o
fibula	fibul/o	iris	ir/o, irid/o
fire	pyr/o	irrational fear	phob/o
flesh (muscular substance)	sarc/o	ischium	ischi/o
fluorescence	fluor/o	jejunum	jejun/o
foot	ped/o, pod/o	joint	arthr/o, articul/o
forgetfulness	amnes/o	ketones	ket/o, keton/o
front	anter/o	kidney	nephr/o, ren/o
fungus	myc/o	labyrinth	labyrinth/o
gall	chol/e	inner ear	labyrinth/o
gallbladder	cholecyst/o	lamina	lamin/o
genital region	pub/o	larynx	laryng/o
genitals	genit/o	leg	crur/o
gland	aden/o	lens	phac/o
glans penis	balan/o	lessening	mi/o

Definition	Combining Form
lice	pedicul/o
to lie back	recumb/o
life	bi/o
light	phot/o
lip	labi/o
liver	hepat/o
lobe	lob/o
loin	lumb/o
to look at	specul/o
low back	lumb/o
luminous	fluor/o
lung	pulmon/o, pneum/o, pneumon/o
lymph	lymph/o
lymph node	lymphaden/o
lymph vessel	lymphangi/o
macula lutea	macul/o
male	andr/o
mandible	mandibul/o
maxilla	maxill/o
meatus	meat/o
medicine	iatr/o
medulla oblongata	medull/o
meninges	mening/o, meningi/o, thec/o
menses	men/o
menstruation	men/o
metacarpals	metacarp/o
metatarsals	metatars/o
middle	medi/o
milk	lact/o
mind	ment/o, phren/o, psych/o
minerals	mineral/o
mouth	or/o
movement	kinesi/o
mucus	muc/o
muscle	my/o, myos/o, muscul/o
nail	onych/o, ungu/o
near to	proxim/o
neck	cervic/o
nerve	neur/o
nerve root	radicul/o
neutral	neutr/o
night	noct/I, nyctal/o
nitrogenous waste	azot/o
nose	nas/o, rhin/o
nucleus	nucle/o
oil	seb/o
old age	presby/o
outer portion	cortic/o
ovary	oophor/o, ovari/o
oxygen	ox/o, ox/i
palate	palat/o
pancreas	pancreat/o
parathyroid gland	parathyroid/o
part of vertebra	lamin/o
patella	patell/o
pelvis	pelv/o
penis	pen/o
perineum	perine/o
peritoneum	peritone/o
phalanges	phalang/o
pharynx	pharyng/o
physician	iatr/o
pineal gland	pineal/o
pituitary gland	pituitar/o
pleura	pleur/o
plug	embol/o
point	stigmat/o
poison	tox/o, toxic/o
polyp	polyp/o
pons	pont/o
potassium	kal/i
pouch	diverticul/o, cyst/o
pouring	fus/o
to press down	depress/o
profuse sweating	diaphor/o
proper	emmetr/o
prostate gland	prostat/o
protection	immun/o
protein	protein/o
pubis	pub/o
pulse	sphygm/o
pupil	pupill/o
pus	py/o
pylorus	pylor/o
radius	radi/o
rapid contracting and relaxing	clon/o
ray (X-ray)	radi/o
rectum	rect/o
rectum and anus	proct/o
red	erythr/o
renal pelvis	pyel/o
retina	retin/o

Definition	Combining Form
to revolve	rotat/o
rib	cost/o
root	radic/o
rosy red	eosin/o
sac	burs/o, cyst/o
sacrum	sacr/o
salivary gland	sialaden/o
sameness	home/o
scaly	ichthy/o
scanty	olig/o
scapula	scapul/o
sclera	scler/o
to secrete	crin/o
seminal vesicle	vesicul/o
to send back	miss/o
sensation	esthes/o
sense of pain	alges/o
sex glands	gonad/o
shape	morph/o
sheath (meninges)	thec/o
side	later/o
sigmoid colon	sigmoid/o
sinus	sinus/o
skin	cutane/o, derm/o, dermat/o
skull	crani/o
sleep	somn/o
to slide back	laps/o
small intestine	enter/o
society	soci/o
sodium	natr/o
sole of foot	plant/o
sound	phon/o, son/o
specific area	topic/o
sperm	spermat/o
spinal cord	myel/o
spine	spin/o
spleen	splen/o
split	schiz/o
stapes	staped/o
star	astr/o
to steal	klept/o
sternum	stern/o
stiff joint	ankyl/o
stomach	gastr/o
stone	lith/o
straight	orth/o
to stretch out	extens/o
sugar	glyc/o, glycos/o
swallow	phag/o
sweat	hidr/o
synovial membrane	synov/o, synovi/o
systems	system/o
tail	caud/o
tarsus	tars/o
tear duct	dacry/o
tears	dacry/o, lacrim/o
tendon	ten/o, tend/o, tendin/o
testes	orch/o, orchi/o, orchid/o, testicul/o
thalamus	thalam/o
thorax	thorac/o
throat	pharyng/o
thymus gland	thym/o
thyroid gland	thyr/o, thyroid/o
tibia	tibi/o
tissue	hist/o
tone	ton/o
tongue	gloss/o, lingu/o
tonsils	tonsill/o
tooth	dent/o, odont/o
trachea	trache/o
treatment	iatr/o
tumor	onc/o
to turn	vers/o
tympanic membrane	myring/o, tympan/o
ulna	uln/o
underarm	axill/o
upright	orth/o
ureter	ureter/o
urethra	urethr/o
urine	ur/o, urin/o
uterine tubes	salping/o
uterus	hyster/o, metr/o, uter/o
vagina	colp/o, vagin/o
valve	valv/o, valvul/o
vas deferens	vas/o
vein	phleb/o, ven/o
ventricle	ventricul/o
vertebra	vertebr/o, spondyl/o
vessel	angi/o, vas/o
vision	opt/o, optic/o
voice box	laryng/o
vulva	episi/o, vulv/o
wall	sept/o
water	aque/o, hydr/o

Definition	Combining Form	Definition	Combining Form
weight	bar/o	work	erg/o
white	albin/o, leuk/o	worry	anxi/o
to widen	dilat/o	wrinkle	rhytid/o
widening	mydr/i	wrist	carp/o
windpipe	trache/o	X-ray	roentgen/o
woman	gynec/o	yellow	cirrh/o

Definition	Suffix
abnormal condition	-iasis, -osis
abnormal decrease	-penia
abnormal flow condition	-rrhagia
abnormal flow	-rrhage
abnormal flow (pertaining to)	-rrhagic
abnormal softening	-malacia
action	-ion
appetite	-orexia
attracted to	-phil, -philia
to bear (offspring)	-para
beginning	-arche
blood condition	-emia
breathing	-pnea
carbon dioxide	-capnia
carry away	-apheresis
carrying	-phoresis
cell	-cyte
chest	-thorax
childbirth	-partum, -tocia
condition	-ion, -ia
condition of sperm	-spermia
condition of stones	-lithiasis
condition of the urine	-uria
cut (instrument to)	-tome
cutting into	-otomy
destruction	-lytic, -lysis
development	-plasia, -trophy, -plasm
development (pertaining to)	-plastic, -trophic
digestion	-pepsia
dilation	-ectasis
discharge	-rrhea
disease	-pathy
drooping	-ptosis
ear condition	-otia
eat	-phagia
embryonic	-blast
enlargement	-megaly
excessive flow	-rrhage
fallopian tube	-salpinx
fear	-phobia
flow	-rrhea
formation	-poiesis, -plasia, -plasm
frenzy	-mania
fuse	-desis
generates	-genesis
growth	-plasia, -plasm
hardening	-sclerosis
hearing	-cusis
hernia	-cele
immature	-blast
inflammation	-itis
pressure (instrument to measure)	-manometer
involuntary muscle contraction	-spasm
to kill	-cide
labor	-tocia
large	-megaly
laws (pertaining to)	-nomics
mass	-oma
meal (pertaining to a)	-prandial
measuring (instrument for)	-meter
measuring (process of)	-metry
medical treatment	-iatry
more than the normal number of cells	-cytosis
movement	-kinesia
muscle coordination	-taxia
narrowing	-stenosis
nontransparent	-opaque
nourishment	-trophy
one who studies	-logist
pain	-algia, -dynia
paralysis	-plegia
pertaining to	-ac, -al, -an, -ar, -ary, -atic, -eal, -ia, -iac, -ic, -ical, -ile, -ine, -ior, -nic, -ory, -ose, -ous, -tic
physician	-iatrist

Definition	Suffix
porous	-porosis
pregnancy	-gravida
pregnancy (state of)	-cyesis
pressure	-tension
to press down	-pressin
produced by	-genic
produces	-genesis
producing	-genic
protection	-phylaxis
protein	-globin, -globulin
protrusion	-cele
puncture to withdraw fluid	-centesis
record or picture	-gram
recording (instrument for)	-graph
recording (process of)	-graphy
removal	-apheresis
resembling	-oid
rupture	-rrhexis
separation of	-crit
to shine through	-lucent
skin condition	-derma
slipping	-listhesis
small	-ole, -ule
smell	-osmia
specialist	-ician, -ist
specialist in measuring	-metrist
specialty of	-istry
speech	-phasia
spitting	-ptysis
stabilize	-desis
standing still	-stasis, -stat
state	-ia
state of	-ism

Definition	Suffix
to stimulate	-tropin
stone	-lith
studying (pertaining to)	-logic
study of	-logy
study of (pertaining to the)	-logical
surgical fixation	-pexy
surgical removal	-ectomy
surgical repair	-plasty
to surgically break	-clasia
surgically create an opening	-ostomy
suture	-rrhaphy
swallow	-phagia
swelling	-edema, -oma
that which produces	-gen
thirst	-dipsia
tone	-tonia
tone (pertaining to)	-tonic
too few	-penia
treatment	-therapy
tumor	-oma
turned condition	-tropia
uterine tube	-salpinx
viewing (instrument for)	-scope
view of	-opsy
vision condition	-opia, -opsia
visually examining (pertaining to)	-scopic
visually examining (process of)	-scopy
voice	-phonia
vomit	-emesis
weakness	-asthenia, -paresis

Appendix III
Abbreviations

Abbreviation	Meaning
@	at
5-FU	5-fluorouracil
^{67}Ga	radioactive gallium
^{99m}Tc	radioactive technetium
^{131}I	radioactive iodine
^{133}Xe	radioactive xenon
^{201}Tl	radioactive thallium
α	alpha
$\bar{a}$	before
AAROM	active assistive range of motion
AB	abortion
ABGs	arterial blood gases
ac	before meals
ACTH	adrenocorticotropic hormone
ad lib	as desired
AD	Alzheimer's disease, right ear
ADD	attention-deficit disorder
ADH	antidiuretic hormone
ADHD	attention-deficit/hyperactivity disorder
ADL	activities of daily living
AE	above elbow
AF	atrial fibrillation
AGN	acute glomerulonephritis
AI	artificial insemination
AIDS	acquired immunodeficiency syndrome
AK	above knee
ALL	acute lymphocytic leukemia
ALS	amyotrophic lateral sclerosis
ALT	alanine transaminase
AMI	acute myocardial infarction
AML	acute myelogenous leukemia
Angio	angiography
ANS	autonomic nervous system
ante	before
AP	anteroposterior
APAP	acetaminophen (Tylenol™)
aq	aqueous (water)
ARC	AIDS-related complex
ARDS	adult (or acute) respiratory distress syndrome
ARF	acute renal failure
ARMD	age-related macular degeneration
AROM	active range of motion
AS	arteriosclerosis, left ear
ASA	aspirin
ASD	atrial septal defect
ASHD	arteriosclerotic heart disease
ASL	American Sign Language
AST	aspartate transaminase
Astigm	astigmatism
ATN	acute tubular necrosis
AU	both ears
AV, A-V	atrioventricular
β	beta
Ba	barium
BaE	barium enema
basos	basophils
BBB	bundle branch block (L for left; R for right)
BC	bone conduction
BCC	basal cell carcinoma
BDT	bone density testing
BE	barium enema, below elbow
bid	twice a day
BK	below knee
BM	bowel movement
BMD	bone mineral density
BMR	basal metabolic rate
BMT	bone marrow transplant
BNO	bladder neck obstruction
BP	blood pressure
BPD	bipolar disorder
BPH	benign prostatic hyperplasia
bpm	beats per minute
Bronch	bronchoscopy
BS	bowel sounds
BSE	breast self-examination
BUN	blood urea nitrogen
BX, bx	biopsy
$\bar{c}$	with
C1, C2, etc.	first cervical vertebra, second cervical vertebra, etc.
Ca	calcium, cancer
CA	chronological age
CABG	coronary artery bypass graft
CAD	coronary artery disease
cap(s)	capsule(s)
CAPD	continuous ambulatory peritoneal dialysis
CAT	computerized axial tomography
cath	catheterization
CBC	complete blood count
CBD	common bile duct
CC	cardiac catheterization, chief complaint, clean catch urine specimen
CCU	coronary care unit

Abbreviation	Meaning
c.gl.	correction with glasses
chemo	chemotherapy
CHF	congestive heart failure
Ci	curie
CIS	carcinoma in situ
Cl^-	chloride
CLL	chronic lymphocytic leukemia
CML	chronic myelogenous leukemia
CNS	central nervous system
CO_2	carbon dioxide
CoA	coarctation of the aorta
COPD	chronic obstructive pulmonary disease
CP	cerebral palsy, chest pain
CPK	creatine phosphokinase
CPR	cardiopulmonary resuscitation
CRF	chronic renal failure
C&S	culture and sensitivity
CS, C-section	cesarean section
CSD	congenital septal defect
CSF	cerebrospinal fluid
CT	calcitonin, computerized tomography
CTA	clear to auscultation
CTS	carpal tunnel syndrome
CV	cardiovascular
CVA	cerebrovascular accident
CVD	cerebrovascular disease
CVS	chorionic villus sampling
Cx	cervix
CXR	chest X-ray
cysto	cystoscopy
d	day
D	diopter (lens strength)
dB	decibel
D & C	dilation and curettage
d/c, DISC	discontinue
DC, disc	discontinue
DEA	Drug Enforcement Agency
decub	decubitus ulcer, lying down
Derm, derm	dermatology
DI	diabetes insipidus, diagnostic imaging
diff	differential
dil	dilute
disp	dispense
DJD	degenerative joint disease
DM	diabetes mellitus
DOE	dyspnea on exertion
DPT	diphtheria, pertussis, tetanus injection
DRE	digital rectal exam
DSA	digital subtraction angiography

Abbreviation	Meaning
DSM	*Diagnostic and Statistical Manual of Mental Disorders*
dtd	give of such a dose
DTR	deep tendon reflex
DVA	distance visual acuity
DVT	deep vein thrombosis
Dx	diagnosis
DXA	dual-energy absorptiometry
e-stim	electrical stimulation
ECC	extracorporeal circulation
ECCE	extracapsular cataract extraction
ECG, EKG	electrocardiogram
ECHO	echocardiogram
ECT	electroconvulsive therapy
ED	erectile dysfunction
EDC	estimated date of confinement
EEG	electroencephalogram, electroencephalography
EENT	eye, ear, nose, and throat
EGD	esophagogastroduodenoscopy
ELISA	enzyme-linked immunosorbent assay
EM	emmetropia
EMB	endometrial biopsy
EMG	electromyogram
Endo	endoscopy
ENT	ear, nose, and throat
EOM	extraocular movement
eosins, eos	eosinophils
ERCP	endoscopic retrograde cholangiopancreatography
ERT	estrogen replacement therapy
ERV	expiratory reserve volume
ESR, SR, sed rate	erythrocyte sedimentation rate
ESRD	end-stage renal disease
ESWL	extracorporeal shockwave lithotripsy
et	and
EU	excretory urography
EUA	exam under anesthesia
FBS	fasting blood sugar
FDA	Federal Drug Administration
FEKG	fetal electrocardiogram
FHR	fetal heart rate
FHT	fetal heart tone
FOBT	fecal occult blood test
FRC	functional residual capacity
FS	frozen section
FSH	follicle-stimulating hormone
FTND	full-term normal delivery
FX, Fx	fracture
GA	gallium, general anesthesia

Abbreviation	Meaning
GB	gallbladder, gallbladder X-ray
GC	gonorrhea
GERD	gastroesophageal reflux disease
GH	growth hormone
GI, grav I	first pregnancy
GI	gastrointestinal
gm	gram
GOT	glutamic oxaloacetic transaminase
gr	grain
gt	drop
gtt	drops
GTT	glucose tolerance test
GU	genitourinary
GVHD	graft versus host disease
GYN, gyn	gynecology
H_2O	water
HA	headache
HAV	hepatitis A virus
HBV	hepatitis B virus
HCG, hCG	human chorionic gonadotropin
HCl	hydrochloric acid
HCO_3^-	bicarbonate
HCT, Hct, crit	hematocrit
HCV	hepatitis C virus
HD	Hodgkin's disease, hemodialysis
HDN	hemolytic disease of the newborn
HDV	hepatitis D virus
HEENT	head, ears, eyes, nose, throat
HEV	hepatitis E virus
Hgb, Hb, HGB	hemoglobin
HIV	human immunodeficiency virus
HMD	hyaline membrane disease
HNP	herniated nucleus pulposus
HPV	human papilloma virus
HRT	hormone replacement therapy
hs	at bedtime
HSG	hysterosalpingography
HSV-1	herpes simplex virus type 1
HSV	herpes simplex virus
HTN	hypertension
Hz	hertz
$\bar{i}$	one
$\bar{ii}$	two
$\bar{iii}$	three
IBD	inflammatory bowel disease
IBS	irritable bowel syndrome
IC	inspiratory capacity
ICCE	intracapsular cataract extraction
ICP	intracranial pressure
ICU	intensive care unit
I&D	incision and drainage
ID	intradermal
IDDM	insulin-dependent diabetes mellitus
Ig	immunoglobulins (IgA, IgD, IgE, IgG, IgM)
IM	intramuscular
inj	injection
I&O	intake and output
IOP	intraocular pressure
IPD	intermittent peritoneal dialysis
IPPB	intermittent positive pressure breathing
IRDS	infant respiratory distress syndrome
IRV	inspiratory reserve volume
IU	international unit
IUD	intrauterine device
IV	intravenous
IVC	intravenous cholangiogram, intravenous cholangiography
IVF	*in vitro* fertilization
IVP	intravenous pyelogram
JRA	juvenile rheumatoid arthritis
K^+	potassium
kg	kilogram
KS	Kaposi's sarcoma
KUB	kidney, ureter, bladder
L1, L2, etc.	first lumbar vertebra, second lumbar vertebra, etc.
L	liter
LASIK	laser-assisted in-situ keratomileusis
LAT, lat	lateral
LBW	low birth weight
LE	lower extremity
LGI	lower gastrointestinal series
LH	luteinizing hormone
LL	left lateral
LLE	left lower extremity
LLL	left lower lobe
LLQ	left lower quadrant
LMP	last menstrual period
LP	lumbar puncture
LUE	left upper extremity
LUL	left upper lobe
LUQ	left upper quadrant
LVAD	left ventricular assist device
LVH	left ventricular hypertrophy
lymphs	lymphocytes
MA	mental age
mA	milliampere
MAO	monoamine oxidase

Abbreviation	Meaning
mcg	microgram
mCi	millicurie
MD	muscular dystrophy
MDI	metered-dose inhaler
mEq	milliequivalent
mets	metastases
mg	milligram
MI	myocardial infarction, mitral insufficiency
mL	milliliter
mm Hg	millimeters of mercury
MM	malignant melanoma
MMPI	Minnesota Multiphasic Personality Inventory
mono	mononucleosis
monos	monocytes
MR	mitral regurgitation
MRA	magnetic resonance angiography
MRI	magnetic resonance imaging
MS	mitral stenosis, multiple sclerosis, musculoskeletal
MSH	melanocyte-stimulating hormone
MTX	methotrexate
MUA	manipulation under anesthesia
MVP	mitral valve prolapse
Na^+	sodium
NB	newborn
NG	nasogastric (tube)
NHL	non-Hodgkin's lymphoma
NIDDM	non-insulin-dependent diabetes mellitus
NK	natural killer cells
NMR	nuclear magnetic resonance
no sub	no substitute
noc	night
non rep	do not repeat
NPH	neutral protamine Hagedorn (insulin)
NPO	nothing by mouth
NS	nephrotic syndrome, normal saline
NSAID	nonsteroidal anti-inflammatory drug
n&v	nausea and vomiting
O_2	oxygen
OA	osteoarthritis
OB	obstetrics
OCD	obsessive–compulsive disorder
OCPs	oral contraceptive pills
od	overdose
OD	right eye
oint	ointment

Abbreviation	Meaning
OM	otitis media
O&P	ova and parasites
Ophth.	ophthalmology
OR	operating room
ORIF	open reduction–internal fixation
Orth, ortho	orthopedics
OS	left eye
OT	occupational therapy
OTC	over the counter
Oto	otology
OU	each eye/both eyes
oz	ounce
$\bar{p}$	after
P	pulse
PA	pernicious anemia, posteroanterior
PAC	premature atrial contraction
Pap	Papanicolaou test
PARR	postanesthetic recovery room
PBI	protein-bound iodine
pc	after meals
PCA	patient-controlled administration
PCP	pneumocystis pneumonia
PCV	packed cell volume
PDA	patent ductus arteriosus
PDR	*Physician's Desk Reference*
PE tube	pressure equalizing tube
per	with
PERRLA	pupils equal, round, react to light and accommodation
PET	positron emission tomography
PFT	pulmonary function test
pH	acidity or alkalinity of urine
PI, para I	first delivery
PID	pelvic inflammatory disease
PMN, polys	polymorphonuclear neutrophil
PMS	premenstrual syndrome
PNS	peripheral nervous system
PO, po	by mouth
PORP	partial ossicular replacement prosthesis
pp	postprandial
PPD	purified protein derivative
preop, pre-op	preoperative
prep	preparation, prepared
PRK	photorefractive keratectomy
PRL	prolactin
prn	as needed
PROM	passive range of motion
prot	protocol
PSA	prostate-specific antigen
PT, pro-time	prothrombin time
pt	patient

Abbreviation	Meaning
PT	physical therapy
PTC	percutaneous transhepatic cholangiography
PTCA	percutaneous transluminal coronary angioplasty
PTH	parathyroid hormone
PUD	peptic ulcer disease
PVC	premature ventricular contraction
q	every
qam	every morning
qh	every hour
qhs	at bedtime
qid	four times a day
qs	quantity sufficient
R	respiration, roentgen
Ra	radium
RA	rheumatoid arthritis, room air
rad	radiation-absorbed dose
RAI	radioactive iodine
RBC	red blood cell
RDS	respiratory distress syndrome
REM	rapid eye movement
Rh+	Rh-positive
Rh–	Rh-negative
RIA	radioimmunoassay
RL	right lateral
RLE	right lower extremity
RLL	right lower lobe
RLQ	right lower quadrant
RML	right middle lobe
ROM	range of motion
RP	retrograde pyelogram
RPR	rapid plasma reagin (test for syphilis)
RRT	registered radiologic technologist, registered respiratory therapist
RUE	right upper extremity
RUL	right upper lobe
RUQ	right upper quadrant
RV	reserve volume
Rx	take
$\bar{s}$	without
$\overline{ss}$	one-half
S1	first heart sound
S2	second heart sound
SA, S-A	sinoatrial
SAD	seasonal affective disorder
SARS	severe acute respiratory syndrome
SC	subcutaneous
SCC	squamous cell carcinoma
SCI	spinal cord injury
SCIDS	severe combined immunodeficiency syndrome
segs	segmented neutrophils
s.gl.	without correction or glasses
SG, sp. gr.	specific gravity
SG	skin graft
SIDS	sudden infant death syndrome
Sig	label as follows/directions
SK	streptokinase
sl	under the tongue
SLE	systemic lupus erythematosus
SMAC	sequential multiple analyzer computer
SMD	senile macular degeneration
SOB	shortness of breath
sol	solution
SOM	serous otitis media
SPP	suprapubic prostatectomy
ST	esotropia
st	stage
stat	at once/immediately
STD	sexually transmitted disease
STSG	split-thickness skin graft
Subc, SubQi subcu, SC, sc, subq	subcutaneous
suppos, supp	suppository
susp	suspension
syr	syrup
T & A	tonsillectomy and adenoidectomy
T, tbsp	tablespoon
t, tsp	teaspoon
T1, T2, etc.	first thoracic vertebra, second thoracic vertebra, etc.
T_3	triiodothyronine
T_4	thyroxine
tab	tablet
TAH-BSO	total abdominal hysterectomy–bilateral salpingo-oophorectomy
TAH	total abdominal hysterectomy
TB	tuberculosis
TENS	transcutaneous electrical stimulation
TFT	thyroid function test
THA	total hip arthroplasty
THR	total hip replacement
TIA	transient ischemic attack
tid	three times a day
TKA	total knee arthroplasty
TKR	total knee replacement
TLC	total lung capacity
TNM	tumor, nodes, metastases

Abbreviation	Meaning
TO	telephone order
top	apply topically
TORP	total ossicular replacement prosthesis
tPA	tissue-type plasminogen activator
TPN	total parenteral nutrition
TPR	temperature, pulse, and respiration
TSH	thyroid-stimulating hormone
TSS	toxic shock syndrome
TUR	transurethral resection
TURP	transurethral resection of the prostate
TV	tidal volume
u	unit
U/A, UA	urinalysis
UC	urine culture, uterine contractions

Abbreviation	Meaning
UE	upper extremity
UGI	upper gastrointestinal series
URI	upper respiratory infection
US	ultrasound
UTI	urinary tract infection
UV	ultraviolet
VA	visual acuity
VC	vital capacity
VCUG	voiding cystourethrography
VD	venereal disease
VF	visual field
Vfib	ventricular fibrillation
VO	verbal order
VSD	ventricular septal defect
VT	ventricular tachycardia
WBC	white blood cell
wt	weight
x	times
XT	exotropia

Appendix IV

The Common Core Connection

About the Common Core State Standards

In 2010, the National Governors Association Center for Best Practices and the Council of Chief State School Officers released the Common Core State Standards (CCSS) in English language arts (ELA) and mathematics. These standards are designed as a set of standard expectations for all students in the United States.

> "The Common Core State Standards provide a consistent, clear understanding of what students are expected to learn, so teachers and parents know what they need to do to help them. The standards are designed to be robust and relevant to the real world, reflecting the knowledge and skills that our young people need for success in college and careers. With American students fully prepared for the future, our communities will be best positioned to compete successfully in the global economy."
> (National Governors Association Center for Best Practices, Council of Chief State School Officers, Washington D.C. 2010)

The CCSS are intended to help all students achieve at higher levels so when you enter college it won't be necessary to take remedial courses or struggle to complete college-level work. There are CCSS for all grades from kindergarten through high school. They are taught primarily in ELA classes and mathematics classes, but they are reinforced through instruction in all other core classes as well as in health science programs of study.

The Common Core State Standards for ELA are organized into six categories:

For all grades K-12

- Reading (literature and information)
- Writing
- Speaking and Listening
- Language

For grades 6-12 only

- Reading for literacy in History/Social Studies
- Reading and Writing for literacy in Science and Technical Subjects

The Common Core State Standards for mathematics are organized into six categories at the high school level:

- Number and Quantity
- Algebra
- Functions
- Modeling
- Geometry
- Statistics and Probability

The importance of these Common Core State Standards cannot be overstated. In a recent survey of more than 400 employers from across the U.S., when asked to identify the skills needed to succeed in the workplace by recently hired graduates from high school, two-year colleges, and four-year colleges, oral communications and reading comprehension are in the top five and written communication rated number 1 as the primary deficiency of high school students recently hired. See Table 1 for the complete rating.

Table 1.

1. Top Five Most Important Skills

	High School Graduates	Two-Year College Graduates	Four-Year College Graduates
Professionalism	80.3%	83.4%	93.8%
Teamwork	74.7%	82.7%	94.4%
Oral Communications	70.3%	82.0%	95.4%
Ethics & Social Responsibility	63.4%		
Reading Comprehension	62.5%	71.6%	

2. Primary deficiencies of high school students recently hired

Written Communication	81%
Leadership	73%
Work Ethic	70%
Critical Thinking and Problem Solving	70%
Self-Direction	58%

(Employers' Perspectives on the Basic Knowledge and Applied Skills of New Entrants to the 21st Century U.S. Workforce, 2006, The Conference Board, Corporate Voices for Working Families, P21 and SHRM)

Building Common Core Strength through Medical Terminology

Whether you choose to enter a health care career immediately after high school, prepare for a technical career that will require at least a certificate or two-year college program, or choose to go on to a professional-level career that will take at least four years of college and perhaps even more, competency in all kinds of communication and computational skills will be needed. Health care requires postsecondary preparation for nearly all careers. Blending medical terminology and body systems study with the CCSS will help you succeed as you continue your studies and begin your career.

Careers in health care demand high levels of reading, writing, and oral communication as well as technology accuracy and mathematical skills to ensure safe patient care. For example, health care workers must be capable of interpreting statistics, understanding measurement, comprehending charts and research reports, communicating with patients, families, colleagues, and co-workers, and utilizing Electronic Health Records (EHRs). Although neither science, health care, nor medical terminology is specifically identified in the CCSS, the standards are intended to transfer to all areas of study. In other words, mastering ELA and mathematics is fundamental to mastering medical terminology.

One set of CCSS ELA standards was developed specifically for use in Science and Technical Subjects. Many of the standards in this set align with the National Healthcare Standards for *Health Informatics*. One example is shown in Table 2. Both of these standards are met by learning, understanding, and utilizing EHR coding systems such as the International Classification of Diseases (ICD), 9th Revision, Clinical Modification, which is an international coding and classification system that groups diseases, disorders and procedures into similar categories. For example, ICD-9 code 796.2 would indicate a diagnosis of high blood pressure in these international locations.

Table 2.

English Language Arts	
CCSS ELA-Literacy. RST.11-12.4	Health Informatics Pathway Standard 3
Determine the meaning of symbols, key terms, and other domain-specific words and phrases as they are used in a specific scientific or technical context	Know how to read and interpret a medical record or other medical document applying knowledge of medical terminology and codes. They will extract required information from a medical record and other medical documents for a variety purposes, upon regulatory or legal request.

Through completion of the *Medical Terminology: A Living Language* (MED TERM) coursework, the Common Core Standards for both ELA and mathematics will be enhanced and reinforced. When completing your ELA and mathematics coursework you will see the connections that help you gain the knowledge and skills needed. Table 3 provides examples showing the connections between your MED TERM text and the CCSS.

Table 3.

English Language Arts	
Reading Standards for Literacy in Science and Technical Subjects Grades 11-12	
Standard 3	MED TERM Practice
Follow precisely a complex multistep procedure when carrying out experiments, taking measurements, or performing technical tasks.	Figure 5.21 (page 162) The process of placing a stent in a blood vessel. (A) A catheter is used to place a collapsed stent next to an atherosclerotic plaque; (B) stent is expanded; (C) catheter is removed, leaving the expanded stent behind.
Standard 4	MED TERM Practice
Determine the meaning of symbols, key terms, and other domain-specific words and phrases as they are used in a specific scientific or technical context	**Tissues** (page 25) **connective tissue** **epithelial tissue** (ep-ih-THEE-lee-al) **muscle tissue** **histology** (hiss-TALL-oh-jee) **nervous tissue** **Histology** is the study of tissues. A tissue is formed when like cells are grouped together and function together to form a specific activity. The body has four types of tissue: **muscle tissue**, **epithelial tissue**, **connective tissue** and **nervous tissue**.

(continued)

Table 3. ***(cont)***

Mathematics	
Interpret functions that arise in applications in terms of the context	
Standard 6	MED TERM Practice
Calculate and interpret the average rate of change of a function (represented symbolically or as a table) over a specified interval. Estimate the rate of change from a graph	MED TERM TIP (page 146) The electrocardiogram, referred to as an EKG or ECG is a measurement of the electrical activity of the heart. This can give the physician information about the health of the heart, especially the myocardium.
Making inferences and justifying conclusions	
Standard 1	MED TERM Practice
Understand statistics as a process for making inferences about population parameters based on a random sample from that population	Pharmacology Terms (page 497) Placebo-Inactive, harmless substance used to satisfy a patient's desire for medication. This is also used in research when given to a control group of patients in a study in which another group receives a drug. The effect of the placebo versus the drug is then observed.

Activities

Search and Find Activity 1

English Language Arts

In teams of two or three read the following ELA standards and see if you can find an example of applying the standard to a *MED TERM Practice* *from your text.*

Reading Standards for Literacy in Science and Technical Subjects Grades 11-12

Standard 6

Analyze the author's purpose in providing an explanation, describing a procedure or discussing an experiment in a text, identifying important issues that remain unsolved

MED TERM Practice

Title ______________________________ Page #__________

Content ______________________________

____

____

Why do you consider this a match?

____

____

Standard 7

Integrate and evaluate multiple sources of information presented in diverse formats and media in order to address a question or solve a problem

MED TERM Practice

Title ______________________________ Page #__________

Content ______________________________

____

____

Why do you consider this a match?

____

____

Writing Standards for Literacy in History/Social Studies, Science and Technical Subjects Grades 11-12

Standard 4

Provide clear and coherent writing in which the development, organization and style are appropriate to task, purpose and audience

MED TERM Practice

Title ______________________________ Page #__________

Content ______________________________

____

____

Why do you consider this a match?

____

____

Standard 6

Use technology, including the Internet, to produce, publish and update individual and shared writing products in response to ongoing feedback, including new arguments or information

MED TERM Practice

Title ______________________________ Page #__________

Content ______________________________

____

____

Why do you consider this a match?

____

____

Search and Find Activity 2

Mathematics

In teams of two or three read the following mathematics standards and see if you can find an example of applying the standard to a MED TERM Practice from your text.

Reason quantitatively and use units to solve problems

Standard 3

Choose a level of accuracy appropriate to limitations on measurement when reporting quantities

MED TERM Practice

Title ______________________________ Page # ____________

Content ______________________________

____

____

Why do you consider this a match?

____

____

Apply geometric concepts in modeling situations

Standard 1

Use geometric shapes, their measures and other properties to describe objects (e.g., modeling a human torso as a cylinder)

MED TERM Practice

Title ______________________________ Page # ____________

Content ______________________________

____

____

Why do you consider this a match?

____

____

Making inferences and justifying conclusions

Standard 6

Evaluate reports based on data

MED TERM Practice

Title ______________________________ Page # ____________

Content ______________________________

____

____

Why do you consider this a match?

____

____

Use probability to evaluate outcomes of decisions

Standard 7
Analyze decisions and strategies using probability concepts (e.g., medical testing)

MED TERM Practice
Title ______________________________ Page #__________
Content ______________________________

____

____

Why do you consider this a match?

____

____

Future Think Activity
Read the following essay and then use the information to complete the activity.

As you think about how the future of health care will impact the work you do, it will be helpful to explore the changes that are in process and others that are being predicted. There are two major changes that are impacting health status around the globe: advances in technology and an aging population in the most-developed countries. The need for a highly educated health care workforce is essential if the U.S. is to remain a leading nation in providing quality of life for its' citizens.

Note: terms italicized represent new processes, procedures, or terminology

---

According to GLOBAL TRENDS 2030: ALTERNATIVE WORLDS, a publication of the National Intelligence Council, "By 2030 we expect to see continued progress on health—including extending the quality of life for those aging. Even in the face of the HIV/AIDS epidemic the global disease burden has be shifting rapidly for several decades from communicable to non-communicable diseases—including AIDS, diarrhea, malaria, and respiratory infections—are projected to decline by nearly 30 percent by 2030.

Technological breakthroughs pertaining to the security of vital resources will be necessary to meet the food, water and energy needs of the world's population. (new) health technologies will continue to extend the average age of populations around the world, ameliorating debilitating physical and mental conditions, and improving overall well-being."

"Disease management technologies in development promise significant healthy longevity gains throughout the world while *human augmentation* technologies will likely transform life, particularly for the elderly and mobility-impaired populations. (diagnostic) and *pathogen-detection devices* will be key in enabling technologies for disease management; the future accuracy of *molecular diagnostics* has the power to transform medicine.

Theranostics, the combination of a diagnostic and therapeutic approach in one treatment, may become an important discipline for disease management, reducing hospital costs by accelerating patient's recovery time and complications caused by invasive surgery. Advances in *synthetic biology* will likely result in production facilities making novel treatments and diagnostics agents. Advances in *regenerative medicine* almost certainly parallel these developments in diagnostic and treatment protocols. For example replacement organs, such as kidneys and livers, could be developed by 2030."

"Spanning a wide gamut of technologies, ranging from implants and prosthetics to *powered exoskeletons*, human augmentation enhances innate human abilities, or replaces missing or defective functions such as damaged limbs.

Future retinal eye implants could enable night vision, and *neuro-enhancements* could provide superior memory recall or speed of thought. *Neuro-pharmaceuticals* will allow people to maintain concentration for longer periods of time to enhance their learning abilities."

Select a practice from the predictions stated. Think of someone you might know, a family member, friend, someone you have read about, or even yourself. Describe how you think this practice would bring an improved quality to their life and how you would like to be part of implementing the practice.

(Use a separate sheet of paper if needed.)

Share your response in a class discussion.

Glossary/Index

A

Agranulocytes, nongranular leukocyte; this is one of two types of leukocytes found in plasma that are classified as either monocytes or lymphocytes, 181, 181*t*

AIDS-related complex (ARC), early stage of AIDS; there is a positive test for virus but only mild symptoms of weight loss, fatigue, skin rash, and anorexia, 202

Alanine transaminase (ALT), enzyme normally present in blood; blood levels are increased in persons with liver disease, 276

Albinism, condition in which person is not able to produce melanin; albino person has white hair and skin and pupils of eye are red, 63

Albumin, protein normally found circulating in bloodstream; it is abnormal for albumin to be in urine, 180, 303

Aldosterone, hormone produced by adrenal cortex; regulates levels of sodium and potassium in body and as a side effect volume of water lost in urine, 380*t*, 382

Alimentary canal, also known as gastrointestinal system or digestive system; system covers area between mouth and anus and includes 30 feet of intestinal tubing; has a wide range of functions; system serves to store and digest food, absorb nutrients, and eliminate waste; major organs of system are mouth, pharynx, esophagus, stomach, small intestine, colon, rectum, and anus, 258

Allergen, antigen capable of causing a hypersensitivity or allergy in body, 201

Allergist, physician who specializes in testing for and treating allergies, 200

Allergy, hypersensitivity to a substance in environment or medication, 201

Allograft, skin graft from one person to another; donor is usually a cadaver, 70

Alopecia, absence or loss of hair, especially of head, 69

Alveolar, pertaining to alveoli,

Alveoli, tiny air sacs at end of each bronchiole; alveoli are surrounded by capillary network; gas exchange takes place as oxygen and carbon dioxide diffuse across alveolar and capillary walls, 223, 224*f*

Alzheimer's disease (AD), chronic, organic mental disorder consisting of dementia that is more prevalent in adults between 40 and 60; involves progressive disorientation, apathy, speech and gait disturbances, and loss of memory, 424, 501

Amblyopia, loss of vision not as a result of eye pathology; usually occurs in patients who see two images; in order to see only one image, brain will no longer recognize image being sent to it by one of eyes; may occur if strabismus is not corrected; commonly referred to as lazy eye, 456

Ambulatory care center, facility that provides services that do not require overnight hospitalization; services range from simple surgeries, to diagnostic testing, to therapy; also called a surgical center or outpatient clinic, 13

Amenorrhea, absence of menstruation, which can be result of many factors, including pregnancy, menopause, and dieting, 342

American Sign Language (ASL), nonverbal method of communicating in which hands and fingers are used to indicate words and concepts; used by people who are deaf and speech impaired, 475, 475*f*

Amino acids, organic substances found in plasma, used by cells to build proteins, 180

Amnesia, loss of memory in which people forget their identity as a result of head injury or disorder, such as epilepsy, senility, and alcoholism; can be either temporary or permanent, 501

Amniocentesis, puncturing of amniotic sac using a needle and syringe for purpose of withdrawing amniotic fluid for testing; can assist in determining fetal maturity, development, and genetic disorders, 348

Amnion, inner of two membranous sacs surrouding fetus; amniotic sac contains amniotic fluid in which baby floats, 338, 340

Amniorrhea, discharge of amniotic fluid, 342

Amniotic, pertaining to amnion, 340

Amniotic fluid, fluid inside amniotic sac, 336, 337*f*, 338

Amniotomy, incision into amniotic sac, 349

Amplification device, 475

Amputation, partial or complete removal of a limb for a variety of reasons, including tumors, gangrene, intractable pain, crushing injury, or uncontrollable infection, 107

Amylase, digestive enzyme found in saliva that begins digestion of carbohydrates, 264

Amyotrophic lateral sclerosis (ALS), disease with muscular weakness and atrophy due to degeneration of motor neurons of spinal cord; also called *Lou Gehrig's disease,* after New York Yankees' baseball player who died from disease, 427

Anacusis, total absence of hearing; unable to perceive sound; also called *deafness,* 472

Anal, pertaining to anus, 267

Anal fistula, abnormal tubelike passage from surface around anal opening directly into rectum, 272

Anal sphincter, ring of muscle that controls anal opening, 263

Analgesia, reduction in perception of pain or sensation due to neurological condition or medication, 422

Analgesic, substance that relieves pain without loss of consciousness; may be either narcotic or non-narcotic; narcotic drugs are derived from opium poppy and act on brain to cause pain relief and drowsiness, 432, 523

Anaphylactic shock, life-threatening condition resulting from ingestion of food or medications that produce severe allergic response; circulatory and respiratory problems occur, including respiratory distress, hypotension, edema, tachycardia, and convulsions, 201

Anaphylaxis, severe reaction to antigen, 201

Anastomosis, creating a passageway or opening between two organs or vessels, 279

Anatomical position, used to describe positions and relationships of a structure in human body; for descriptive purposes assumption is always that person is in anatomical position; body is standing erect with arms at side of body, palms of hands facing forward, and eyes looking straight ahead; legs are parallel with feet and toes pointing forward, 31, 32*f*

Ancillary reports, report in patient's medical record from various treatments and therapies patient has received, such as rehabilitation, social services, respiratory therapy, or from dietician, 12

Androgen, class of steroid hormones secreted by adrenal cortex; these hormones, such as testosterone, produce a masculinizing effect, 380*t*, 382

Androgen therapy, replacement male hormones to treat patients who produce insufficient hormone naturally, 362

Anemia, reduction in number of red blood cells (RBCs) or amount of hemoglobin in blood; results in less oxygen reaching tissues, 186

Anesthesia, partial or complete loss of sensation with or without loss of consciousness as a result of drug, disease, or injury, 422, 520, 521*t*

Anesthesiologist, physician who has specialization in practice of administering anesthetics, 422, 520

Anesthesiologist's report, medical record document that relates details regarding drugs given to patient and patient's response to anesthesia and vital signs during surgery, 12

Anesthesiology, branch of medicine specializing in all aspects of anesthesia, including for surgical procedures, resuscitation measures, and management of acute and chronic pain; physician is *anesthesiologist*, 422

Anesthetic, substance that produces a lack of feeling that may be of local or general effect, depending on type of administration, 72, 432, 523

Anesthetic ophthalmic solution, eyedrops for pain relief associated with eye infections and corneal abrasions, 463

Aneurysm, weakness in wall of artery that results in localized widening of artery, 157, 157*f*

Aneurysmectomy, surgical removal of aneurysm, 162

Angiitis, inflammation of vessels, 153

Angina pectoris, severe chest pain with sensation of constriction around heart; caused by a deficiency of oxygen to heart muscle, 154, 155*f*

Angiogram, record of a vessel, 159

Angiography, process of taking X-ray of blood or lymphatic vessels after injection of a radiopaque substance, 159

Angioplasty, surgical repair of blood vessels, 163, 163*f*

Angiospasm, involuntary muscle contraction of a vessel, 153

Angiostenosis, narrowing of a vessel, 153

Anhidrosis, abnormal condition of no sweat, 58

Ankylosing spondylitis, inflammatory spinal condition that resembles rheumatoid arthritis; results in gradual stiffening and fusion of vertebrae; more common in men than women, 103

Anorchism, congenital absence of one or both testes, 358

Anorexia, loss of appetite that can accompany other conditions such as gastrointestinal (GI) upset, 269

Anorexia nervosa, type of eating disorder characterized by severe disturbance in body image and marked refusal to eat, 501, 501*f*

Anorexiant, substance that treats obesity by suppressing appetite, 281

Anosmia, loss of sense of smell, 230

Anoxia, lack of oxygen, 230

Antacid, substance that neutralizes acid in stomach, 281

Antagonistic pairs, pair of muscles arranged around a joint that produce opposite actions, 115, 116–18*t*

Anteflexion, while uterus is normally in this position, exaggeration of forward bend of uterus is abnormal; forward bend is near neck of uterus; position of cervix, or opening of uterus, remains normal, 334

Antepartum, before birth, 341

Anterior, directional term meaning near or on front or belly side of body, 34*f*, 37*t*

Anus, terminal opening of digestive tube, 263, 264*f*
Anvil, 467*f*, 468
Anxiety, feeling of apprehension or worry, 500
Anxiety disorders, characterized by persistent worry and apprehension; includes panic attacks, anxiety, phobias, and obsessive-compulsive disorder, 500
Aorta, largest artery in body; located in mediastinum and carries oxygenated blood away from left side of heart, 35*t*, 140*f*, 141*f*, 142*f*, 144, 145*f*, 146*f*, 195*f*, 384*f*
Aortic, pertaining to aorta, 152
Aortic arch, 148*f*
Aortic semilunar valve, 144*f*
Aortic valve, semilunar valve between left ventricle of heart and aorta in heart; prevents blood from flowing backwards into ventricle, 142*f*, 143, 144*f*, 145*f*
Apex, directional term meaning tip or summit; an area of lungs and heart, 37*t*, 141, 141*f*, 145*f*, 224, 225*f*
Apgar score, evaluation of neonate's adjustment to outside world; observes color, heart rate, muscle tone, respiratory rate, and response to stimulus, 348
Aphagia, not eating, 269
Aphasia, inability to communicate through speech; often after effect of stroke (CVA), 422
Aphonia, no voice, 230
Aphthous ulcers, painful ulcers in mouth of unknown cause; commonly called *canker sores*, 270
Aplastic anemia, severe form of anemia that develops as consequence of loss of functioning red bone marrow; results in decrease in number of all formed elements; treatment may eventually require bone marrow transplant, 186
Apnea, condition of not breathing, 230
Apocrine gland, type of sweat gland that opens into hair follicles located in pubic, anal, and mammary areas; glands secrete substance that can produce odor when it comes into contact with bacteria on skin causing what is commonly referred to as body odor, 56
Appendectomy, surgical removal of appendix, 279
Appendicitis, inflammation of appendix, 272
Appendicular skeleton, appendicular skeleton consists of bones of upper and lower extremities, shoulder, and pelvis, 89, 92, 93*f*
Appendix, 36*t*, 263*f*, 264*f*
Aqueous, pertaining to water or being water-like, 454
Aqueous humor, watery fluid filling spaces between cornea and lens, 448*f*, 449
Arachnoid layer, delicate middle layer of meninges, 417, 417*f*
Areola, pigmented area around nipple of breast, 336, 336*f*
Arrector pili, small slip of smooth muscle attached to hairs; when this muscle contracts hair shaft stands up and results in "goose bumps," 53*f*, 55, 55*f*
Arrhythmia, irregularity in heartbeat or action, 154
Arterial, pertaining to artery, 152
Arterial anastomosis, surgical joining together of two arteries; performed if artery is severed or if damaged section of artery is removed, 162
Arterial blood gases (ABG), lab test that measures amount of oxygen, carbon dioxide, and nitrogen in blood, and pH, 238
Arteries, blood vessels that carry blood away from heart, 28*t*, 87*f*, 140, *147*, *147f*, 148*f*
Arteriole, smallest branch of arteries; carries blood to capillaries, 147, 152, 193*f*
Arteriorrhexis, ruptured artery, 157
Arteriosclerosis (AS), condition with thickening, hardening, and loss of elasticity of walls of arteries, 157
Arthralgia, pain in a joint, 100
Arthrocentesis, removal of synovial fluid with needle from joint space, such as in knee, for examination, 107
Arthroclasia, surgically breaking loose a stiffened joint, 107
Arthrodesis, surgical fusion or stiffening of a joint to provide stability; sometimes done to relieve pain of arthritis, 107
Arthrogram, record of a joint, 106
Arthrography, visualization of joint by radiographic study after injection of contrast medium into joint space, 106
Arthroscope, instrument to view inside joint, 3, 106
Arthroscopic surgery, use of arthroscope to facilitate performing surgery on joint, 107
Arthroscopy, examination of interior of joint by entering joint with arthroscope; arthroscope contains small television camera allowing physician to view interior of joint on monitor during procedure, 107
Arthrotomy, surgically cutting into a joint, 97
Articular, pertaining to a joint, 98
Articular cartilage, layer of cartilage covering ends of bones forming synovial joint, 86, 87*f*, 96*f*
Articulation, another term for a joint, point where two bones meet, 95
Artificial tears, medications, many of them over-the-counter, to treat dry eyes, 463
Asbestosis, type of pneumoconiosis developing from collection of asbestos fibers in lungs; may lead to development of lung cancer, 234
Ascending colon, section of colon following cecum; ascends right side of abdomen, 263, 263*f*, 264*f*

Autonomic nervous system (ANS), portion of nervous system consisting of nerves to internal organs that function involuntarily; regulates functions of glands (especially salivary, gastric, and sweat glands), adrenal medulla, heart, and smooth muscle tissue; system is divided into two parts: sympathetic and parasympathetic, 145, 418, 419–20

Axial skeleton, axial skeleton includes bones in head, spine, chest, and trunk, 89–92, 90*f*

Axillary, pertaining to armpit; there is a collection of lymph nodes in this area that drains each arm, 194*t*, 195*f*

Axon, single projection of a neuron that conducts impulse away from nerve cell body, 412, 413*f*

Azotemia, accumulation of nitrogenous waste in bloodstream; occurs when kidney fails to filter these wastes from blood, 305

B

B cells, common name for B lymphocytes, responds to foreign antigens by producing protective antibodies, 198

B lymphocytes, humoral immunity cells, which respond to foreign antigens by producing protective antibodies; simply referred to as *B cells,* 198

Babinski's reflex, reflex test to determine lesions and abnormalities in nervous system; Babinski reflex is present if great toe extends instead of flexes when lateral sole of foot is stroked; normal response to this stimulation would be flexion, or upward movement, of toe, 431

Bacteria, primitive, single-celled microorganisms that are present everywhere; some are capable of causing disease in humans, 197

Bacteriuria, bacteria in urine, 305

Balanic, pertaining to glans penis, 357

Balanitis, inflammation of skin covering glans penis, 359

Balanoplasty, surgical repair of glans penis, 361

Balanorrhea, discharge from glans penis, 358

Balloon angioplasty, 163*f*

Bariatric surgery, group of surgical procedures such as stomach stapling and restrictive banding to reduce size of stomach; treatment for morbid (extreme) obesity, 279

Barium (Ba), soft metallic element from earth used as radiopaque X-ray dye, 507

Barium enema (BE), 277, 277*f*

Barium swallow, 278

Barrier contraception, prevention of pregnancy using a device to prevent sperm from meeting ovum; examples include condoms, diaphragms, and cervical caps, 349

Bartholin's glands, glands located on either side of vaginal opening that secrete mucus for vaginal lubrication, 335

Basal cell carcinoma (BCC), tumor of basal cell layer of epidermis; frequent type of skin cancer that rarely metastasizes or spreads; these cancers can arise on sun-exposed skin, 63, 63*f*

Basal layer, deepest layer of epidermis; this living layer constantly multiplies and divides to supply cells to replace cells that are sloughed off skin surface, 53

Base, directional term meaning bottom or lower part, 37*t*, 224, 225*f*

Basilic vein, 150*f*

Basophil (Basos), granulocyte white blood cell that releases histamine and heparin in damaged tissues, 181*f*, 181*t*, 184

Bell jar apparatus, 226*f*

Bell's palsy, one-sided facial paralysis with unknown cause; person cannot control salivation, tearing of eyes, or expression; patient will eventually recover, 428

Benign, not cancerous; benign tumor is generally not progressive or recurring, 526

Benign prostatic hypertrophy (BPH), enlargement of prostate gland commonly seen in males over 50, 358

Beta blocker drugs, medication that treats hypertension and angina pectoris by lowering heart rate, 164

Biceps, arm muscle named for number of attachment points; *bi-* means two and biceps have two heads attached to bone, 115

Bicuspid valve, valve between left atrium and ventricle; prevents blood from flowing backwards into atrium; has two cusps or flaps; also called mitral valve, 143

Bicuspids, premolar permanent teeth having two cusps or projections that assist in grinding food; humans have eight bicuspids, 260*f*, 260

Bilateral, 4

Bile, substance produced by liver and stored in gallbladder; added to chyme in duodenum and functions to emulsify fats so they can be digested and absorbed; cholesterol is essential to bile production, 265

Bile duct, 265*f*, 276*f*

Bilirubin, waste product produced from destruction of worn-out red blood cells; disposed of by liver, 181

Bronchography, process of taking X-ray of lung after radiopaque substance has been placed into trachea or bronchial tree, 238

Bronchoplasty, surgical repair of a bronchial defect, 241

Bronchoscope, instrument to view inside a bronchus, 238, 239*f*

Bronchoscopy (Bronch), using bronchoscope to visualize bronchi; instrument can also be used to obtain tissue for biopsy and to remove foreign objects, 238, 239*f*

Bronchospasm, involuntary muscle spasm in bronchi, 230

Bronchus, distal end of trachea splits into left and right main bronchi as it enters each lung; each main bronchus is subdivided into smaller branches; smallest bronchi are bronchioles; each bronchiole ends in tiny air sacs called alveoli, 223, 223*f*

Buccal, (1) pertaining to cheeks; (2) drugs that are placed under lip or between cheek and gum, 267, 494, 496*t*

Buccolabial, pertaining to cheeks and lips, 267

Buffers, chemicals that neutralize acid, particularly stomach acid, 265

Bulbourethral gland, also called *Cowper's gland*; these two small male reproductive system glands are located on either side of urethra just distal to prostate; secretion from these glands neutralizes acidity in urethra and vagina, 30*t*, 353*f*, 354, 354*f*, 356

Bulimia, eating disorder characterized by recurrent binge eating and then purging of food with laxatives and vomiting, 502

Bundle branch block (BBB), occurs when electrical impulse is blocked from travelling down bundle of His or bundle branches; results in ventricles beating at a different rate than atria; also called a *heart block*, 154

Bundle branches, part of conduction system of heart; electrical signal travels down interventricular septum, 145, 146*f*, 154

Bundle of His, bundle of His is located in interventricular septum; receives electrical impulse from atrioventricular node and distributes it through ventricular walls, causing them to contract simultaneously, 145, 146*f*, 154

Bunion, inflammation of bursa of the great toe, 105

Bunionectomy, removal of bursa at joint of great toe, 107

Burn, full-thickness burn exists when all layers are burned; also called *third-degree burn;* partial-thickness burn exists when first layer of skin, epidermis, is burned, and second layer of skin, dermis, is damaged; also called *second-degree burn; first-degree burn* damages only epidermis, 64, 64*f*

Bursa, saclike connective tissue structure found in some joints; protects moving parts from friction; some common bursa locations are elbow, knee, and shoulder joints, 96

Bursectomy, excision of a bursa, 108

Bursitis, inflammation of bursa between bony prominences and muscles or tendons; common in shoulder and knee, 96, 100

C

Cachexia, loss of weight and generalized wasting that occurs during a chronic disease, 269

Calcitonin (CT), hormone secreted by thyroid gland; stimulates deposition of calcium into bone, 381*t*, 388

Calcium (Ca^+), inorganic substance found in plasma; is important for bones, muscles, and nerves, 180, 384

Calcium channel blocker drugs, medication that treats hypertension, angina pectoris, and congestive heart failure by causing heart to beat less forcefully and less often, 164

Calcium supplements, maintaining high blood levels of calcium in association with vitamin D helps maintain bone density and treats osteomalacia, osteoporosis, and rickets, 109

Calculus, stone formed within organ by accumulation of mineral salts; found in kidney, renal pelvis, bladder, or urethra; plural is *calculi,* 306, 306*f*

Callus, mass of bone tissue that forms at fracture site during its healing, 100

Calyx, duct that connects renal papilla to renal pelvis; urine flows from collecting tubule through calyx and into renal pelvis, 298, 299*f*

Cancellous bone, bony tissue found inside a bone; contains cavities that hold red bone marrow; also called *spongy bone,* 86, 87, 87*f*

Cancerous tumors, malignant growths in the body, 197

Candidiasis, yeastlike infection of skin and mucous membranes that can result in white plaques on tongue and vagina, 344

Canines, also called cuspid teeth or eyeteeth; permanent teeth located between incisors and biscuspids that assist in biting and cutting food; humans have four canine teeth, 260, 260*f*

Canker sores, 270

Capillaries, smallest blood or lymphatic vessels; blood capillaries are very thin to allow gas, nutrient, and waste exchange between blood and tissues; lymph capillaries collect lymph fluid from tissues and carry it to larger lymph vessels, 139*f*, 140, 149, 194, 224*f*

Colon, also called *large intestine;* functions to reabsorb most of fluid in digested food; material that remains after water reabsorption is feces; sections of colon are cecum, ascending colon, transverse colon, descending colon, and sigmoid colon, 26*f,* 29*t,* 35*t,* 36*t,* 258, 263, 264*f,*

Colonic, pertaining to colon, 267

Colonoscope, instrument to view inside colon, 278

Colonoscopy, flexible fiberscope passed through anus, rectum, and colon is used to examine upper portion of colon; polyps and small growths can be removed during procedure, 278

Color vision tests, use of polychromic (multicolored) charts to determine ability of patient to recognize color, 460, 460*f*

Colorectal, pertaining to colon and rectum, 267

Colorectal carcinoma, cancerous tumor originating in the colon or rectum, 272

Colostomy, surgical creation of opening in some portion of colon through abdominal wall to outside surface; fecal material (stool) drains into bag worn on abdomen, 280, 280*f*

Colostrum, thin fluid first secreted by breast after delivery; does not contain much protein, but is rich in antibodies, 341

Colposcope, instrument to view inside vagina, 347

Colposcopy, visual examination of cervix and vagina using colposcope or instrument with magnifying lens, 347

Coma, profound unconsciousness resulting from illness or injury, 422

Combining form, word root plus combining vowel; is always written with a / between word root and combining vowel; for example, in combining form *cardi/o, cardi* is word root and */o* is combining vowel, 3–4

Combining vowel, vowel inserted between word parts that makes it possible to pronounce long medical terms; is usually the vowel *o,* 2, 3–4

Comedo, medical term for blackhead; is an accumulation of sebum in sebaceous gland that has become blackened, 58

Comminuted fracture, fracture in which bone is shattered, splintered, or crushed into many pieces or fragments; fracture is completely through bone, 101

Common bile duct (CBD), duct that carries bile from gallbladder to duodenum, 265, 265*f*, 276*f*

Common iliac artery, 148*f*

Common iliac vein, 150*f*

Compact bone, hard exterior surface bone; also called *cortical bone,* 86, 87*f*, 96*f*

Complemental air, 225*t*

Complete blood count (CBC), blood test consisting of five tests; red blood cell count (RBC), white blood count (WBC), hemoglobin (Hg), hematocrit (Hct), and white blood cell differential, 187

Compound fracture, open fracture in which skin has been broken through by fracture, 101, 101*f*

Compression fracture, fracture involving loss of height of vertebral body, 101

Computed tomography scan (CT scan, CAT), imaging technique able to produce cross-sectional view of body; X-ray pictures are taken at multiple angles through body and computer uses all images to construct composite cross-section, 508

Conception, fertilization of ovum by a sperm, 333, 334

Concussion, injury to brain resulting from blow or impact from object; can result in unconsciousness, dizziness, vomiting, unequal pupil size, and shock, 426

Conductive hearing loss, loss of hearing as a result of blocking of sound transmission in middle ear and outer ear, 469

Condyle, refers to rounded portion at end of a bone, 88, 88*f*

Cones, sensory receptors of retina that are active in bright light and see in color, 449

Confidentiality, 14

Congenital anomalies, 337

Congenital septal defect (CSD), defect, present at birth, in wall separating two chambers of heart; results in a mixture of oxygenated and deoxygenated blood being carried to surrounding tissues; there can be atrial septal defect (ASD) and ventricular septal defect (VSD), 155

Congestive heart failure (CHF), pathological condition of heart in which there is reduced outflow of blood from left side of heart; results in weakness, breathlessness, and edema, 155

Conization, surgical removal of core of cervical tissue; also refers to partial removal of cervix, 349

Conjunctiva, protective mucous membrane lining on underside of each eyelid and across anterior surface of each eyeball, 448, 448*f*, 450*f*, 451, 459

Conjunctival, pertaining to conjunctiva, 454

Conjunctivitis, also referred to as *pinkeye* or inflammation of conjunctiva, 459

Conjunctivoplasty, surgical repair of conjunctiva, 462

Connective tissue, supporting and protecting tissue in body structures; examples are fat or adipose tissue, cartilage, and bone, 25, 26*f*

Conscious, condition of being awake and aware of surroundings, 422

Constipation, experiencing difficulty in defecation or infrequent defecation, 269

Consultation reports, document in patient's medical record; reports given by specialists who physician has requested to evaluate patient, 12

Contracture, abnormal shortening of muscle, making it difficult to stretch muscle, 120

Contraindication, condition in which particular drug should not be used, 496

Contrast studies, radiopaque substance is injected or swallowed; X-rays are then taken that outline body structure containing radiopaque substance, 509, 509*f*

Controlled substances, drugs that have potential for being addictive (habit forming) or can be abused, 492, 492*t*

Contusion, injury caused by blow to body; causes swelling, pain, and bruising; skin is not broken, 58

Conversion reaction, somatoform disorder in which patient unconsciously substitutes physical signs or symptoms for anxiety; most common physical signs or symptoms are blindness, deafness, and paralysis, 503

Convulsions, severe involuntary muscle contractions and relaxations; these have a variety of causes, such as epilepsy, fever, and toxic conditions, 422

Corium, living layer of skin located between epidermis and subcutaneous tissue; also referred to as *dermis,* it contains hair follicles, sweat glands, sebaceous glands, blood vessels, lymph vessels, nerve fibers, and muscle fibers, 54

Cornea, portion of sclera that is clear and transparent and allows light to enter interior of eye; also plays role in bending light rays, 447*f*, 448, 448*f*, 452*f*

Corneal, pertaining to cornea, 454

Corneal abrasion, scraping injury to cornea; if it does not heal, it may develop into ulcer, 456

Coronal plane, vertical plane that divides body into front (anterior or ventral) and back (posterior or dorsal) sections; also called *frontal plane,* 32*f*, 33

Coronal section, sectional view of body produced by cut along frontal plane; also called *frontal section,* 33

Coronary, pertaining to heart, 147, 152

Coronary arteries, group of three arteries that branch off aorta and carry blood to myocardium, 147, 147*f*

Coronary artery bypass graft (CABG), open-heart surgery in which blood vessel is grafted to route blood around point of constriction in diseased coronary artery, 162

Coronary artery disease (CAD), insufficient blood supply to heart muscle due to obstruction of one or more coronary arteries; may be caused by atherosclerosis and may cause angina pectoris and myocardial infarction, 155, 155*f*

Corpus, body or central portion of uterus, 332*f*, 334

Corpus (uterus), 332*f*

Corpus albicans, 333*f*

Corpus luteum, 333*f*

Cortex, outer layer of organ; in endocrine system, it refers to outer layer of adrenal glands; in urinary system, outer layer of kidney, 298, 299*f*, 382, 382*f*

Cortical, pertaining to cortex, 98

Cortical bone, hard exterior surface bone; also called *compact bone,* 86, 87*f*

Corticosteroid cream, powerful anti-inflammatory cream, 72

Corticosteroids, general term for group of hormones secreted by adrenal contex; they include mineralocorticoid hormones, glucocorticoid hormones, and steroid sex hormones; used as medication for its strong anti-inflammatory properties, 109, 205, 243, 382, 397

Cortisol, steroid hormone secreted by adrenal cortex; regulates carbohydrate metabolism, 382

Costal, pertaining to ribs, 98

Cowper's glands, also called *bulbourethral glands;* these two small male reproductive system glands are located on either side of urethra just distal to prostate; secretion from these glands neutralizes acidity in urethra and vagina, 356

Crackles, abnormal sound made during inspiration; usually indicates presesnce of fluid or mucus in small airways; also called *rales*, 230

Cranial, pertaining to skull, 39, 98

Cranial bones, 91*t*

Cranial cavity, dorsal body cavity; is within skull and contains brain, 34, 34*f*, 35*t*

Cranial nerves, nerves that arise from brain, 412, 418*t*

Craniotomy, incision into skull, 108

Cranium, skull; bones that form protective covering over brain, 89, 90*f*

Creatine phosphokinase (CPK), muscle enzyme found in skeletal muscle and cardiac muscle; blood test becomes elevated in disorders such as heart attack, muscular dystrophy, and other skeletal muscle pathologies, 122

Creatinine, waste product of muscle metabolism, 180, 311

Creatinine clearance, test of kidney function; creatinine is waste product cleared from bloodstream by kidneys; for this test, urine is collected for 24 hours and amount of creatinine in urine is compared to amount of creatinine that remains in bloodstream, 311

Crepitation, sound of broken bones rubbing together, 100

Cytologic testing, examination of cells to determine structure and origin; pap smears are considered a form of cytologic testing, 529
Cytology, study of cells, 24, 39
Cytoplasm, watery internal environment of a cell, 24
Cytotoxic, pertaining to poisoning cells, 197, 198

D

Dacryoadenitis, inflammation of lacrimal gland, 459
Dacryocystitis, inflammation of tear sac, 459
Day surgery, type of outpatient surgery in which patient is discharged on same day he or she is admitted; also called ambulatory surgery, 523
Deafness, inability to hear or having some degree of hearing impairment, 472
Debridement, removal of foreign material and dead or damaged tissue from wound, 71, 516
Decibel (dB), measures intensity or loudness of sound; zero decibels is quietest sound measured and 120 dB is loudest sound commonly measured, 473
Deciduous teeth, 20 teeth that begin to erupt around age of 6 months; eventually pushed out by permanent teeth, 260, 261
Decongestant, substance that reduces nasal congestion and swelling, 243
Decubitus ulcer (decub), bedsore or pressure sore caused by pressure over bony prominences on body; caused by lack of blood flow, 65
Deep, directional term meaning away from surface of body, 37*t*
Deep tendon reflex (DTR), muscle contraction in response to stretch caused by striking muscle tendon with reflex hammer; test used to determine if muscles are responding properly, 122
Defecation, evacuation of feces from rectum, 263
Defibrillation, procedure that converts serious irregular heartbeats, such as fibrillation, by giving electric shocks to heart, 161, 161*f*
Delirium, state of mental confusion with lack of orientation to time and place, 423
Delivery, emergence of baby from birth canal, 338, 338*f*
Delusion, false belief held with conviction even in face of strong evidence to contrary, 503
Dementia, progressive impairment of intellectual function that interferes with performing activities of daily living; patients have little awareness of their condition; found in disorders such as Alzheimer's, 423, 501
Dendrite, branched process off a neuron that receives impulses and carries them to cell body, 412, 413*f*
Dental, pertaining to teeth 267
Dental caries, gradual decay and disintegration of teeth caused by bacteria that can result in inflamed tissue and abscessed teeth; commonly called a *tooth cavity*, 270
Dentalgia, tooth pain, 269
Dentin, main bulk of tooth; is covered by enamel, 260, 261, 261*f*
Dentist, practitioner of dentistry, 268
Dentistry, branch of healthcare involved with prevention, diagnosis, and treatment of conditions involving teeth, jaw, and mouth; dentistry is practiced by *dentist* or *oral surgeon*, 268
Denture, partial or complete set of artificial teeth that are set in plastic materials; substitute for natural teeth and related structures, 279
Deoxygenated, blood in veins that is low in oxygen content, 140
Depigmentation, loss of normal skin color or pigment, 59
Depression, downward movement, as in dropping shoulders, 88–89, 118*t*
Dermabrasion, abrasion or rubbing using wire brushes or sandpaper, 71
Dermal, pertaining to skin, 57
Dermatitis, inflammation of skin, 65
Dermatologist, physician specialized in diagnosis and treatment of diseases of integumentary system, 58
Dermatology (Derm, derm), branch of medicine specializing in conditions of integumentary system, 27*t*, 39, 58
Dermatome, instrument for cutting skin or thin transplants of skin, 70
Dermatoplasty, surgical repair of skin, 71, 520
Dermatosis, abnormal condition of skin, 65
Dermis, living layer of skin located between epidermis and subcutaneous tissue; also referred to as corium or *true skin;* contains hair follicles, sweat glands, sebaceous glands, blood vessels, lymph vessels, nerve fibers, and muscle fibers, 52, 53*f*, 54, 54*f*
Descending aorta, 145*f*
Descending colon, section of colon that descends left side of abdomen, 263, 263*f*, 264*f*
Descending tracts, nerve tracts carrying motor signals down spinal cord to muscles, 416, 417
Diabetes insipidus (DI), disorder caused by inadequate secretion of hormone by posterior lobe of pituitary gland; there may be polyuria and polydipsia; is more common in young, 385, 393
Diabetes mellitus (DM), serious disease in which pancreas fails to produce insulin or insulin does not work properly; consequently, patient has very high blood sugar; kidney will attempt to lower high blood sugar level by excreting excess sugar in urine, 385, 392

E

Echocardiography (ECHO), noninvasive diagnostic method using ultrasound to visualize internal cardiac structures; cardiac valve activity can be evaluated using this method, 160
Echoencephalography, recording of ultrasonic echoes of brain; useful in determining abnormal patterns of shifting in brain, 430
Eclampsia, convulsive seizures and coma that can occur in woman between twentieth week of pregnancy and first week of postpartum; often associated with hypertension, 345
Ectopic pregnancy, 333
Eczema, superficial dermatitis accompanied by papules, vesicles, and crusting, 65
Edema, condition in which body tissues contain excessive amounts of fluid, 390
Effacement, thinning of cervix during labor, 338
Efferent, 299
Efferent arteriole, arteriole that carries blood away from glomerulus, 299, 300*f*, 302*f*
Efferent neurons, nerves that carry impulses away from brain and spinal cord to muscles and glands; also called *motor neurons,* 418, 419*f*
Egg cell, 333*f*, 334*f*
Ejaculation, impulse of forcing seminal fluid from male urethra, 355
Elastin fibers, 224*f*
Elbow, 88
Elective abortion, legal termination of pregnancy for nonmedical reasons, 349
Electrocardiogram (ECG,EKG), record of electrical activity of heart; useful in diagnosis of abnormal cardiac rhythm and heart muscle (myocardium) damage, 146*f,* 160
Electrocardiography, process of recording electrical activity of heart, 160
Electrocautery, to destroy tissue with electric current, 71, 524
Electroconvulsive therapy (ECT), procedure occasionally used for cases of prolonged major depression in which electrode is placed on one or both sides of patient's head and current is turned on briefly causing convulsive seizure; low level of voltage is used in modern ECT, and patient is administered a muscle relaxant and anesthesia; advocates of treatment state that it is a more effective way to treat severe depression than with use of drugs; is not effective with disorders other than depression, such as schizophrenia and alcoholism, 504
Electroencephalogram (EEG), record of brain's electrical activity, 431
Electroencephalography (EEG), recording electrical activity of brain by placing electrodes at various positions on scalp; also used in sleep studies to determine if there is a normal pattern of activity during sleep, 431
Electrolyte, chemical compound that separates into charged particles, or ionizes, in solution; sodium chloride (NaCl) and potassium (K) are examples of electrolytes, 301
Electromyogram (EMG), record of muscle electricity, 122, 516
Electromyography, recording of electrical patterns of muscle in order to diagnose diseases, 122, 516
Elephantiasis, inflammation, obstruction, and destruction of lymph vessels that results in enlarged tissues due to edema, 201
Elevation, muscle action that raises body part, as in shrugging the shoulders, 118*t*
Embolectomy, surgical removal of embolus or clot from a blood vessel, 162
Embolus, obstruction of blood vessel by blood clot that moves from another area, 153, 153*f*
Embryo, term to describe developing infant from fertilization until end of eighth week, 336, 337, 337*f*
Embryonic, pertaining to embryo, 340
Emesis, vomiting, usually with some force, 269
Emmetropia (EM), state of normal vision, 455
Emphysema, pulmonary condition that can occur as result of long-term heavy smoking; air pollution also worsens this disease; patient may not be able to breathe except in sitting or standing position, 235
Empyema, pus within pleural space, usually result of infection, 237
Emulsification, to make fats and lipids more soluble in water, 265
Enamel, hardest substance in body; covers outer surface of teeth, 260, 261, 261*f*
Encapsulated, growth enclosed in sheath of tissue that prevents tumor cells from invading surrounding tissue, 527
Encephalic, pertaining to brain, 421
Encephalitis, inflammation of brain due to disease factors such as rabies, influenza, measles, or smallpox, 426
Endarterectomy, removal of inside layer of an artery, 162
Endings
  plural, 10
  singular, 10
Endocarditis, inflammation of inner lining layer of heart; may be due to microorganisms or to abnormal immunological response, 142, 155
Endocardium, inner layer of heart, which is very smooth and lines chambers of heart, 142, 142*f*
Endocervicitis, inflammation of inner aspect of cervix, 343

F

Farsightedness, 457, 457*f*
Fascia, connective tissue that wraps muscles; it tapers at each end of a skeletal muscle to form tendons, 114
Fascial, pertaining to fascia, 119
Fasciitis, inflammation of fascia, 121
Fasciotomy, incision into fascia, 122
Fasting blood sugar (FBS), blood test to measure amount of sugar circulating throughout body after 12-hour fast, 395
Fats, lipid molecules transported throughout body dissolved in blood, 180
Fecal occult blood test (FOBT), laboratory test on feces to determine if microscopic amounts of blood are present; also called *hemoccult* or *stool guaiac*, 276
Feces, food that cannot be digested becomes waste product and is expelled or defecated as feces, 263
Federal Drug Administration (FDA), 498
Female reproductive system, system responsible for producing eggs for reproduction and provides place for growing baby; organs include ovaries, fallopian tubes, uterus, vagina, and mammary glands, 30*t*, 331*f*, 332*f*
  abbreviations, 351
  anatomical terms, 340–41
  anatomy and physiology, 332–39
  breast, 336, 336*f*
  diagnostic procedures, 347–48
  internal genitalia, 332–35
  pathology, 342–46
  pharmacology, 351
  terminology, 339–48
  therapeutic procedures, 349–50
  vulva, 335–36
Female urethra, 301*f*
Femoral, pertaining to femur or thigh bone, 98
Femoral artery, 148*f*
Femoral vein, 150*f*
Femur, also called *thigh bone;* is a lower extremity bone, 85*f*, 88*f*, 92, 93*f*, 94, 95*f*, 95*t*
Fertility drug, medication that triggers ovulation; also called *ovulation stimulant*, 351
Fertilization, also called *impregnation;* fusion of ova and sperm to produce embryo, 332
Fetal, pertaining to fetus, 340
Fetal monitoring, using electronic equipment placed on mother's abdomen to check baby's heart rate and strength during labor, 348
Fetus, term to describe developing newborn from end of eighth week until birth, 336, 337, 337*f*
Fever blisters, 271
Fibrillation, abnormal quivering or contractions of heart fibers; when this occurs within fibers of ventricle of heart, arrest and death can occur; emergency equipment to defibrillate, or convert heart to a normal beat, is necessary, 156
Fibrin, whitish protein formed by action of thrombin and fibrinogen, which is basis for clotting of blood, 182
Fibrinogen, blood protein that is essential for clotting to take place, 180
Fibrinous, pertaining to being fibrous, 184
Fibrocystic breast disease, benign cysts forming in breast, 345, 345*f*
Fibroid tumor, benign tumor or growth that contains fiberlike tissue; uterine fibroid tumors are most common tumors in women, 343, 343*f*
Fibromyalgia, condition with widespread aching and pain in muscles and soft tissue, 121
Fibrous joints, joint that has almost no movement because ends of bones are joined together by thick fibrous tissue; sutures of skull are example, 95, 96, 96*f*
Fibula, one of the lower leg bones in lower extremity, 85*f*, 92, 93*f*, 94, 95*f*, 95*t*
Fibular, pertaining to fibula, a lower leg bone, 98
Fibular vein, 150*f*
Film, thin sheet of cellulose material coated with light-sensitive substance used in taking photographs; there is a special photographic film that is sensitive to X-rays, 507
Film badge, badge containing film that is sensitive to X-rays; is worn by all personnel in radiology to measure amount of X-rays to which they are exposed, 507
Filtration, first stage of urine production during which waste products are filtered from blood, 302, 302*f*
Fimbriae, fingerlike extensions on end of fallopian tubes; drape over each ovary in order to direct ovum into fallopian tube after it is expelled by ovary, 333, 333*f*, 334, 334*f*, 383*f*
Fine motor skills, use of precise and coordinated movements in such activities as writing, buttoning, and cutting, 515
First-degree burn, 64, 64*f*
Fissure, deep groove or slit-type opening, 59, 59*f*, 88, 89
Fistulectomy, excision of a fistula, 280
Fixation, procedure to stabilize fractured bone while it heals; *external fixation* includes casts, splints, and pins inserted through skin; *internal fixation* includes pins, plates, rods, screws, and wires that are applied during an *open reduction*, 109
Flat bone, type of bone with thin flattened shape; examples include scapula, ribs, and pelvic bones, 86, 87*f*
Flexion, act of bending or being bent, 116*t*, 116*f*

G

H

Homeostasis, steady state or state of balance within body; kidneys assist in maintaining this regulatory, steady state, 301, 380
Homologous transfusion, replacement of blood by transfusion of blood received from another person, 189
Hordeolum, a *stye* (or sty), a small purulent inflammatory infection of a sebaceous gland of eye, treated with hot compresses and surgical incision, 459
Horizontal plane, horizontal plane that divides body into upper (superior) and lower (inferior) sections; also called *transverse plane,* 32, 33
Hormonal contraception, use of hormones to block ovulation and prevent contraception; may be in pill form, patch or implant under skin, or injection, 349
Hormone, chemical substance secreted by endocrine gland; enters blood stream and is carried to target tissue; hormones work to control functioning of target tissue; given to replace loss of natural hormones or to treat disease by stimulating hormonal effects, 380
Hormone replacement therapy (HRT), artificial replacement of hormones in patient who is unable to produce sufficient hormones; example is estrogen replacement in menopausal women, 351, 396
Hormone therapy, treatment of cancer with natural hormones or with chemicals that produce hormonelike effects, 529
Hospice, organized group of healthcare workers who provide supportive treatment to dying patients and their families, 13
Human growth hormone therapy, therapy with human growth hormone in order to stimulate skeletal growth; used to treat children with abnormally short stature, 397
Human immunodeficiency virus (HIV), virus that causes AIDS; also known as a retrovirus, 202, 202*f*, 360
Human papilloma virus (HPV), 343
Humanistic psychotherapy, form of psychological counseling in which therapist does not delve into patients' past; it is believed that patients can learn how to use their own internal resources to deal with their problems, 505
Humeral, pertaining to humerus or upper arm bone, 98
Humerus, upper arm bone in upper extremity, 85*f*, 87*f*, 92, 93*f*, 94, 94*f*, 94*t*
Humoral immunity, immunity that responds to antigens, such as bacteria and foreign agents, by producing antibodies; also called *antibody-mediated immunity,* 197
Humpback, 104
Hunchback, 104
Hyaline membrane disease (HMD), 235
Hydrocele, accumulation of fluid within testes, 358
Hydrocephalus, accumulation of cerebrospinal fluid within ventricles of brain, causing head to be enlarged; treated by creating artificial shunt for fluid to leave brain, 426, 426*f*
Hydrochloric acid (HCl), acid secreted by stomach lining; aids in digestion, 262
Hydronephrosis, distention of pelvis due to urine collecting in kidney resulting from obstruction, 308
Hydrotherapy, using water for treatment purposes, 517
Hymen, thin membranous tissue that covers external vaginal opening or orifice; membrane is broken during first sexual encounter of female; can also be broken prematurely by use of tampons or during some sports activities, 335
Hymenectomy, surgical removal of hymen; performed when hymen tissue is particularly tough, 350
Hyoid bone, single, U-shaped bone suspended in neck between mandible and larynx; a point of attachment for swallowing and speech muscles, 89, 221*f*
Hypercalcemia, condition of having excessive amount of calcium in blood, 390
Hypercapnia, excessive carbon dioxide, 231
Hyperemesis, excessive vomiting, 270
Hyperemia, redness of skin caused by increased blood flow to skin, 59
Hyperesthesia, having excessive sensation, 423
Hyperglycemia, having excessive amount of glucose (sugar) in blood, 390
Hyperhidrosis, abnormal condition of excessive sweat, 59
Hyperkalemia, condition of having excessive amount of potassium in blood, 391
Hyperkinesia, excessive amount of movement, 120
Hyperlipidemia, condition of having too high a level of lipids such as cholesterol in bloodstream; risk factor for developing atherosclerosis and coronary artery disease, 185
Hyperopia, with this condition a person can see things in the distance but has trouble reading material at close vision; also known as *farsightedness,* 457, 457f
Hyperparathyroidism, state of excessive thyroid, 393
Hyperpigmentation, abnormal amount of pigmentation in skin, which is seen in diseases such as acromegaly and adrenal insufficiency, 59

I

Immunization, providing protection against communicable diseases by stimulating immune system to produce antibodies against that disease; children can now be immunized for: hepatitis B, diphtheria, tetanus, pertussis, tetanus, *Haemophilus influenzae* type b, polio, measles, mumps, rubella, and chickenpox; also called *vaccination,* 196, 197, 204

Immunocompromised, having immune system unable to respond properly to pathogens, 203

Immunodeficiency disorder, 203

Immunoglobulins (Ig), antibodies secreted by B cells; all antibodies are immunoglobulins; assist in protecting body and its surfaces from invasion of bacteria; for example, immunoglobulin IgA in colostrum, first milk from mother, helps to protect newborn from infection, 199

Immunologist, physician who specializes in treating infectious diseases and other disorders of immune system, 200

Immunology, branch of medicine specializing in conditions of lymphatic and immune systems, 28*t*, 200

Immunosuppressants, substances that block certain actions of immune system; required to prevent rejection of transplanted organ, 205

Immunotherapy, production or strengthening of patient's immune system in order to treat disease, 204, 529

Impacted fracture, fracture in which bone fragments are pushed into each other, 102

Impetigo, highly contagious staphylococcal skin infection, most commonly occurring on faces of children; begins as blisters that then rupture and dry into thick, yellow crust, 66, 66*f*

Implant, prosthetic device placed in jaw to which a tooth or denture may be anchored, 279

Implantable cardiovert-defibrillator, device implanted in heart that delivers electrical shock to restore normal heart rhythm; particularly useful for persons who experience ventricular fibrillation, 161

Impulse control disorders, inability to resist impulse to perform some act harmful to individual or others; includes kleptomania, pyromania, explosive disorder, and pathological gambling, 502

Incision and drainage (I&D), making incision to create opening for drainage of material such as pus, 71

Incisors, biting teeth in very front of mouth that function to cut food into smaller pieces; humans have eight incisors, 259*f*, 260, 260*f*

Incus, one of three ossicles of middle ea; also called *anvil,* 467*f*, 468, 468*f*

Infant respiratory distress syndrome (IRDS), lung condition most commonly found in premature infants characterized by tachypnea and respiratory grunting; also called *hyaline membrane disease* (HMD) and *respiratory distress syndrome of the newborn,* 235

Infarct, area of tissue within organ that undergoes necrosis (death) following loss of blood supply, 153

Inferior, directional term meaning toward feet or tail, or below, 34*f*, 37*t*

Inferior vena cava, branch of vena cava that drains blood from abdomen and lower body, 142*f*, 144, 145*f*, 150*f*, 157*f*, 382*f*

Infertility, inability to produce children; generally defined as no pregnancy after properly timed intercourse for one year, 346

Inflammation, tissue response to injury from pathogens or physical agents; characterized by redness, pain, swelling, and feeling hot to touch, 200, 200*f*

Inflammatory bowel disease (IBD), 275

Influenza, viral infection of respiratory system characterized by chills, fever, body aches, and fatigue; commonly called the *flu,* 235

Informed consent, medical record document, voluntarily signed by patient or responsible party, that clearly describes purpose, methods, procedures, benefits, and risks of diagnostic or treatment procedure, 12

Inguinal, pertaining to groin area; there is a collection of lymph nodes in this region that drain each leg, 194*t*, 199

Inguinal hernia, hernia or outpouching of intestines into inguinal region of body, 273, 274*f*

Inguinal nodes, 195*f*

Inhalation, (1) to breathe air into lungs; also called *inspiration;* (2) to introduce drugs into body by inhaling them, 220, 494*t*, 495*f*, 520, 521*t*

Innate immunity, 197

Inner ear, innermost section of ear; contains cochlea, semicircular canals, saccule, and utricle, 466*f*, 467, 467*f*, 468, 469*f*

Inner ear infection, 473

Innominate bone, also called os coxae or hip bone; pelvis portion of lower extremity; consists of ilium, ischium, and pubis and unites with sacrum and coccyx to form pelvis, 92, 94

Insertion, attachment of skeletal muscle to more movable bone in joint, 115

Insomnia, sleeping disorder characterized by marked inability to fall asleep, 503

Inspiration, 220, 226*f*

Inspiratory capacity (IC), volume of air inhaled after normal exhale, 225*t*

Inspiratory reserve volume (IRV), air that can be forcibly inhaled after normal respiration has taken place; also called *complemental air*, 225*t*

Insulin, hormone secreted by pancreas; regulates level of sugar in blood stream; the more insulin present in blood, the lower blood sugar will be, 381*t*, 383, 397

Insulin-dependent diabetes mellitus (IDDM), also called type 1 diabetes mellitus; develops early in life when pancreas stops insulin production; persons with IDDM must take daily insulin injections, 392

Insulinoma, tumor of islets of Langerhans cells of pancreas that secretes excessive amount of insulin, 392

Integument, another term for skin, 52

Integumentary system, skin and its appendages including sweat glands, oil glands, hair, and nails; sense organs that allow us to respond to changes in temperature, pain, touch, and pressure are located in skin; largest organ in body, 27*t*, 49–82, 51*f*

Interatrial, pertaining to between atria, 152

Interatrial septum, wall or septum that divides left and right atria, 143

Intercostal muscles, muscles between ribs; when they contract, they raise ribs, which helps to enlarge thoracic cavity, 226

Intercostal nerve, 419*f*

Intermittent claudication, attacks of severe pain and lameness caused by ischemia of muscles, typically calf muscles; brought on by walking even very short distances, 120

Intermittent positive pressure breathing (IPPB), method for assisting patients to breathe using mask connected to a machine that produces increased pressure, 240

Internal genitalia, 332–35

Internal iliac artery, 148*f*, *315f*

Internal iliac vein, 148*f*, *315f*

Internal medicine, branch of medicine involving diagnosis and treatment of diseases and conditions of internal organs such as respiratory system; physician is *internist*, 229

Internal respiration, process of oxygen and carbon dioxide exchange at cellular level when oxygen leaves bloodstream and is delivered to tissues, 220

Internal sphincter, ring of involuntary muscle that keeps urine within bladder, 300

Internist, physician specialized in treating diseases and conditions of internal organs such as respiratory system, 229

Internodal pathway, 146*f*

Interstitial cystitis, disease of unknown cause in which there is inflammation and irritation of bladder; most commonly seen in middle-aged women, 310

Interventricular, pertaining to between ventricles, 152

Interventricular septum, wall or septum that divides left and right ventricles, 143, 145*f*, 146*f*

Intervertebral, pertaining to between vertebrae, 98

Intervertebral disk, fibrous cartilage cushion between vertebrae, 89, 91

Intracavitary, injection into body cavity such as peritoneal and chest cavity, 495*t*

Intracoronary artery stent, placing a stent within coronary artery to treat coronary ischemia due to atherosclerosis, 162

Intracranial, pertaining to inside skull, 98

Intradermal (ID), (1) pertaining to within skin; (2) injection of medication into skin, 57, 495*t*

Intramuscular (IM), injection of medication into muscle, 123, 495*t*

Intraocular, pertaining to within eye, 454

Intraoperative, period of time during operation, 524

Intrathecal, (1) pertaining to within meninges; (2) injection into meninges space surrounding brain and spinal cord, 421, 495*t*

Intrauterine device (IUD), device inserted into uterus by physician for purpose of contraception, 349, 349*f*

Intravenous (IV), injection into veins; this route can be set up so that there is continuous administration of medication, 496*t*, 520

Intravenous cholecystography, dye is administered intravenously to patient that allows for X-ray visualization of gallbladder, 277

Intravenous pyelogram (IVP), injecting contrast medium into vein and then taking X-ray to visualize renal pelvis, 316

Intussusception, intestinal condition in which one portion of intestine telescopes into adjacent portion causing obstruction and gangrene if untreated, 274, 274*f*

Invasive disease, tendency of malignant tumor to spread to immediately surrounding tissue and organs, 527

Inversion, directional term meaning turning inward or inside out, 117*t*, 117*f*

J

K

L

Lower extremity (LE), the leg, 33, 94, 95*f,* 95*t,* 515
Lower gastrointestinal series (lower GI series), x-ray image of colon and rectum is taken after administration of barium by enema; also called *barium enema,* 277, 277*f*
Lumbar, pertaining to five low back vertebrae, 98
Lumbar puncture (LP), puncture with needle into lumbar area (usually fourth intervertebral space) to withdraw fluid for examination and for injection of anesthesia; also called *spinal puncture* or *spinal tap,* 431, 431*f*
Lumbar vertebrae, five vertebrae in low back region, 89, 91, 92*t*
Lumbosacral plexus, 419*f*
Lumen, space, cavity, or channel within tube or tubular organ or structure in body, 146, 147*f*
Lumpectomy, excision of only a breast tumor and tissue immediately surrounding it, 350
Lung metastases, 528*f*
Lung volumes/capacities, 225, 225*t*
Lungs, major organs of respiration; consist of air passageways, bronchi and bronchioles, and air sacs, alveoli; gas exchange takes place within alveoli, 29*t,* 36*t,* 140*f,* 218, 219*f,* 220, 224–25
Lunula, lighter-colored, half-moon region at base of a nail, 55
Luteinizing hormone (LH), hormone secreted by anterior pituitary; regulates function of male and female gonads and plays a role in releasing ova in females, 333, 381*t,* 385
Lymph, clear, transparent, colorless fluid found in lymphatic vessels and cisterna chyli, 193
Lymph glands, another name for *lymph nodes;* small organs composed of lymphatic tissue located along route of lymphatic vessels; remove impurities from lymph and manufacture lymphocytes and antibodies, 194
Lymph nodes, small organs in lymphatic system that filter bacteria and other foreign organisms from body fluids, 28*t,* 193*f,* 194, 194*t,* 195*f*
Lymphadenectomy, excision of the lymph node; this is usually done to test for malignancy, 205
Lymphadenitis, inflammation of lymph glands; referred to as swollen glands, 201
Lymphadenopathy, disease of lymph nodes, 201
Lymphangial, pertaining to lymph vessels, 199
Lymphangiogram, x-ray taken of lymph vessels after injection of dye; lymph flow through chest is traced, 203
Lymphangiography, process of taking X-ray of lymph vessels after injection of radiopaque material, 203
Lymphangioma, lymph vessel tumor, 199
Lymphatic, pertaining to lymph, 200
Lymphatic and immune system, 28*t,* 192*f*
  abbreviations, 205
  anatomical terms, 199–200
  anatomy and physiology, 193–98
  diagnostic procedures, 203–04
  immunity, 196–98
  lymph nodes, 194, 194*t,* 195*f*
  pathology, 200–03
  pharmacology, 205
  spleen, 196, 196*f*
  terminology, 199–205
  therapeutic procedures, 204–05
  thymus gland, 196, 196*f*
  tonsils, 196, 196*f*
Lymphatic capillaries, smallest lymph vessels; they collect excessive tissue fluid, 193, 194
Lymphatic ducts, two largest vessels in lymphatic system, right lymphatic duct and thoracic duct, 193, 194, 195*f*
Lymphatic system, system that helps body fight infection; organs include spleen, lymph vessels, and lymph nodes, 28*t,* 192*f*
Lymphatic vessels, extensive network of vessels throughout entire body; conduct lymph from tissue toward thoracic cavity, 28*t,* 193*f,* 193–94, 194*f,* 195*f*
Lymphedema, edema appearing in extremities due to obstruction of lymph flow through lymphatic vessels, 201
Lymphocytes (lymphs), agranulocyte white blood cell that provides protection through immune response, 181*t,* 195*f*
Lymphoma, tumor of lymphatic tissue, 202

M

Macrophage, phagocytic cells found in large quantities in lymph nodes; they engulf foreign particles, 196, 197*f*
Macrotia, abnormally large ears, 471
Macula lutea, area of retina onto which straight ahead images are projected, 449
Macular, pertaining to macula lutea, 454
Macular degeneration, deterioration of macular area of retina of eye; may be treated with laser surgery to destroy blood vessels beneath macula, 457
Macule, flat, discolored area flush with skin surface; example would be freckle or birthmark, 60, 60*f*
Magnetic resonance imaging (MRI), medical imaging that uses radio-frequency radiation as its source of energy; does not require injection of contrast medium or exposure to ionizing radiation; technique is useful for visualizing large blood vessels, heart, brain, and soft tissues, 104*f,* 509, 509*f*

Melanocyte-stimulating hormone (MSH), hormone secreted by anterior pituitary; stimulates pigment production in skin, 381*t*, 385

Melanocytes, special cells in basal layer of epidermis; they contain black pigment melanin that gives skin its color and protects against ultraviolet rays of sun, 53

Melanoma, also called *malignant melanoma;* dangerous form of skin cancer caused by overgrowth of melanin in melanocyte; may metastasize or spread; exposure to ultraviolet light is a risk factor for developing melanoma, 66, 66*f*

Melatonin, hormone secreted by pineal gland; plays a role in regulating body's circadian rhythm, 384

Melena, passage of dark tarry stools; color is result of digestive enzymes working on blood in stool, 270

Menarche, first menstrual period, 334, 335

Ménière's disease, abnormal condition within labyrinth of inner ear that can lead to progressive loss of hearing; symptoms are dizziness or vertigo, hearing loss, and tinnitus (ringing in ears), 473

Meningeal, pertaining to meninges, 421

Meninges, three connective tissue membrane layers that surround brain and spinal cord; three layers are dura mater, arachnoid layer, and pia mater; dura mater and arachnoid layer are separated by subdural space; arachnoid layer and pia mater are separated by subarachnoid space, 413, 417, 417*f*, 429

Meningioma, slow-growing tumor in meninges of brain, 429

Meningitis, inflammation of membranes of spinal cord and brain caused by microorganism, 429

Meningocele, congenital hernia in which meninges, or membranes, protrude through opening in spinal column or brain, 427, 428*f*

Menometrorrhagia, excessive bleeding during menstrual period and at intervals between menstrual periods, 344

Menopause, cessation or ending of menstrual activity; generally between ages of 40 and 55, 334, 335

Menorrhagia, excessive bleeding during menstrual period; can be either in total number of days or amount of blood or both, 342

Menstrual cycle, 28-day fertility cycle in women; includes ovulation and sloughing off endometrium if pregnancy does not occur, 382

Menstrual period, another name for menstrual cycle, 334, 335

Menstruation, loss of blood and tissue as endometrium is shed by uterus; flow exits body through cervix and vagina; flow occurs approximately every 28 days, 334, 335

Mental health, 499–05
- abbreviations, 505
- disciplines, 500
- pathology, 500–04
- psychiatry, 500
- psychology, 500
- therapeutic procedures, 504–05

Mental retardation, disorder characterized by diminished ability to process intellectual functions, 501

Metacarpal, pertaining to hand bones, 99

Metacarpals, hand bones in upper extremity, 92, 93*f*, 94, 94*t*

Metastacized, 194

Metastases (mets), spreading of cancerous tumor from original site to different locations of body; singular is metastasis, 526, 526*f*

Metastasis (mets), movement and spread of cancer cells from one part of body to another; metastases is plural, 528, 528*f*

Metastasize, when cancerous cells migrate away from tumor site; commonly move through lymphatic system and become trapped in lymph nodes, 194

Metatarsal, pertaining to foot bones, 99

Metatarsals, ankle bones in lower extremity, 92, 93*f*, 94, 95*f*, 95*t*

Metered dose inhaler (MDI), 240

Metrorrhagia, rapid (menstrual) blood flow from uterus, 342

Metrorrhea, discharge from uterus, 342

Microtia, abnormally small ears, 471

Micturition, another term for urination, 300

Midbrain, portion of brain stem, 385*f*, 414, 414*f*, 415–416

Middle ear, middle section of ear; contains ossicles, 466*f*, 467, 467*f*, 468, 469*f*, 472

Middle ear infection, 472

Midline organs, 36*t*

Midsagittal plane, when sagittal plane passes through middle of body, dividing it into equal right and left halves, also called *median plane*, 32

Migraine, specific type of headache characterized by severe head pain, photophobia, vertigo, and nausea, 427

Miner's lung, 234

Mineralocorticoids, group of hormones secreted by adrenal cortex; regulate electrolytes and fluid volume in body; aldosterone is an example, 380*t*, 382

Minnesota Multiphasic Personality Inventory (MMPI), 505

Minor tranquilizers, medications that are central nervous system depressants and are prescribed for anxiety, 504

Miotic drops, substance that causes pupil to constrict, 463

N

O

Paranoid personality disorder, personality disorder characterized by exaggerated feelings of persecution, 502
Paraplegia, paralysis of lower portion of body and both legs, 423
Parasympathetic branch, branch of autonomic nervous system; serves as counterbalance for sympathetic nerves; therefore, it causes heart rate to slow down, lower blood pressure, constrict eye pupils, and increase digestion, 419
Parathyroid glands, four small glands located on back surface of thyroid gland; parathyroid hormone secreted by these glands regulates amount of calcium in blood, 30*t*, 378, 379*t*, 380, 381*t*, 384, 384*f*
Parathyroid hormone (PTH), hormone secreted by parathyroid glands; the more hormone, the higher the calcium level in blood and lower the level stored in bone; low hormone level will cause tetany, 381*t*, 384
Parenteral, route for introducing medication other than through gastrointestinal tract; most commonly involves injection into body through needle and syringe, 494, 495*t*
Parathyroidal, pertaining to parathyroid glands, 389
Parathyroidectomy, excision of one or more of parathyroid glands; performed to halt progress of hyperparathyroidism, 397
Parenteral administration of drugs, 495*t*
Paresthesia, abnormal sensation such as burning or tingling, 423
Parietal bone, cranial bone, 89, 91*f*, 91*t*
Parietal layer, outer pleural layer around lungs; lines inside of chest cavity, 34, 35
Parietal lobe, one of four cerebral hemisphere lobes; receives and interprets nerve impulses from sensory receptors, 414, 415, 415*f*
Parietal pericardium, outer layer of pericardium surrounding heart, 142
Parietal peritoneum, outer layer of serous membrane sac lining abdominopelvic cavity, 34, 35
Parietal pleura, outer layer of serous membrane sac lining thoracic cavity, 34, 35, 224
Parkinson's disease, chronic disorder of nervous system with fine tremors, muscular weakness, rigidity, and shuffling gait, 427
Paronychia, infection around nail, 69, 69*f*
Parotid duct, 264*f*
Parotid glands, pair of salivary glands located in front of ears, 264, 264*f*
Passive acquired immunity, immunity that results when person receives protective substances produced by another human or animal; may take form of maternal antibodies crossing placenta to baby or antitoxin injection, 196, 197
Passive aggressive personality, personality disorder in which person expresses feelings or anger or hostility through indirect or covert actions, 503
Passive range of motion (PROM), therapist putting patient's joints through full range of motion without assistance from patient, 517
Patella, also called *kneecap;* lower extremity bone, 85, 94, 95*f*, 95*t*
Patellar, pertaining to patella or kneecap, 99
Patent, open or unblocked, such as patent airway, 232
Patent ductus arteriosus (PDA), congenital heart anomaly in which opening between pulmonary artery and aorta fails to close at birth; condition requires surgery, 158
Pathogenic, pertaining to microscopic organisms, such as bacteria, capable of causing disease, 201
Pathogens, disease-bearing organisms, 52, 181
Pathologic fracture, fracture caused by diseased or weakened bone, 102
Pathological gambling, impulse control disorder in which patient is unable to control urge to gamble, 502
Pathologist, physician who specializes in evaluating specimens removed from living or dead patients, 527
Pathologist's report, medical record report given by pathologist who studies tissue removed from patient (for example: bone marrow, blood, or tissue biopsy), 12
Pathology, branch of medicine specializing in studying how disease affects body, 200
Pectoral girdle, consists of clavicle and scapula; functions to attach upper extremity to axial skeleton, 92, 93*f*, 94, 94*f*
Pediculosis, infestation with lice, 67
Pedophilia, sexual disorder characterized by having sexual interest in children, 503
Pelvic, pertaining to pelvis, 99
Pelvic cavity, inferior portion of abdominopelvic cavity, 34, 34*f*, 35*t*
Pelvic examination, physical examination of vagina and adjacent organs performed by physician placing fingers of one hand into vagina; visual examination is performed using speculum, 348
Pelvic girdle, consists ofilium, ischium, and pubis; functions to attach lower extremity to axial skeleton, 93*f*, 95*f*, 95*t*
Pelvic inflammatory disease (PID), any inflammation of female reproductive organs, generally bacterial in nature, 344
Pelvic region, lowest anterior region of trunk, 33, 34*f*

Pelvic ultrasonography, use of ultrasound waves to produce image or photograph of organ, such as uterus, ovaries, or fetus, 347

Pelvis, 96*f*

Penile, pertaining to penis, 357

Penis, male sex organ; composed of erectile tissue that becomes erect during sexual stimulation, allowing it to be placed within female vagina for ejaculation of semen; larger, soft tip is referred to as glans penis, 30*t*, 353*f*, 354, 355

Peptic ulcer disease (PUD), ulcer occurring in lower portion of esophagus, stomach, and duodenum and thought to be caused by acid of gastric juices, 272, 272*f*

Percussion, use of fingertips to tap body lightly and sharply; aids in determining size, position, and consistency of underlying body part, 242

Percutaneous diskectomy, thin catheter tube is inserted into intervertebral disk through skin and herniated or ruptured disk material is sucked out or a laser is used to vaporize it, 108

Percutaneous transhepatic cholangiography (PTC), contrast medium is injected directly into liver to visualize bile ducts; used to detect obstructions, 277

Percutaneous transluminal coronary angioplasty (PTCA), method for treating localized coronary artery narrowing; balloon catheter is inserted through skin into coronary artery and inflated to dilate narrow blood vessel, 163

Perforated ulcer, 272

Pericardial cavity, cavity formed by serous membrane sac surrounding heart, 34, 35, 35*t*

Pericarditis, inflammatory process or disease of pericardium, 10, 157

Pericardium, double-walled outer sac around heart; inner layer of pericardium is called epicardium, outer layer is heart itself; this sac contains pericardial fluid that reduces friction caused by heart beating, 141*f*, 142, 142*f*

Perimetritis, inflammation around uterus, 344

Perimetrium, outer layer of uterus, 334, 334*f*

Perineal, pertaining to perineum, 341

Perineum, in male, external region between scrotum and anus; in female, external region between vagina and anus, 335, 336, 337*f*, 354, 355

Periodontal disease, disease of supporting structures of teeth, including gums and bones, 271

Periodontal ligaments, small ligaments that anchor root of tooth in socket of jaw, 260, 261, 261*f*

Periodontics, branch of dentistry concerned with treating conditions involving gums and tissues surrounding teeth; specialist is a *periodontist*, 269

Periodontist, dental specialist in treating conditions involving gums and tissues surrounding teeth, 269

Perioperative, period of time that includes before, during, and after surgical procedure, 524

Periosteum, membrane that covers most bones; contains numerous nerves and lymphatic vessels, 86, 87*f*

Peripheral nervous system (PNS), portion of nervous system that contains cranial nerves and spinal nerves; these nerves are mainly responsible for voluntary muscle movement, smell, taste, sight, and hearing, 412, 418–20

Peripheral neuropathy, damage to nerves in lower legs and hands as a result of diabetes mellitus; symptoms include either extreme sensitivity or numbness and tingling, 392

Peripheral vascular disease (PVD), any abnormal condition affecting blood vessels outside heart; symptoms may include pain, pallor, numbness, and loss of circulation and pulses, 158

Peristalsis, wavelike muscular movements in wall of digestive system tube—esophagus, stomach, small intestines, and colon—that function to move food along tube, 261

Peritoneal, pertaining to peritoneum, 40

Peritoneal dialysis, removal of toxic waste substances from body by placing warm chemically balanced solutions into peritoneal cavity; used in treating renal failure and certain poisonings, 314, 314*f*

Peritoneoscopy, 278

Peritoneum, membranous sac that lines abdominal cavity and encases abdominopelvic organs; kidneys are exception since they lay outside peritoneum and alongside vertebral column, 34, 35

Peritubular capillaries, capillary bed surrounding renal tubules, 300*f*, 302, 302*f*

Permanent teeth, 32 permanent teeth begin to erupt at about age 6; generally complete by age sixteen, 260, 261

Pernicious anemia (PA), anemia associated with insufficient absorption of vitamin B_{12} by digestive system, 186

Peroneal artery, 148*f*

Peroneal nerve, 419*f*

Personality disorders, inflexible or maladaptive behavior patterns that affect person's ability to function in society; includes paranoid personality disorder, narcissistic personality disorder, antisocial personality disorder, and passive aggressive personality, 502

Perspiration, another term for sweating, 56

Pneumocystis pneumonia (PCP), Pneumonia with a nonproductive cough, very little fever, and dyspnea caused by fungus *Pneumocystis jiroveci;* opportunistic infection often seen in those with weakened immune systems, such as AIDS patients, 203, 236

Pneumonia, inflammatory condition of lung, which can be caused by bacterial and viral infections, diseases, and chemicals, 236

Pneumothorax, collection of air or gas in pleural cavity, which can result in collapse of lung, 237, 237*f*

Podiatrist, 100

Podiatry, healthcare profession specializing in diagnosis and treatment of disorders of feet and lower legs; healthcare professional is *podiatrist*, 100

Poliomyelitis, acute viral disease that causes inflammation of gray matter of spinal cord, resulting in paralysis in some cases; has been brought under almost total control through vaccinations, 427

Polyarteritis, inflammation of many arteries, 158

Polycystic kidneys, formation of multiple cysts within kidney tissue; results in destruction of normal kidney tissue and uremia, 309, 309*f*

Polycythemia vera, production of too many red blood cells in bone marrow, 186

Polydipsia, condition of having excessive amount of thirst, such as in diabetes, 391

Polymyositis, disease involving muscle inflammation and weakness from unknown cause, 121

Polyneuritis, inflammation of many nerves, 429

Polyp, small tumor with pedicle or stem attachment; commonly found in vascular organs such as nose, uterus, and rectum, 274, 275*f*

Polyphagia, to eat excessively, 270

Polyposis, small tumors that contain pedicle or footlike attachment in mucous membranes of large intestine (colon), 274, 275*f*

Polysomnography, monitoring a patient while sleeping to identify sleep apnea; also called *sleep apnea study*, 239

Polyuria, condition of having excessive urine production; can be a symptom of disease conditions such as diabetes, 307, 391

Pons, this portion of brain stem forms bridge between cerebellum and cerebrum; also where nerve fibers cross from one side of brain to control functions and movement on other side of brain, 414, 414*f*, 415, 415*f*

Pontine, pertaining to pons, 421

Popliteal artery, 148*f*

Popliteal vein, 150*f*

Positron emission tomography (PET), use of positive radionuclides to reconstruct brain sections; measurements can be taken of oxygen and glucose uptake, cerebral blood flow, and blood volume, 431, 510, 510*f*

Posterior, directional term meaning near or on back or spinal cord side of body, 37*f*, 37*t*

Posterior lobe, posterior portion of pituitary gland; secretes antidiuretic hormone and oxytocin, 385

Posterior pituitary gland, 384*f*

Posterior tibial artery, 148*f*

Posterior tibial vein, 150*f*

Posteroanterior (PA) view, positioning patient so that X-rays pass through body from back to front, 507

Postoperative, period of time immediately following surgery, 524

Postpartum, period immediately after delivery or childbirth, 341

Postprandial (PP), pertaining to after a meal, 270

Postural drainage, draining secretions from bronchi by placing patient in position that uses gravity to promote drainage; used for treatment of cystic fibrosis and bronchiectasis, and before lobectomy surgery, 240

Postural drainage with clapping, drainage of secretions from bronchi or a lung cavity by having patient lie so that gravity allows drainage to occur; clapping is using hand in cupped position to perform percussion on chest; assists in loosening secretions and mucus, 517

Potassium, inorganic substance found in plasma; important for bones and muscles, 180

Potentiation, giving patient second drug to boost (potentiate) effect of another drug; total strength of drugs is greater than sum of strength of individual drugs, 497

Preeclampsia, toxemia of pregnancy that, if untreated, can result in true eclampsia; symptoms include hypertension, headaches, albumin in urine, and edema, 346

Prefix, word part added in front of word root; frequently gives information about location of organ, number of parts or time (frequency); not all medical terms have prefix, 2, 3, 4–6
  number, 6

Pregnancy, time from fertilization of ovum to birth of newborn, 314, 336–39
  labor and delivery, 338–39

Pregnancy test, chemical test that can determine pregnancy during first few weeks; can be performed in physician's office or with home-testing kit, 347

Premature, infant born prior to 37 weeks of gestation, 337

Premenstrual syndrome (PMS), symptoms that develop just prior to onset of menstrual period, which can include irritability, headache, tender breasts, and anxiety, 344

Proton pump inhibitor, blocks stomach's ability to secrete acid; used to treat peptic ulcers and gastroesophageal reflux disease, 281

Protozoans, single-celled organisms that can infect body, 196, 197

Proximal, directional term meaning located closest to point of attachment to body, 37*f*, 37*t*

Proximal convoluted tubule, portion of renal tubule, 299, 300*f*, 302*f*

Pruritus, severe itching, 61

Pseudocyesis, false pregnancy, 346

Pseudohypertrophic muscular dystrophy, one type of inherited muscular dystrophy in which muscle tissue is gradually replaced by fatty tissue, making muscle look strong, 121

Psoriasis, chronic inflammatory condition consisting of crusty papules forming patches with circular borders, 67, 67*f*

Psychiatric nurse, nurse with additional training in care of patients with mental, emotional, and behavioral disorders, 500

Psychiatric social work, social worker with additional training in care of patients with mental, emotional, or behavioral disorders, 500

Psychiatrist (MD or DO), physician with specialized training in diagnosing and treating mental disorders; prescribes medication and conducts counseling, 500

Psychiatry, branch of medicine that deals with the diagnosis, treatment, and prevention of mental disorders, 500

Psychoanalysis, method of obtaining a detailed account of past and present emotional and mental experiences from patient to determine source of problem and eliminate effects, 505

Psychology, study of human behavior and thought process; behavioral science is primarily concerned with understanding how human beings interact with their physical environment and with each other, 500

Psychopharmacology, study of effects of drugs on mind and particularly use of drugs in treating mental disorders; main classes of drugs for treatment of mental disorders are antipsychotic drugs, antidepressant drugs, minor tranquilizers, and lithium, 504

Psychotherapy, method of treating mental disorders by mental rather than chemical or physical means; includes psychoanalysis, humanistic therapies, and family and group therapy, 505

Pterygium, hypertrophied conjunctival tissue in inner corner of eye, 459

Puberty, beginning of menstruation and ability to reproduce; usually occurs around age 16, 334, 335

Pubic, pertaining to pubis; one of pelvic bones, 99

Pubic region, genital region of body, 33, 33*f*

Pubis, one of three bones that form os coxae or innominate bone, 94, 95*f*, 95*t*

Pulmonary, pertaining to lung, 229

Pulmonary angiography, injecting dye into blood vessel for purpose of taking X-ray of arteries and veins of lungs, 238

Pulmonary artery, large artery that carries deoxygenated blood from right ventricle to lung, 140*f*, 144, 145*f*

Pulmonary capillaries, network of capillaries in lungs that tightly encase each alveolus; site of gas exchange, 223

Pulmonary circulation, pulmonary circulation transports deoxygenated blood from right side of heart to lungs where oxygen and carbon dioxide are exchanged; then it carries oxygenated blood back to left side of heart, 140

Pulmonary edema, condition in which lung tissue retains excessive amount of fluid; results in labored breathing, 236

Pulmonary embolism, blood clot or air bubble in pulmonary artery or one of its branches, 236

Pulmonary fibrosis, formation of fibrous scar tissue in lungs, which leads to decreased ability to expand lungs; may be caused by infections, pneumoconiosis, autoimmune diseases, and toxin exposure, 236

Pulmonary function test (PFT), group of diagnostic tests that give information regarding air flow in and out of the lungs, lung volumes, and gas exchange between the lungs and bloodstream, 225, 225*t*, 239

Pulmonary semilunar valve, 144*f*

Pulmonary trunk, 142*f*

Pulmonary valve, semilunar valve between right ventricle and pulmonary artery in heart; prevents blood from flowing backwards into ventricle, 142*f*, 143, 144*f*, 145*f*

Pulmonary vein, large vein that returns oxygenated blood from lungs to left atrium, 140*f*, 144, 145*f*

Pulmonologist, physician specialized in treating diseases and disorders of respiratory system, 229

Pulmonology, branch of medicine specializing in conditions of respiratory system, 29*t*, *229*

Pulp cavity, hollow interior of tooth; contains soft tissue made up of blood vessels, nerves, and lymph vessels, 260, 261, 261*f*

Pulse (P), expansion and contraction produced by blood as it moves through artery; pulse can be taken at several pulse points throughout body where artery is close to surface, 149

Pupil, hole in center of iris; size of pupil is changed by iris dilating or constricting, 447*f*, 448*f*, 449, 452*f*

Pupillary, pertaining to pupil, 454
Purified protein derivative (PPD), 239
Purkinje fibers, part of conduction system of heart; found in ventricular myocardium, 144, 146*f*
Purpura, hemorrhages into skin and mucous membranes, 61, 61*f*,
Purulent, pus-filled sputum, which can be result of infection, 61
Pustule, raised spot on skin containing pus, 62, 62*f*
Pyelitis, inflammation of renal pelvis, 309
Pyelogram, x-ray record of the pelvis after injection of radiopaque dye, 311
Pyelonephritis, inflammation of renal pelvis and kidney; one of most common types of kidney disease; may be result of lower urinary tract infection that moved up to kidney by way of ureters; may be large quantities of white blood cells and bacteria in urine, and blood (hematuria) may even be present in urine in this condition; can occur with any untreated or persistent case of cystitis, 309
Pyeloplasty, surgical repair of renal pelvis, 315
Pyloric, pertaining to pylorus, 268
Pyloric sphincter, sphincter at distal end of stomach; controls passage of food into duodenum, 262, 262*f*, 265*f*
Pyoderma, pus producing skin infection, 62
Pyosalpinx, condition of having pus in fallopian tubes, 343
Pyothorax, condition of having pus in chest cavity, 232, 237
Pyromania, impulse control disorder in which patient is unable to control impulse to start fires, 502
Pyrosis, heartburn, 270
Pyuria, presence of pus in urine, 307

Q

Quadriplegia, paralysis of all four extremities; same as tetraplegia, 423

R

Radial, pertaining to radius; lower arm bone, 99
Radial artery, 148*f*
Radial keratotomy, spokelike incisions around cornea that result in it becoming flatter; surgical treatment for myopia, 463
Radial nerve, 419*f*
Radial vein, 150*f*
Radiation therapy, use of X-rays to treat disease, especially cancer, 529
Radical mastectomy, surgical removal of breast tissue plus chest muscles and axillary lymph nodes, 350
Radical surgery, extensive surgery to remove as much tissue associated with tumor as possible, 529
Radiculitis, nerve root inflammation, 429
Radiculopathy, disease of nerve root, 429
Radioactive implant, embedding radioactive source directly into tissue to provide highly localized radiation dosage to damage nearby cancerous cells; also called *brachytherapy,* 529
Radiography, making of X-ray pictures, 106, 507
Radioimmunoassay (RIA), test used to measure levels of hormones in plasma of blood, 396
Radioisotope, radioactive form of element, 507
Radiologist, physician who practices diagnosis and treatment by use of radiant energy; responsible for interpreting X-ray films, 507
Radiology, branch of medicine that uses radioactive substances such as X-rays, isotopes, and radiation to prevent, diagnose, and treat diseases, 510
Radiolucent, structures that allow X-rays to pass through and expose photographic plate, making it appear as black area on X-ray, are termed radiolucent, 507
Radiopaque, structures impenetrable to X-rays, appearing as light area on radiograph (X-ray), 507
Radius, one of forearm bones in upper extermity, 92, 93*f*, 94, 94*f*
Range of motion (ROM), range of movement of a joint, from maximum flexion through maximum extension; measured as degrees of a circle, 516
Raynaud's phenomenon, periodic ischemic attacks affecting extremities of body, especially fingers, toes, ears, and nose; affected extremities become cyanotic and very painful; attacks are brought on by arterial constriction due to extreme cold or emotional stress, 158
Reabsorption, second phase of urine production; substances needed by body are reabsorbed as filtrate passes through kidney tubules, 302
Recklinghausen disease, excessive production of parathyroid hormone, which results in degeneration of bones, 393
Rectal, (1) pertaining to rectum; (2) substances introduced directly into rectal cavity in form of suppositories or solution; drugs may have to be administered by this route if patient is unable to take them by mouth due to nausea, vomiting, and surgery, 268, 494, 496*t*

S

Schedule III, drugs with moderate-to-low potential for addiction and abuse; examples are butabarbital, anabolic steroids, and acetaminophen with codeine, 492*t*

Schedule IV, drugs with lower potential for addiction and abuse than Schedule III drugs; examples are chloral hydrate, phenobarbital, and diazepam, 492*t*

Schedule V, drugs with low potential for addiction and abuse; example is low-strength codeine combined with other drugs to suppress coughing, 492*t*

Schizophrenia, mental disorders characterized by distortions of reality such as delusions and hallucinations, 503

Schwann cell, 413*f*

Sciatic nerve, 419*f*

Sclera, tough protective outer layer of eyeball; commonly referred to as white of eye, 447*f*, 448, 448*f*

Scleral, pertaining to sclera, 454

Scleral buckling, placing a band of silicone around outside of sclera to stabilize detaching retina, 463

Scleritis, inflammation of sclera, 458

Scleroderma, disorder in which skin becomes taut, thick, and leatherlike, 62

Scleromalacia, softening of sclera, 456

Sclerotomy, incision into sclera, 453

Scoliosis, abnormal lateral curvature of spine, 104*f*, 105

Scratch test, form of allergy testing in which body is exposed to allergen through light scratch in skin, 204, 204*f*

Scrotum, sac that serves as container for testes; sac, which is divided by septum, supports testicles and lies between legs and behind penis, 354, 355

Scrub nurse, surgical assistant who hands instruments to surgeon; person wears sterile clothing and maintains sterile operative field, 524

Sebaceous cyst, sac under skin filled with sebum or oil from sebaceous gland; can grow to large size and may need to be excised, 67

Sebaceous glands, also called oil glands; produce substance called sebum that lubricates skin surface, 27*t*, 50, 55, 55*f*, 451

Seborrhea, excessive discharge of sebum, 62

Sebum, thick, oily substance secreted by sebaceous glands that lubricates skin to prevent drying out; when sebum accumulates, it can cause congestion in sebaceous glands and whiteheads or pimples may form; when sebum becomes dark it is referred to as comedo or blackhead, 55

Second-degree burn, 64, 64*f*

Secretion, third phase of urine production; additional waste products are added to filtrate as it passes through kidney tubules, 302

Sedative, produces relaxation without causing sleep, 433

Seizure, sudden attack of severe muscular contractions associated with loss of consciousness; seen in grand mal epilepsy, 423

Self-innoculation, infection that occurs when person becomes infected in different part of body by pathogen from another part of his or her own body, such as intestinal bacteria spreading to urethra, 198

Semen, semen contains sperm and fluids secreted by male reproductive system glands; leaves body through urethra, 354

Semen analysis, procedure used when performing fertility workup to determine if male is able to produce sperm; semen is collected by patient afer abstaining from sexual intercourse for a period of three to five days; sperm in semen are analyzed for number, swimming strength, and shape; also used to determine if vasectomy has been successful; after a period of six weeks, no sperm should be present in sample from patient, 360

Semicircular canals, portion of labyrinth associated with balance and equilibrium, 467

Semiconscious, state of being aware of surroundings and responding to stimuli only part of time, 423

Semilunar valve, heart valves located between ventricles and great arteries leaving heart; pulmonary valve is located between right ventricle, and pulmonary artery and aortic valve are located between left ventricle and aorta, 143

Seminal vesicles, two male reproductive system glands located at base of bladder; secrete fluid that nourishes sperm into vas deferens; fluid plus sperm constitutes much of semen, 30*t*, 35*t*, 96*f*, 353*f*, 354, 356

Seminiferous tubules, network of coiled tubes that make up bulk of testes; sperm development takes place in walls of tubules and mature sperm are released into tubule in order to leave testes, 354, 355

Sensorineural hearing loss, type of hearing loss in which sound is conducted normally through external and middle ear but there is a defect in inner ear or with cochlear nerve, resulting in inability to hear; hearing aid may help, 469

Sensory neurons, nerves that carry sensory information from sensory receptors to brain; also called *afferent neurons*, 418, 419*f*

T

Thyroid echography, ultrasound examination of thyroid that can assist in distinguishing thyroid nodule from cyst, 396

Thyroid function test (TFT), blood tests used to measure levels of T_3, T_4, and TSH in blood stream to assist in determining thyroid function, 396

Thyroid gland, endocrine gland located on either side of trachea; shape resembles butterfly with large left and right lobe connected by narrow isthmus; gland produces hormones thyroxine (also known as T_4 and triiodothyronine (also known as T_3), 30*t,* 221*f,* 379*f,* 380, 381*t,* 387–88, 388*f*

Thyroid replacement hormone, given to replace thyroid in patients with hypothyroidism or who have had thyroidectomy, 398

Thyroid replacement therapy, 398

Thyroid scan, test in which radioactive element is administered that localizes in thyroid gland; gland can then be visualized with scanning device to detect pathology such as tumors, 396

Thyroid-stimulating hormone (TSH), hormone secreted by anterior pituitary; regulates function of thyroid gland, 381*t,* 385

Thyroidal, pertaining to thyroid gland, 389

Thyroidectomy, removal of entire thyroid or portion (partial thyroidectomy) to treat variety of conditions, including nodes, cancer, and hyperthyroidism, 397

Thyromegaly, enlarged thyroid, 391

Thyrotoxicosis, condition that results from overproduction of thyroid glands; symptoms include rapid heart action, tremors, enlarged thyroid gland, exophthalmos, and weight loss, 395

Thyroxine (T_4), hormone produced by thyroid gland; also known as T_4 and requires iodine for production; hormone regulates level of cell metabolism; the greater the level of hormone in the bloodstream, the higher cell metabolism will be, 381*t,* 387

Tibia, also called *shin bone;* lower extremity bone, 85*f,* 92, 93*f,* 94, 95*f,* 95*t*

Tibial, pertaining to tibia or shin bone, 99

Tidal volume (TV), amount of air that enters lungs in single inhalation or leaves lungs in single exhalation of quiet breathing, 225*t*

Tinea, fungal skin disease resulting in itching, scaling lesions, 68

Tinea capitis, fungal infection of scalp; commonly called *ringworm,* 68

Tinea pedis, fungal infection of foot; commonly called *athlete's foot,* 68

Tinnitus, ringing in ears, 472

Tissues, formed when cells of same type are grouped to perform one activity; for example, nerve cells combine to form nerve fibers; there are four types: nerve, muscle, epithelial, and connective, 25
  connective, 25

epithelial, pertaining to epithelium, 25
  muscle, 25
  nervous, 25

Tolerance, development of capacity for withstanding large amount of substance, such as foods, drugs, or poison, without any adverse effect; decreased sensitivity to further doses will develop, 497

Tongue, muscular organ in floor of mouth; works to move food around inside mouth and is also necessary for speech, 221*f,* 258, 264*f*

Tonic-clonic seizure, type of severe epileptic seizure characterized by loss of consciousness and convulsions; seizure alternates between strong continuous muscle spasms (tonic) and rhythmic muscle contraction and relaxation (clonic); also called *grand mal seizure,* 424

Tonometry, measurement of intraocular pressure of eye using tonometer to check for condition of glaucoma; generally part of normal eye exam for adults, 461

Tonsillar, pertaining to tonsils, 200

Tonsillectomy, surgical removal of tonsils, 205

Tonsillitis, inflammation of tonsils, 202

Tonsils, collections of lymphatic tissue located in pharynx to combat microorganisms entering body through nose or mouth; include pharyngeal tonsils, palatine tonsils, and lingual tonsils, 28*t,* 192*f,* 193, 196, 196*f*

Tooth cavity, 270

Topical, applied directly to skin or mucous membranes; distributed in ointment, cream, or lotion form; used to treat skin infections and eruptions, 494, 496*t*

Topical anesthesia, topical anesthesia is applied using either liquid or gel placed directly onto specific area; patient remains conscious; this type of anesthetic is used on skin, cornea, and mucous membranes in dental work, 520, 521*t*

Torticollis, severe neck spasms pulling head to one side; commonly called *wryneck* or *crick in the neck,* 121

Total abdominal hysterectomy - bilateral salpingo-oophorectomy (TAH-BSO), removal of entire uterus, cervix, both ovaries, and both fallopian tubes, 350

Total calcium, blood test to measure total amount of calcium to assist in detecting parathyroid and bone disorders, 396

U

V

W

X

Y

Z